Basic
Histology

Many of the illustrations in this book were prepared with financial aid from the
Fundação de Amparo à Pesquisa do Estado de São Paulo.

Basic Histology

Luis C. Junqueira, MD
Head, Laboratory of Morphology
Ludwig Institute for Cancer Research
São Paulo Branch, Brazil

Honorary Research Associate in Biology
Harvard College, Boston

Formerly Research Associate
Medical School, University of Chicago

José Carneiro, MD
Professor of Histology & Embryology
Institute of Biomedical Sciences, University of São Paulo, Brazil

Formerly Research Associate, Department of Anatomy
Medical School, McGill University, Montreal, Canada

Formerly Visiting Associate Professor, Department of Anatomy
Medical School, University of Virginia, Charlottesville, Virginia

John A. Long, PhD
Associate Professor, Department of Anatomy
University of California, San Francisco

Fifth Edition

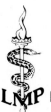 **LANGE Medical Publications/Los Altos, California**

APPLETON-CENTURY-CROFTS/Norwalk, Connecticut

Copyright © 1986 by Appleton-Century-Crofts
A Publishing Division of Prentice-Hall
Copyright © 1983, 1980, 1977, 1975 by Lange Medical Publications

Italian Edition: *Piccin Nuova Libraria, S.p.A., Via Altinate, 107, 35121 Padua, Italy*
Dutch Edition: *Kooyker Scientific Publications B.V., Postbus 24,*
2300 AA Leiden, The Netherlands
Indonesian Edition: *CV. E.G.C. Medical Publisher, P.O. Box 4276,*
10711 Jakarta, Indonesia
Japanese Edition: *Hirokawa Publishing Company, 27-14, Hongo 3, Bunkyo-ku,*
Tokyo 113, Japan
German Edition: *Springer-Verlag GmbH & Co. KG, Postfach 10 52 80,*
6900 Heidelberg 1, West Germany

86 87 88 89 90 / 10 9 8 7 6 5 4 3 2 1

Prentice-Hall of Australia, Pty. Ltd., Sydney
Prentice-Hall Canada, Inc.
Prentice-Hall Hispanoamericana, S.A., Mexico
Prentice-Hall of India Private Limited, New Delhi
Prentice-Hall International (UK) Limited, London
Prentice-Hall of Japan Inc., Tokyo
Prentice-Hall of Southeast Asia (Pte.) Ltd., Singapore
Whitehall Books Ltd., Wellington, New Zealand
Editora Prentice-Hall do Brasil Ltda., Rio de Janeiro

ISBN: 0-8385-0570-8

PRINTED IN THE UNITED STATES OF AMERICA

Table of Contents

Preface

This fifth edition of *Basic Histology* continues to be a compact and well illustrated exposition of the basic facts and interpretation of histology for medical students and others in the biologic sciences. Bearing in mind that the information contained in this book is the foundation on which pathology and pathophysiology are built, we emphasize the relationships between structure and function. We present the facts that the student must know, but we also stress concepts based on these facts.

In revising *Basic Histology* we aimed to provide our readers with the most modern and useful text possible. This we did in two ways: by describing the most important recent developments in the science of histology, and by recognizing that our readers are faced with the task of learning an ever-increasing number of facts in an ever-shortening period of time.

Organization of the Book

Today, the study of histology requires a firm foundation in cell biology. Thus, *Basic Histology* begins with an accurate, up-to-date description of the structure and functions of cells and their products. We assume that the student has an elementary knowledge of biochemistry.

This foundation is followed by a description of the four major tissues of the body, pointing out how cells are specialized to perform the specific functions of these tissues.

Finally, we devote a chapter to each of the organs and organ systems of the human body. Here, the emphasis is on the spatial arrangement of the several tissues, which provides the key to understanding the functions of the organ. Again, we emphasize cell biology as the most fundamental approach to the study of structure and function.

The illustrations are an outstanding feature of the book. Numerous photomicrographs and electron micrographs exemplify and amplify the text and remind the reader of structures studied in the histology laboratory. We place particular emphasis on diagrams that summarize morphologic and functional features of cells, tissues, and organs.

Changes in the Fifth Edition

All chapters have been revised to reflect new findings and interpretations, and the emphasis on human histology has been strengthened. We present new information on the origin and functions of peroxisomes, a completely rewritten section on protein secretion, and the most recent model of the structure of membranes and the membrane skeleton. The material on intercellular junctions has been updated, and the modern concept of the structure and functions of the basal lamina has been introduced. The role of endothelial cells in the secretion of a clotting factor and in the metabolism of several hormones is discussed. Storage and secretion of an atrial natriuretic hormone is described. Rapid advances in cellular immunology have dictated extensive reorganization and revision of the chapter on the lymphoid system, which now includes new information on antigen-presenting cells. A new section on the development of teeth has been added to the chapter on the digestive tract.

Some existing diagrams have been revised, and several new diagrams have been drawn for this edition. About 75 new light and electron micrographs have been provided to supplant or supplement the existing figures.

We are pleased to announce that Italian, Dutch, Indonesian, Japanese, and German translations have been published and Serbo-Croatian, French, and Greek translations are in process.

—LCJ
—JC
April, 1986   —JAL

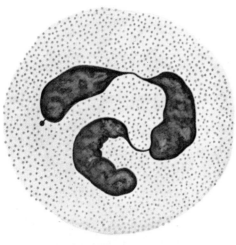

Neutrophilic granulocyte

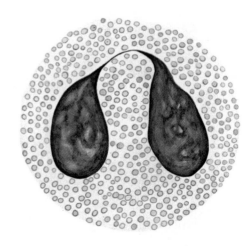

Eosinophilic granulocyte

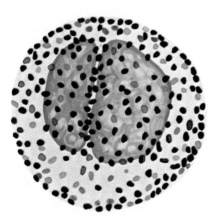

Basophilic granulocyte

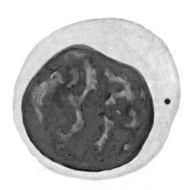

Lymphocyte

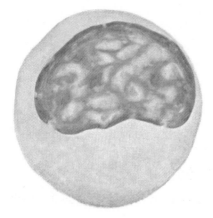

Monocyte

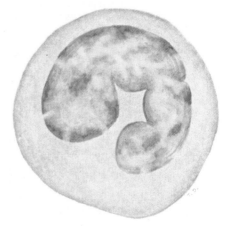

Monocyte

The 5 Types of Human Leukocytes. (See Fig 13-7.)

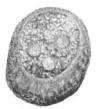

Proerythroblast

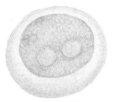

Myeloblast

Basophilic
erythroblast

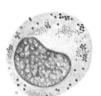

Early neutrophilic
myelocyte

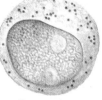

Promyelocyte

Early basophilic
myelocyte

Polychromatophilic
erythroblast

Late neutrophilic
myelocyte

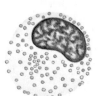

Early eosinophilic
myelocyte

Orthochromatophilic
erythroblast

Neutrophilic
metamyelocyte

Late eosinophilic
myelocyte

Late basophilic
myelocyte

Reticulocyte

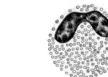

Band cell

Eosinophilic
metamyelocyte

Erythrocyte

Mature neutrophil

Mature eosinophil

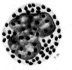

Mature basophil

Stages of Development of Erythrocytes and Granulocytes. (See Fig 14–5.)

Methods of Study

Familiarity with the tools and methods of any branch of science is essential for proper understanding of the subject. Some of the more common methods used to study cells and tissues and the principles involved in these methods will be reviewed here: units of measurement, preparation of tissues for examination, light microscopy, phase contrast microscopy, polarizing microscopy, electron microscopy, problems in interpretation of tissue sections, cryofracture, radioautography, examination of living cells and tissues, isolation and study in vitro of pure cell strains, and cell fractionation.

The most important units of measurement used in histology are given in Table 1 – 1. The **Ångström unit** (Å; 10^{-10} meter) is no longer recognized in the international system of units (Système International), and the **nanometer** (nm, 10^{-9} meter) is used in its stead (1 nm = 10 Å). The term **micrometer** (μm) has replaced the **micron** (μ) but has the same value (10^{-6} meter).

Table 1–1. Units of measurement used in light and electron microscopy.

Système International (SI) Unit	Symbol and Value
Micrometer	μm = 0.001 mm, 10^{-6} m
Nanometer	nm = 0.001 μm, 10^{-9} m

PREPARATION OF TISSUES FOR MICROSCOPIC EXAMINATION

The most common procedure used in the study of tissues is the preparation of histologic sections that can be studied with the aid of the light microscope. Under the light microscope, tissues are examined by transillumination. Since tissues and organs are usually too thick for transillumination, techniques have been developed for obtaining thin, translucent sections. In some cases, very thin layers of tissues or transparent membranes of living animals (eg, the mesentery, the tail of a tadpole, the wall of a hamster's cheek pouch) can be observed in the microscope without first sectioning the tissue. In such instances, it is possible to study these structures for long periods and under varying physiologic or experimental conditions. If a permanent preparation is desired, small fragments of these thin structures can be fixed, spread on a glass slide,

stained and mounted with resin, and examined under the microscope. In most cases, however, tissues must be sliced into thin sections before they can be examined. These sections are cut by precision fine cutting instruments called **microtomes,** and the organ or tissue must be preserved and prepared for sectioning. (See Table 1 – 2.)

The ideal microscope tissue preparation would of course be preserved with suitable chemicals so that the tissue on the slide would have the same structure and molecular composition as it had in the body. This is sometimes possible but, as a practical matter, seldom feasible, and artifacts resulting from the preparation process are almost always present.

Fixation

In order to avoid tissue digestion by enzymes (autolysis) or bacteria and to preserve physical structure, pieces of organs should be promptly and adequately treated prior to or as soon as possible following removal from the animal's body. This treatment—fixation—usually consists of submerging the tissues in stabilizing or cross-linking agents or perfusing them with these substances in order to pre-

Table 1–2. Typical sequence of procedures in preparing tissues for observation under the light microscope. Following embedding in paraffin blocks, the tissues can be sectioned with a microtome (Fig 1–1).

Stage	Purpose	Duration
1. Fixation in simple or compound fixatives (Bouin's, Zenker's formalin)	To preserve tissue morphology and molecular composition	About 12 h, according to the fixative and the size of the piece of tissue
2. Dehydration in graded concentrated ethyl alcohol (70% up to 100% alcohol)	To replace tissue water with organic solvents	6–24 h
3. Clearing in benzene, xylene, or toluene	To impregnate the tissues with a paraffin solvent	1–6 h
4. Embedding in melted paraffin at 58–60 °C	Paraffin penetrates all intercellular spaces and even into the cells, making the tissues more resistant to sectioning	½–6 h

serve as much as possible of their morphologic and molecular characteristics.

The chemical substances used to preserve tissues are called **fixatives.** Some fixatives (eg, mercuric chloride, picric acid) promote the precipitation or clumping of proteins. Others (eg, formalin, glutaraldehyde) promote cross-linking but not coarse precipitation of proteins. All fixatives have both desirable and undesirable effects. The goal of combining the desirable effects and minimizing the undesirable ones has led to the development of several mixtures. The most commonly used mixtures are **Bouin's fluid,** composed of picric acid, formalin (a saturated solution—37% by weight of formaldehyde gas in water), acetic acid, and water; and **Zenker's formalin (Helly's fluid),** containing formalin, potassium dichromate, mercuric chloride, and water. The simple fixatives most commonly used are a 10% solution of formalin in saline and a 2–6% solution of buffered glutaraldehyde.

The chemistry of the process involved in fixation is complex and not well understood. However, for-maldehyde and glutaraldehyde are known to react with the amine groups (NH_2) of tissue proteins. In the case of glutaraldehyde, the fixing action is reinforced by the fact that it is a dialdehyde and can cross-link.

In view of the high resolution afforded by the electron microscope, greater care is necessitated in fixation in order to preserve ultrastructural detail. Toward that end, a double fixation procedure, using a buffered glutaraldehyde solution first, followed by a second fixation in buffered osmium tetroxide, has become a standard procedure in preparations for fine structural studies. The glutaraldehyde cross-links proteins, while the effect of osmium tetroxide is to preserve and stain lipids and proteins.

Embedding

In order to obtain thin sections with the microtome, tissues must be infiltrated after fixation with embedding substances that impart a rigid consistency to the tissue. Embedding materials include gelatin, celloidin, paraffin, and the more recently developed plastic resins. Paraffin is used routinely for light microscopy;

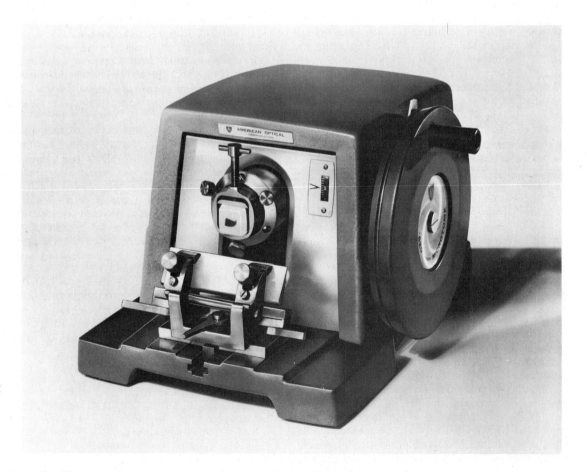

Figure 1–1. Microtome for sectioning paraffin-embedded tissues. Rotation of the drive wheel—seen with a handle on the right side of the instrument—moves the tissue block holder up and down. Each turn of the drive wheel advances the specimen holder a controlled distance, generally 3–8 μm, and the embedded tissue passes over the knife edge, cutting the sections. The sticky paraffin sections adhere to each other, producing a ribbon of sections that is collected and affixed to a slide. (Courtesy of American Optical Corp.)

resins of the epoxy type (Epon or Araldite) are more commonly employed for electron microscopy.

The process of embedding or tissue impregnation is usually preceded by 2 main steps: **dehydration** and **clearing.** The water of the fragments to be embedded is first extracted by bathing successively in a graded series of mixtures of ethanol with water (usually from 70% to 100% ethanol). The ethanol is then replaced by a solvent miscible with the embedding medium. (In paraffin embedding, the solvent used is xylene.) As the tissues become infiltrated with the solvent, they usually become transparent in a step called **clearing.** Once the tissue is impregnated with the solvent, it is placed in melted paraffin in the oven, usually at 58–60 °C. The heat causes the solvent to evaporate, and the space becomes filled with paraffin. Tissues to be embedded for electron microscopy are also dehydrated in ethanolic solutions and subsequently infiltrated with plastic solvents such as propylene oxide. These solvents are miscible with and later replaced by plastic solutions (eg, Epon, Araldite) hardened by means of cross-linking polymerizers and heat. This is the infiltration or embedding procedure.

The small blocks of paraffin containing the tissues are sectioned by the steel blade of the microtome to a thickness of 1–20 μm (Fig 1–1). The sections are floated on warm water and transferred to glass slides. For electron microscopy, much thinner sections are necessary (0.02–0.1 μm); embedding is therefore performed in a hard epoxy plastic. The blocks thus obtained are so hard that glass or diamond knives are usually necessary to section them. Since the electron beam in the microscope cannot penetrate glass, the extremely thin plastic sections are collected on small metal (usually etched copper) grids. Those portions of the sections spanning the holes in the mesh of the grid can be examined in the microscope.

Immersion of tissues in solvents such as xylene dissolves the tissue lipids, which is an undesirable effect when these compounds are to be studied. To avoid loss of lipids, a **freezing microtome** has been devised in which the tissues are hardened at low temperatures in order to provide the rigidity necessary to permit sectioning. The freezing microtome—and its more elaborate and efficient successor, the **cryostat**—permit sections to be obtained quickly without going through the embedding procedure described above.

They are often used in hospitals, for they allow rapid study of pathologic specimens during surgical procedures. They are also effective in the histochemical study of very sensitive enzymes or small molecules, since freezing does not inactivate enzymes and hinders the diffusion of small molecules.

Staining

With few exceptions, most tissues are colorless, so that observing them unstained in the light microscope is difficult. Methods of staining tissues have therefore been devised that not only make various tissue components conspicuous but also permit distinctions to be made between them. This is done by using mixtures of dyes that stain tissue components more or less selectively. Most dyes used in histologic studies behave like acidic or basic compounds and have a tendency to form electrostatic (salt) linkages with ionizable radicals of the tissues. Tissue components that stain more readily with basic dyes are termed **basophilic;** those with an affinity for acid dyes are termed **acidophilic.**

Examples of basic dyes are toluidine blue and methylene blue. Hematoxylin behaves in the manner of a basic dye; ie, it stains the basophilic tissue components. The main tissue components that ionize and react with basic dyes do so because of acids in their composition (nucleoproteins and glycosaminoglycans). Acid dyes (eg, orange G, eosin, acid fuchsin) stain mostly the basic components present in cytoplasmic proteins.

Of all dyes, the combination of hematoxylin and eosin (H&E) is most commonly used. Many other dyes are used in different histologic procedures. Although they are useful in visualizing the different tissue components, they usually provide no insight into the chemical nature of the tissue being studied. Besides tissue staining with dyes, impregnation with such metals as silver and gold is a much used technique, especially in studies of the nervous system. Table 1–3 summarizes some staining techniques used in preparing microscope slides.

In electron microscopy, the image formed is due to the capacity of the tissue or stains to absorb or scatter electrons. Heavy metal salts such as lead citrate and uranium acetate exhibit a high electron-absorbing or -scattering capacity and are the primary stains used in electron microscopy.

Table 1–3. Examples of staining techniques commonly used in histology.

Techniques	Components	Nucleus	Cytoplasm	Collagen	Elastic Fibers	Reticular Fibers
H&E	Hematoxylin and eosin	Blue	Pink	Pink	Variable	. . .
Masson's trichrome	Iron hematoxylin, acid fuchsin, Ponceau 2R, light green	Black	Red	Green	. . .	Green
Weigert's elastic stain	Resorcin and fuchsin, HCl, hematoxylin, Ponceau's picric acid, glacial acetic acid	Gray	Yellow	Red	Black	. . .
Silver impregnation for reticular fibers	Silver salt solution	. . .	. . .	Dark brown	. . .	Black

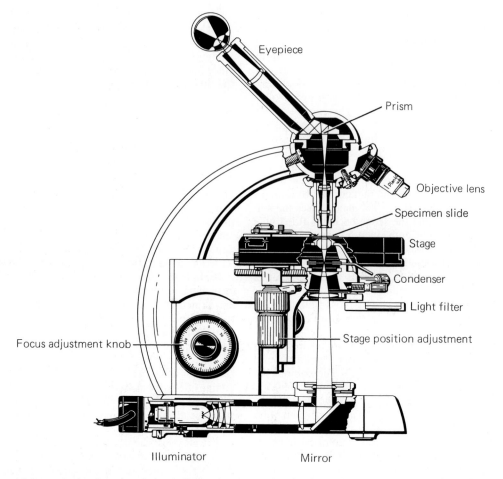

Eyepiece

Prism

Objective lens

Specimen slide

Stage

Condenser

Light filter

Focus adjustment knob

Stage position adjustment

Illuminator

Mirror

Figure 1–2. Schematic drawing of a student's light microscope showing its main components and the pathway of light from the source (substage lamp) to the eye of the observer. (Courtesy of Carl Zeiss Co.)

LIGHT MICROSCOPY

With the light microscope, stained preparations are usually examined by transillumination. The microscope is composed of both mechanical and optical parts. The mechanical components are illustrated in Fig 1–2. The optical components consist of 3 systems of lenses: condenser, objective, and ocular. The **condenser** collects and focuses the illumination to produce a cone of light that illuminates the object to be observed. The role of the condenser is usually underestimated because it does not contribute to the magnification; however, its proper use influences the quality of the image observed. The **objective** lens enlarges and projects the illuminated image of the object in the direction of the ocular lens. The **ocular** lens further magnifies this image and projects it onto the viewer's retina or onto a phosphorescent screen or photographic plate. The total magnification is obtained by multiplying the magnifying power of the objective and ocular lenses.

Resolution

The critical factor in obtaining a good image with the microscope is the resolution, which is the smallest distance between 2 particles when the 2 particles can be seen as separate objects. For example, 2 particles will appear distinct if they are separated by a distance of 0.2 μm and the microscope has a resolution of 0.2 μm. However, if the same particles are examined with a microscope that has a resolution of only 0.5 μm, they will appear as a single point. The resolving power of the best light microscopes is approximately 0.2 μm.

The quality of an image—its clarity and richness of detail—depends on the microscope's resolving power. The **magnification** is independent of its resolving power and is only of value when accompanied by a high resolution capacity. The resolving power of a microscope depends mainly on its objective lens. The ocular lens only enlarges the image obtained by the objective; it does not improve resolution. Thus, high magnification with low resolution gives blurred images of little value.

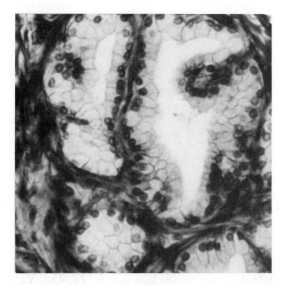

Figure 1–3. Drawing of the light beam that enters the objective lens to show the semiangle of aperture (α) from which the numerical aperture can be calculated.

Numerical Aperture

One of the main characteristics of an objective lens is its numerical aperture (NA), for resolution (R) is a function of NA and of the light wavelength employed (Fig 1–3). NA can be defined as the smallest refractive index (n)* observed between the micro-

---

*The refractive index (n) is the ratio between the speed of light in a vacuum and the speed of light in any other medium.

    Air   n = 1.000
    Water n = 1.333
    Glass n = 1.520

scopic preparation and the objective multiplied by the sine of the semiangle of aperture of the lens (α): NA = n × sin α (Fig 1–3).

The resolution of an objective can be defined by the following equation:

$$R = \frac{0.61 \times \lambda}{NA}$$

where λ is the wavelength. Resolution is directly proportionate to the wavelength used and inversely proportionate to the NA. To calculate the resolution when working with white light, a wavelength of 0.55 μm is most often used. This corresponds to yellowish-green, a color to which the human eye is very sensitive. Fig 1–4 is an example of the importance of resolution in microscopy.

An objective lens system often has several numbers engraved on it (Fig 1–5). The first number (upper left) refers to the enlargement; to its right is the NA. The number on the left in the second line is the tube length in millimeters; the number on the right indicates the thickness (in millimeters) of the coverslip for which the objective is corrected. The thickness of the coverslip is important in dry field examination, but when oil immersion is used the oil equalizes the refractive index of the light path between the coverslip and the objective, and the thickness of the coverslip becomes irrelevant.

Objective & Ocular Lenses

Objective and ocular lenses are formed by systems of lenses put together in order to achieve partial correction of their individual defects (aberrations). Al-

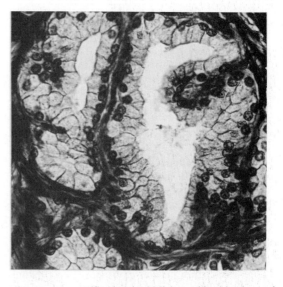

Figure 1–4. Photomicrographs of the same microscopic field at the same magnification (× 350) but with objectives of different numerical apertures (NA). The photomicrograph on the left was made with an objective of NA = 0.22; the one on the right was made with an objective of NA = 1.0. Dog prostate gland stained by Masson's trichrome stain. Observe that the picture at right (NA = 1.0) shows more detail and is sharper than the one on the left.

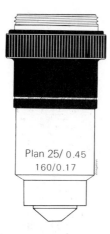

Figure 1-5. Drawing of an objective with following characteristics: magnification × 25, NA = 0.45, planachromatic, corrected for 160-mm tube and for 0.17-mm coverslips.

though a perfect lens system has not been developed, it is possible to devise objective lenses with increasing optical perfection.

Three common aberrations are as follows:

A. Chromatic Aberration: This type of aberration occurs because spherical lenses bring light of shorter wavelength into focus closer to the retina than light of longer wavelength. Consequently, several slightly separate images of the object are formed and details are blurred. In the **achromatic** lens system, this aberration is corrected to a large extent.

B. Spherical Aberration: In spherical aberration, the quality of the image is hindered because the optical properties of the center of a lens are somewhat different from those of its periphery. In **apochromatic** objective lens systems, complete correction of chromatic and spherical aberrations has been achieved.

C. Curvature of Field: Lenses with this aberration produce an image in which the central field is in focus while the peripheral field is out of focus, or vice versa. **Planar** lenses are corrected to provide "flat field" focus, in which the entire field is in focus.

PHASE CONTRAST MICROSCOPY

Unstained biologic specimens are usually transparent and difficult to view in detail, since all parts of the specimen have almost the same optical density. However, phase contrast microscopy employs a lens system that produces visible images from transparent objects (Fig 1-6).

The principle of phase contrast microscopy is based on the fact that light passing through a medium with different refractive indexes slows down and changes direction. Within a cell, different organelles (such as the nucleus, mitochondria, and secretion granules) exhibit different refractive indexes that variably alter the light passing through them. As light passes through

a cell, these refractive index differences are, by means of a special optical system, transformed into differences in light intensity, so that the image becomes visible (Fig 1-6). The examination of fresh tissue and living cells has been facilitated by the development of phase contrast microscopy.

POLARIZING MICROSCOPY

When normal light passes through a **Nicol prism** or a **Polaroid filter,** it exits vibrating in only one direction. Polaroid filters are most often used at present. They contain organic compounds so disposed as to have the same effect on light as a Nicol prism. If a second Polaroid filter is placed in the microscope above the first one, with its main axis in a perpendicular position, no light passes through. In a polarizing microscope, the first Polaroid filter is usually

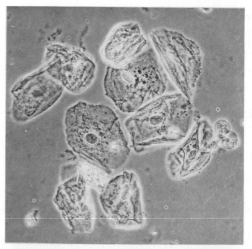

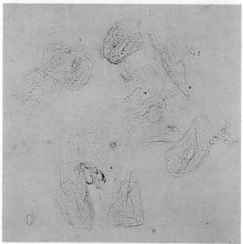

Figure 1-6. Desquamated cells from the oral mucosa (unstained fresh preparation). The top photomicrograph was taken with the phase contrast microscope; the bottom photomicrograph with the standard light microscope. × 300.

located below the condenser and is called the **polarizer.** A second filter (**analyzer**) is placed between the objective and the eyepiece. When polarizer and analyzer are disposed with their main axes perpendicular, no light passes, resulting in a darkfield effect. If, however, substances containing oriented molecules (such as cellulose, collagen, cilia, or muscle fibers) are located between the polarizer and analyzer, their repetitive molecular structure allows them to rotate the axis of the light emerging from the polarizer. Consequently, they appear as bright structures against a dark background (Figs 5 – 9 and 8 – 11). The capacity to rotate the direction of the vibration of the polarized light is called **birefringency** and is present in crystalline substances or substances containing oriented molecules as noted above.

ELECTRON MICROSCOPY

The principle upon which electron microscopy is based can be understood by referring to the following equation (used above to calculate the resolution in the light microscope):

$$R = \frac{0.61 \times \lambda}{NA}$$

The wavelength (λ) of an electron beam accelerated by 60 kV is approximately 0.005 nm, which gives a very high theoretic resolution. However, very small numerical apertures must be used because of large, uncorrectable aberrations in electron lenses. In practice, a resolution of 1 nm in tissue sections is considered to be quite satisfactory. This by itself permits enlargements to be obtained up to 200 times greater than those achieved with the light microscope.

The electron microscope functions on the principle that a beam of electrons can be deflected by electromagnetic fields in a manner similar to light deflection in glass lenses. Electrons are produced by high-temperature heating of a metallic filament (cathode) in a vacuum. The electrons emitted are then submitted to a potential difference of approximately 60 – 100 kV or more between the cathode and the anode (Fig 1 – 7). The anode is a metallic plate with a small hole in its center. Electrons are accelerated from the cathode to the anode. Some of these particles pass through the central orifice of the anode, forming a constant stream (or beam) of electrons. This beam is deflected by electromagnetic lenses in a way roughly analogous to that which occurs in the optical microscope. Thus, the condenser focuses the beam at the object plane and the objective forms an image of the object. The image obtained is further enlarged by 1 – 2 projecting lenses and is finally projected on a fluorescent screen or photographic plate (Figs 1 – 7 and 1 – 8).

Differences Between Electron & Light Microscopes

In contrast to the light microscope, the enlarge-

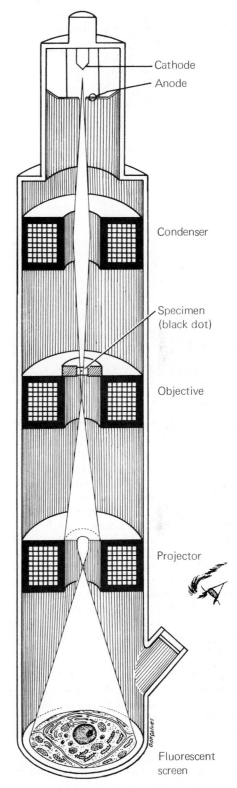

Cathode
Anode
Condenser
Specimen (black dot)
Objective
Projector
Fluorescent screen

Figure 1–7. Pathway of the electron beam in the electron microscope. The ultrathin section is placed just over the objective electromagnetic lens. The image is projected on a fluorescent screen and observed directly or through a × 10 magnifying optical system.

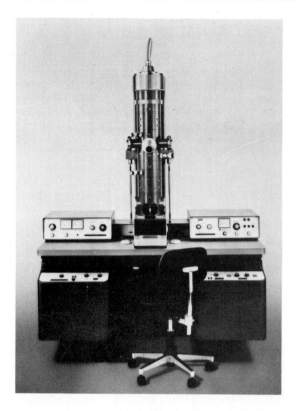

Figure 1–8. Photograph of the Zeiss model EM 10 electron microscope. (Courtesy of Carl Zeiss Co.)

ment produced by the objective lens in the electron microscope is fixed (or unvariable). Enlargements are produced by changes in the magnetic field of the projecting lenses, which are analogous to the "zoom" ocular lens in the light microscope.

Since electrons are easily scattered or absorbed by the object, very thin sections of tissue—usually $0.02-0.1$ μm—must be used. Another characteristic of the electron microscope is that the electrons are scattered or absorbed by portions of the object with high molecular weight, whereas in the light microscope light is absorbed by stained structures. The scattered electrons are absorbed by the aperture of the objective lens (usually a diameter of $25-100$ μm). This aperture filters out the scattered electrons which therefore do not contribute to image formation. The structures that scatter electrons thus appear in the fluorescent screen as dark bodies (electron-dense regions). The capacity to scatter electrons depends on the molecular weight (and therefore the density) of a given stain. Heavy metals (eg, uranium, lead) are therefore used to stain tissue sections, thereby increasing the contrast.

Limitations in the Use of the Electron Microscope

The nature of the electron beam requires that work with the electron microscope be done in high vacuum

with very thin sections. These conditions preclude the use of living material. Additionally, an electron beam focused on an object can damage it and can produce unwanted changes in tissue structures. Electron microscopy is a rapidly developing field, however. Advances include the use of high-voltage $(500,000-1,000,000$ V) transmission electron microscopes in which the high-velocity electron beam allows the penetration and consequently the visualization of tissues within relatively thick plastic sections $(1-5$ μm). The development of a high-resolution scanning transmission electron microscope (Crewe) has permitted direct visualization of atoms. Other recent advances in electron microscopy include instruments that provide higher resolution, permit the localization of specific ions in tissues, and allow the use of live specimens.

SCANNING ELECTRON MICROSCOPY

A variant of electron microscopy called scanning electron microscopy, in use since 1965, permits pseudo–3-dimensional views of surfaces of cells, tissues, and organs. The very narrow (10 nm) electron beam is moved sequentially from point to point across the surface to be examined. At each point, the primary electron beam interacts with atoms of the material being observed, giving rise to backscattered (reflected) electrons, x-rays characteristic of the irradiated atoms, and low-energy **secondary electrons.** These secondary electrons are used to form an image of the topography of the surface, since elevations of the surface give rise to more secondary electrons and depressions yield fewer secondary electrons. This fluctuation in electron signal is captured by a detector that, in turn, modulates the brightness of a cathode ray tube whose electron beam is being moved (scanned) in synchrony with the primary electron beam of the miscroscope. The resulting photographs are easily understood, since they present a view that appears to be illuminated from above, just as our ordinary macroscopic world is filled with highlights and shadows due to illumination from above.

Scanning electron micrographs illustrating the surface of the oocyte before and after fertilization and the initial stages of the formation of a morula are shown in Fig 24–16. Other scanning electron micrographs are shown in Figs 15–7, 17–17A, 17–17C, and 18–17.

PROBLEMS IN THE INTERPRETATION OF TISSUE SECTIONS

During the study and interpretation of stained tissue sections in microscope preparations, it should be remembered that the observed product is the end result of a series of processes which considerably distort the image observable in the living tissue, mainly through shrinking and retraction. As a consequence of these processes, the spaces frequently seen between the cells and other tissue components are artifacts. Furthermore, there is a tendency to think in terms of only 2 dimensions when examining thin sections, whereas in actuality the structures from which the sections are made have 3 dimensions. In order to understand the architecture of an organ, it is therefore necessary to study sections made in different planes and to reason accordingly (Fig 1–9).

The **serial sectioning technique** is often used in the study of organ and tissue structure. In this technique, sequential serial sections of a whole organ or an organ fragment are prepared and studied. By analysis of each section in the sequence in which it was prepared, information on the 3-dimensional architecture of the organ can be gained.

Another difficulty in the study of microscope preparations is the impossibility of differentially staining all tissue components on only one slide. It is therefore necessary to examine several preparations stained by different methods before a general idea of the composition and structure of any type of tissue can be obtained.

CRYOFRACTURE

The technique of cryofracture (freeze fracture) is an important technical development in electron microscopy that permits examination of tissues without fixation and embedding. Although it is not free of artifacts, this technique is useful for verifying the results obtained with the conventional technique in which ultrathin sections of fixed tissue are examined under the electron microscope. The cryofracture technique confirmed what we already knew about cell ultrastructure and has furnished new information regarding the structure of the cell membrane and associated structures.

The technique of cell fracture consists of freezing a fragment of tissue at very low temperatures and then fracturing it with a sharp metal blade. The fractured tissue is kept at low temperature in a high-vacuum environment. During this step, water sublimates, leaving behind nonsublimable cellular constituents (such as proteins and lipids) that protrude above the aqueous surface. Still in a vacuum environment, platinum or another heavy metal is deposited from a low angle,

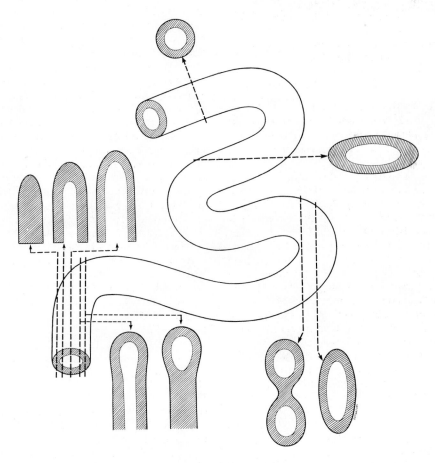

Figure 1–9. Some of the aspects a tube-shaped organ might exhibit when sectioned. The arrows indicate what is seen under the microscope in each particular section plane.

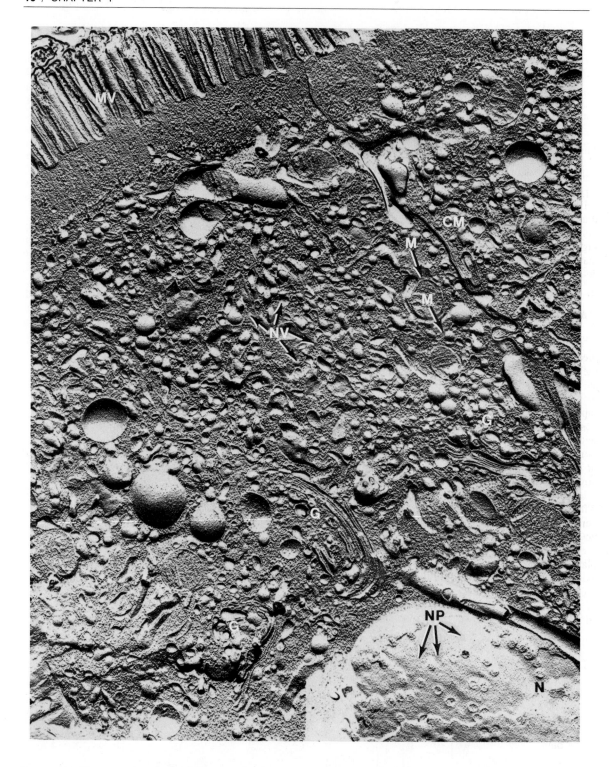

Figure 1–10. Electron micrograph of a mouse intestinal epithelial cell. The tissue was prepared by a process called cryofracture. It consists of freezing a fragment of tissue to very low temperatures and fracturing it with a sharpened metal blade. The fractured surface is kept at low temperature in a vacuum environment. A portion of the water in the surface sublimates, giving a bas-relief effect (etching). A replica of this surface is then obtained by coating it with a layer of platinum and carbon. In this picture, one can observe in material that has not been submitted to the processes of embedding and sectioning the presence of the various cell components described by classic transmission electron microscopy, eg, microvilli (MV), cell membrane (CM), mitochondria (M), Golgi complex (G), nucleus (N), and nuclear pores (NP). × 24,000. (Courtesy of LS Staehelin.)

producing a shadowing effect; ie, more heavy metal is deposited on the side of the protuberance closest to the source of the heavy metal. Next, a thick layer of carbon is deposited on the surface from directly above. This serves to strengthen and stabilize the surface. Subsequently, the whole assembly is brought to atmospheric pressure, and the underlying tissue is destroyed by use of sodium hypochlorite or acids. This frees the platinum-carbon replica, which is then picked up on a standard copper grid and studied in the transmission electron microscope. Fig 1–10 shows the replica of a freeze-fractured mouse intestinal epithelial cell in which most of the cell organelles can be seen, thus confirming their structure as shown by conventional transmission electron microscopy (compare with Fig 16–30). An important feature of cryofracture is that cellular membranes are often split open, revealing details of their internal structure (see Chapter 3).

RADIOAUTOGRAPHY

Radioautography permits the localization of radioactive substances in cells or tissues by means of the effect of emitted radiation on photographic emulsions. Silver bromide crystals present in the emulsion act as microdetectors of radioactivity. In radioautography, tissue sections obtained from animals previously treated with radioactive compounds are covered with photographic emulsion by dipping mounted sections in a glass container filled with a warmed mixture of gelatin and silver bromide (Fig 1–11). The slide, now covered with this thin layer of emulsion, is then dried and stored in a light-proof box in a refrigerator. After different exposure times depending on the experiment and the radioactive element, the slides are developed photographically and examined. All silver bromide crystals hit by radiation are reduced to small black granules of elemental silver, which reveal the existence of radioactivity in the structures in close proximity to these granules. The location and amount of radiation are thus determined, and the quantity of silver granules is proportionate to the intensity of the radioactivity present. The tissue is then stained with regular stains, and the preparation is mounted in resin and covered with a coverslip. This procedure can be employed in electron microscopy by using thin sections of resin-embedded, radioactively labeled tissue. With the resolution provided by the electron microscope, the silver granules usually appear as short, coiled filaments (Fig 1–12).

In light microscopy, radioautography permits distinction of radioactive particles that are 1 μm apart. It therefore has a resolving power (or resolution) of 1 μm; in electron microscopy, this resolution is increased 5–10 times.

Radioautography is often used to study important dynamic biologic phenomena. As soon as it became possible to synthesize radioactive isotopes of normal metabolites with the aid of carbon 14 and tritium, it was possible to study not only different metabolic pathways in tissue specimens but also the speed with which metabolic processes occurred. For example, the metabolism of proteins and nucleic acids can be studied by injecting labeled amino acids (eg, ^{14}C-leucine for studies of protein synthesis) and nucleosides (eg, ^{3}H-thymidine for studies of DNA synthesis) into animals. In both cases, the precursors are incorporated within the tissues and cells into protein or nucleic acids and can be localized and quantitated with the aid of radioautography. If a fixed unit of time is used in the experiments, it is possible to estimate the speed of the metabolic process under study. The metabolism of proteins, carbohydrates, lipids, and nucleic acids has been localized and analyzed using this procedure. Specific examples include localization of the site and time of DNA synthesis in the nucleus and in mitochondria as well as the sulfation of glycoproteins in the Golgi complex of goblet cells and fibroblasts.

EXAMINATION OF LIVING CELLS & TISSUES

Living cells from an animal can be suspended in an appropriate liquid (saline solution, serum) and ex-

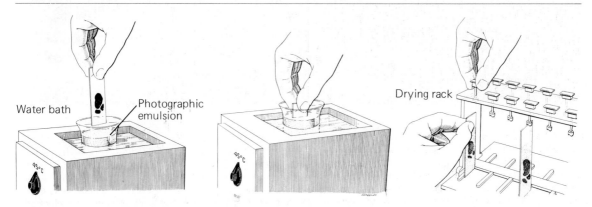

Figure 1–11. Radioautographs are usually made by dipping labeled tissue sections mounted on slides in photographic emulsion. All steps shown above are done in the darkroom under a dark red safelight.

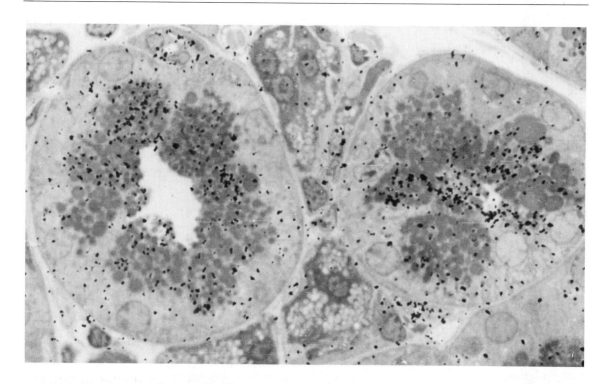

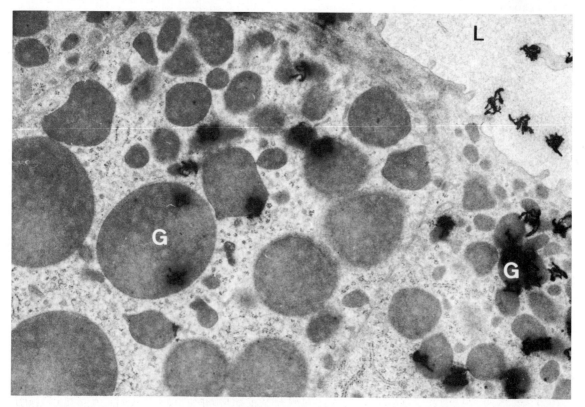

Figure 1–12. Radioautographs from the submandibular gland of a mouse injected 8 hours before sacrifice with ³H-fucose. *Top:* Photomicrograph showing black silver grains indicating radioactive regions in the cells. Most radioactivity is in the granules of the cells of the granular ducts of this gland. × 500. *Bottom:* The same cells in an electron micrograph. Observe the silver grains that, in this enlargement, appear as coiled structures localized mainly over the granules (G) and in the tubular lumen (L). × 9000. (Courtesy of TG Lima and A Haddad.)

amined under the light microscope. Such cells, however, will soon die by a process known as autolysis (described on p 42) if they are not provided with an appropriate medium and gaseous atmosphere.

Prolonged study of living cells and tissues can be achieved by culturing them in solutions that contain the necessary nutrients to keep them alive. The culture medium should be changed frequently, since the nutrients become depleted and toxic products of metabolism accumulate. Rigorous aseptic technique is necessary during the process of cell cultivation in order to avoid contamination of the culture medium with bacteria and molds.

The first culture media used consisted of blood plasma and an extract from embryonic tissues. The composition of this fluid was complicated and difficult to control. Synthetic media of rigidly defined chemical composition are now available. In preparing cultures, cells can be dispersed mechanically or by prior treatment with enzymes such as trypsin or collagenase.

Once isolated, the cells can be cultivated either in a suspension or spread out on a culture plate to which they can adhere as a single layer of cells (Fig 1–13).

Organs can also be cultured, starting from their respective embryonic rudiments. For example, a small bone can be maintained in a culture and allowed to grow. This technique permits study of the factors that influence the development of the organs in conditions much simpler than those that exist inside the living organism. The term **organ culture** means primarily the culture of fragments of organs maintained in conditions such that the architecture of the organ is kept intact. The term **in vitro** is applied to cells and tissue fragments isolated and maintained in culture, in order to distinguish this type of controlled cellular environment from that which the cells experience **in vivo** as an integral part of their parent organism.

Cultures have been used for the study of the metabolism of normal and cancerous cells. This technique is most useful in experiments with viruses that proliferate only in the interior of cells. Some parasitic protozoa have also been studied in tissue culture to observe their development inside the cytoplasm of fibroblasts (Fig 1–13).

In cytogenetic research, tissue cultures permit the study of mitoses and of chromosomes in human cells. Determination of human karyotypes (the number and morphology of an individual's chromosomes) is accomplished by the short-term cultivation of blood lymphocytes or of skin fibroblasts. In examining these cells during mitotic division, one can detect anomalies in the number and morphology of the chromosomes, thus perhaps establishing the diagnosis of certain diseases caused by these anomalies.

THE ISOLATION & STUDY IN VITRO OF PURE CELL STRAINS

Techniques have been developed that permit the isolation of pure suspensions of one cell type, such

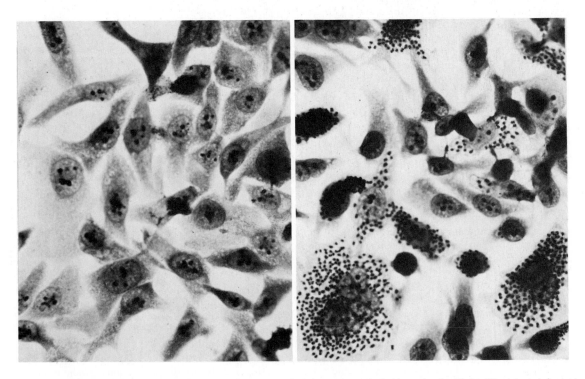

Figure 1–13. Photomicrographs of chicken fibroblasts grown in tissue culture. *Left:* Normal cells. *Right:* Fibroblasts infected by *Trypanosoma cruzi.* Giemsa staining was used. × 340. (Courtesy of S Yoneda.)

as the pancreatic acinar cell, the liver cell, and the parietal cell of the stomach. In vivo, these cells are mixed with other cell types, which adversely influences biochemical and cytophysiologic analyses. Isolated cancer cells, which are usually mixed with blood vessels and connective tissue cells, can now be studied as homogeneous cell preparations.

All methods used are based on the enzymatic digestion of the cellular and extracellular components that bind cells together. The most used enzymes are proteases, collagenase, and hyaluronidase. Incubation of tissue with these enzymes loosens the cells, and they are then separated by weak shearing forces (agitation, pipetting, etc). The cell suspension with different cell types is then purified by centrifugal fractionation or by gravity sedimentation. This last procedure may consist of gently depositing a cell suspension on the surface of a gradient of albumin. The cells slowly settle in the solution of albumin, stopping at different levels within the gradient, reflecting differences in cell density.

CELL FRACTIONATION

Cell fractionation is the physical process by which centrifugal force is used to separate organelles and cellular inclusions as a function of their sedimentation coefficients. The sedimentation coefficient of a particle depends on its size, form, and density and on the viscosity of the medium. If a cell is subjected to an adequate centrifugal force, the organelles inside the cell will be distributed in different layers (Fig 1–14). In each layer, one finds only one type of organelle, and its position inside the cell depends on its coefficient of sedimentation. By means of differential centrifugation, certain cellular organelles can be isolated and their chemical composition and functions determined in vitro.

Differential centrifugation is achieved by subjecting a suspension of cellular components, obtained by disrupting the cells in a process called **homogenization,** to the action of different centrifugal forces (Fig 1–15). The organ or tissue from a recently killed animal is cut into very small fragments, which are then immersed in an appropriate solution. Sucrose in a 0.25 mol/L concentration is often used, but the density, viscosity, and composition of the medium can vary. The fragments of the organ in the solution of sucrose are placed in a homogenizer, often consisting of a glass cylinder within which is a rod that turns with great velocity (Fig 1–15). The fragments of the tissues are crushed by the friction of the rod on the wall of the cylinder, breaking the cell membranes and liberating the organelles and inclusions into the solution.

After homogenization is complete, the suspension is allowed to rest for a few minutes so that the fibers of connective tissue, large cell remnants, and intact cells can settle out. The supernatant is then centrifuged, and the more dense particles (organelles or

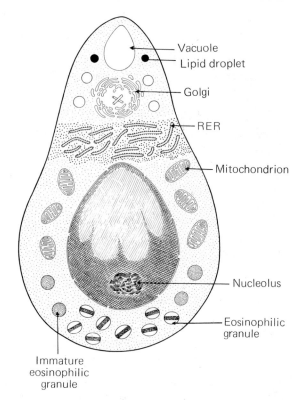

Figure 1–14. Stratification seen in an immature eosinophil after centrifugation. Cell components of higher density (eosinophilic granules, nucleus) accumulate at the bottom of the cell, whereas lighter organelles (Golgi, rough endoplasmic reticulum [RER]) are displaced to the opposite side. (Redrawn and reproduced, with permission, from Bessis in: *The Cell.* Vol 5. Brachet J, Mirsky AE [editors]. Academic Press, 1961.)

inclusions) sediment first. The supernatant from each centrifugation is subjected again to greater centrifugal force, thus separating out the different cellular components, in decreasing order of their density, as shown in Fig 1–15.

An improvement in the technique of differential centrifugation is **centrifugation against a gradient, or density gradient centrifugation.** The gradient consists of a sucrose solution whose concentration (density) is maximal at the bottom of the tube and minimal at the top, with a gradual increase in concentration from top to bottom. The homogenate is placed on top of this stabilized gradient and centrifuged. The particles penetrate the gradient but only to a level where an equilibrium exists between the action of the centrifugal force and the tendency of the particle to float (the buoyant density). This technique permits one to obtain purer fractions of organelles.

In contrast to the continuous gradient just described, one can use a discontinuous, or step, gradient, which is made up of superimposed zones whose den-

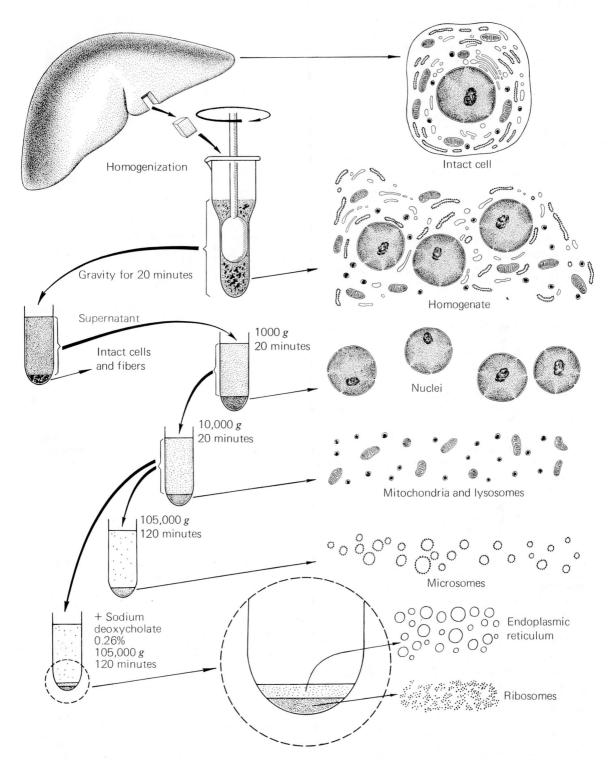

Figure 1–15. Isolation of cell constituents by differential centrifugation. The supernatant of each tube is again centrifuged at higher speeds. The drawings at right show the cellular organelles at the bottom of each tube after centrifugation. Centrifugal force is expressed by *g*, which is equivalent to the force of gravity (1000 *g* means a force 1000 times stronger than that of the gravitational field). (Redrawn and reproduced, with permission, from Bloom W, Fawcett DW: *A Textbook of Histology,* 9th ed. Saunders, 1968.)

Labels in figure:

Homogenization

Intact cell

Gravity for 20 minutes

Homogenate

Supernatant

Intact cells and fibers

1000 *g* 20 minutes

Nuclei

10,000 *g* 20 minutes

Mitochondria and lysosomes

105,000 *g* 120 minutes

Microsomes

+ Sodium deoxycholate 0.26% 105,000 *g* 120 minutes

Endoplasmic reticulum

Ribosomes

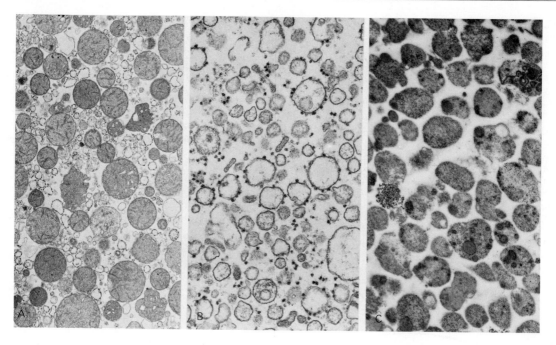

Figure 1–16. Electron micrographs of 3 cell fractions isolated by density gradient centrifugation. *A:* Mitochondrial fraction, contaminated with microsomes. × 13,000. *B:* Microsomal fraction. × 42,500. *C:* Lysosomal fraction. × 25,000. (Courtesy of P Baudhuin.)

sity decreases from one zone to the other, starting from the bottom and proceeding to the top of the centrifuge tube.

All of the stages of the techniques described are carried out at a temperature slightly higher than the freezing point in order to inhibit the action of lytic enzymes that would disrupt the organelles during the separation.

The homogeneity of the fractions thus obtained is examined with the light microscope (for nuclei, mitochondria, and secretory granules), with the electron microscope (for ribosomes, microsomes, etc [Fig 1–16]), or with biochemical methods. For example, the fraction containing the lysosomes can be identified by the quantity of acid phosphatase, an enzyme usually found in these particles, while the fraction containing the nuclei can be identified by the quantity of DNA it possesses.

The isolation of cellular components by differential centrifugation represents a great technical advance and allows the detailed study of cellular components that have been obtained in a relatively pure state, ie, nuclei, nucleoli, mitochondria, rough endoplasmic reticulum, ribosomes, secretory granules, and pigment granules. An example of the application of this method is the study of the physiology of mitochondria; after much discussion, it was established by the isolation of these organelles and subsequent biochemical study that they are the "powerhouses of the cell" where the energy of ingested foods is converted to the common energy currency of the cell—adenosine triphosphate (ATP).

REFERENCES

Bancroft JD, Stevens A: *Theory and Practice of Histological Techniques.* Churchill Livingstone, 1977.

Baserga R, Malamud D: *Autoradiography: Techniques and Application.* Harper & Row, 1969.

Crewe AV: High-resolution scanning transmission electron microscopy. *Science* 1983;**221**:325.

DeDuve C, Beaufay H: A short history of tissue fractionation. *J Cell Biol* 1981;**91**:293s.

Everhart TE, Hayes TL: The scanning electron microscope. *Sci Am* (Jan) 1972;**226**:54.

Glauert AM (editor): *Practical Methods in Electron Microscopy.* North-Holland/American Elsevier, 1975–1980.

Goldstein JI et al: *Scanning Electron Microscopy and X-Ray Microanalysis.* Plenum, 1981.

Hayat MA: *Fixation for Electron Microscopy.* Academic Press, 1981.

Hayat MA: *Introduction to Biological Scanning Electron Microscopy.* University Park Press, 1978.

James J: *Light Microscopic Techniques in Biology and Medicine.* Martinus Nijhoff, 1976.

Paul J: *Cell and Tissue Culture.* Churchill Livingstone, 1975.

Rogers AW: *Techniques of Autoradiography,* 3rd ed. Elsevier, 1979.

Spencer M: *Fundamentals of Light Microscopy.* Cambridge Univ Press, 1982.

Stolinski C, Breathnack AS: *Freeze-Fracture Replication of Biological Tissues.* Academic Press, 1975.

Wischnitzer S: *Introduction to Electron Microscopy.* Pergamon, 1981.

2

Histochemistry & Cytochemistry

The chemistry of tissues and cells is studied by both microscopic and chemical analytic methods. Chemical substances in tissues and cells can be identified by chemical reactions that produce insoluble colored compounds—observed with the light microscope—or electron-scattering precipitates that can be observed with the electron microscope. In Perls's reaction, for example, potassium ferrocyanide reacts with ferric ions in tissues to produce an insoluble dark blue precipitate of ferric ferrocyanide.

In addition to the chemical reactions that take place in tissues, other methods—chiefly physical ones—are frequently used. Examples are interference microscopy, which permits determination of the mass of cells or tissues; and microspectrophotometry, which permits, by means of ultraviolet light, localization and quantitation of DNA and RNA in cells.

BASIC HISTOCHEMICAL & CYTOCHEMICAL PRINCIPLES

For a histochemical reaction to be recognized as valid and meaningful, it must fulfill the following basic requirements:

(1) The substances being analyzed must not diffuse out of their original sites. This problem is easily solved when macromolecules (eg, DNA, proteins) are analyzed. However, when the substance is soluble in the fixative used or in the medium where the reaction is taking place—as in the case of urea and glycogen and of sodium, potassium, or chloride ions—special care must be exercised in the interpretation of the results. Fixatives should preserve the structure of the cell and prevent diffusion of compounds to be studied. For example, fixatives used to study lipids should not contain lipid solvents, and acid fixatives should not be used in techniques for identifying calcium phosphate, since calcium phosphate is soluble in an acid medium. The fixatives most commonly used are formaldehyde (formalin) for light microscopic and glutaraldehyde for electron microscopic histochemical procedures.

(2) The product of the reaction should be insoluble and colored or electron-scattering. Insolubility prevents diffusion of the product of the reaction into the fluid reagent or its spread to a different site in the specimen. Colored or electron-scattering products can be studied with the light or electron microscope, respectively.

(3) The method employed should be specific for the substance or chemical groups being studied.

(4) The procedure must not denature or block reactive groups.

In some histochemical reactions, the intensity of color produced is directly proportionate to the concentration of the substance being analyzed. Under these conditions, concentration of the substances under study can be determined by **microspectrophotometry.** This procedure is carried out by use of a microspectrophotometer, a combination microscope and spectrophotometer. By measuring the light absorbed by small areas of a cell or a tissue, it is possible to quantitate chemical substances in this region. This method was improved by the introduction of scanning devices that analyze with great precision the optical density of the images produced by the cytochemical method and relay the information to a computer that processes the results. This method is of great importance for it permits the analysis of a specific cell type in tissues that contain several cell types—a frequent occurrence in nature.

SOME EXAMPLES OF HISTOCHEMICAL METHODS FOR SUBSTANCES OF BIOLOGIC INTEREST

Ions

A. Iron: When sections of tissues containing ferric ions (Fe^{3+}) are incubated in a mixture of potassium ferrocyanide and hydrochloric acid, iron can be detected by the formation of a highly insoluble, dark blue precipitate of ferric ferrocyanide (Perls's reaction). This method not only allows localization of cells that catabolize hemoglobin but also permits diagnosis of diseases in which deposits of iron occur in the tissues.

B. Phosphates: Phosphates are demonstrated by their reaction with silver nitrate. The silver phosphate formed is reduced by hydroquinone in the next phase of the reaction, producing a black precipitate of reduced silver (Fig 2–1). This reaction is frequently used to study bone and the ossification process, because the only insoluble phosphate found abundantly in the body is calcium phosphate, which is present in large amounts in bone tissue.

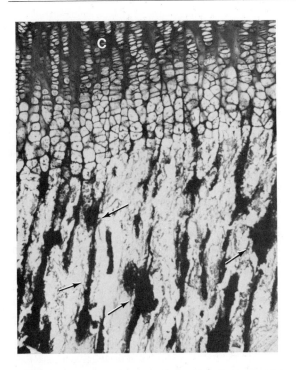

Figure 2–1. Photomicrograph of a section from the epiphysis of an undecalcified bone treated with silver nitrate and subsequently reduced by hydroquinone. The black precipitate in the ossified tissue (arrows) indicates the presence of calcium phosphate. Nonreacting cartilage tissue (C) lies in the upper portion of the section. × 120.

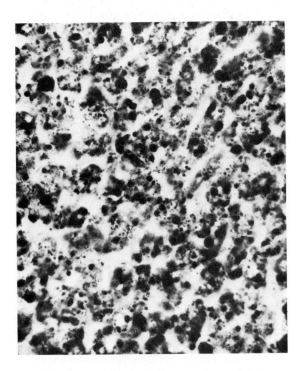

Figure 2–2. Photomicrograph of a section of puppy liver stained by Sudan black. Observe the stained intracellular lipid droplets. × 200.

Lipids

Lipids are best revealed with dyes that are more soluble in the lipids than in the medium in which the dye is dissolved.

In this process, frozen sections are immersed in alcoholic solutions saturated with the appropriate dye. The stain then migrates from the alcohol to the cellular lipid droplets. The dyes most commonly used for this purpose are Sudan IV and Sudan black; they confer on lipids red and black colors, respectively (Fig 2–2).

Additional methods used for the localization of cholesterol and its esters, phospholipids, and glycolipids are useful in the diagnosis of metabolic diseases in which intracellular accumulations of different kinds of lipids occur.

Nucleic Acids

A. Deoxyribonucleic Acid (DNA): DNA is studied chiefly with Feulgen's reaction, a method that starts with the hydrolysis of DNA by hydrochloric acid. This process separates purine bases from sugar, promoting the formation of aldehyde groups in deoxyribose. The free aldehyde groups then react with the Schiff reagent (basic fuchsin bleached by sodium metabisulfite), producing an insoluble red substance. By using this staining procedure in conjunction with microspectrophotometry, it is possible to quantitate the content of DNA in the nuclei of cells.

B. Ribonucleic Acid (RNA): RNA can be identified in tissues by virtue of its great affinity for basic stains (basophilia)—eg, it stains intensely with toluidine blue or methylene blue. Since RNA is not the only basophilic substance in the tissue, it is necessary to incubate a control slide with ribonuclease, an enzyme that removes RNA. Any structure that loses its basophilia as a result of pretreatment with ribonuclease is considered to contain RNA.

Proteins

Nonspecific reactions for the demonstration of proteins in tissues and cells are based chiefly on methods of identifying amino acids. Localization and, sometimes, quantitation of proteins in tissues can be accomplished by means of reactions that produce a color with tyrosine (Millon reaction), tryptophan (tetrazotized benzidine; Fig 2–3), or arginine (Sakaguchi reaction). The Sakaguchi reaction is used frequently in the study of the distribution of basic proteins in nuclei (eg, histones and protamines, which are both rich in arginine). There are also methods for studying the S–H and S–S groups abundant in certain proteins such as keratin.

Polysaccharides & Oligosaccharides

Polysaccharides in the body occur either in a free state or combined with proteins. In the combined state, they constitute an extremely complex heterogeneous group. A ubiquitous polysaccharide in the body, not bound to protein, is **glycogen,** which can be demonstrated by the periodic acid–Schiff (PAS) reaction. The PAS reaction, based on the oxidative action of

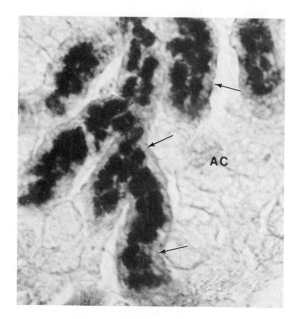

Figure 2–3. Section of mouse submandibular gland stained by the tetrazotized benzidine method for proteins containing tryptophan. The acinar cells (AC) show no reaction, while the tubular cells (arrows) are filled with strongly reacting secretory granules. × 300. (Courtesy of LC Bruschi.)

A variety of anionic, unbranched long-chain polysaccharides composed of aminated monosaccharides (amino sugars) constitute the **glycosaminoglycans** (formerly known as mucopolysaccharides). These substances contain chains of repeating disaccharide units containing an N-acetylated hexosamine. Complexes of covalently bound glycosaminoglycans inserted at regular intervals along a protein core constitute the **proteoglycans.** In proteoglycans, which are significant constituents of connective tissue matrices (see Chapters 5 and 7), the carbohydrate moieties constitute the major component of the molecule.

Interest in the wide variety of sugar-containing macromolecules in the body gave rise to the general term **glycoconjugates** for these substances. This term is applied to **glycoproteins** and **glycolipids** as well as proteoglycans. Although both contain protein and carbohydrate residues, glycoproteins differ in 4 major ways from proteoglycans. (1) Glycoproteins are generally smaller molecules than proteoglycans. (2) The carbohydrate moieties of glycoproteins contain fewer sugar residues and are usually termed **oligosaccharides** rather than polysaccharides. (3) The oligosaccharide chains of glycoproteins are often branched, whereas the polysaccharides of proteoglycans are more likely to be unbranched. (4) The oligosaccharides of glycoproteins are characterized by wide variability in the types and order of the individual sugars in the chain, while the polysaccharides of proteoglycans generally take the form of regular repeating units of disaccharides containing one amino sugar each.

Glycoproteins such as thyroglobulin present in thyroid gland and gonadotropins of the pituitary contain a high proportion of protein. Other glycoproteins with a low protein content, such as those produced by some epithelial cells, are identified as **mucous substances.** Some glycoproteins contain no acidic groups (ie, neutral glycoproteins); others have limited amounts of carboxyl or sulfate radicals (ie, acid mucous substances). The carbohydrate moiety of proteoglycans and glycoproteins containing sulfate and carboxyl groups reacts strongly with the alcian blue dye (Figs 2–4 and 2–5). Neutral glycoproteins can be identified in tissue sections by the fact that they react with the PAS method but are not digested by prior incubation with a glycogenolytic enzyme. Using specific enzymes that digest proteoglycans and some glycoprotein components, one can distinguish these substances in tissue sections.

periodic acid (HIO_4) on 1,2-glycol groups present in the glucose residues, gives rise to aldehyde groups, as shown in the equation below.

As in Feulgen's reaction, these aldehyde groups react with bleached fuchsin (Schiff's reagent), producing a new complex compound having a purple or magenta color. This can be seen in the light microscope, and we call such substances PAS-positive. Since other PAS-positive substances occur in cells, the specificity of this reaction depends on pretreatment with a glycogenolytic enzyme (eg, salivary amylase). Structures that stain intensely with the PAS reaction but fail to do so after pretreatment with amylase are considered to contain glycogen. Using this method, glycogen can be demonstrated in normal liver and striated muscle. It also permits the diagnosis of several diseases in which abnormal intracellular accumulations of glycogen are observed.

Glucose moiety in glycogen $+ HIO_4 \longrightarrow$ Aldehyde moiety

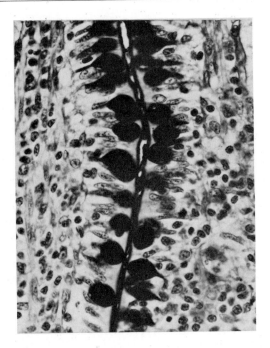

Glycolipids are characteristic constituents of most cell membranes and are significant components of the plasma membranes of nerve cells (eg, gangliosides, cerebrosides). The carbohydrate moieties of glycolipids are oligosaccharides similar to those described for glycoproteins. In analyzing the results of sugar-specific histochemical localization of glycoconjugates, the presence of glycolipids must be taken into account.

Catecholamines

The fact that formaldehyde reacts with catecholamines to produce fluorescent compounds makes it possible to localize epinephrine (adrenaline) and norepinephrine (noradrenaline) in tissue. This method is founded on the observation that ring hydroxylated phenylethylamines, indolealkylamines, and their corresponding amino acids are converted to fluorescent complexes in the presence of relatively dry formaldehyde vapor at 60–80 °C. This reaction has been helpful in studying the distribution of catecholamines and their precursors in neuronal pathways, cell bodies, and nerve endings.

Enzymes

Many histochemical methods are used to reveal

Figure 2–4. Photomicrograph of an intestinal villus stained by alcian blue. The goblet cells stain intensely because of their high content of glycosaminoglycans. × 400.

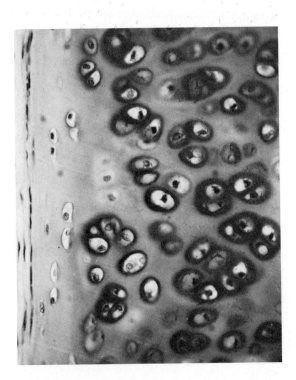

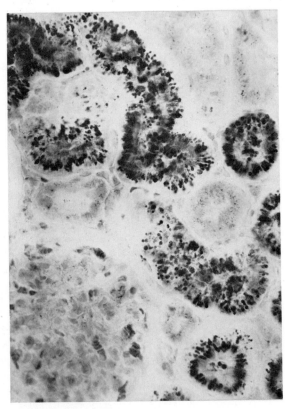

Figure 2–5. Photomicrograph of a section of hyaline cartilage stained with PAS and alcian blue. The region of the matrix close to the cartilage cells contains an abundance of acidic proteoglycans and stains blue with the alcian blue method. The rest of the matrix contains neutral glycoproteins which stain red using the PAS method. × 200.

Figure 2–6. Photomicrograph of a rat kidney section treated by the lead acid phosphatase method. The lysosomes stain intensely as dark granules present in the proximal convoluted tubule cells. × 400.

and identify enzymes. When unstable enzymes are studied, sections of frozen, unfixed material must be used. However, many enzymes may retain a portion of their activity in tissues fixed with aldehyde fixatives such as formalin or glutaraldehyde. Most enzymatic histochemical procedures are based on the production of intensely stained or electron-dense precipitates at the site of enzymatic activity. Three examples of enzymes that can be demonstrated by either the light or the electron microscope are described below.

A. Acid Phosphatase: The Gomori method of demonstrating acid phosphatase activity consists of incubating formalin-fixed tissue sections in a solution containing sodium glycerophosphate and lead nitrate buffered to pH 5.0. The enzyme hydrolyzes the glycerophosphate, liberating phosphate ions that react with lead nitrate to produce an insoluble, colorless precipitate of lead phosphate at the site of the enzymatic activity. In a second step, the preparation is immersed in a solution of ammonium sulfide that reacts with the colorless lead phosphate to produce a black precipitate of lead sulfide. This method permits the localization of this enzyme's activity and is frequently used to demonstrate **lysosomes,** cytoplasmic organelles that contain acid phosphatase (Figs 2–6 and 2–7). The ammonium sulfide step is omitted when the tissue is to be examined in the electron microscope.

B. Dehydrogenases: These enzymes remove hydrogen from one substrate and transfer it to another. There are many different dehydrogenases in the body; they play an important role in several metabolic processes and can be distinguished by means of the substrate on which they act. The histochemical demonstration of dehydrogenases consists of incubating nonfixed tissue sections in a substrate solution containing **tetrazole,** a weakly colored soluble H^+ acceptor. The enzyme transports hydrogen from the substrate to tetrazole and reduces it to an intensely colored insoluble compound called **formazan,** which precipitates at the site of the enzymatic activity. By this method, succinate dehydrogenase—a key enzyme in the citric acid (Krebs) cycle—can be localized in mitochondria (Fig 2–8).

C. Peroxidase: This enzyme, which is present in several types of cells, promotes the oxidation of certain substrates with the transfer of hydrogen ions to hydrogen peroxide, forming molecules of water.

$$\begin{array}{c}OH \\ | \\ OH\end{array} \; + \; \begin{array}{c}OH \\ | \\ R \\ | \\ OH\end{array} \; \boxed{\text{PEROXIDASE}} \longrightarrow \; 2H_2O \; + \; \begin{array}{c}O \\ \| \\ R \\ \| \\ O\end{array}$$

Hydrogen   Substrate   Insoluble and
peroxide   electron-dense
                                                   precipitate

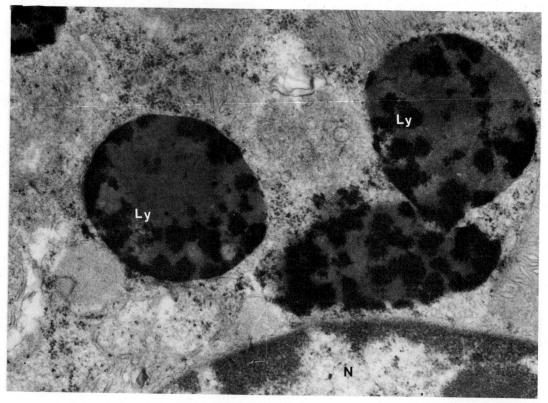

Figure 2–7. Electron micrograph of a rat kidney cell previously treated by the Gomori method for acid phosphatase. The 3 dark, rounded structures above the nucleus (N) are lysosomes (Ly). The denser heterogeneous precipitate within these structures is the lead phosphate that scatters the electrons. The information in this electron micrograph is equivalent to that in the light micrograph illustrated in Fig 2–6. × 25,000. (Courtesy of E Katchburian.)

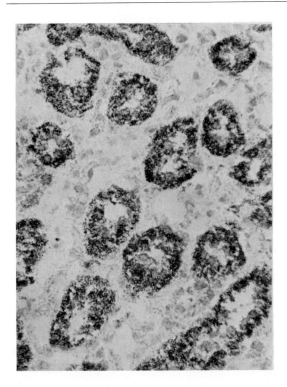

Figure 2–8. Photomicrograph of a frozen section of fresh, unfixed kidney previously incubated in succinate plus monotetrazole (MTT). The dark precipitate seen in the tubules indicates the activity of succinate dehydrogenase. × 400. (Courtesy of AGE Pearse.)

In this method, sections of adequately fixed tissue are incubated in a solution containing hydrogen peroxide and 3,3′-diaminoazobenzidine. In the presence of peroxidase, the latter compound is oxidized, resulting in an insoluble black, electron-dense precipitate that permits the localization of peroxidase activity in the optical and electron microscopes. Since the enzyme is extremely active, it produces an appreciable amount of insoluble precipitate in a short time, making this procedure a very sensitive histochemical assay.

FLUORESCENCE MICROSCOPY

This technique is based on the fact that when certain fluorescent substances are irradiated by light of a proper wavelength, they emit light with a longer wavelength. In fluorescence microscopy, tissue sections are usually irradiated with ultraviolet light so that the emission is in the visible portion of the spectrum. The fluorescent substances appear as brilliant shiny particles on a dark background. In this procedure, a microscope with a strong ultraviolet light source is used. Special filters that eliminate ultraviolet light are employed to protect the observer's eyes.

Fluorescent Compounds

Some naturally fluorescent substances are normal constituents of cells, eg, vitamin A, vitamin B₂, and porphyrins. Other fluorescent compounds that have an affinity for tissues and cells are used as fluorescent stains. Acridine orange is most widely used, because it can combine with DNA and RNA. When observed in the fluorescence microscope, the DNA–acridine orange complex emits a yellowish-green light, whereas the RNA–acridine orange complex emits a reddish-orange light. Thus, it is possible to identify and localize nucleic acids in the cells (Fig 2–9). Since cancer cells usually contain larger amounts of RNA than normal cells, acridine orange can be used to identify them in smears obtained from patients.

Fluorescence spectroscopy is a method of analyzing the light emitted by a fluorescent compound in a microspectrophotometer. It can be used to characterize several compounds present in cells and is of particular importance in the study of catecholamines.

IMMUNOCYTOCHEMISTRY

Specific amino acids or reactive groups can be identified by conventional cytochemical methods, but these techniques cannot localize specific proteins. The fluorescent antibody method has proved most useful

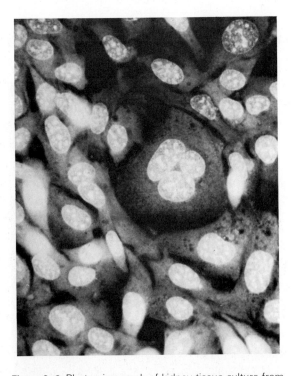

Figure 2–9. Photomicrograph of kidney tissue culture from an embryonic hamster transformed by simian virus 40, stained with acridine orange, and photographed with the fluorescence microscope. A green fluorescence (shown as white in photo) appears in the regions containing DNA (nucleus); a reddish-orange color (shown as gray) is characteristic of the RNA-rich cytoplasm. In the center is a giant cell. × 1000. (Courtesy of A Geraldes and JMV Costa.)

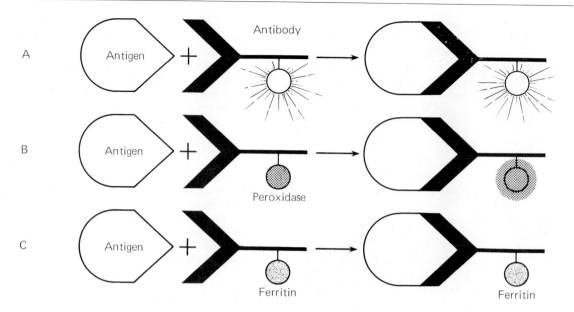

Figure 2–10. Three current methods of labeling and identifying specific proteins by immunocytochemistry. *A:* The antibody is coupled to a fluorescent compound, such as fluorescein isothiocyanate (green) or rhodamine (red). After incubation, the sections containing the antigen exposed to the labeled antibody solution are studied in the fluorescence microscope. *B:* The antibody is coupled to peroxidase. After the antigen-antibody reaction, the section is submitted to the histochemical method for peroxidase and studied with the light or electron microscope (see text). *C:* The antibody is coupled to ferritin. After the antigen-antibody reaction, this material is studied with the electron microscope, in which the electron-scattering iron atoms of ferritin can be visualized.

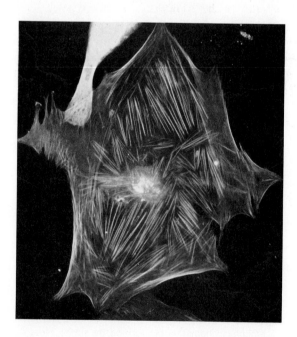

Figure 2–11. Actin fibrils composed of aggregates of actin filaments in the cytoplasm of a cultured human fibroblast preincubated in fluorescent actin antibody. × 1767. (Reproduced, with permission, from E Lazarides: Tropomyosin antibody: The specific localization of tropomyosin in nonmuscle cells. *J Cell Biol* 1975;**65:**549.)

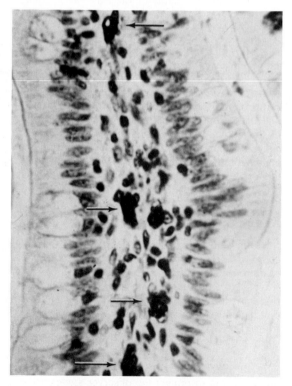

Figure 2–12. Photomicrograph of an intestinal villus showing macrophages stained by the immunoperoxidase method using antilysozyme antibodies (arrows). × 400.

in localizing specific proteins and certain other macromolecules. This test is based on the reaction of the body when exposed to foreign substances called **antigens** or **immunogens.** The body will respond by producing **antibodies** that react specifically and bind strongly to the antigen and result in neutralization of the foreign substance. Antibodies are proteins of the globulin group (immunoglobulins) that appear in plasma and tissue fluids after antigen injection. Their production enables the organism to oppose invasion by foreign microorganisms and to eliminate certain proteins and other foreign matter not recognized as self. Immunocytochemistry is based on the coupling of immunoglobulins to substances that render them visible in the microscope without causing loss of biologic activity of the antibody. Since the labeled immunoglobulins bind specifically to their antigens, these compounds permit localization of specific antigens in tissue specimens. When a tissue section containing certain antigens is incubated in a solution containing labeled antibodies to these antigens, the antibodies bind specifically to the antigens, whose location can then be visualized with either the light or electron microscope.

Three methods of labeling antibodies are frequently used (Fig 2–10):

(1) Coupling with fluorescent compounds: This permits one to identify the site of specific antigens using a fluorescence microscope (Fig 2–11).

(2) Coupling with an enzyme: This permits detection of the labeled antibody by conventional enzyme cytochemistry. The enzyme most often used is peroxidase, which can be detected by the method described above, using either the light or electron microscope (Fig 2–12).

(3) Coupling to an electron-scattering compound that can be detected in the electron microscope: An iron-rich protein called **ferritin** or gold particles are often used as antibody markers. In the electron microscope, the location of electron-dense ferritin- or gold-bound antibodies can be easily identified.

There are both direct and indirect methods for antigen localization by immunocytochemistry.

(1) Direct method: Sections of a tissue suspected of containing an antigen (protein X) are incubated with a labeled antibody to X, and the antibody will specifically combine with X. The excess antibodies are washed off, and the tissue is processed according to the methods outlined above (Fig 2–13A). The location of the antigen is then detected in either the light or electron microscope.

(2) Indirect method: Antibodies to protein X (the antigen) are produced in an animal, eg, a rabbit. Rabbit immunoglobulins are, in turn, capable of inducing an antibody response in another animal, such as a sheep or goat. A tissue section containing protein X is incubated with unlabeled rabbit anti-X antibodies. After washing, labeled antirabbit antibodies are added, and the location of protein X can be visualized by a microscopic technique appropriate for the label. This method has the advantage that the sensitivity of the technique is considerably increased (Fig 2–13B) over the direct method (Fig 2–13A).

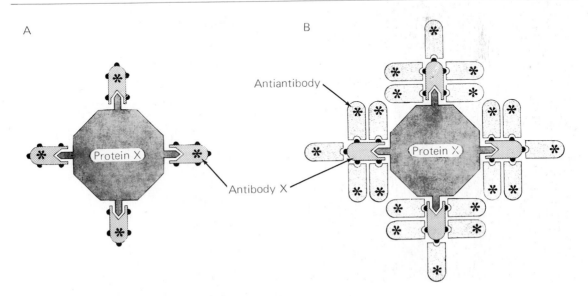

Figure 2–13. The direct *(A)* and indirect *(B)* techniques of immunofluorescence. In the direct technique, fluorescently tagged antibody binds to the antigen present in the cells. Observe that in this hypothetical case each antigen molecule binds only a small number of antibody molecules. In the indirect technique, nonfluorescent antibody is first bound to the antigen, and fluorescent antiantibody (also called fluorescent immunoglobulin) then binds to the antibody. Because each antibody molecule binds 5 molecules of fluorescent antiantibody, the indirect procedure is more sensitive in that each antigen molecule indirectly binds a large number of fluorescent antibody molecules.

REFERENCES

Cuello ACC: *Immunocytochemistry*. Wiley, 1983.

Hayat MA: *Electron Microscopy of Enzymes*. Vols 1–5. Van Nostrand-Reinhold, 1973–1977.

Kuhlmann WD: Ultrastructural immunoperoxidase cytochemistry. *Prog Histochem Cytochem* 1977;**10**:1.

Martin DW Jr et al: *Harper's Review of Biochemistry*, 20th ed. Lange, 1985.

Pearse AGE: *Histochemistry: Theoretical and Applied*, 4th ed. Churchill Livingstone, 1980.

Polak JM, VanNoorden S (editors): *Immunocytochemistry: Practical Applications in Pathology and Biology*. PSG, 1983.

Sternberger LA: *Immunocytochemistry*, 2nd ed. Wiley, 1979.

The Cell

3

Cells are the structural units of all living organisms. It has been recognized for some time that there exist 2 fundamentally different types of cells, at least from the structural point of view. So many biochemical similarities exist between the 2 types that many investigators have postulated that one group evolved from the other.

The **prokaryotic** cell is typified by bacteria. These cells are small ($1-5$ μm long), may have a cell wall outside the limiting membrane (cell membrane, plasmalemma), and do not have a nuclear envelope separating the genetic material (DNA) from other cellular constituents. In addition, prokaryotes have no histones (specific basic proteins) bound to their DNA, and membranous organelles are usually not present.

In contrast, **eukaryotic** cells are larger (> 10 μm in diameter) and have a distinct nucleus surrounded by a nuclear envelope (Fig 3–1). Histones are associated with the genetic material, and numerous membrane-limited organelles are found in the cytoplasm. Eukaryotic cells are characteristic of protozoa (eg, amebas) and their presumed evolutionary offspring, ie, all other plants and animals (metazoa). This chapter is concerned almost exclusively with eukaryotic cells.

CELLULAR FUNCTIONS & DIFFERENTIATION

During the process of evolution, the cells of metazoa gradually became modified and specialized, resulting in increased efficiency of function. Through phylogenetic development, undifferentiated primitive cells exhibiting several functional activities, each with little efficiency, were transformed into a variety of differentiated cells that were collectively able to perform some specific functions with much greater efficiency. This process of cell specialization is known as **cell differentiation.**

For example, the muscle cell during its differentiation elongates into a spindle-shaped cell that synthesizes and accumulates myofibrillar proteins. The resulting cell acts to efficiently convert chemical energy into contractile force. Another example is the pancreatic cell, which is specialized to synthesize and secrete digestive enzymes.

Morphologic modifications during differentiation are accompanied by chemical changes, and the quantitative synthesis of specific proteins by each differentiated cell type characterizes this process. Examples

Table 3–1. Cellular functions in some specialized cells.

Function	Specialized Cell(s)
Movement	Muscle cell
Conductivity	Nerve cell
Synthesis and secretion of enzymes	Pancreatic acinar cells
Synthesis and secretion of mucous substances	Mucous gland cells
Synthesis and secretion of steroids	Some adrenal gland, testis, and ovary cells
Ion transport	Cells of the kidney and salivary gland ducts
Intracellular digestion	Macrophages and some white blood cells
Transformation of physical and chemical stimuli into nervous impulses	Sensory cells
Metabolite absorption	Cells of the intestine, kidney, etc

are the synthesis of the proteins actin and myosin by the muscle cell or of several digestive enzymes by pancreatic acinar cells. Cellular functions performed by specialized cells in the body are listed in Table 3–1.

Cells are not always restricted to a single, specialized function and frequently are capable of performing 2 or more functions. Thus, the cells of the proximal convoluted tubules of the kidney not only transport ions but also reabsorb metabolites and digest proteins. Similarly, the intestinal epithelial cells reabsorb metabolites and synthesize digestive enzymes (proteins) such as disaccharidases and peptidases (see Chapter 16).

It will be seen that the morphology of a cell varies predictably according to its functions.

CELL COMPONENTS

The cell is composed of 2 basic parts: **cytoplasm** and **nucleus.** Individual cytoplasmic components are usually not clearly distinguishable in common hematoxylin and eosin–stained preparations; the nucleus, however, appears intensely stained dark blue or black (Fig 4–1).

Cytoplasm

The outermost organelle of the cell, separating the cytoplasm from its extracellular environment, is the plasma membrane (plasmalemma). The cytoplasm it-

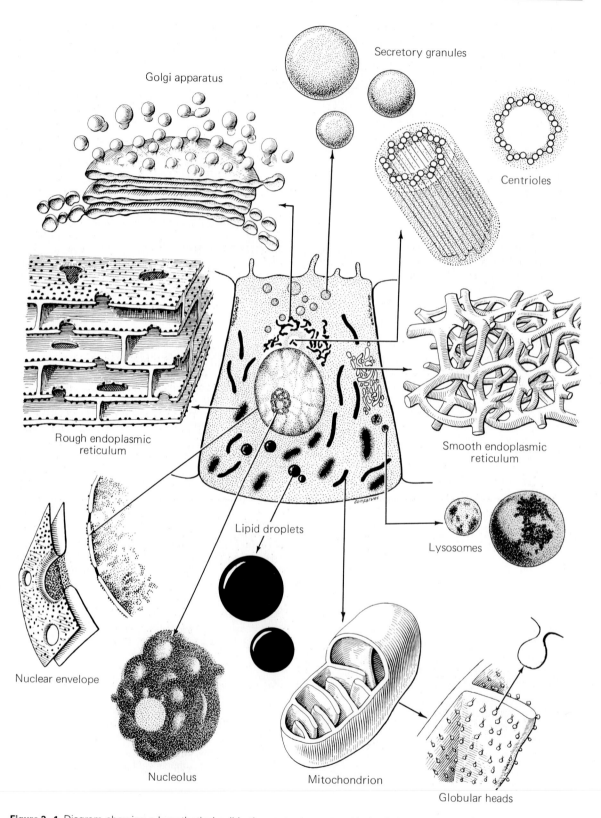

Golgi apparatus

Secretory granules

Centrioles

Rough endoplasmic reticulum

Smooth endoplasmic reticulum

Nuclear envelope

Lipid droplets

Lysosomes

Nucleolus

Mitochondrion

Globular heads

Figure 3–1. Diagram showing a hypothetical cell in the center as seen with the light microscope. It is surrounded by its various structures as seen with the electron microscope. (Redrawn and reproduced, with permission, from Bloom W, Fawcett DW: *A Textbook of Histology,* 9th ed. Saunders, 1968.)

self is composed of a matrix in which are embedded several structures classified into 3 groups: organelles, inclusions, and other components. The structures known as **organelles** are present in all eukaryotic cells, have a limiting membrane, and contain enzymes that participate in cellular metabolic activity. They are permanent components of the cytoplasm. Examples include the endoplasmic reticulum, mitochondria, the Golgi complex, and lysosomes. **Cytoplasmic inclusions** generally are temporary components of certain cells and usually are accumulations of pigment, lipids, proteins, or carbohydrates that may or may not be enclosed in a membrane. The other components cannot be classified as one of the 2 preceding classes and have different structures and functions. They are not enclosed in a membrane and do not participate directly in cellular metabolism. This group comprises the centriole, microtubules, microfilaments, and intermediate filaments. Taken together, these other components are often referred to as the cytoskeleton and act as a dynamic supportive network within the cytoplasm.

Plasma Membrane

All eukaryotic cells are enveloped by a limiting membrane composed of lipids (phospholipids and cholesterol), protein, and oligosaccharides covalently linked to some of the lipids and proteins. The cell membrane (plasmalemma) functions as a selective barrier that regulates the passage of certain materials into and out of the cell. In addition, membranes may *facilitate* the transport of specific materials through this limiting barrier. Membranes also carry out a number of specific recognition and regulatory functions, to be discussed later. For these reasons, the plasma membrane plays an important role in the way a cell interacts with its environment.

Cell membranes range from 7.5 to 10 nm in thickness and consequently are visible only in the electron microscope. Micrographs reveal that the plasmalemma—and, for that matter, almost all other organellar membranes—exhibit a trilaminar structure after fixation in osmium tetroxide (Fig 3–2). Based on the universality of this appearance, this 3-layered structure has been designated the **unit membrane** (Fig 3–3).

Membrane phospholipids, such as phosphatidylcholine (lecithin) and phosphatidylethanolamine (cephalin), consist of 2 long, nonpolar (hydrophobic) hydrocarbon chains linked to a charged (hydrophilic) head group. Cholesterol is also a constituent of most membranes. Within the membrane, lipids are most stable when organized into a double layer with their hydrophobic (nonpolar) chains directed toward the center of the membrane and their charged (hydrophilic) heads directed outward (Fig 3–2). The lipid composition of each half of the bilayer is different. In the erythrocyte, phosphatidylcholine and sphingomyelin are more abundant in the outer half of the membrane, while phosphatidylserine and phosphatidylethanolamine are more concentrated in the inner half. Some of the lipids, known as glycolipids, possess oligosaccharide chains that extend outward from the surface of the cell membrane and thus contribute to the lipid asymmetry (Fig 3–4A). The trilaminar appearance of membranes in the electron microscope is apparently due to the deposition of reduced osmium on the hydrophilic groups on each side of the lipid bilayer.

The proteins, which are a major molecular constituent of membranes (> 50% w/w), can be divided into 2 groups. **Integral proteins** represent a class of proteins that are directly incorporated within the lipid bilayer, while **peripheral proteins** exhibit a looser association with membrane surfaces. The loosely bound peripheral proteins can be easily extracted from cell membranes by use of salt solutions, whereas integral proteins can only be extracted by drastic methods involving the use of detergents.

From freeze-fracture electron microscopic studies, it appears that many integral proteins are distributed

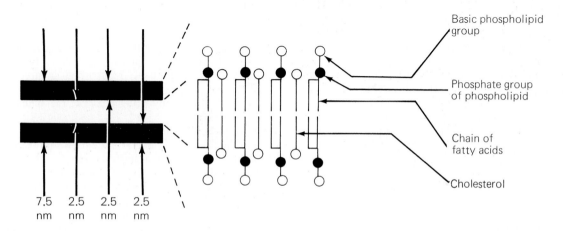

7.5 nm 2.5 nm 2.5 nm 2.5 nm

Basic phospholipid group

Phosphate group of phospholipid

Chain of fatty acids

Cholesterol

Figure 3–2. The ultrastructure *(left)* and molecular structure *(right)* of the cell membrane. The dark lines at left represent the 2 dense layers observed in the electron microscope due to deposition of osmium in the hydrophilic portions of the lipid molecules.

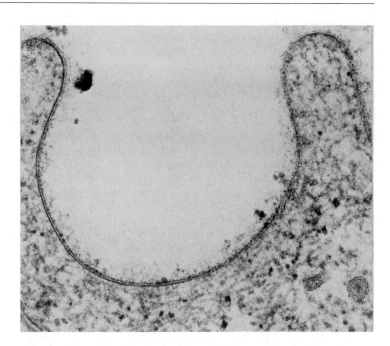

Figure 3–3. Electron micrograph of a section of the surface of an epithelial cell, showing the unit membrane with its 2 dark lines limiting a clear band. On the surface of the membrane is a layer of granular material forming the cell coat. × 100,000.

as globular molecules intercalated among the lipid molecules (Fig 3–4B). Some of these proteins are only partially embedded in the lipid bilayer, so that they may protrude from either the outer or inner surfaces. Other proteins are large enough to extend across the 2 lipid layers and protrude from both membrane surfaces. Some of the proteins that completely cross the membrane are believed to provide for a channel through which water-soluble substances, such as ions, can pass back and forth between the extracellular and intracellular compartments. These protein channels correspond to the membrane pores postulated by cell physiologists to account for the data generated by permeability experiments. Other proteins, which may possess lipid (lipoproteins) or carbohydrate (glycoproteins and proteoglycans) side chains, are arranged as mosaics within the cell membrane (Fig 3–4). The carbohydrate moieties of glycoproteins and glycolipids project from the external surface of the plasma membrane and have been implicated as mediators of important cellular interactions such as adhesion and recognition.

Integration of the proteins within the lipid bilayer is the result of hydrophobic interactions between the lipids and nonpolar (hydrophobic) regions on the surface of the membrane proteins (Fig 3–4A). However, the integral proteins are not bound rigidly in place and are able to move by diffusing within the plane of the cell membrane. Under certain circumstances, these proteins can accumulate at one region of the plasma membrane, occasionally forming a localized aggregation of proteins. This process, called **capping,** has been observed in several cell types and appears to be a general phenomenon. Experiments have also revealed that movement of some membrane proteins is not random but is probably controlled by intracellular mechanisms involving microfilaments. The associa-

tion of actin-containing microfilaments with integral membrane proteins, via one to several peripheral membrane proteins, is becoming better understood, especially in the erythrocyte (red blood cell). At the inner surface of the plasma membrane of erythrocytes, a lattice, composed of a protein called **spectrin,** is found. Spectrin consists of 2 copies each of an α subunit (MW 240,000) and a β subunit (MW 225,000). The subunits are coiled around each other and associate head-to-head, forming a tetramer 200 nm in length. Spectrin binds to cytoplasmic actin-containing microfilaments and also binds to another protein known as **ankyrin.** Ankyrin, in turn, binds to an erythrocyte integral membrane protein referred to as **protein 3 tetramer.** The latter serves as an anion channel in the erythrocyte membrane (Fig 3–4A). If spectrin is extracted, the erythrocyte membrane breaks up into small vesicles, thus demonstrating the importance of this protein as part of the membrane skeleton. Recently, spectrinlike proteins have been found in cells such as neurons and intestinal epithelial cells. These proteins have been given other names (eg, fodrin, TW260/240), but they are probably related both in structure and function to spectrin. They also help maintain the shape of these cells by being a part of the submembrane skeleton.

Fig 3–5 illustrates an experiment that demonstrates the fluidity of integral proteins within the cell membrane. The above-described "mosaic" disposition of membrane proteins, in conjunction with the fluid nature of the lipid bilayer, constitutes the basis of the presently accepted **fluid mosaic model** for membrane structure, as illustrated in Fig 3–4A.

The plasma membrane is the site where materials are exchanged between the cell and its environment. Some ions, such as Na^+, K^+, and Ca^{2+}, are actively transported across the cell membrane using channels that are integral membrane proteins. Mass transfers of material also occur through the intervention of the plasma membrane. A general name for uptake of material is **endocytosis;** the corresponding name for release of material is **exocytosis.** Several varieties of endocytosis are recognized.

(1) Fluid phase pinocytosis: Small invaginations of the cell membrane form and entrap extracellular fluid and anything in solution in the fluid. **Pinocytotic vesicles** (about 80 nm in diameter) pinch off from the cell surface (Fig 4–20), and most eventually fuse with lysosomes (see p 38). However, in the lining cells of capillaries (endothelial cells), pinocytotic vesicles may move to the surface opposite their origin. Here they fuse with the plasma membrane and release their contents onto the cell surface, thus accomplishing bulk transfer of material across the cell (see Fig 4–22 and p 261).

(2) Receptor-mediated endocytosis: Receptors for many substances, such as low-density lipoproteins and protein hormones, are located at the cell surface. The receptors are either originally widely dispersed over the surface or are aggregated in special regions called **coated pits.** Binding of the ligand to its receptor causes widely dispersed receptors to accumulate in coated pits. The "coat" on the cytoplasmic surface of the membrane is composed of several polypeptides, the major one being **clathrin** (MW 180,000). These proteins form a lattice composed of pentagons and hexagons very similar in arrangement to the struts in a geodesic dome. It is believed that this arrangement produces a force which causes the coated pit to invaginate and pinch off, forming a **coated vesicle** that carries the ligand and its receptor into the cell. Recently, an intermediate structure was discovered be-

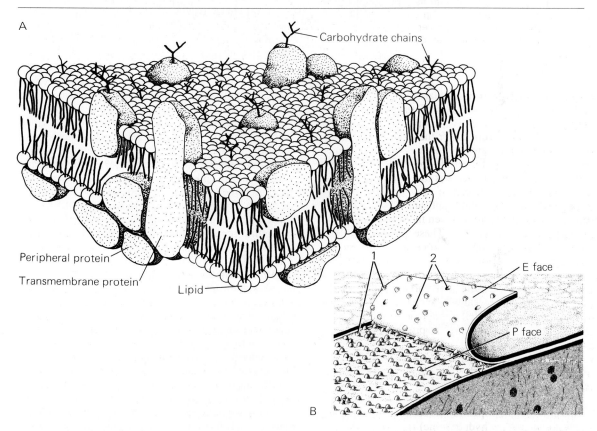

Figure 3–4. *A:* The fluid mosaic model of membrane structure. The membrane consists of a bimolecular lipid layer with proteins inserted in it or bound to the cytoplasmic surface. Integral membrane proteins are firmly embedded in the lipid layers. Some of these proteins completely span the bilayer and are called transmembrane proteins, while others are embedded in either the outer or inner leaflet of the lipid bilayer. Loosely bound to the inner surface of the membrane are the peripheral proteins. Many of the proteins and lipids have externally exposed oligosaccharide chains. *B:* Membrane cleavage occurs when a cell is frozen and fractured (cryofracture). Most of the membrane particles (1), generally thought to represent proteins or aggregates of proteins, remain attached to the half of the membrane adjacent to the cytoplasm (P, or protoplasmic, face of the membrane). Fewer particles are found attached to the outer half of the membrane (E, or extracellular, face). For every protein particle that bulges on one surface, a corresponding depression (2) appears in the opposite surface. Membrane splitting occurs along the line of weakness formed by the fatty acid tails of membrane phospholipids. Only weak hydrophobic interactions serve to bind the 2 halves of the membrane together along this line. The study of these protein particles by cryofracture has contributed significantly to our knowledge of cell membranes. (Modified and reproduced, with permission, from Krstić RV: *Ultrastructure of the Mammalian Cell.* Springer-Verlag, 1979.)

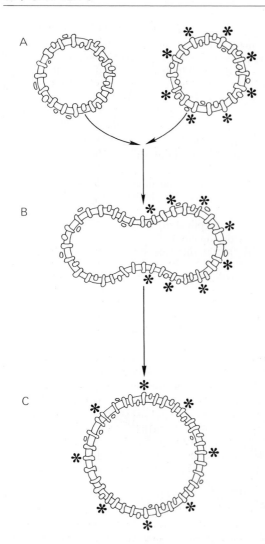

Figure 3–5. Experiment demonstrating the fluid nature of proteins within the cell membrane. The plasmalemma is shown as 2 parallel lines (representing the lipid portion) in which proteins are embedded. Some of these particles are characteristic of the cell at top right and are identified by asterisks. In this experiment, 2 different types of cells derived from tissue cultures (one with a fluorescent marker [right] and one without) are fused *(A → B)* owing to the action of Sendai virus. Minutes after the fusion of the membranes, the fluorescent marker of the labeled cell spreads to the entire surface of the fused cells and finally covers it uniformly *(C)*.

tween the coated vesicle and the lysosome. This is the **endosome,** a larger vesicle without the clathrin coat. The membrane of the endosome contains proton pumps, and its internal pH is 5.0 or less. Most ligands dissociate from their receptors at this pH. Short tubular extensions of the endosome membrane seem to segregate the membrane-bound receptors from the now soluble ligands. Some workers have called this structure **CURL,** an acronym denoting *c*ompartment of

*u*ncoupling of *r*eceptor and *l*igand. The receptors are recycled to the cell surface, while the ligands are directed to lysosomes (see p 38).

(3) Phagocytosis: This term literally means "cell eating" and can be compared to pinocytosis, which means "cell drinking." Certain cell types, such as macrophages and polymorphonuclear leukocytes, are specialized for taking up and disposing of invading bacteria, protozoa, fungi, damaged cells, and unneeded extracellular constituents. For example, after a bacterium becomes bound to the surface of a macrophage, cytoplasmic processes of the macrophage are extended and ultimately surround the bacterium. The edges of these processes fuse, resulting in the bacterium being enclosed in an intracellular **phagocytic vacuole** (Fig 5– 18). Lysosomes will then fuse with the vacuole, resulting in destruction of the bacterium (see also p 38 and Chapter 13).

Exocytosis is the term used to describe the fusion of a membrane-limited organelle with the plasma membrane, resulting in the release of the contents of the organelle into the extracellular space without compromising the integrity of the plasma membrane. A typical example is the release of stored products from secretory cells such as the exocrine pancreas or neurons (Fig 4– 23).

The structures of other membranes (nuclear envelope, endoplasmic reticulum, Golgi complex, secretory granules, and lysosomes)—although not identical—are similar to those of the plasma membrane. The structural and functional differences observed are at present being actively investigated. Chemical differences have been noted, and structural differences have been associated with the presence of different structural proteins, lipids, enzymes, and receptors on them.

Mitochondria

Mitochondria are present in all eukaryotic cells, at least in the early stages of differentiation. They are organelles that transform with high efficiency the chemical energy of the metabolites present in cytoplasm into energy that is easily accessible to the cell. This energy is stored as high-energy phosphate bonds in several compounds. These compounds, the most important of which is adenosine triphosphate (ATP), promptly release energy when required by the cell to perform any type of work, whether it be of osmotic, mechanical, electrical, or chemical nature.

Mitochondria are spherical or filamentous organelles 0.5– 1 μm wide that can attain a length of up to 10 μm. Their distribution in cells varies. They tend to accumulate in parts of the cytoplasm where metabolic activity is more intense, such as at the apical ends of ciliated cells (Fig 4– 14), in the middle piece of spermatozoa (Fig 23– 4), or at the base of iontransferring cells (Fig 4– 20). In instances where they are not polarized, they have a tendency to be oriented along the long axis of long cells, or radially in round cells.

Cells contain great numbers of mitochondria—an

estimated 2500 in one liver cell—but always in a characteristic number for that cell. Mitochondria are composed mainly of protein. Lipids are present to a lesser degree, along with small quantities of DNA and RNA. Like most cell components, mitochondria have a short life span, and their proteins are constantly being renewed. The average half-life of mitochondrial proteins in rat liver cells is 10 days. The ultrastructure of mitochondria varies with the organ and species from which the tissue is obtained for examination.

Mitochondria generally have a characteristic structure under the electron microscope (Figs 3–1 and 3–6). They are composed of an **outer mitochondrial membrane** and an **inner mitochondrial membrane,** and the latter projects folds into the interior of mitochondria, which are termed **cristae.** These membranes enclose 2 spaces. The outer space, located between the 2 membranes, is termed the **intramembrane space** and is continuous with the **intracristal spaces** that penetrate the cristae. The other space is the **intercristal,** or **matrix, space,** which is enclosed by the inner membrane and is in turn penetrated by the cristae. Filling the matrix space is a fine granular material of variable electron density. Most mitochondria have flat, shelflike cristae in their interiors (Figs 3–1 and 3–6), whereas cells that secrete steroids (eg, adrenal and gonadal cells; see Chapter 4) frequently contain tubular cristae (Fig 4–30). The cristae increase the internal surface area of mitochondria, and it is on these structures that enzymes and other compounds involved in the oxidative phosphorylation and electron transport systems are located. The ADP to ATP phosphorylating system is localized in globular structures connected to the membrane via cylindric stalks (Fig 3–1). The other electron transport enzymes are found embedded within the membrane.

The number of mitochondria and the number of cristae in each mitochondrion are proportionate to the metabolic activity of the cells in which they reside. Thus, cells with a high rate of metabolism (eg, cardiac muscle or kidney tubule cells) have abundant mitochondria with a large number of closely packed cristae, whereas others with low metabolism have few mitochondria with short cristae.

Between the cristae is an amorphous **matrix** rich in protein and some DNA. In a great number of cell types, the mitochondrial matrix also exhibits rounded electron-dense granules rich in cations such as calcium and magnesium. Although their function is not completely understood, the granules are apparently related to the mitochondrion's ability to concentrate cations. Enzymes for the citric acid (Krebs) cycle and fatty acid β-oxidation are found to reside within the matrix space.

The DNA isolated from the mitochondrial matrix has been shown to have a circular structure. DNA strands are synthesized within the mitochondrion, and their duplication is independent of nuclear DNA replication. Particles resembling ribosomes are present in mitochondria. Mitochondria are known to contain the 3 types of RNA (ribosomal RNA [rRNA], messenger RNA [mRNA], and transfer RNA [tRNA]) usually present in cells and necessary for protein synthesis. Protein synthesis occurs in mitochondria, but owing to the reduced amount of mitochondrial DNA only a small proportion of the mitochondrial proteins are produced locally. Most of the mitochondrial proteins are coded by nuclear DNA and synthesized in polysomes present in the cytosol. The proteins are then transported into mitochondria by mechanisms which are not fully understood but which require energy.

Metabolites within the cell are utilized within mitochondria by the catalytic activity of the enzymes of the citric acid (Krebs) cycle, and the energy liberated in this process is captured through oxidative phos-

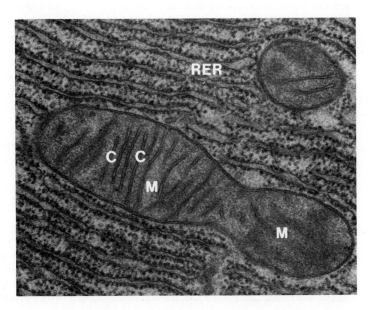

Figure 3–6. Electron micrograph of a section of pancreas from the rat. A mitochondrion with its membranes, cristae (C), and matrix (M) is seen in the center. Numerous flattened cisternae of rough endoplasmic reticulum (RER) with ribosomes on their cytoplasmic surfaces are also visible. × 50,000.

phorylation. The end product of these reactions is the high-energy compound ATP. In addition, CO_2 and water are concurrently produced.

The initial degradation of proteins, carbohydrates, and fats is carried out in the cytosol—that portion of the cell outside the mitochondria. The metabolic end product of these extramitochondrial metabolic pathways is acetyl-CoA, which then enters the mitochondria. Within the mitochondria, acetyl-CoA combines with oxaloacetate to form citric acid. Within the citric acid cycle, there are several reactions of decarboxylation producing CO_2, and 4 pairs of hydrogen atoms are removed by specific reactions catalyzed by dehydrogenases. The H atoms react ultimately with oxygen to form H_2O. The **electron transport system,** which is known to be located in the inner mitochondrial membrane, is capable, by virtue of the action of cytochromes a, b, and c, coenzyme Q, and cytochrome oxidase, of releasing energy that is captured at 3 points of this system through the formation of ATP from ADP and inorganic phosphate. Under aerobic conditions, the combined activity of extramitochondrial glycolysis and the citric acid cycle as well as the electron transport system gives rise to 36 molecules of ATP per mole of glucose. This is 18 times the energy obtainable under anaerobic circumstances, when only the glycolytic pathway can be utilized.

Origin & Evolution of Mitochondria

In the process of mitosis, each daughter cell receives approximately half of the mitochondria originally present in the parent cell just before division. New mitochondria originate from preexisting mitochondria by accretion of material that leads to growth and subsequent division (fission) of the organelle itself.

The fact that mitochondria have some characteristics in common with bacteria has led to speculation regarding the possible origin of mitochondria from an ancestral prokaryote that became adapted to a symbiotic life within a eukaryotic host cell.

Ribosomes

Ribosomes are small electron-dense particles, about 20 × 30 nm in size. They are composed of 4 types of ribosomal RNA (rRNA) and almost 80 different proteins. Ribosomes are found in all cells, at least early in differentiation, but each cell type has a characteristic number and distribution of these particles.

There are 2 classes of ribosomes: one class is found in prokaryotes, chloroplasts, and mitochondria, and the other is found in eukaryotic cells. Both classes of ribosomes are composed of 2 different-sized subunits. The properties of eukaryotic ribosomes are shown in Table 3-2.

In eukaryotic cells, the RNAs of both subunits are synthesized within the nucleoli of the nucleus. The numerous proteins, synthesized in the cytoplasm, enter the nucleus and associate with the RNAs. Subunits then leave the nucleus, via nuclear pores, to enter the cytoplasm and participate in protein synthesis.

Ribosomes, which are intensely basophilic owing to the presence of numerous phosphate groups of the constituent rRNAs acting as polyanions, react with such basic stains as methylene blue, toluidine blue, and hematoxylin. Thus, sites in the cytoplasm that are rich in ribosomes stain intensely with these dyes. These basophilic regions were described as early as the 19th century and were named according to the cell being studied. In glandular cells, they were known as **ergastoplasm;** in neurons, as **Nissl bodies;** and in other cells as **basophilic bodies** or **basophilic components.** Although ribosomes are below the resolution of the light microscope, they can be visualized indirectly because of their staining characteristics.

Ribosomes occur as individual granules or in clusters called **polyribosomes.** The individual ribosomes of a polyribosome, or **polysome** (Fig 3-7A), are held together by a strand of messenger RNA (mRNA). The "message" carried by mRNA is a code for the amino acid sequence of proteins being synthesized by the cell. Ribosomes play a crucial role in decoding or "translating" the message during protein synthesis. Proteins synthesized for use within the cell and destined to remain diffusely distributed throughout the cytosol (eg, hemoglobin in immature red blood cells) are synthesized on free or unattached polyribosomes—polyribosomes existing as isolated clusters within the cytoplasm. Polyribosomes that are attached to the membranes of the endoplasmic reticulum (via their large subunit) translate mRNAs which code for proteins that are segregated into the cisternae of the reticulum (Fig 3-7B). These proteins can be secreted (eg, pancreatic and salivary enzymes) or stored in the cell (eg, enzymes of lysosomes and proteins within granules of white blood cells). In addition, most integral membrane proteins are synthesized on polyribosomes attached to membranes of the endoplasmic reticulum.

It should be emphasized that there are no intrinsic chemical differences between free and attached ribosomes. As seen below, it is the mRNA that possesses a signal which will cause ribosomes to attach to membranes of the endoplasmic reticulum.

Endoplasmic Reticulum (ER)

This predominantly membranous organelle may appear as elongated, flattened, rounded, or tubular vesicles in electron micrographs. The endoplasmic reticulum takes its name from the manner in which these structures anastomose with one another to form

Table 3-2. Properties of eukaryotic ribosomes.

	Sedimentation Coefficient	Mass (daltons)	RNA	Proteins
Intact ribosome	80S	4.5×10^6		
Small subunit	40S	1.5×10^6	18S	~ 33
Large subunit	60S	3.0×10^6	28S 5.8S 5S	~ 45

A

Free polysome showing protein
synthesis with no segregation

B

Bound polysomes showing protein
synthesis and segregation

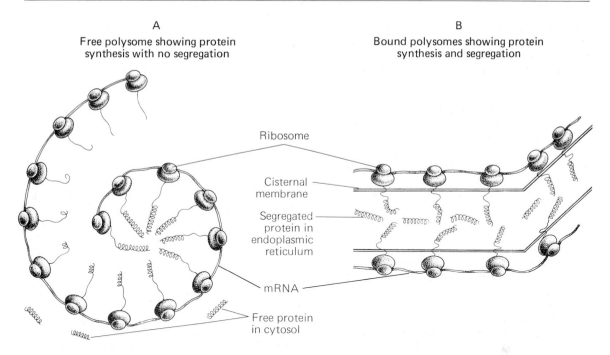

Ribosome

Cisternal
membrane

Segregated
protein in
endoplasmic
reticulum

mRNA

Free protein
in cytosol

Figure 3–7. This diagram illustrates (in *A*) the concept expressed in the text that cells synthesizing proteins (represented here by spirals) which are to remain within the cytosol possess (free) polysomes (nonadherent to the endoplasmic reticulum). In *B,* where the proteins are segregated in the endoplasmic reticulum and may eventually be extruded from the cytoplasm (export proteins), not only do the polysomes adhere to the membranes of rough endoplasmic reticulum but also the proteins produced by them are injected into the interior of the organelle across its membrane. In this way, the proteins—especially enzymes such as ribonucleases and proteases, which could have undesirable effects on the cytoplasm—are separated from it.

an intracellular network (reticulum). The disposition of endoplasmic reticulum membranes varies considerably from cell to cell and even from region to region within the same cell. Endoplasmic reticulum appears very early in the differentiation of embryonic cells and gradually develops a specialized appearance that varies with the size and functional state of different cell types. In fully differentiated cells, there are essentially 2 specialized types of endoplasmic reticulum: **rough** (granular) and **smooth** (agranular).

The 2 types of endoplasmic reticulum show differences in function as described below. However, these differences are quantitative; for example, the enzymes required for smooth endoplasmic reticulum function are synthesized in the rough endoplasmic reticulum. Thus, there can be no absolute differences in the composition of these membranes. A probable exception to this statement is the presence of ribophorins I and II only in rough endoplasmic reticulum (see below).

As a generalization, some of the functions of the endoplasmic reticulum follow. Certain of these functions are much more conspicuous in one type of reticulum than the other. (1) Segregation of newly synthesized proteins destined for export. (2) Limited proteolysis of newly synthesized proteins. (3) Core glycosylation. (4) Posttranslational modifications of

amino acids. (5) Assembly of multichain proteins. (6) Lipid synthesis. (7) Breakdown of endogenous and exogenous compounds.

Rough endoplasmic reticulum (RER): This form of endoplasmic reticulum is prominent in cells specialized for protein secretion, such as pancreatic acinar cells (digestive enzymes), fibroblasts (collagen), and plasma cells (immunoglobulins). The rough endoplasmic reticulum consists of tubules as well as parallel stacks of flattened cisternae (Figs 3–1 and 3–6), limited by membranes that are sometimes continuous with the outer membrane of the nuclear envelope (Fig 3–25). Although not obvious in a single thin section, the lumen of the rough endoplasmic reticulum is a single membrane-limited compartment within the cell. The name rough endoplasmic reticulum alludes to the presence of ribosomes and polyribosomes on the cytoplasmic surfaces of the endoplasmic reticulum membranes that give them a rough or granular appearance (Figs 3–1 and 3–6). The presence of ribosomes also confers basophilic staining properties on this organelle when viewed with the light microscope.

The principal function of the rough endoplasmic reticulum is to segregate proteins destined for export from the other components of the cytoplasm. Additional functions include the initial (core) glycosylation of glycoproteins having N-linked oligosaccharides, phospholipid synthesis, assembly of multichain proteins, and certain posttranslational modifications of newly formed polypeptides.

All protein synthesis begins on unattached (free) ribosomes. Messenger RNAs of proteins destined for export contain an additional sequence of bases at their 5' end that code for approximately 20–25 mainly hydrophobic amino acids termed the **signal sequence.** Upon translation, the signal sequence interacts with a complex of 6 nonidentical polypeptides plus a 7S RNA molecule that is referred to as the **signal recognition particle (SRP).** SRP acts to inhibit further polypeptide elongation until the SRP-polyribosome complex binds to a receptor in the rough endoplasmic reticulum called the **docking protein.** Upon binding to the docking protein, SRP is released from polyribosomes, allowing continuation of translation. Also present in membranes of rough endoplasmic reticulum, but lacking in smooth endoplasmic reticulum, are 2 integral membrane proteins designated **ribophorins I** and **II.** Ribophorins may provide attachment sites for the large subunits of ribosomes. In addition, ribophorins may form hydrophilic channels through the hydrophobic core of rough endoplasmic reticulum membranes, thus allowing passage of newly synthesized proteins into the lumen of the rough endoplasmic reticulum. This process is termed **vectorial discharge** to emphasize its unidirectional nature.

Once inside the lumen of the rough endoplasmic reticulum, the signal sequence is removed by a specific enzyme, **signal peptidase,** localized at the inner surface of the rough endoplasmic reticulum. Translation of the protein continues, accompanied by secondary and tertiary structural changes as well as certain posttranslational modifications.

The most important posttranslational modification is core glycosylation, wherein high-mannose oligosaccharides are added to most proteins destined for export. Proteins synthesized in the rough endoplasmic reticulum can have several destinations—extracellular and lysosomal and as components of other membranes. A widely accepted hypothesis is that complex oligosaccharides may form a signal for directing proteins to their appropriate destination.

Core glycosylation begins in the endoplasmic reticulum with the synthesis of a branched high-mannose core oligosaccharide on a lipid carrier called **dolichol phosphate.** The oligosaccharide is transferred, as a unit, to specific asparagine residues in the protein. This unit is referred to as an N-linked oligosaccharide, since it is attached to the amide group of asparagine. Removal of glucose residues occurs in the rough endoplasmic reticulum, but further trimming and carbohydrate addition occur in the Golgi complex (see below).

Smooth endoplasmic reticulum (SER): This type of endoplasmic reticulum also takes the form of a membranous network within the cell; however, its ultrastructure differs from that of rough endoplasmic reticulum in 2 important ways. First, smooth endoplasmic reticulum lacks the associated ribosomes that characterize rough endoplasmic reticulum, and thus smooth endoplasmic reticulum membranes appear smooth rather than granular. Second, its cisternae are more tubular and more likely to appear as a profusion of interconnected channels of variable shape and size than as stacks of flattened cisternae (Figs 3–1 and 4–30). Smooth endoplasmic reticulum membranes arise from rough endoplasmic reticulum, so that it is not surprising to see membrane continuity between the 2 forms.

Smooth endoplasmic reticulum not only exhibits a diversity of morphologic appearances in different cell types but also is associated with a variety of specialized functional capabilities. For example, in cells that synthesize steroid hormones (eg, cells of the adrenal cortex), smooth endoplasmic reticulum occupies a large portion of the cytoplasm and contains some of the enzymes required for steroid synthesis (Figs 4–30 and 4–31). It is abundant in liver cells, where it is responsible for the oxidation, conjugation, and methylation processes employed by the liver to neutralize or detoxify certain hormones and noxious substances, such as alcohol and insecticides. Smooth endoplasmic reticulum is also involved in the breakdown of glycogen in liver cells, where the enzyme glucose-6-phosphatase is a constituent of its membranes. This enzyme is also found in rough endoplasmic reticulum—an example of the lack of absolute partition of functions between these 2 organelles. Smooth endoplasmic reticulum participates in the contraction process in muscle cells, where it appears in a specialized form called **sarcoplasmic reticulum** that is involved in the sequestration and release of the calcium ions that regulate muscular contraction (see Chapter 11).

The term **microsome,** as used in cytology and biochemistry, denotes vesicles generated by fragmentation of the endoplasmic reticulum during the process of homogenization that precedes differential or density-gradient centrifugation. This term should never be applied to intact cells. The broken ends of membrane fragments generated during homogenization fuse to produce small vesicles that may have ribosomes attached. These microsomes can then be isolated for biochemical analyses via centrifugation. It is now possible to fractionate the microsomes further and even to separate the attached ribosomes from their membranes (Figs 1–15 and 1–16).

Golgi Complex (Golgi Apparatus)

This organelle, present in most cells, is composed of 3 distinct smooth-membrane limited compartments (Figs 3–1, 3–8, and 3–9). The most obvious is a slightly curved stack of 3–10 flattened **cisternae.** Second, numerous small **vesicles** are seen around the periphery of the stack. Third, usually at one pole of the Golgi complex are a few larger **vacuoles.** In highly polarized cells, such as columnar epithelial cells lining the intestine, the Golgi complex occupies a characteristic position in the cytoplasm between the nucleus and the apical plasma membrane. Because the Golgi complex is functionally an intermediate between the endoplasmic reticulum and the rest of the cell, it is sometimes difficult to exactly demarcate its boundaries.

In most cells, there is also polarity in Golgi structure and function. Near the Golgi complex, one can sometimes see that the rough endoplasmic reticulum is budding off small vesicles which serve to shuttle newly synthesized proteins to the Golgi for further processing. The Golgi cisterna nearest this point is called the forming, convex, or *cis* face. On the opposite side of the Golgi complex—the maturing, con-

cave, or *trans* face—large Golgi vacuoles accumulate. These are sometimes called **condensing vacuoles.**

A compositional heterogeneity exists across the stack of Golgi cisternae (Fig 3–9). Thus, mannose 6-phosphate receptors are found in *trans* cisternae, N-acetylglucosamine transferase and nicotinamide adenine dinucleotide phosphatase are found in the middle cisternae, and acid phosphatase, thiamine pyrophosphatase, and galactosyltransferase are located in *cis* cisternae. It is believed that this heterogeneity is important in sorting and directing proteins to specific

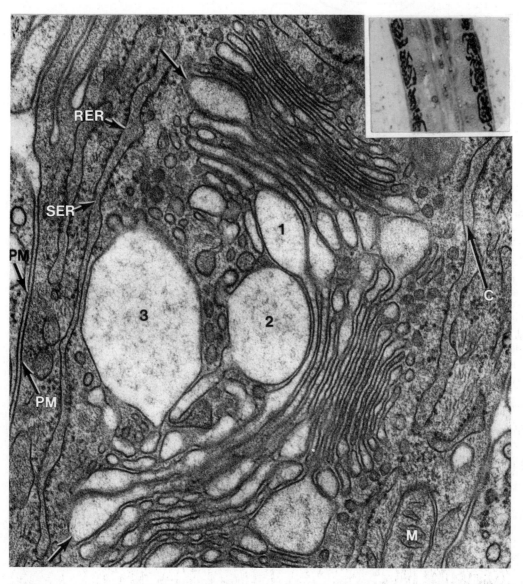

Figure 3–8. Electron micrograph of a Golgi complex of a mucous cell. To the right is a cisterna (C) of the rough endoplasmic reticulum containing granular material. Close to it are small vesicles containing this material. In the center are flattened and stacked cisternae of the Golgi complex. Dilatations can be observed extending from the ends of the cisternae. These dilatations gradually detach themselves from the cisternae and fuse, forming the secretory granules (1, 2, and 3). PM is the plasma membrane of 2 neighboring cells. Near the plasma membrane is endoplasmic reticulum with a smooth section (SER) and a rough section (RER). × 30,000. *Inset:* The Golgi complex as seen in 1-μm sections of epididymis cells impregnated by silver. × 1200.

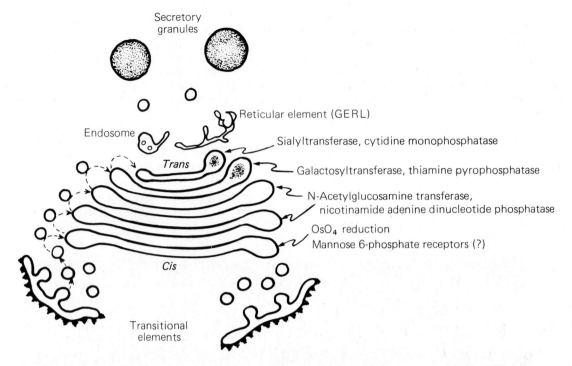

Figure 3–9. Diagram of the Golgi complex. The membrane components that have been localized in situ by immunocytochemical methods are listed on the right. The flow of biosynthetic products through the Golgi complex is diagrammed on the left. (Reproduced, with permission, from Farquhar MG: Progress in unraveling pathways of Golgi traffic. *Annu Rev Cell Biol* 1985;1:447.)

destinations such as lysosomes, the plasmalemma, or secretory granules.

A wide variety of activities take place in the Golgi complex. Concentration and packaging of secretory proteins is a prominent function. In cells whose secretion is periodic, the product is concentrated in Golgi vacuoles and stored until the appropriate signal for release is received. Thus, the vacuole membrane becomes the membrane surrounding the secretory granule. When secretory granules fuse with the plasmalemma, the granule membrane is incorporated into the plasma membrane. A process of membrane recycling serves to retrieve small vesicles from the plasma membrane and return them to the Golgi complex. Concentration does not involve ion pumps; rather, it appears that proteins become complexed with high-molecular-weight sulfated polyanions, thereby losing their osmotic activity. Then, water flows out of the vacuole, accomplishing the concentration step.

It was mentioned above that additional stages in protein glycosylation occur in the Golgi complex. These steps include further trimming of mannose residues until only 3 remain. Then, a group of enzymes, each with a specificity for a different sugar, progressively add carbohydrate residues until the complete oligosaccharide is formed. These enzymes have the general name of **glycosyltransferases.**

In some cells, a long, straight cisterna of smooth membranes is found near the *trans* face of the Golgi complex. This has been called **GERL,** an acronym for *G*olgi *e*ndoplasmic *r*eticulum *l*ysosome. The presence of lysosomal enzymes can be demonstrated by histochemical methods in GERL, and many workers believe this is a special site for directing lysosomal enzymes to their storage granules.

Radioautographic studies using ^{35}S reveal that, in cells which secrete sulfated proteoglycans (such as cartilage cells), the Golgi complex is the site of sulfation.

Many cells synthesize proteins that are larger than the product ultimately secreted. These larger precursors are called **proproteins.** Insulin is a good example. This hormone is synthesized as a large precursor. A large segment in the middle of the molecule is removed, leaving the 2 ends which then associate via disulfide bonds to form the active insulin molecule. Conversion of proproteins to their mature state occurs in the Golgi complex. Recently, a type of human diabetes has been described in which conversion of proinsulin to insulin does not occur.

Lysosomes

Lysosomes are membrane-limited vesicles that contain a large variety of hydrolytic enzymes (more than 40) whose main function is intracytoplasmic digestion (Figs 3–10, 3–11, 3–12, and 3–13). Lysosomes are present in almost all cells, but they are particularly abundant in cells exhibiting phagocytic activity (eg, macrophages, kidney tubule cells, and neutrophilic leukocytes). Although the nature and activity of lysosomal enzymes varies depending on the cell type being studied, the most common enzymes are acid phosphatase, ribonuclease, deoxyribonuclease, cathepsins (proteases), sulfatases, lipases, and β-glucuronidase. As can be seen from this list, lysosomal enzymes are capable of breaking down all classes of macromolecules. Generally, lysosomal enzymes are active at an acid pH.

Lysosomes are usually spherical, range in diameter from 0.05 to 0.5 μm, and present a uniformly granular electron-dense appearance in electron micrographs. The enveloping single unit membrane serves to separate the lytic enzymes from the cytoplasm, an important role in that it prevents the lysosomal enzymes from attacking and digesting cytoplasmic organelles.

Lysosomal enzymes are synthesized and segregated in the rough endoplasmic reticulum and subsequently transferred to the Golgi complex, where the enzymes are modified and packaged as lysosomes. These enzymes have oligosaccharides attached to them, as described earlier but with an important modification. One or more of the mannose residues is phosphorylated at the 6′ position. There are receptors for mannose 6-phosphate–containing proteins in the rough endoplasmic reticulum and Golgi complex that allow these proteins to be diverted from the main secretory pathway and segregated in lysosomes. This is the first indication of how the cell manages to sort out proteins going to different destinations.

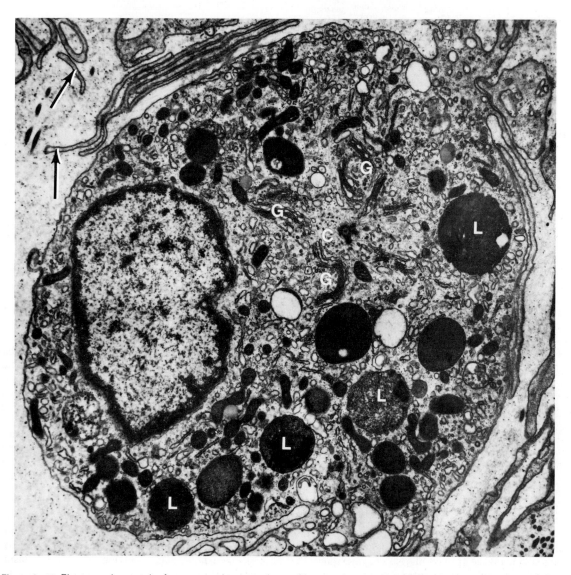

Figure 3–10. Electron micrograph of a mesenteric macrophage. Observe the presence of abundant cytoplasmic extensions (arrows). In the center is a centriole (C) surrounded by Golgi cisternae (G). Secondary lysosomes (L) are abundant. × 15,000.

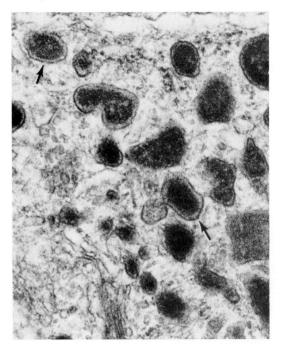

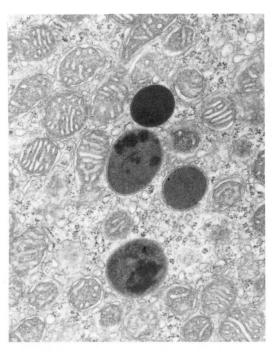

Figure 3–11. Electron micrograph of the cytoplasm of a macrophage showing primary lysosomes (arrows) characterized by uniform granular content and a limiting membrane. × 45,000.

Figure 3–12. Electron micrograph showing 4 dark secondary lysosomes surrounded by numerous mitochondria.

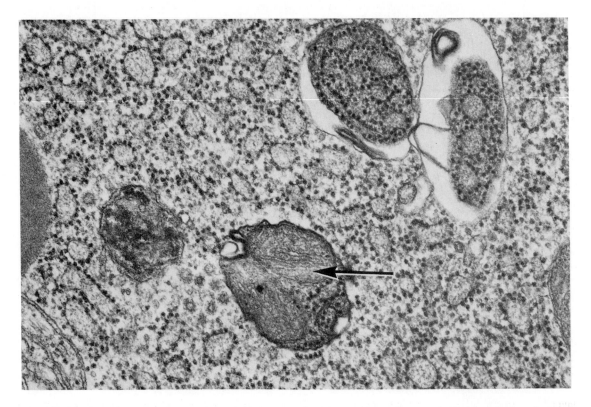

Figure 3–13. Section of a pancreatic acinar cell showing autophagosomes. *Above:* Two portions of the rough endoplasmic reticulum segregated by a membrane. *Below:* An autophagosome containing mitochondria (arrow) plus rough endoplasmic reticulum. *Left:* A secondary lysosome with undigestible material, or residual body.

Lysosomes that have not entered into a digestive event are identified as **primary lysosomes** (Fig 3–11). They can be very small (0.05 μm in diameter) membrane-limited vesicles with a clathrin coat and may be impossible to identify with certainty in the absence of a histochemical test of their content. This is the appearance of primary lysosomes in most cells. In a few cells, such as macrophages and neutrophilic leukocytes, primary lysosomes are larger, up to 0.5 μm in diameter, and thus just visible with the light microscope.

Secondary lysosomes are those in which digestion is occurring. They are generally 0.2–0.5 μm in di-

ameter and, in electron micrographs, present a heterogenous appearance owing to the wide variety of materials they may be digesting (Fig 3–12). Again, the only sure guide to their identification is histochemical methods to detect the presence of hydrolytic enzymes (eg, acid phosphatase) within these structures (Fig 2–7).

Following digestion of the contents of the secondary lysosome, nutrients diffuse through the lysosomal limiting membrane and enter the cytoplasm. The remaining undigestible compounds are retained within the vacuoles, which are now called **residual bodies** (Fig 3–13). In some long-lived cells (eg, neu-

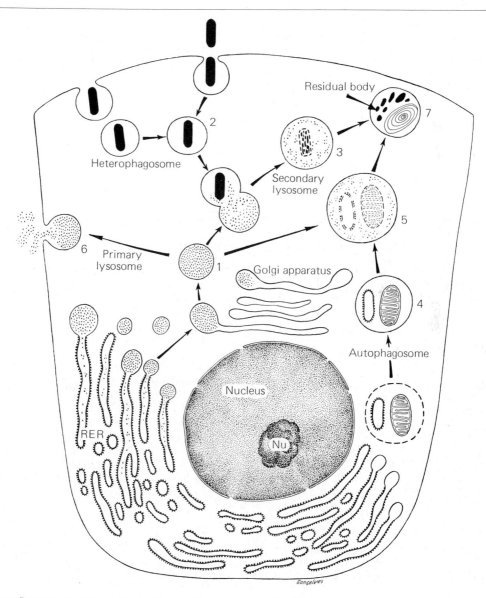

Figure 3–14. Present concepts of the functions of the lysosomes. Synthesis occurs in the rough endoplasmic reticulum (RER), and the enzymes are packaged in the Golgi complex. 1, 2, and 3 represent digestion of extracellular substance segregated into a heterophagosome; 1, 4, and 5, digestion of segregated cytoplasmic material (autophagosome); 1 and 6, extrusion of lysosomal enzymes that will act extracellularly (eg, collagenase); and 7, a residual body.

rons, heart muscle, hepatocytes), large quantities of residual bodies accumulate and are referred to as **lipofuscin** or **age pigment.**

Lysosomes can digest materials taken into the cell from its environment, a process called **heterophagy.** The material is taken into a phagocytic vacuole (see p 32); primary lysosomes then fuse with the membrane of the phagosome and empty their hydrolytic enzymes into the vacuole. Digestion ensues, and the composite structure is now termed a secondary lysosome.

Another function of lysosomes concerns the turnover of cytoplasmic organelles. Under certain conditions, organelles or portions of the cytoplasm may become enclosed by a membrane. Primary lysosomes fuse with this structure and initiate the lysis of the enclosed cytoplasm (Fig 3–13). The resulting secondary lysosomes are known as **autophagosomes,** indicating that their contents are of intracellular origin. The digested products of this hydrolysis are recycled by the cell to permit renewal, rearrangement, and reconstruction of the cytoplasmic contents. In certain pathologic conditions, or when cellular damage occurs, the lysosomes may rupture, release their enzymes, and ultimately destroy the cell from within. This process is called **autolysis.**

In some cases, primary lysosomes release their contents extracellularly, in which case their enzymes act in the extracellular milieu. An example is the destruction of bone matrix by collagenases synthesized and released by osteoclasts. This type of reaction plays a significant role in an inflammatory or injury response. Several possible pathways relating to lysosome activities are schematically illustrated in Fig 3–14.

Lysosomes play an important role in the metabolism of several substances in the human body, and consequently many diseases have been ascribed to deficiencies of lysosomal enzymes. In **metachromatic leukodystrophy,** there is an intracellular accumulation of sulfated cerebrosides caused by lack of lysosomal sulfatase. In most of these diseases, a specific lysosomal enzyme is absent or inactive, and the digestion of certain substances (glycogen, cerebrosides, gangliosides, sphingomyelin, etc) does not occur. As a result, these substances accumulate in the cell and interfere with normal cell function.

Peroxisomes, or Microbodies

Peroxisomes are spherical membrane-limited organelles whose diameter ranges from 0.5 to 1.2 μm (Fig 3–21). Their homogeneous matrix contains D- and L-amino oxidases and hydroxyacid oxidase. In some species, but not humans, a crystalline "nucleoid" is present that is composed of urate oxidase. All of these enzymes oxidize their substrate and reduce O_2 to H_2O_2. Peroxisomes also contain catalase, an enzyme that decomposes hydrogen peroxide to water and oxygen ($2 H_2O_2 \rightarrow 2 H_2O + O_2$). Peroxisomes function to protect the cell from the effects of hydrogen peroxide, which could cause irreversible damage to numerous important cellular constituents.

Recent investigations have provided evidence that peroxisomes contain several enzymes involved in lipid metabolism. The most prominent of these is 3-hydroxy-3-methylglutaryl–coenzyme A reductase (HMG-CoA reductase), which is the rate-limiting enzyme in cholesterol biosynthesis. This enzyme was formerly thought to be confined to membranes of the endoplasmic reticulum. β-Oxidation of long-chain fatty acids (18 carbons and longer) is preferentially accomplished by peroxisomal enzymes that differ from their mitochondrial counterparts. Certain hydroxylation reactions leading to the formation of bile acids also have been localized in highly purified peroxisomal fractions.

Much smaller **microperoxisomes** (0.2 μm in diameter) have been identified in a variety of tissues. They also contain catalase, but other functions have not yet been established.

The biogenesis of peroxisomes is controversial. The traditional view is that the constituent enzymes are synthesized on ribosomes attached to membranes of the rough endoplasmic reticulum and then transferred to the lumen of the endoplasmic reticulum. In other words, the synthesis of peroxisomal enzymes is not different from the synthesis of secretory proteins. It was suggested that portions of the endoplasmic reticulum containing peroxisomal enzymes would pinch off to give rise to mature peroxisomes. Recently, it has been established that some peroxisomal enzymes (catalase, enzymes of β-oxidation) are synthesized on free ribosomes and posttranslationally transferred to peroxisomes by an unknown mechanism. This is not consistent with the traditional view but is similar to the way in which certain proteins are incorporated into mitochondria. In addition, it is now believed that new peroxisomes are formed by the fission of preexisting peroxisomes.

Secretory Granules

Secretory granules are found in those cells that store a product until its release is signaled by a metabolic, hormonal, or neural message (regulated secretion). Secretory granules range in size from 30 nm to 800 nm in diameter. These granules are surrounded by a typical unit membrane and contain a concentrated form of the secretory product (Fig 3–15). The contents of some secretory granules may be up to 200 times more concentrated than in the rough endoplasmic reticulum. In addition, binding proteins, nucleotides, or glycosaminoglycans may be present. These constituents are thought to form complexes with the principal secretory product, thus rendering it less osmotically active. Secretory granules permit the storage of substances that could destroy the cell, such as digestive enzymes; in this case, the granules are usually referred to as **zymogen granules.**

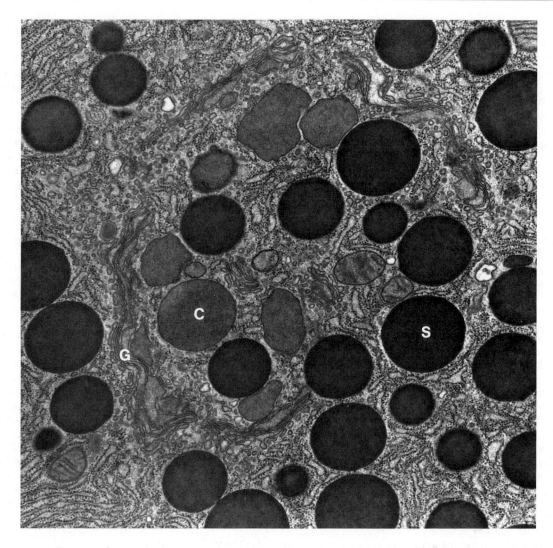

Figure 3–15. Electron micrograph of a pancreatic acinar cell from the rat. Numerous mature secretory granules (S) are seen in association with condensing vacuoles (C) and the Golgi complex (G). × 18,900.

MICROTUBULES, MICROFILAMENTS, & INTERMEDIATE FILAMENTS

In addition to the membrane-bound organelles, the cytoplasmic matrix contains a complex network consisting of microtubules, microfilaments, and intermediate filaments (Fig 3–16). These structural proteins not only provide for the form and shaping of cells but also play an important role in cytoplasmic and cellular movement.

Microtubules

Within the cytoplasmic matrix of most eukaryotic cells are rodlike or pipelike organelles known as microtubules. Generally, they have an outer diameter of 24 nm consisting of a dense wall 5 nm thick and a less dense (possibly hollow) core 14 nm wide. Mi-

crotubule lengths are variable, and individual tubules have often been observed to attain lengths of several micrometers (Fig 3–16). Normally, a clear zone, probably composed of glycoproteins, isolates the tubules from the adjacent cytoplasm. Occasionally, arms or bridges are found linking 2 or more tubules together (Figs 3–17, 3–18, and 3–19).

The subunit of a microtubule is a heterodimer composed of α and β **tubulin** molecules, each with a molecular weight of about 50,000. Tubulins are closely related in amino acid composition, and it is probable that the 2 tubulin monomers evolved from a single prototubulin molecule.

Under appropriate conditions either in vivo or in vitro, tubulin subunits polymerize to form typical microtubules. Using special staining procedures, tubulin appears to organize into **protofilaments** that run par-

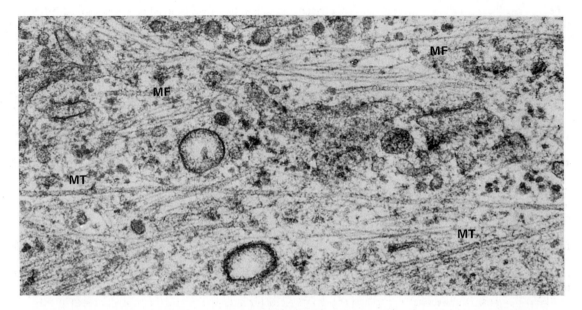

Figure 3–16. Electron micrograph of rat fibroblast cytoplasm. Observe the microfilaments (MF) and microtubules (MT). × 60,000. (Courtesy of E Katchburian.)

allel to the length of the tubule. A total of 13 protofilaments generally comprise the wall of a microtubule (Figs 3–17 and 3–19).

Polymerization of tubulins to form microtubules is believed to be directed by a variety of structures collectively known as microtubule organizing centers (MTOCs). These structures include basal bodies, centrioles, and the centromeres of chromosomes. Microtubule growth, via subunit polymerization, generally occurs more rapidly at the free end of existing tubules. This end is referred to as the fast-growing (+) end. If either colchicine or podophyllotoxin (antimitotic alkaloids that bind to tubulin heterodimers) is administered, microtubule growth will be blocked because of the unavailability of heterodimers. Microtubules will eventually be broken down because the constant exchange of polymerized heterodimers with soluble heterodimers will proceed, but heterodimers with bound colchicine cannot polymerize. Another alkaloid, vinblastine, acts by inducing the formation of paracrystalline arrays of tubulin heterodimers.

Modulation in microtubule number and length is believed to reflect the alteration of a tubulin dimer-polymer equilibrium. New tubule formation or increase in length of existing tubules would result from the polymerization of free dimers. The dissolution or shortening of tubules would return subunits to the dimer pool (Fig 3–19).

Within the cytoplasm, microtubules may exist in states ranging from an apparently random distribution to highly complex organized subcellular structures. Functions attributed to microtubules are usually based on 2 criteria: (1) the process must be sensitive to the pharmacologic agents known to interact with tubulin, and (2) morphologic data (numbers and orientation of

tubules) must be sufficient to implicate tubules with a given cellular process.

Microtubules have been considered to play a significant role in the development and maintenance of cell form based on the observation that tubules in intact cells or from cell-free preparations are normally quite straight and never exhibit oblique bends. These observations suggest that microtubules are rigid and lend support to the implication that they serve as a cytoskeletal element. Morphologic studies indicate a structural role, since microtubules are usually present in a proper orientation either to effect development of or to maintain a given cellular asymmetry. Procedures known to disrupt microtubules generally result in the loss of this cellular asymmetry.

Microtubules have also been implicated in the intracellular transport of other organelles. Time-lapse cinematography of living cells reveals a significant movement and redistribution of cytoplasmic components (eg, mitochondria, vesicles). Examples include axoplasmic transport in neurons, melanin dispersion in pigment cells, chromosome movements along the mitotic spindle, and vesicle movements between the endoplasmic reticulum and Golgi complex and between the Golgi complex and the cell membrane. In each of these examples, movement is related to the presence of complex microtubule networks, and such activities are suspended if microtubules are disrupted.

Microtubules also provide the basis for several complex cytoplasmic organelles, including centrioles, cilia, and flagella. **Centrioles** are cylindric structures (0.15 μm in diameter and 0.3–0.5 μm in length) primarily composed of highly organized microtubules (Fig 3–19). Each centriole is composed of 9 sets of microtubule triplets arranged in the fashion of a "pinwheel.'' The tubules are so close together that adjacent tubules of a triplet share a common wall. A single pair of centrioles is normally found in nondividing cells. In each pair, the long axes of the centrioles are at right angles to each other. Prior to cell division, more specifically during the S period of the interphase, each centriole duplicates itself; and during mitosis, the resulting 2 pairs move to opposite poles of the cell and become organizing centers for the developing mitotic spindles (Fig 3–37).

Centrioles duplicate by the growth of a **procentriole** that forms on the surface of, and at right angles to, the original centriole. At first, the procentriole consists of 9 single tubules; later, 9 pairs of tubules arise in close association with the original tubules, completing the centriolar organization.

In nondividing cells, centriole pairs are usually found in a juxtanuclear position and in association with the Golgi complex. Associated with the centrioles are dense **pericentriolar bodies** from which microtubules seem to arise, suggesting that these bodies represent the microtubule organizing center for microtubule formation. This is confirmed by the observation that when isolated centrioles are added in vitro to depolymerized microtubular dimers, polymerization of microtubules occurs at these structures in a radial disposition. The pair of centrioles in conjunction with the Golgi complex constitute the **cytocenter** of the cell.

Cilia and **flagella** are motile processes that have a highly organized microtubule core and extend from the surface of many different cell types. Ciliated cells usually possess a large number of cilia that range from 2 to 10 μm in length. Flagellated cells normally have only one or 2 flagella, which range in length from 100 to 200 μm. Cilia and flagella both have a diameter of $0.3-0.5$ μm and possess the same complexly organized core of microtubules.

This core consists of 9 pairs of microtubules surrounding 2 central tubules. This sheaf of tubules, possessing the characteristic ''9+2 pattern,'' is called an **axoneme.** Each of the 9 peripheral pairs of **doublets** shares a common wall of $2-3$ protofilaments. The central pair of tubules are separated from each other and are enclosed within a **central sheath.** Adjacent doublets are linked to each other via protein

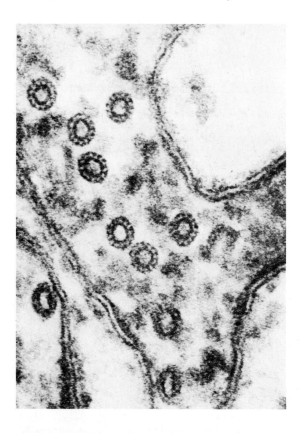

Figure 3–17. Section of a Sertoli cell of the testis of *Rana polypedatus.* This material was fixed with glutaraldehyde containing tannic acid. This compound makes the dimers of the microtubules visible, and they are shown here in cross section of the microtubules. Each dimer appears as a small white dot surrounded by a dark collar. × 247,000. (Courtesy of V Mizuhira.)

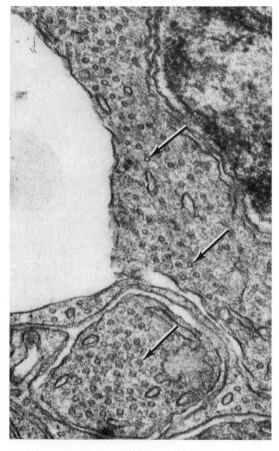

Figure 3–18. Electron micrograph of a section of a photosensitive retinal cell of a monkey. Observe the accumulation of transversely sectioned microtubules (arrows). Reduced slightly from × 80,000.

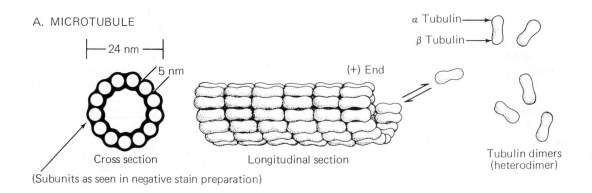

A. MICROTUBULE

24 nm

5 nm

Cross section

(Subunits as seen in negative stain preparation)

(+) End

Longitudinal section

α Tubulin

β Tubulin

Tubulin dimers
(heterodimer)

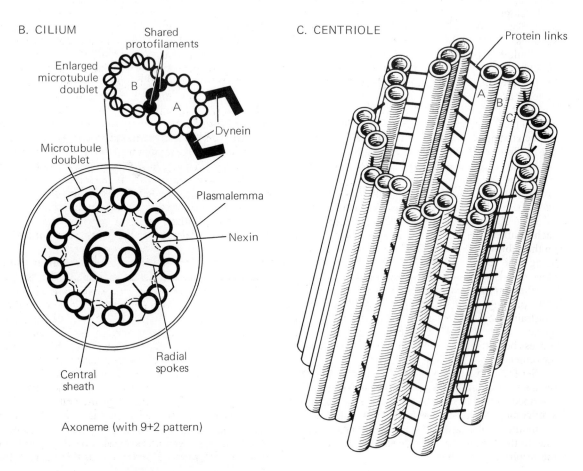

B. CILIUM

Shared
protofilaments

Enlarged
microtubule
doublet

B

A

Dynein

Microtubule
doublet

Plasmalemma

Nexin

Central
sheath

Radial
spokes

Axoneme (with 9+2 pattern)

C. CENTRIOLE

Protein links

A B
C

Figure 3–19. Schematic representation of microtubules, cilia, and centrioles. *A:* Microtubules as seen in the electron microscope following fixation with tannic acid in glutaraldehyde. The unstained tubulin subunits are delineated by the dense tannic acid. Cross sections of tubules reveal a ring of 13 subunits, while in longitudinal section the tubules appear to be composed of 13 linear protofilaments. Changes in microtubule length are due to the addition or loss of individual tubulin subunits. The (+) end is defined as the fast-growing end. *B:* A cross section through a cilium reveals a core of microtubules called an **axoneme.** The axoneme consists of 2 central microtubules surrounded by 9 microtubule doublets. In the doublets, microtubule A is complete and consists of 13 subunits, while microtubule B shares 2–3 protofilaments with A. When activated, the dynein arms link adjacent tubules and provide for the sliding of tubules in the presence of ATP. *C:* Centrioles consist of 9 microtubule triplets linked together in a pinwheellike arrangement. In the triplets, microtubule A is complete and consists of 13 subunits, whereas tubules B and C share tubulin subunits. Under normal circumstances, these organelles are found in pairs with the centrioles disposed at right angles to one another.

bridges called **nexins** and are also linked to the central sheath by **radial spokes.** The tubule units of each doublet are identified as subfibers A and B. Subfiber A is a complete microtubule with 13 protofilaments, while subfiber B has only 10 or 11 protofilaments. Extending from the surface of subfiber A are pairs of arms formed by a protein known as **dynein** that has ATPase activity (Fig 3–19).

At the base of each cilium or flagellum is a **basal body.** A basal body is essentially identical to a centriole except at its basal end, which has a complex central organization resembling a cartwheel. At the apical end of the basal body, the C tubule ends, while the A and B tubules are continuous with the corresponding tubules of the ciliary or flagellar axoneme. In developing cilia or flagella, the basal bodies act as a template to control the assembly of the axoneme subunits.

While basal bodies and centrioles have the same structure, they differ in the way in which they control the polymerization of tubulin monomers. Ciliary and flagellar axonemes are doublets that arise directly from the distal end of the basal body. In contrast, centrioles control the polymerization of single microtubules that characteristically radiate from the centriole and are not in direct contact with this organelle.

Recent experimental investigations show that the undulating motion exhibited by cilia and flagella is propagated by sliding of adjacent doublets within the axoneme. This sliding mechanism is mediated by the dynein (ATPase) arms that extend from subfiber A of each doublet. It is currently thought that the dynein on the subfiber A of one doublet binds to and "walks along" the surface of subfiber B of the adjacent doublet.

The sliding process occurring between adjacent pairs of microtubules does not occur freely and is constrained by the presence of the nexin and radial spokes. Thus, forces developed during the sliding process bend the cilia or flagella and account for their movements.

Several mutations occurring in humans result in the absence of dynein arms in cilia and flagella. This is termed the **immotile cilia syndrome (Kartagener's syndrome),** characterized by male infertility (due to nonmotile sperm) and chronic respiratory infections (due to the absence of the cleansing action of cilia in the respiratory tract).

Microfilaments

Contractile activity in muscle cells primarily results from an interaction between 2 proteins: **actin** and **myosin.** In muscle, actin is present as a thin (5–7 nm in diameter) filament composed of globular subunits organized into a double-stranded helix. Structural and biochemical studies reveal that actin may be an important component of the total protein of *all* cells. In nonmuscle cells, actin is usually present in the form of microfilament (5–7 nm in diameter) networks.

Biochemical analyses reveal that nonmuscle cells normally contain several species of actin, with some actins differing only by a single amino acid substitution. The close similarities of actin within a given cell, as well as between cells of far-ranging species on the evolutionary scale, attest to the highly conserved nature of this protein. The differences in amino acid composition appear to be related to specific functional and stability characteristics of the various actins found within a cell. Within cells, microfilaments can be organized in many different forms: (1) In skeletal muscle, they assume a paracrystalline array integrated with thick (16-nm) myosin filaments. (2) In most cells, microfilaments are present as a thin sheath just beneath the plasmalemma. These filaments appear to be associated with membrane activities such as endocytosis and exocytosis, contraction of microvilli (fingerlike projections on some cell surfaces), and cell migratory activity. Microfilaments are often found as an irregular lattice at the leading end of the cell as well as constituting the primary structural component of migratory (pseudopodial and filopodial) processes. (3) Microfilaments are intimately associated with a number of cytoplasmic organelles, vesicles, and granules. The filaments are believed to play a role in moving and shifting cytoplasmic components (cytoplasmic streaming). (4) Microfilaments form a "purse string" ring of filaments whose constriction results in the cleavage of mitotic cells. (5) In most cells, microfilaments are found scattered in what appears to be an unorganized fashion within the cytoplasm. It is currently thought that such actin networks provide part of the "cytoskeleton" or structural framework within the cell (Fig 3–16).

While actin filaments in muscle cells are structurally stable, microfilaments in nonmuscle cells are readily able to dissociate and reassemble. Microfilament polymerization appears to be under the direct control of minute changes in Ca^{2+} and cAMP levels. A large number of actin-binding proteins have been demonstrated in a wide variety of cells. Much current research is focused on how these proteins regulate the state of polymerization and lateral aggregation of microfilaments. Their importance can be deduced from the fact that only about half of the cell's actin is in the form of microfilaments. In vitro, all cellular actin can be polymerized, demonstrating that other proteins (the actin-binding proteins) regulate the degree to which actin is polymerized to form microfilaments within the cell.

Presumably, most microfilament-related activities depend upon the simultaneous presence of **myosin,** a protein that binds actin. The structure and activity of the "thick" myosin filaments are described in the section on muscle tissues. A soluble form of myosin has been isolated from most motile nonmuscle cells. The myosin apparently functions by complexing with the microfilaments, forming contractile "actomyosin." The myosin in normal preparations is not evident in electron micrographs but may be visualized utilizing special procedures that alter the ionic balance, pH, or temperature of the cell before fixation. Myosin-actin

Table 3—3. Examples of types of intermediate filaments found in eukaryotic cells.

Filament Type	Cell Type	Examples
Cytokeratins (tonofilaments)	Epithelium	Both keratinizing and non-keratinizing epithelia
Vimentin	Mesenchymal cells	Fibroblasts, chondroblasts, macrophages, endothelial cells, vascular smooth muscle
Desmin	Muscle	Striated and smooth muscle (except vascular smooth muscle)
Glial fibrillary acidic proteins	Glial cells	Astrocytes and Bergmann's glia
Neurofilaments	Neurons	Most but probably not all neurons

interactions are described in detail in the discussion of muscle tissue.

Intermediate Filaments

Recent ultrastructural and immunocytochemical investigations reveal that a third major filamentous structure is present in almost all eukaryotic cells. In addition to the thin (actin) and thick (myosin) filaments, cells contain a class of intermediate-sized filaments with a diameter of 10 nm. The study of these **intermediate filaments** is a rapidly developing field. Different proteins that form intermediate filaments have been isolated and localized by immunocytochemical means. (1) **Cytokeratins (tonofilaments)** are found in most epithelia and consist of a family of approximately 20 polypeptides (MW 40,000–68,000). (2) **Vimentin** filaments are characteristic of cells of mesenchymal origin. Vimentin is a single protein (MW 56,000–58,000). Vimentin may copolymerize with desmin or glial fibrillary acidic protein. (3) **Desmin (skeletin)** is found in smooth muscle and in the Z disks of skeletal and cardiac muscle (MW 53,000–55,000). (4) **Glial filaments (glial fibrillary acidic protein, GFA)** are characteristic of astrocytes but are not found in neurons, muscle, mesenchymal cells, or epithelia (MW 51,000). (5) **Neurofilaments** consist of at least 3 high-molecular-weight polypeptides (MW 68,000, 140,000, and 210,000). These intermediate filament proteins have different chemical structures and very probably different (but not yet clearly defined) roles in cellular function. They form part of the cytoskeleton (microtubules, microfilaments, and intermediate filaments).

Cytoplasmic Inclusions

These are usually transitory components of the cytoplasm, composed mainly of accumulated metabolites or deposits of varied nature. The accumulated

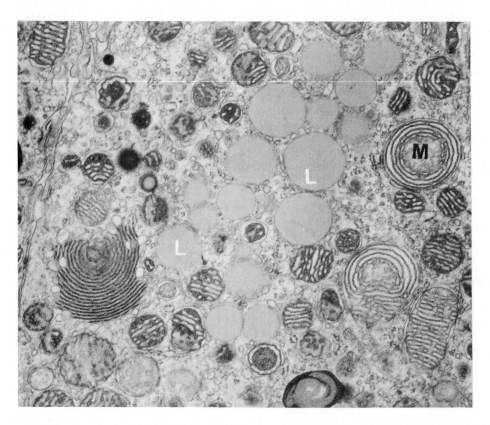

Figure 3—20. Section of adrenal gland showing lipid droplets, L, and abundant mitochondria, M. × 19,000.

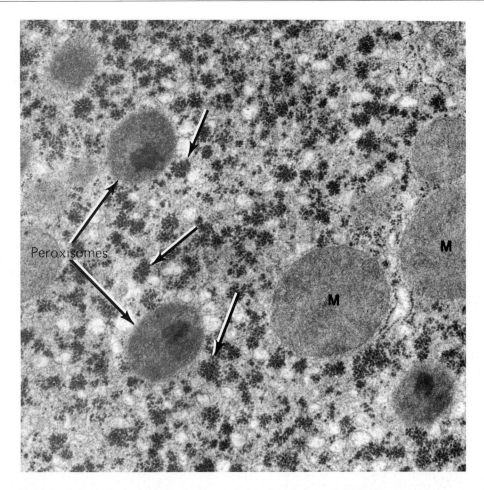

Figure 3–21. Electron micrograph of a section of a liver cell showing glycogen inclusions appearing as accumulations of electron-dense particles (arrows). The dark structures with a dense core are peroxisomes. Mitochondria (M). × 30,000.

metabolites occur in several forms, one of them being lipid droplets present in adipose tissue, adrenal cortex cells, and liver cells (Fig 3–20). Carbohydrate accumulations are also visible in several cells in the form of glycogen. After impregnation with lead salts, this substance appears as collections of coarse, irregular electron-dense particles (Fig 3–21). Proteins are stored in glandular cells as **secretory granules** (Fig 3–15); these are periodically released into the extracellular medium. In some cells, protein crystalloids of unknown significance have been described (Fig 3–22).

Deposits of colored substances—**pigment**—are often found in cells. They may be synthesized by the cell (eg, in the skin melanocytes) or may come from outside the body (eg, vitamin A). One of the most common pigments is **lipofuscin,** a yellowish-brown substance that increases in quantity in cells with age. Its chemical constitution is complex. It is believed that granules of lipofuscin derive from secondary lysosomes and represent deposits of undigestible substances (Fig 3–23). Another widely distributed pig-

ment, **melanin,** is abundant in the epidermis of the skin and in the pigment layer of the retina in the form of dense, intracellular, membrane-limited granules (Fig 3–24).

Cytomatrix

Until recently, it was believed that the cytoplasm intervening between the discrete organelles and inclusions was unstructured and consisted of soluble enzymes, low-molecular-weight metabolites, ions, and water. This belief was reinforced by the widespread application of the techniques of homogenization and centrifugation of the homogenates to yield fractions consisting of recognizable organelles. The final supernatant contains the soluble components of the cell and is called the **cytosol,** or soluble ground substance.

It now seems probable that homogenization of cells disrupts a delicate **microtrabecular lattice** that incorporates filaments, microtubules, and perhaps enzymes and other ''soluble'' constituents into a structured cytomatrix. This matrix may coordinate intracellular movements of organelles as well as provide

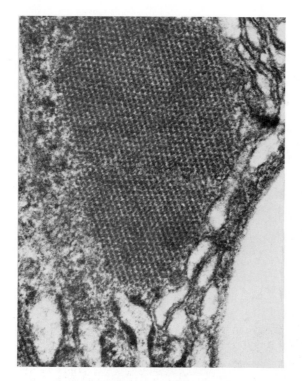

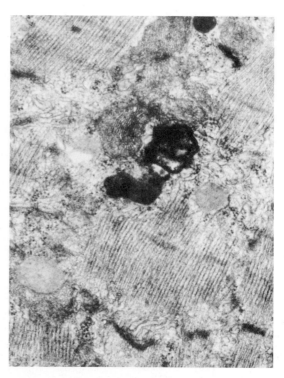

Figure 3 –22. Electron micrograph of a crystalloid inclusion body from a human adrenal cell. Most of these inclusions are composed of proteins. (Courtesy of M Magalhães.)

Figure 3 –23. Section of heart muscle with a granule containing lipofuscin.

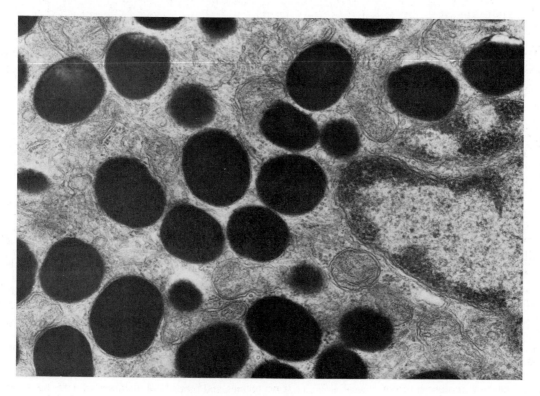

Figure 3 –24. Section of a melanophore. The nucleus is shown at right. The cytoplasm is full of dense, membrane-bound melanin granules. Mitochondria are also numerous. × 20,000.

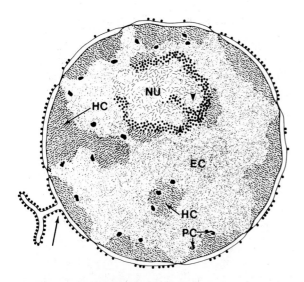

Figure 3–25 (at left). Structure of a nucleus. The nuclear envelope merges with the endoplasmic reticulum (arrow). HC, heterochromatin; EC, euchromatin. The dark heavy dots (PC) are perichromatin granules. In the nucleolus (NU), fibrillar and granular portions can be distinguished. The heterochromatin surrounding the nucleolus forms the **nucleolus-associated chromatin.** Portions of euchromatin appear interspersed with nucleolar material (arrowhead). This latter chromatin contains the genes specifying rRNAs.

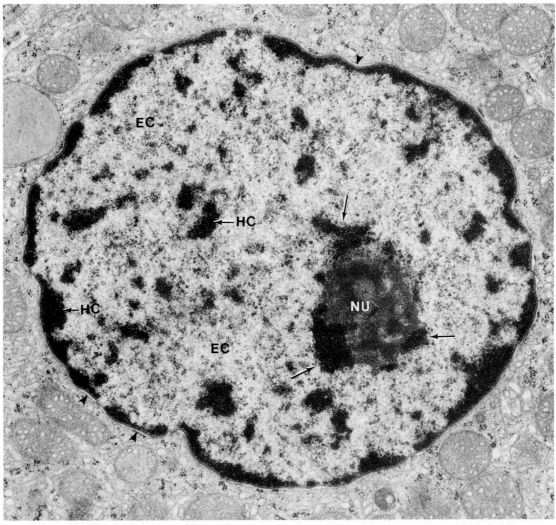

Figure 3–26. Electron micrograph of a nucleus. HC, heterochromatin; EC, euchromatin. Arrows point to the nucleolus-associated chromatin around the nucleolus (NU). Arrowheads indicate the perinuclear cisterna. × 26,000. (Courtesy of J James.)

an explanation for the viscosity of the cytoplasm. It has been suggested that soluble enzymes, such as those of the glycolytic pathway, might function more efficiently if they were organized in a sequence rather than if they rely on random collisions with their substrates. The cytomatrix may provide a framework for this organization.

THE NUCLEUS

The nucleus of the cell appears as a rounded or elongated structure, usually in the center of the cell. In mammalian tissues, its diameter usually varies between 5 and 10 μm. The nucleus is composed of the nuclear envelope, chromatin, the nucleolus, and nucleoplasm (Fig 3–25).

Nuclear Envelope

A nuclear ''membrane'' can be observed under the light microscope as a thin line surrounding the

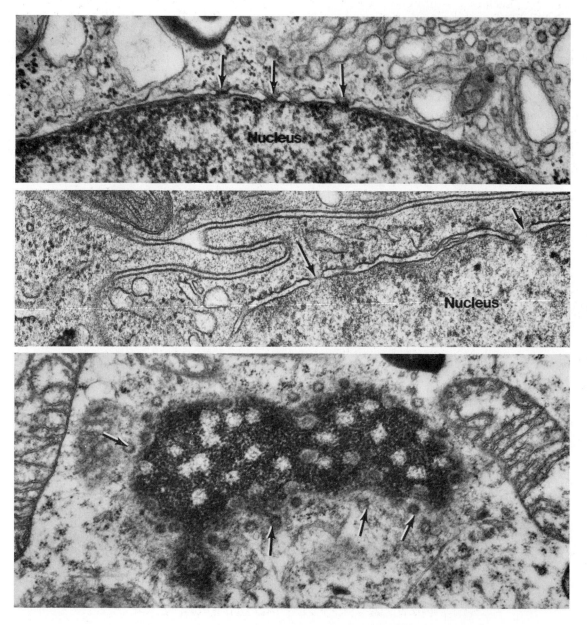

Figure 3–27. Electron micrographs of nuclei showing their envelopes composed of 2 membranes and the nuclear pores (arrows). The 2 upper pictures are of transverse sections. The lower one is of a tangential section. Chromatin, frequently condensed below the nuclear envelope, is not usually seen in the pore regions. × 80,000.

nucleus. Electron microscopy has revealed that the nucleus is actually surrounded by 2 parallel unit membranes separated by a narrow (40–70 nm) space called the **perinuclear cisterna.** Together, the paired membranes and the intervening space make up the nuclear envelope. What is seen in the light microscope as the nuclear "membrane" is mainly a layer of heterochromatin that lines and binds to the internal surface of the nuclear envelope (Figs 3–26 and 3–27). Closely associated with the internal membrane of the nuclear envelope is the **fibrous lamina,** which varies in thickness from 80 to 300 nm depending on the cell examined. Nuclear pores are not blocked by this structure. The fibrous lamina is composed of 3 main polypeptides, called **lamins,** which form part of the nuclear matrix. During interphase, the chromatin adjacent to the centromeres of chromosomes is associated with the fibrous lamina. The pattern of association is very regular from cell to cell within a tissue. This finding has given rise to the idea that chromatin has a definite organization within the nucleus. This organization could have an effect on the way in which genes are expressed. Ribosomes are frequently attached to the outer membrane, and this portion of the nuclear envelope is sometimes continuous with the rough endoplasmic reticulum (Fig 3–25). When covered with ribosomes, the nuclear envelope functions as rough endoplasmic reticulum, synthesizing polypeptide chains and segregating them in the perinuclear cistern between its 2 membranes. Around the nuclear envelope, at sites where the inner and outer membranes fuse, there are circular gaps, the **nuclear pores** (Fig 3–28), that provide pathways between the nucleus and the cytoplasm. Nuclear pores have an average diameter of 70 nm and are composed of 8 subunits. The pores are not open but are bridged by an electron-dense membrane forming a single-layered diaphragm of protein. This structure is thinner than the membranes comprising the nuclear envelope. The permeability of the nucleus to molecules is variable, but all pores are permeable to some macromolecules (eg, mRNA).

Chromatin

Two types of chromatin can be distinguished with both the light and the electron microscopes (Figs 3–25 and 3–26). **Heterochromatin,** which is electron-dense and appears as coarse granules in the electron microscope, is visible in the light microscope (after appropriate staining) as basophilic clumps of nucleoprotein. **Euchromatin** is visible as an organized structure only in the electron microscope. However, when viewed with the light microscope, lightly stained areas in the nucleus correspond to euchromatin recognized by electron microscopy. The proportion of heterochromatin to euchromatin accounts for the light-to-dark appearance of nuclei in light and electron microscopic tissue sections. The intensity of nuclear staining resulting from the chromatin is frequently used to differentiate and identify different tissues and cell types in the light microscope. Consequently, the morphology of chromatin in cell nuclei is mentioned throughout this book with respect to the study and identification of cells and tissues.

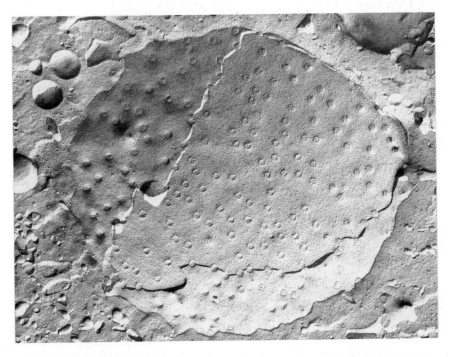

Figure 3–28. Electron micrograph of rat intestine preparation obtained by cryofracture, showing the 2 membranous components of the nuclear envelope and the nuclear pores. (Courtesy of A Pinto da Silva.)

Chromatin is composed mainly of coiled strands of DNA bound to basic proteins (histones); its structure is schematically presented in Fig 3–29. The basic structural unit of chromatin is the nucleosome. This consists of a core of histones (4 types; 2 copies each of histones H2A, H2B, H3, and H4) around which are wrapped 166 DNA base pairs. A further 48-base-pair segment forms a link between adjacent nucleosomes, and another type of histone (H1 or H5) is bound to this DNA. This organization of chromatin has been referred to as "beads-on-a-string." Non-histone proteins are also associated with chromatin, but their arrangement is less well understood.

The next higher order of organization of chromatin is the 30-nm fiber commonly referred to as a "sele-noid." In this structure, nucleosomes become coiled around an axis, with 6 nucleosomes per turn, to form the 30-nm chromatin fiber. Higher orders of coiling must be necessary, especially in the condensation of chromatin into chromosomes during mitosis and meiosis, but details are lacking at this time.

Chromatin DNA represents the major form of DNA in the cell and consequently carries most of the genetic information. Within the chromatin, the precursors of the messenger, ribosomal, and transfer ribonucleic acids (mRNA, rRNA, and tRNA) are synthesized.

The nucleoprotein of chromatin is coiled, and the degree of coiling varies during cell activity. The chromatin pattern of a nucleus has been considered a guide to the cell's activity. In lightly staining nuclei (with few heterochromatin clumps), more DNA surface is available for the transcription of genetic information. In darkly staining nuclei, less surface is available as a result of the coiling of DNA. In general, cells with light nuclei are more active than those with condensed, dark nuclei.

Careful study of the chromatin of mammalian cell nuclei has revealed the presence of a heterochromatin

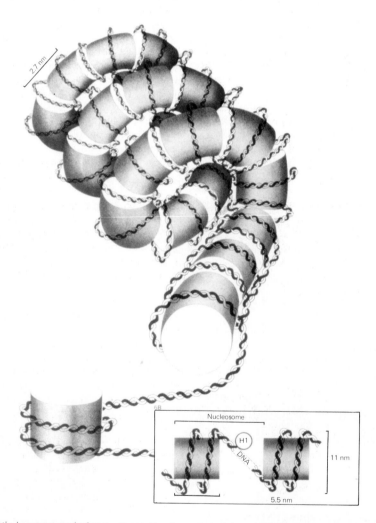

Figure 3–29. Chromatin is composed of repeating units of small particles visible with the electron microscope in suitable preparations. These units (**nucleosomes**) contain a core of histones. DNA surrounds these particles and binds them together. The strands that resemble beads on a string form a superhelix. (Reproduced, with permission, from Bradbury EM: La chromatine. *La Recherche* 1978;9:466.)

THE CELL / 55

mass frequently observed in female cells but not in male cells. This chromatin clump is the **sex chromatin.** It was first observed in nerve cells obtained from female cats and is present in cells of most mammals, including humans. This heterochromatin mass is one of the pair of X chromosomes that exists in female cells. It remains tightly coiled and is visible during interphase, while the other X chromosome is uncoiled and not visible. The coiling of this chromosome explains why it is easily stained and can be observed with the light microscope. Evidence suggests that the coiled X chromosome comprising the sex chromatin is genetically inactive. The male has one X chromosome and one Y chromosome as sex determinants; the X chromosome is uncoiled, and therefore no sex chromatin is visible. In human epithelial cells, sex chromatin appears as a small granule attached to the nuclear envelope. The cells lining the internal surface of the cheek are frequently used to study sex chromatin. Blood smears are also often used, in which case the sex chromatin appears as a drumsticklike appendage to the nuclei of the neutrophilic leukocytes (Fig 3–30).

The study of sex chromatin has wide applicability in medicine, because it permits analysis of genetic sex in doubtful cases (hermaphroditism, pseudohermaphroditism). It is essential for the study of other anomalies involving the sex chromosomes—eg, Klinefelter's syndrome, in which testicular abnormalities, azoospermia, and other symptoms are associated with the presence of XXY chromosomes in the cell.

The study of chromosomes of animals, and particularly of humans, made considerable progress after the discovery of methods of inducing cells to divide, then arresting mitotic cells during metaphase and subsequently causing cellular rupture, which permits the separation, detailed observation, and analysis of the chromosomes. Mitosis can be induced by phytohemagglutinin and can be arrested in metaphase by colchicine. Rupture of cells is brought about by initial immersion in a hypotonic solution, causing swelling,

after which cells are flattened and broken between a glass slide and a coverslip. The pattern of chromosomes obtained with a human cell after staining is illustrated in Fig 3–31. In addition to the 2 sex chromosomes X and Y, it is customary to group the remaining chromosomes according to their morphologic characteristics in 22 successively numbered pairs (Fig 3–31).

Until recently, recognition of individual chromosomes was not possible, because different chromosomes of the same karyotype often had the same general morphology. The development of techniques that reveal segmentation of chromosomes in transverse, differentially stained bands made it possible not only to identify individual chromosomes but also to study in detail phenomena of genetic deletion and translocation. These techniques are based mainly on the appearance of transverse bands in chromosomes previously treated with saline or enzyme solution and stained with fluorescent dyes or Giemsa's blood staining technique (Fig 3–32). (See Chapter 13.) This procedure has revolutionized the field of cytogenetics and has made possible a series of important observations on human cytogenetics.

The number and type of chromosomes encountered in an individual is known as his or her **karyotype** (Fig 3–31). Study of karyotypes has revealed chromosomal alterations associated with several types of diseases, including a form of leukemia.

Nucleolus

The nucleolus is a spherical structure, up to 1 μm in diameter, rich in rRNA and protein. It is usually basophilic when stained with hematoxylin and eosin. As seen with the electron microscope, the nucleolus consists of 3 distinct components. One to several palestaining regions are composed of **nucleolar-organizer DNA**—sequences of bases that code for rRNAs (Fig 3–33). In the human genome, 5 pairs of chromosomes contain nucleolar organizers. Closely associated with the nucleolar organizers are densely packed 5- to 10-nm ribonucleoprotein fibers, the **pars fibrosa** (Fig 3–33). The pars fibrosa is composed of primary transcripts of rRNA genes. The third component of the nucleolus is the **pars granulosa,** consisting of 15- to 20-nm granules, which are maturing ribosomes (Fig 3–33). When tritiated uridine is used as a tracer for rRNA synthesis, the tracer can be detected by autoradiography over these 3 components in sequence. Proteins, synthesized in the cytoplasm, become associated with rRNAs in the nucleolus; ribosome subunits then migrate into the cytoplasm. Heterochromatin (**nucleolus-associated chromatin**) is often seen attached to the nucleolus, but the functional significance of this association is not known (Figs 3–25 and 3–26). The pars fibrosa and the pars granulosa form a threadlike structure called the **nucleolonema** by light microscopists; the pale-staining nucleolar-organizing region has been termed the **pars amorpha.**

Although each human cell has the potential of forming 10 separate nucleoli, only one or 2 are usually

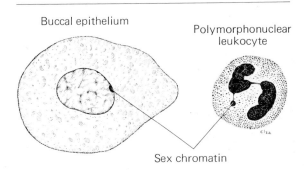

Buccal epithelium

Polymorphonuclear leukocyte

Sex chromatin

Figure 3–30. Morphology of sex chromatin in human female oral epithelium and in a polymorphonuclear leukocyte. In the epithelium, it appears as a small, dense granule adhering to the nuclear envelope. In the leukocyte, it has a drumstick shape.

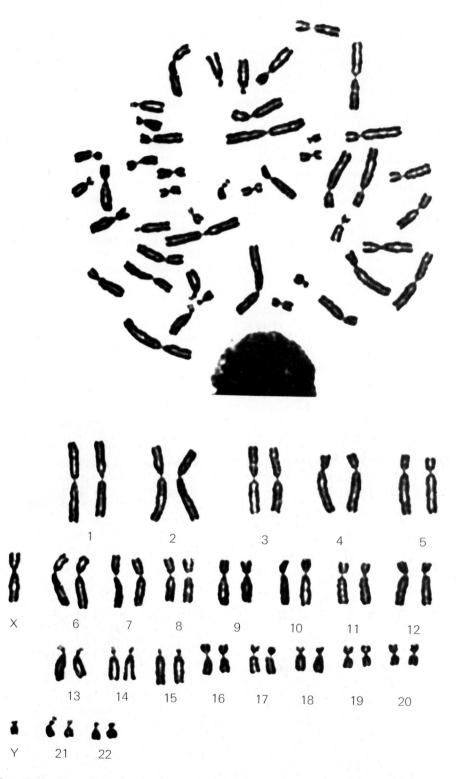

Figure 3–31. *Top:* Photomicrograph of chromosomes of a human cell obtained during metaphase. *Bottom:* Karyotype of a normal human male. The chromosomes are grouped according to their morphologic characteristics. (Courtesy of G Gimenez-Martin.)

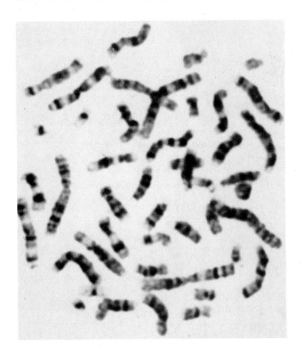

Figure 3–32. Human karyotype preparation using the GTG banding technique (*G* bands by *Trypsin* and *Giemsa* stain). Each chromosome has a particular pattern of banding, permitting identification of not only individual chromosomes but also the relationship of the banding pattern to genetic anomalies. × 2000. (Courtesy of A Wajntal.)

observed. This is because nucleoli tend to fuse during the interphase stage of the cell cycle. When nuclear chromatin becomes very condensed, as in lymphocytes, nucleoli become very difficult to visualize. Large nucleoli are encountered in embryonic cells during their proliferation, in cells that are actively synthesizing proteins, and in rapidly growing malignant tumors. The nucleolus disperses during cell division but reappears in the telophase stage of mitosis.

Nucleoplasm

Nucleoplasm is an amorphous matrix that fills the space between the chromatin and the nucleoli in the nucleus. It is composed mainly of proteins (some of which have enzymatic activity), metabolites, and ions.

Extraction of nuclear nucleic acids shows that nucleoplasm contains a continuous fibrillar structure called **nuclear matrix** that is a nucleoskeletal structure. The fibrous lamina of the nuclear envelope is a part of the nuclear matrix. The functions of the nuclear matrix are still being studied, but the fact that it binds to hormone receptors and to recently synthesized DNA suggests an important role in nuclear functions.

CELL DIVISION

Cell division can be observed with the light microscope. During this process, known as **mitosis,** the parent cell divides and each of the daughter cells

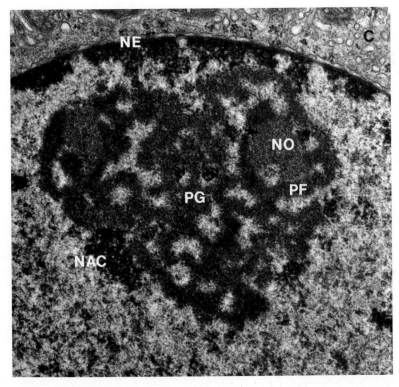

Figure 3–33. Nucleolus in a human adrenocortical cell. NO, nucleolar-organizer DNA; PF, pars fibrosa; PG, pars granulosa; NAC, nucleolus-associated chromatin; NE, nuclear envelope; and C, cytoplasm. × 50,000.

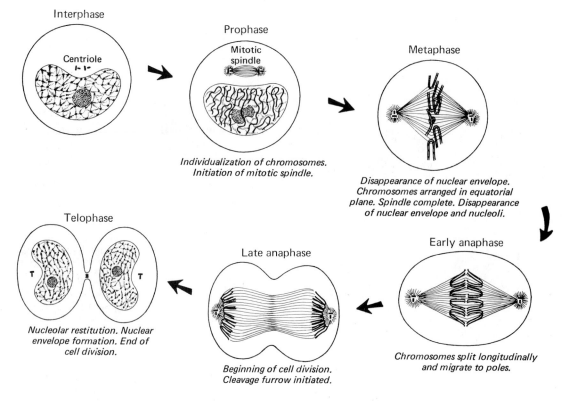

Interphase

Prophase

Metaphase

Centriole

Mitotic spindle

*Individualization of chromosomes.
Initiation of mitotic spindle.*

*Disappearance of nuclear envelope.
Chromosomes arranged in equatorial
plane. Spindle complete. Disappearance
of nuclear envelope and nucleoli.*

Telophase

Late anaphase

Early anaphase

*Nucleolar restitution. Nuclear
envelope formation. End of
cell division.*

*Beginning of cell division.
Cleavage furrow initiated.*

*Chromosomes split longitudinally
and migrate to poles.*

Figure 3–34. Phases of mitosis.

receives a chromosomal karyotype identical to that of the parent cell. Essentially, a longitudinal duplication of the chromosomes takes place, and they are distributed to the daughter cells. The phase during which the cell does not undergo division is called **interphase,** and the nucleus appears as it is normally observed in microscope preparations. The process of mitosis is dynamic and continuous but is subdivided into phases to facilitate its study (Figs 3–34 and 3–35).

The **prophase** is characterized by the gradual coiling of nuclear chromatin, giving rise to several individualized rod-shaped or hairpin-shaped bodies that stain intensely. These are the **chromosomes.** The nuclear envelope remains unaltered, and the chromosomes appear coiled in the nucleus. The centrioles separate, and a pair migrates to each pole of the cell. Simultaneously, the microtubules of the mitotic spindle appear between the 2 pairs of centrioles (Figs 3–34 and 3–35).

During **metaphase,** the nuclear envelope and the nucleolus disappear. The chromosomes migrate to the equatorial plane of the cell, where each divides longitudinally to form 2 chromatids. These attach to the microtubules of the mitotic spindle at a special plaquelike, electron-dense region, the **centromere (kinetochore)** (Figs 3–36 and 3–37).

In **anaphase,** the sister chromatids separate from each other and migrate toward the opposite poles of the cell, following the direction of the spindle microtubules. Throughout this process, the centromeres move from the center, pulling along the remainder of the chromosome (Fig 3–34). It has been shown by immunofluorescence that microtubular protein (tubulin), actin, and myosin occur in the spindle region. It is probable that these proteins participate in the process of chromosome migration to the cell poles, although the mechanism of this process is still a subject of controversy.

Telophase is characterized by the reappearance of nuclei in the daughter cells. The chromosomes revert to their semidispersed state, and the nucleoli, chromatin, and nuclear envelope reappear. While these nuclear alterations are taking place, a constriction develops at the level of the equatorial plane of the parent cell and progresses until it divides the cytoplasm and its organelles in half (Figs 3–34 and 3–38). A beltlike accumulation of microfilaments occurs beneath the cell membrane in the region of mitotic constriction. This and other evidence suggest that the actin and myosin participate in the cytoplasmic component of cell division.

Most tissues undergo a constant turnover because of continuous cell division and continuous death of cells. Nerve tissue and cardiac muscle cells are an exception, since they do not multiply postnatally and consequently cannot regenerate. The turnover rate of the cells varies greatly from one tissue to another— rapid in the epithelium of the alimentary canal and the epidermis, slow in the pancreas and thyroid.

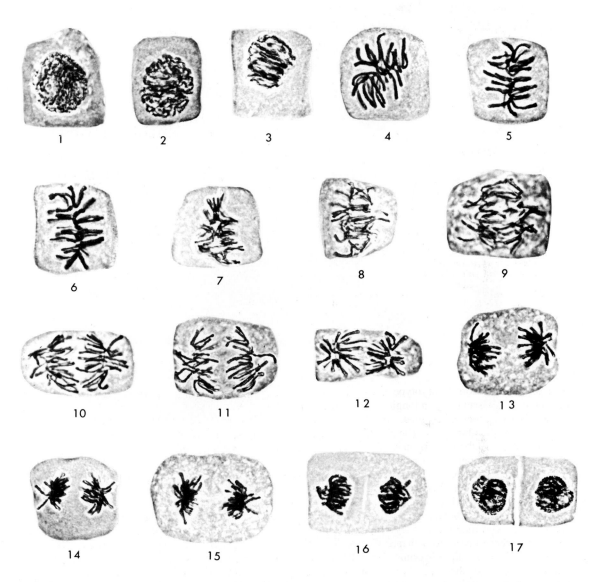

Figure 3−35. Stages of mitosis in the cells of the root of *Allium cepa*. Phase microscopy. 1−3, prophase; 4−7, metaphase; 8−13, anaphase; 14−17, telophase. (Courtesy of G Gimenez-Martin.)

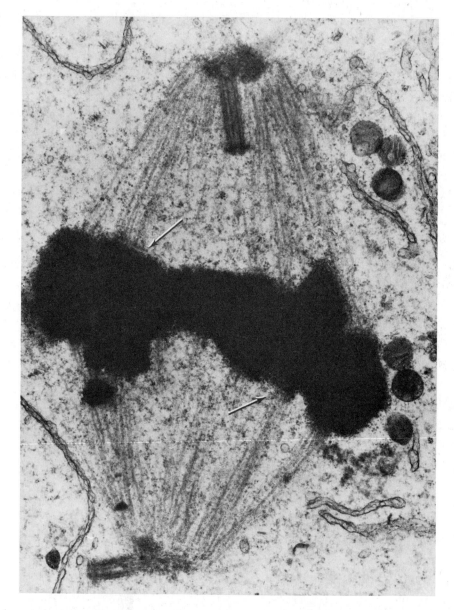

Figure 3–36. Electron micrograph of a section of a rooster spermatocyte in metaphase. Observe the presence of 2 centrioles in each pole, the mitotic spindle formed by microtubules, and the chromosomes in the equatorial plate. The arrows show the insertion of microtubules in the centromeres. × 19,000. (Courtesy of R McIntosh.)

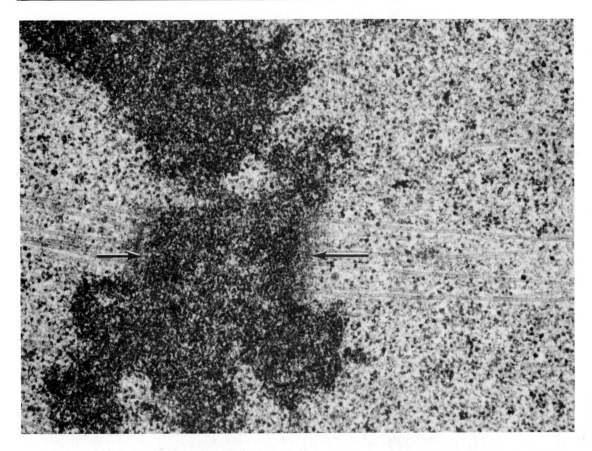

Figure 3 –37. Electron micrograph of the metaphase of a human lung cell in tissue culture. Note the insertion of microtubules in the centromeres (arrows) of the densely stained chromosomes. Reduced from × 50,000. (Courtesy of R McIntosh.)

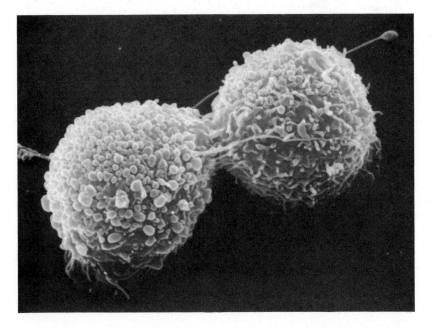

Figure 3 –38. Scanning electron micrograph of cell division in a Chinese hamster ovary cell in cell culture. The numerous blebs are characteristic of the telophase stage of mitosis. × 5000. (Courtesy of J Aggelar.)

THE CELL CYCLE

Mitosis is the visible manifestation of cell division, but there are other processes, not so easily observed with the light microscope, that play a fundamental role in cell multiplication. Principal among these is the phase in which DNA, the main chromosomal component, replicates. This process can be analyzed by the introduction of labeled, radioactive DNA precursors (eg, ^{3}H-thymidine), which are then traced by biochemical and radioautographic methods. DNA replication has been shown to occur during **interphase,** when no visible phenomena of cell division are observable with the microscope. This alternation between mitosis and interphase in all tissues with cellular turnover is known as the cell cycle. A careful study of the cell cycle reveals that it may be divided into 2 stages: mitosis, consisting of the 4 phases already described (prophase, metaphase, anaphase, and telophase), and interphase.

Interphase is itself divided into 3 phases: G_1 (presynthesis), S (DNA synthesis), and G_2 (post DNA duplication) (Fig 3–39). Synthesis and replication of DNA and centrioles take place in the S phase. The sequence of these phases and the time involved are illustrated in Fig 3–39. The G_1 (for gap) phase is the phase during which RNA and protein synthesis occur and the cell volume, previously reduced to one-half by mitosis, is restored to its normal size. In cells that are not continuously dividing, the cell cycle activities may be temporarily or permanently suspended. Cells

in such a stage of development are referred to as being in G_0 (eg, muscle, nerve).

Processes that occur during the G_2 phase are the production and accumulation of energy to be utilized during mitosis and the synthesis of tubulin to be assembled in microtubules during mitosis.

CELL DYNAMICS

Study of the cell by means of the light or electron microscope gives the false impression that the cell is static. However, cinematography at accelerated rates (5–30 times normal) shows considerable activity in cells. Thus, it has been observed that the nucleus can rotate within the cytoplasm up to 270 degrees per minute. Mitochondria demonstrate active wriggling movements in the cytoplasm. In only a few minutes, they can be seen to become fragmented and fuse together again.

Profound cellular changes are also observed during cell differentiation. Depending upon the function of the cell, some organelles become better developed than others and are major features of the cytoplasm. Cytoplasm in striated muscle cells is composed mainly of contractile fibrils, the myofibrils. Cells of the acinar pancreas that synthesize and secrete protein contain cytoplasm almost completely filled with rough endoplasmic reticulum and zymogen granules. Furthermore, in an already differentiated cell, modification of the organelles can be observed according to the

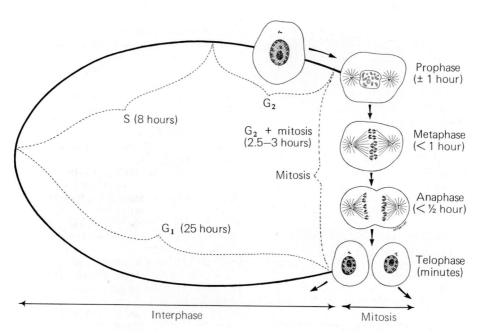

Figure 3–39. Phases of the cell cycle. G_1 (presynthetic) phase is variable and depends on many factors, including the rate of cell division in the tissue. In this particular case of bone tissue, it lasts 25 hours. The S (DNA synthetic) phase lasts about 8 hours. The G_2 plus mitosis phase lasts 2.5–3 hours. The times are from Young RW in: *J Cell Biol* 1962;**14:**357.

phase of cell activity. This depends on whether the cell is hypoactive or hyperactive. Cells that actively secrete protein have a more highly developed rough endoplasmic reticulum and Golgi complex than those that secrete protein in moderate or minimal amounts.

In addition to these morphologic aspects of the cell's continuous activity as reflected in its organelles, it should also be realized that with few exceptions, the cell's chemical components are continually being turned over.

REFERENCES

Afzelius BA, Eliasson R: Flagellar mutants in man: On the heterogeneity of the immotile-cilia syndrome. *J Ultrastruct Res* 1979;**69**:43.

Alberts B et al: *Molecular Biology of the Cell.* Garland, 1983.

Bielka H (editor): *The Eukaryotic Ribosome.* Springer-Verlag, 1982.

Bittar EW (editor): *Membrane Structure and Function.* 4 vols. Wiley, 1980–1981.

Bostock CJ, Sumner AT: *The Eucaryotic Chromosome.* North-Holland, 1978.

Bretscher A: Microfilament organization in the cytoskeleton of the intestinal brush border. In: *Cell and Muscle Motility.* Vol 4. Dowben RM, Shay JW (editors). Plenum, 1983.

Bretscher MS: The molecules of the cell membrane. *Sci Am* (Oct) 1985;**253**:100.

Brinkley BR: Microtubule organizing centers. *Annu Rev Cell Biol* 1985;**1**:145.

Brown MS, Anderson RGW, Goldstein JL: Recycling receptors: The round-trip itinerary of migrant membrane proteins. *Cell* 1983;**32**:663.

Craig SW, Pollard TD: Actin-binding proteins. *Trends in Biochemical Science* 1982;**7**:88.

DeDuve C: Microbodies in the living cell. *Sci Am* (May) 1983;**248**:74.

DePierre JW, Ernster L: Enzyme topology of intracellular membranes. *Annu Rev Biochem* 1977;**46**:201.

Dingle JT (editor): *Lysosomes in Biology and Pathology.* 6 vols. Elsevier/North-Holland, 1969–1979.

Dustin P: *Microtubules,* 2nd ed. Springer-Verlag, 1984.

Fakan S, Puvion E: The ultrastructural visualization of nucleolar and extranucleolar RNA synthesis and distribution. *Int Rev Cytol* 1980;**65**:255.

Farquhar MG: Progress in unraveling pathways of Golgi traffic. *Annu Rev Cell Biol* 1985;**1**:447.

Farquhar MG, Palade GE: The Golgi apparatus (complex)—(1954–1981): Artifact to center stage. *J Cell Biol* 1981;**91**:77s.

Fawcett D: *The Cell,* 2nd ed. Saunders, 1981.

Fuchs E, Hanukoglu I: Unraveling the structure of the intermediate filaments. *Cell* 1983;**34**:332.

Goessens G: Nucleolar structure. *Int Rev Cytol* 1984;**87**:107.

Harrison SC, Kirchhausen T: Clathrin, cages and coated vesicles. *Cell* 1983;**33**:650.

Helenius A et al: Endosomes. *Trends in Biochemical Science* 1983;**8**:245.

Holtzmann E: *Lysosomes: A Survey.* Springer-Verlag, 1976.

Hubbard SC, Ivatt RJ: Synthesis and processing of asparagine-linked oligosaccharides. *Annu Rev Biochem* 1981;**50**:555.

Igo-Kemenes T, Horz W, Zachu HG: Chromatin. *Annu Rev Biochem* 1982;**51**:89.

Inoue S: Cell division and the mitotic spindle. *J Cell Biol* 1981;**91**:132s.

Jordan EG: *The Nucleolus,* 2nd ed. Oxford Univ Press, 1978.

Kornberg RD, Klug A: The nucleosome. *Sci Am* (Feb) 1981;**244**:52.

Kreil G: Transfer of proteins across membranes. *Annu Rev Biochem* 1981;**50**:317.

Krstić RV: *Ultrastructure of the Mammalian Cell.* Springer-Verlag, 1979.

Lake JA: The ribosome. *Sci Am* (Feb) 1981;**245**:84.

Lazarow PB, Fujiki Y: Biogenesis of peroxisomes. *Annu Rev Cell Biol* 1985;**1**:489.

Lloyd D, Poole PK, Edwards SW: *The Cell Division Cycle.* Academic Press, 1982.

McClosky M, Poo MM: Protein diffusion in cell membranes: Some biological implications. *Int Rev Cytol* 1984;**87**:19.

Neupert W, Schatz G: How proteins are transported into mitochondria. *Trends in Biochemical Science* 1981;**6**:1.

Novikoff AB: The endoplasmic reticulum: A cytochemist's view (a review). *Proc Natl Acad Sci USA* 1976;**73**:2781.

Osborn M, Weber K: Intermediate filaments: Cell-type-specific markers in differentiation and pathology. *Cell* 1982;**31**:303.

Palade GE: Intracellular aspects of the process of protein synthesis. *Science* 1975;**189**:347.

Pastan IH, Willingham MC: Receptor-mediated endocytosis of hormones in cultured cells. *Annu Rev Physiol* 1981;**43**:239.

Poisner AM, Trifaro JM (editors): *The Secretory Granule.* Elsevier, 1982.

Pollard TD, Craig SW: Mechanisms of actin polymerization. *Trends in Biochemical Science* 1982;**7**:55.

Porter KR: The cytomatrix: A short history of its study. *J Cell Biol* 1984;**99**(No. 1–Part 2):3s.

Prescott DM, Goldstein L (editors): *Cell Biology: A Comprehensive Treatise.* 4 vols. Academic Press, 1977–1980.

Rothman J: The compartmental organization of the Golgi apparatus. *Sci Am* (Sept) 1985;**253**:74.

Sabatini DD et al: Mechanisms for the incorporation of proteins in membranes and organelles. *J Cell Biol* 1982;**92**:1.

Satir P et al: The mechanochemical cycle of the dynein arm. *Cell Motil* 1981;**1**:303.

Silverstein SC, Steinman RM, Cohn ZA: Endocytosis. *Annu Rev Biochem* 1977;**46**:669.

Singer SJ, Nicolson GL: The fluid mosaic model of the structure of cell membranes. *Science* 1972;**175**:720.

Tolbert NE, Essner E: Microbodies: Peroxisomes and glyoxysomes. *J Cell Biol* 1981;**91**:271s.

Tzagoloff A: *Mitochondria.* Plenum, 1982.

Weber K, Osborn M: The molecules of the cell matrix. *Sci Am* (Oct) 1985;**253**:110.

Weissman G, Claiborne R (editors): *Cell Membranes: Biochemistry, Cell Biology, and Pathology.* HP Publishing Co., 1975.

Wickner W: Assembly of proteins into membranes. *Science* 1980;**210**:861.

Wool IG: The structure and function of eukaryotic ribosomes. *Annu Rev Biochem* 1979;**48**:719.

4

Epithelial Tissue

Tissues are structures formed by collections of cells that frequently have similar morphologic characteristics and similar functions. Despite its complexity, the human body is composed of only **4 basic types of tissue:** epithelial, connective, muscular, and nervous. These tissues do not exist as isolated units but rather in association one with another and in variable proportions, forming different organs and systems of the body.

Connective tissue is characterized by the abundance of intercellular material produced by its cells; muscular tissue is composed of elongated cells that have the specialized function of contraction; and nervous tissue is composed of cells with elongated processes extending from the cell body that have the specialized functions of receiving, generating, and transmitting nervous impulses.

Epithelial tissues are composed of closely aggregated polyhedral cells with very little intercellular substance. Adhesion between these cells is strong. Thus, cellular sheets are formed that cover the surface of the body and line its cavities.

Epithelial tissues have the following principal functions: (1) covering and lining surfaces (eg, skin); (2) absorption (eg, the intestines); (3) secretion (eg, the epithelial cells of glands); (4) sensation (eg, neuroepithelium); and (5) contractility (eg, myoepithelial cells).

Epithelia are derived from all 3 embryonic germ layers. Most of the epithelium lining the skin, mouth, nose, and anus has an ectodermal origin. The lining of the respiratory system, the digestive tract, and the glands of the digestive tract such as the pancreas and the liver are derived from the endoderm. Other epithelia (eg, the endothelial lining of blood vessels) originate from mesoderm.

GENERAL CHARACTERISTICS OF EPITHELIAL TISSUES

Although epithelial tissues have varied morphology depending on their function and position in the body, they possess some common characteristics.

The Forms of Epithelial Cells

The forms and dimensions of epithelial cells are varied, ranging from high columnar to cuboidal to low squamous cells and including all intermediate forms (Fig 4–1). Their common polyhedral form is accounted for by their juxtaposition in cellular layers

or masses. A similar phenomenon might be observed if a large number of inflated rubber balloons were compressed into a limited space. With appropriate stains, the cell nuclei have a distinctive appearance, varying from spherical to elongated or elliptic in shape. The nuclear form often corresponds roughly to the cell shape; thus, cuboidal cells have spherical nuclei whereas squamous cells have flattened, elliptic nuclei. The long axis of the nucleus is always parallel to the main axis of the cell.

Since the boundaries between cells are frequently indistinguishable at the light microscope level, observation of the form of the cell nucleus is of great importance because it is an indirect clue to the shape of the cell. This is of value in determination of cell

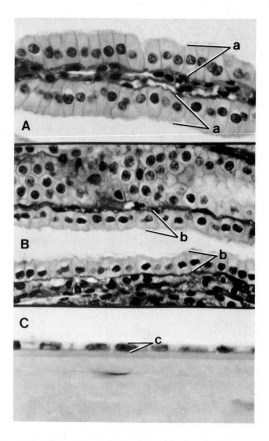

Figure 4–1. Examples of simple epithelia. *A:* Simple columnar type from the intestine (a). *B:* Simple cuboidal epithelium from the kidney (b). *C:* Simple squamous epithelium from the cornea (c). × 300.

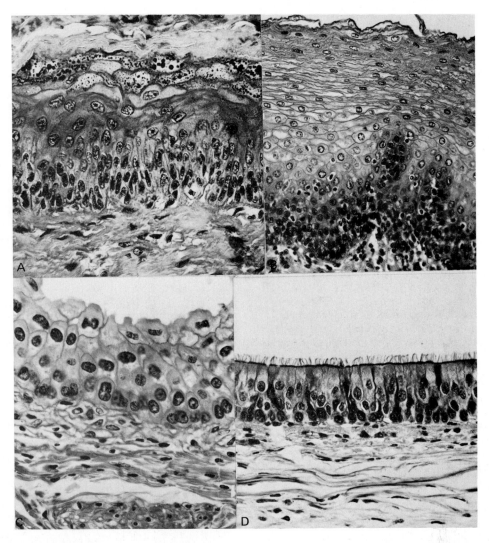

Figure 4–2. Photomicrographs of more complex types of epithelial tissue. *A:* Stratified squamous keratinized epithelium. *B:* Stratified squamous nonkeratinized epithelium. *C:* Transitional epithelium. *D:* Pseudostratified columnar ciliated epithelium. H&E stain, × 500.

disposition—whether or not they are arranged in layers, which is a primary morphologic criterion for classifying epithelia (Fig 4–2).

Presence of a Basal Lamina

All epithelial cells have at their basal surfaces a sheetlike extracellular structure called the basal lamina. This structure is visible only with the electron microscope, where it appears as a dense layer, 20–100 nm thick, consisting of a delicate network of fine fibrils (**lamina densa**). In addition to the lamina densa, basal laminae may have electron-lucent layers on one or both sides of the dense layer that are called **laminae rarae** or **laminae lucidae**. Basal laminae are composed mainly of **type IV collagen,** a glycoprotein called **laminin,** and **proteoglycan** (heparan sulfate). Basal laminae are sometimes attached to the under-

lying connective tissues by **anchoring fibrils** of unknown composition (Figs 4–3B and 4–4A).

A basal lamina is present where cells come into contact with connective tissue; thus, it is present at the base of epithelia (eg, in skin and glands, in the respiratory, urinary, reproductive, and digestive tracts, and around the endothelium of capillaries) as well as around muscle, adipose, and Schwann cells (Fig 4–3B). These basal laminae provide a barrier limiting or regulating exchanges of macromolecules between connective tissue and the other tissues. A basal lamina is also found between adjacent epithelial layers, as in lung alveoli and the renal glomerulus (Fig 4–3A). In these cases, the basal lamina is thicker as a result of fusion of the basal laminae of each epithelial cell layer.

It is now well established that the components of the basal lamina are secreted by epithelial, muscle,

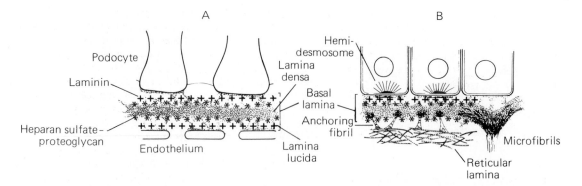

Figure 4–3. Types of basement membranes. *A:* The type of basement membrane that consists of only a basal lamina. The basal lamina is divided into a central **lamina densa** with a **lamina lucida (lamina rara)** on either side. *B:* The more complex basement membrane underlying most epithelia. The right-most cell illustrates the unique basement membrane of lymphatic capillaries. Microfibrils attached to the basal lamina are thought to put tension on the walls of lymphatic capillaries and hold them open.

adipose, and Schwann cells. In some instances, reticular fibers are closely associated with the basal lamina, forming a layer termed the **reticular lamina.** The reticular fibers are produced by connective tissue cells.

One of the functions of the basal lamina is to provide a selective barrier between connective tissue and other cells. The basal lamina also seems to contain the information necessary for certain cell-cell inter-

actions. An example is the reinnervation of denervated muscle cells. Presence of the basal lamina around a muscle cell is necessary for the establishment of new neuromuscular junctions. Another function of the basal lamina is the control of epithelial cell location and movement. When the basal lamina underneath a carcinoma breaks down, cancer cells can invade underlying tissues.

The term "basement membrane" is used to spec-

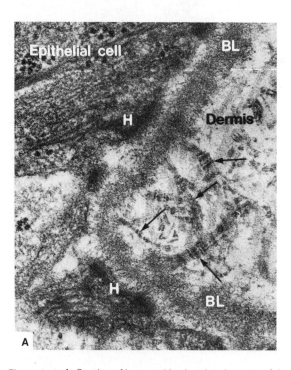

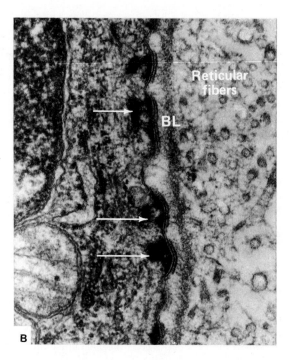

Figure 4–4. *A:* Section of human skin showing the zone of the epithelial–connective tissue junction. Observe the anchoring fibrils (arrows) that apparently insert in the basal lamina (BL). The characteristically irregular spacing of these fibrils distinguishes them from collagen fibrils. × 54,000. (Courtesy of FM Guerra Rodrigo.) *B:* Section of skin showing the basal lamina (BL) and hemidesmosomes (arrows). At top is a portion of an epithelial cell. × 80,000.

ify a PAS-positive layer, visible with the light microscope, beneath epithelia and around muscle, adipose, and Schwann cells. The basement membrane consists of the basal lamina and the reticular lamina. The use of these terms is not agreed upon by all authors. In this book, the term ''basal lamina'' is used to denote the lamina densa and the variable presence of laminae rarae, structures seen with the electron microscope. When referring to thicker structures seen with the light microscope, the term ''basement membrane'' is used.

Cohesion Among Epithelial Cells

Epithelial cells are extremely cohesive, and relatively strong mechanical forces are necessary to separate them. This quality of intercellular adhesion is especially marked in those epithelial tissues usually subjected to traction and pressure (eg, the skin). This is due in part to the binding action of the glycoproteins, which are integral membrane proteins of the plasma membrane, and of a small amount of intercellular proteoglycan. Calcium ions are also important in maintaining this cellular cohesion. Thus, the chelating agent EDTA, which complexes with calcium, is known to decrease cell adhesion and is widely used in cell biology to separate epithelial cells, a necessary step in obtaining a suspension of isolated cells. Intercellular adhesiveness changes with age, as indicated by the cells' different responses to the presence of trypsin or deoxycholate or to the removal of calcium ions.

In addition to the cohesive effects of intercellular macromolecules and ions, the lateral membranes of epithelial cells exhibit several specializations that form **intercellular junctions.** These junctions serve not

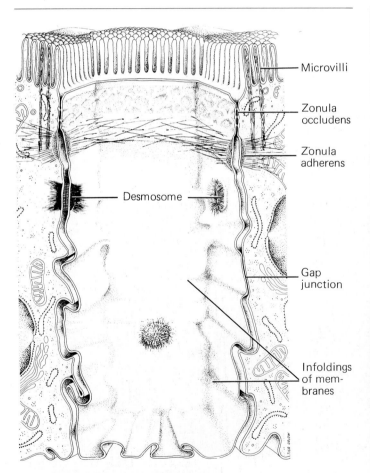

Figure 4–5. The main structures that participate in cohesion among epithelial cells. The drawing shows 3 cells from the intestinal epithelium. The cell in the middle was emptied of its contents to show the inner surface of its membrane. Observe that the zonulae occludens and adherens form a continuous ribbon around the cell apex, while the desmosomes and gap junctions comprise spotlike plaques. The zonula occludens is formed by multiple ridges where the membranes' outer laminae fuse. (Redrawn and reproduced, with permission, from Krstić RV: *Ultrastructure of the Mammalian Cell.* Springer-Verlag, 1979.)

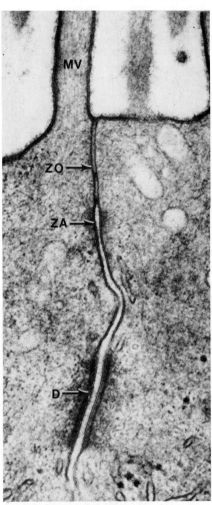

Figure 4–6. Electron micrograph of a section of epithelial cells in the large intestine showing a junctional complex with its zonula occludens (ZO), zonula adherens (ZA), and desmosome (D). Also shown is a microvillus (MV). × 80,000.

only as sites of **adhesion** but also as **seals** to prevent the flow of materials through the intercellular space (paracellular pathway) and to provide a mechanism for **intercellular communication.** The various junctions are usually present in a definite order from apex toward the base of the cell.

Tight junctions, or **zonulae occludentes** (singular, zonula occludens), are the most apical of the junctions. The Latin terminology gives important information about the geometry of the junction. *Zonula* refers to the fact that the junction forms a **band** completely encircling the cell, while *occludens* alludes to the **membrane fusions** which thereby close off the intercellular space. In properly stained thin sections viewed in the electron microscope, the outer leaflets of adjacent unit membranes are seen to fuse, giving rise to a local pentalaminar appearance. One to several of these fusion sites may be observed, depending on the epithelium under observation (Figs 4–5 and 4–6). After cryofracture (Fig 4–7), the replicas show anastomosing lines of ridges (P face) and grooves (E face), the number of which corresponds to the number of fusion sites observed in conventional thin sections. The number of ridges and grooves, or fusion sites, has a high correlation with the ''leakiness'' of the epithelium. Epithelia with one or very few fusion sites are more permeable to water and solutes (eg, proximal renal tubule) than epithelia with numerous (12–15) fusion sites (eg, urinary bladder). Thus, the principal function of the tight junction is to form a more or less tight seal preventing the flow of materials between epithelial cells (paracellular pathway) in either direction (from apex to base or base to apex) (Fig 4–21). In some epithelia, electrical potentials are set up across the epithelium that influence the ability of the epithelium to transport molecules. In these cases, more fusion sites are usually found, but some little-understood exceptions do occur.

In many epithelia, the next junctional type encountered is the **zonula adherens** (Figs 4–5 and 4–6). Less is known about this junction; it encircles the cell and is thought to provide for some of the adhesion of one cell to its neighbor. The distance between adjacent cell membranes may be greater than the usual 20 nm

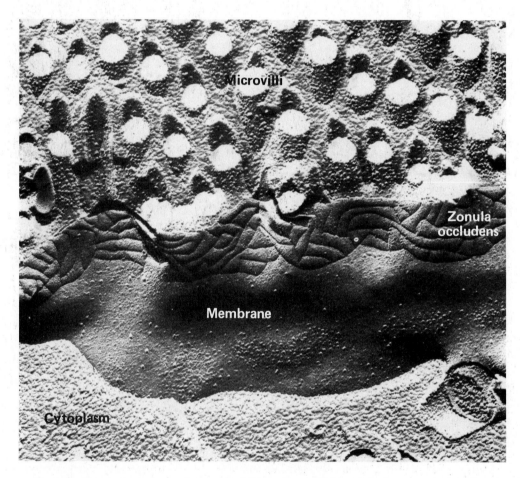

Figure 4–7. Electron micrograph of a freeze-fractured small intestine epithelial cell. In the upper portion, the microvilli are fractured transversely; in the lower portion, the fracture crossed through the cytoplasm of the intestinal epithelial cell. The grooves, which actually lie in the lipid (middle) layer of each plasmalemma, reveal that the membranes of adjoining cells were fused in the zonula occludens. × 100,000. (Courtesy of A Pinto da Silva.)

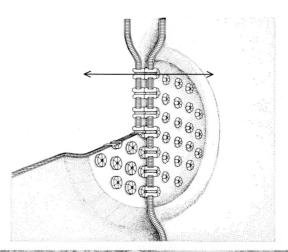

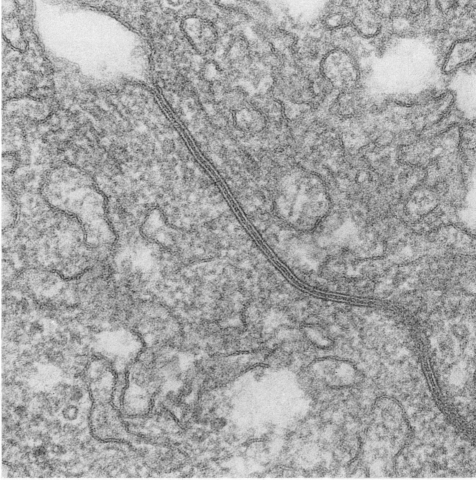

Figure 4–8. Gap junction between 2 rat liver cells. At the junction, 2 apposed membranes are separated by an electron-dense space, or gap, 2 nm wide. In the upper portion (oblique view) is a model of a gap junction depicting the structural elements that allow the exchange of nutrients and signal molecules between cells without loss of material into the intercellular space. The communicating "pipes" are formed by pairs of abutting particles, which are in turn composed of 6 dumbbell-shaped protein subunits that span the lipid bilayer of each cell membrane. The channel passing through the cylindric bridges is about 2 nm in diameter, limiting the size of the molecules that can pass through it. Unlike the tight junction, fluids and tracers in the intercellular space can permeate the gap junction by flowing around the protein bridges. (Illustration at top is from Staehelin LA, Hull BE: Junctions between living cells. *Sci Am* [May] 1978;**238**:41. Copyright © 1978 by Scientific American, Inc. All rights reserved. Illustration at bottom is × 193,000. Courtesy of MC Williams.)

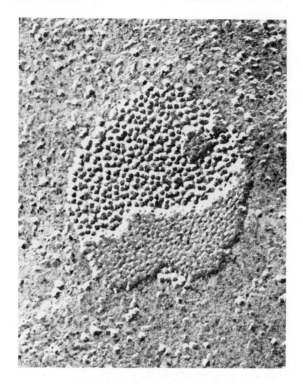

Figure 4–9. Gap junction as seen on cryofracture preparation. It appears as a plaquelike agglomeration of intramembrane protein particles. × 45,000. (Courtesy of A Pinto da Silva.)

in these regions. A noteworthy feature of this junction is the insertion of numerous actin-containing microfilaments into dense plaques of material on the cytoplasmic surfaces of the junctional membranes. The plaques contain myosin, tropomyosin, α actinin, and vinculin, but exactly how the actin filaments interact with the membrane has not yet been determined. The microfilaments arise from a web of filaments of several types in the apical cytoplasm called the **terminal web.** In this region, most cytoplasmic organelles are excluded, and the terminal web is thought to provide a certain rigidity to the apex of the cell.

Both of the above-described junctions are responsible for a structure long known to light microscopists as the **terminal bar** (Figs 4–15 and 4–16).

A **gap junction,** or nexus, can occur almost anywhere along the lateral membranes of most epithelial cells. Gap junctions are characterized, in conventional electron micrographs, by the close (2 nm) apposition of adjacent cell membranes (Fig 4–8). After cryofracture, aggregates of intramembrane particles are found in circular patches in the P face of the plasma membrane (Fig 4–9). If an extracellular tracer such as lanthanum hydroxide is introduced, the tracer cannot penetrate all of the intercellular space at the sites of gap junctions. The areas not penetrated by the tracer are occupied by proteins that connect a cell to its neighbor. Gap junctions have been isolated from liver, lens, and cardiac muscle. The major protein constit-

uent is a polypeptide (MW 26,000–30,000). Detailed study raises the possibility that these proteins may be tissue-specific or at least specific for tissues arising from one or another of the embryonic germ layers (ectoderm, mesoderm, endoderm). Gap junction proteins form hexamers with a hydrophilic pore, about 1.5 nm in diameter in the center. This unit is called a **connexon,** and connexons in adjacent cell membranes are aligned to form a hydrophilic channel between the 2 cells (Fig 4–8, top).

Many cells within tissues of both vertebrates and invertebrates are not independent, isolated units but have intercellular communications that permit the interchange of ions and larger molecules (MW ≤ 1500). This occurs by means of gap junctions present between membranes of neighboring cells. This communication phenomenon has been studied by the following techniques:

A. Following the intracellular microinjection of stains or fluorescent compounds, the injected compounds gradually pass to neighboring cells and then to still other cells.

B. By inserting microelectrodes into neighboring cells, it was shown that an electric current can pass between cells with very slight loss of voltage (Fig 4–10). The curve registered for the electrical stimulus (curve I) was compared with tracings from the 3 microelectrodes (curves II, III, and IV). Analysis led to the following conclusions:

1. The electrical stimulus is transmitted with little loss of its intensity to an electrode inserted in the same cell. The cell cytoplasm is a good conductor and does not hinder the flow of the stimulus curve (curve II).

2. When the stimulus is applied to cell 2, it is not registered in cell 1 (curve IV). This indicates that the plasma membranes between cells 1 and 2 have high resistance.

3. When the stimulus is applied to cell 2, the response registered in the electrode inserted in cell 3 is almost the same (curve III) as the one observed in the electrode of cell 2 (curve II). This is due to the existence of a low-resistance pathway between cells 2 and 3 and suggests that there is communication between these cells.

Careful measurements show that the resistance between communicating cells can be 1000 times lower than between noncommunicating cells. These results are important because they demonstrate that most tissues are not merely aggregates of independent cells but function as integrated units. Cellular communication appears during embryogenesis and is probably important in the coordination of embryonic development.

Gap junctions can be rapidly formed between previously isolated cells. Metabolic inhibitors—especially those blocking oxidative phosphorylation—can inhibit the formation of junctions or undo junctions already present between cells. However, new junctions can be formed in the absence of protein synthesis. In this case, connexons may form from subunits diffusely scattered in the plasma membrane.

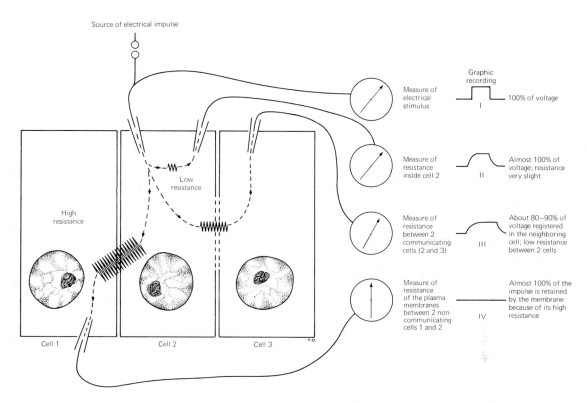

Figure 4–10. Experiments measuring the electrical conductivity between cells with or without communication. Cells 1 and 2 do not communicate, whereas cells 2 and 3 do. In cell 2, two microelectrodes were inserted. One is connected simultaneously to a stimulator (generator of electrical impulse) and to a measuring device. The other electrode is connected to a registering electrode and measures the current that crosses the cell cytoplasm. Electrodes were also inserted in cells 1 and 3 to measure the current that passes from cell 2 to cell 1 and from cell 2 to cell 3. Graphs obtained from the electrical stimulations are shown to the right of the figure. The upper graph expresses the total impulse measured by the electrode to the left of cell 2. The second graph shows only a very small lowering of the current due to the resistance of the cytoplasm. The third and fourth graphs show that most of the current (80–90%) passes from cell 2 to cell 3, while practically no current crosses the membranes that separate cell 2 from cell 1. Cells 2 and 3 have a special junction that lowers the membrane's resistance. This does not occur between cells 1 and 2.

The final junctional type to be considered is the **desmosome,** or **macula adherens** (Figs 4–5, 4–6, and 4–11). The desmosome is a complex disk-shaped structure at the surface of one cell that is matched with an identical structure at the surface of the adjacent cell. The cell membranes are very straight in this region and are usually somewhat farther apart (> 30 nm) than the usual 20 nm. In addition, some desmosomes possess a line of dense material in the intercellular space (Fig 4–11). Inside the membrane of each cell and separated from it by a short distance is a circular plaque of material called an **attachment plaque.** At least 12 different proteins make up the plaque. Groups of intermediate filaments of the cytokeratin (tonofilament) variety are inserted in the attachment plaque or make hairpin turns and return to the cytoplasm. Desmosomes are distributed in patches along the lateral membranes of most epithelial cells and, in the stratified squamous epithelium of the skin, are the only type of junction present. Their only

function appears to be that of providing an especially firm adhesion of one cell to the next.

In the contact zone between certain epithelial cells and the basal lamina, **hemidesmosomes** can often be observed. Morphologically, these structures take the form of half a desmosome on the epithelial cell plasmalemma. They probably serve to bind the epithelial cell to the subjacent basal lamina (Fig 4–4B).

Certain of these types of cell junctions will be encountered again in the discussion of muscle and nervous tissue.

SPECIALIZATIONS OF THE APICAL SURFACES OF EPITHELIA

Microvilli

When viewed in the electron microscope, most cells are seen to have few to numerous projections arising from the surface. These projections may be

Figure 4–11 (at right). A model of a desmosome is outlined in this diagram. The intermediate filaments, 10 nm in diameter, form a tensile network that extends throughout the interior of the cell. They are attached to the plaques of the desmosome through poorly defined filamentous structures. Other filaments, called transmembrane linkers, connect the plaques of the spot desmosome across the intercellular space. The junction therefore serves to couple the tonofilament networks of adjacent cells, allowing the dissipation of shearing stresses throughout the tissue. (Reproduced, with permission, from Staehelin LA, Hull BE: Junctions between living cells. *Sci Am* [May] 1978;**238**:141. Copyright © 1978 by Scientific American, Inc. All rights reserved.)

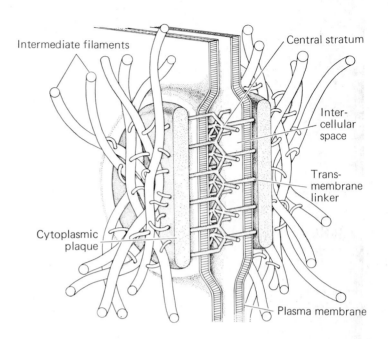

Figure 4–12. Electron micrograph of the apical region of an intestinal epithelial cell. Observe the terminal web composed of a horizontal network of intermediate filaments in which are anchored the vertical microfilaments that constitute the core of the microvilli. An extracellular filamentous **cell coat** (CC) is bound to the plasmalemma of the microvilli. × 45,000.

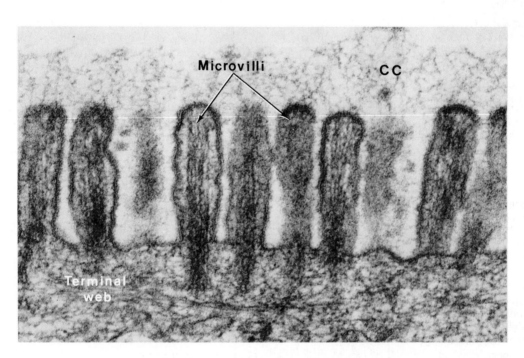

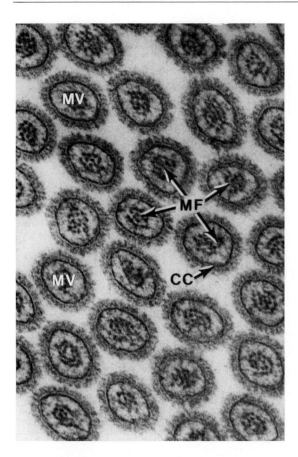

Figure 4–13. Electron micrograph of a section from the apical region of a cell from the intestinal lining showing cross-sectioned microvilli (MV). In their interiors, note the microfilaments (MF) in cross section. The surrounding unit membrane can be clearly discerned and is covered by a layer of cell coat (CC). × 100,000.

linked to each other and to the surrounding plasma membrane by several other proteins. The basal ends of these microfilaments intermingle with the filaments of the terminal web found just beneath the microvilli.

Stereocilia

Stereocilia are long, nonmotile processes of cells of the epididymis and the ''hair cells'' of the inner ear. Stereocilia are actually longer microvilli and should not be confused with true cilia, which are sometimes called kinocilia to emphasize their motility.

Cilia & Flagella

Cilia are elongated, motile structures on the surface of epithelial cells, 5–10 μm long and 0.2 μm in diameter—much longer than and different in structure from the microvilli. Under the electron microscope in cross section, they are observed to be surrounded by the cell membrane and contain a central pair of microtubules and, at the periphery inside the membrane, arranged in a circle, 9 more pairs of microtubules, all of which run in the direction of the long axis (Figs 3–19 and 4–14).

Cilia are inserted into **basal bodies,** which are dense structures present at the apical pole just below the cell membrane (Fig 4–14). They have an internal structure analogous to that of the centrioles (see Chapter 3).

In living organisms, rapid back-and-forth movement can be observed in cilia. Ciliary movement is frequently coordinated to permit a current of fluid or particulate matter to be propelled in one direction *over* the ciliated epithelium. ATP is the source of energy for ciliary motion.

It is estimated that a ciliated cell of the trachea can have about 250 cilia. Flagella, present in the human body only in the spermatozoa, are similar in structure to cilia but are much longer and are limited in most cases to one per cell.

CLASSIFICATION OF EPITHELIA

Epithelia are customarily classified according to their structure and function into 2 main groups: covering epithelia and glandular epithelia. This is an arbitrary division, for there are covering epithelia in which all cells secrete mucus (eg, the surface epithelium of the stomach) or in which glandular cells are very sparse (eg, mucous cells in the small intestine or trachea).

Covering Epithelia

Covering epithelia are tissues whose cells are organized in layers that cover the external surface or line the cavities of the body. They can be classified morphologically according to the number of cell layers and the morphology of the cells in the surface layer (Table 4–1). **Simple** epithelium contains only one layer of cells, and **stratified** epithelium contains more than one layer (Figs 4–1, 4–2, 4–15, and 4–16).

short or long fingerlike extensions or folds that pursue a sinuous course. All the extensions of the cell surface may be called microvilli, although the term ''microplicae'' is sometimes used for the long folds. In absorptive cells, such as the lining epithelium of the small intestine and the cells of the proximal renal tubule, orderly arrays of many hundreds of microvilli are encountered (Figs 4–12 and 4–13). This amplification of the surface increases the efficiency of absorption in these cells. Each microvillus is about 1 μm high and 0.08 μm wide. At the tip of the microvillus is a filamentous coat of variable thickness, the **glycocalyx,** which contains glycoproteins and is thus PAS-positive. The complex of microvilli and glycocalyx is easily seen in the light microscope and is called the **brush** (or striated) **border.**

Each microvillus is an extension of the cytoplasm of the cell and thus is covered by plasma membrane, greatly increasing the surface area of the apex of the cell. In their interiors, microvilli contain a cluster of 20–30 actin-containing microfilaments that are cross-

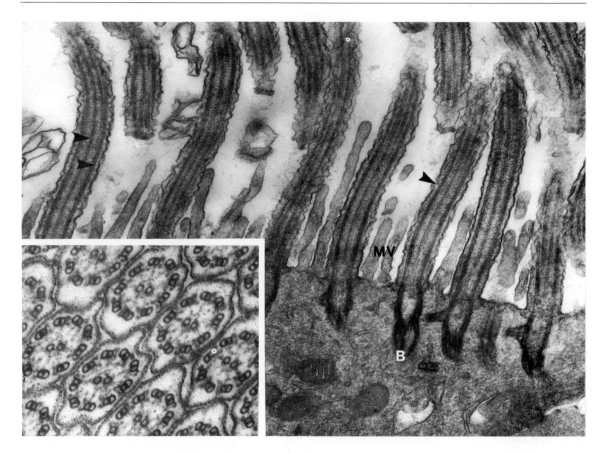

Figure 4–14. Electron micrograph of the apical portion of a ciliated epithelial cell. Cilia are seen in longitudinal section. At the left, arrowheads point to the central and peripheral microtubules of the axoneme. At the right, the arrowhead indicates the plasma membrane surrounding the cilium. Each cilium has a basal body (B) from which it grows. MV, microvilli. × 59,000. The inset shows cilia in cross section. The 9 + 2 array of microtubules in each cilium is evident. × 80,000. (Reproduced, with permission, from Junqueira LCU, Salles LMM: *Ultra-Estrutura e Função Celular.* Edgard Blücher, 1975.)

Table 4–1. Common types of covering epithelia in the human body.

According to the Number of Cell Layers	According to the Form of the Cells	Examples of Distribution	Function
Simple (one layer)	Squamous	Lining of vessels (endothelium). Serous lining of cavities: pericardium, pleura, peritoneum (mesothelia).	Facilitates the movement of the viscera (mesothelium), active transport by pinocytosis.
	Cuboidal	Covering the ovary, thyroid.	Covering, secretion.
	Columnar	Lining of intestine, gallbladder.	Protection, lubrication, absorption, secretion.
Pseudostratified (layers of cells with nuclei at different levels; not all cells reach surface but all adhere to basal lamina)		Lining of trachea, bronchi, nasal cavity.	Protection; transport of particles out of the air passages; secretion.
Stratified (2 or more layers)	Squamous keratinized (dry)	Epidermis.	Protection; prevents water loss.
	Squamous nonkeratinized (moist)	Mouth, esophagus, larynx, vagina, anal canal.	Protection; prevents water loss; secretion.
	Cuboidal	Sweat glands, developing ovarian follicles.	Protection, secretion.
	Transitional	Bladder, ureters, renal calyces.	Protection, distensibility.
	Columnar	Conjunctiva.	Protection.

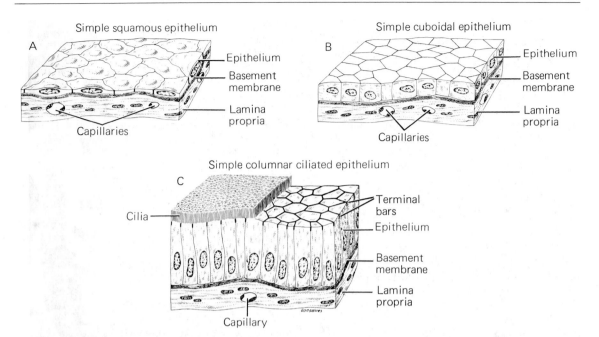

Figure 4–15. Diagrams of epithelial tissue. *A:* Simple squamous epithelium. *B:* Simple cuboidal epithelium. *C:* Simple ciliated columnar epithelium. All are separated from the subjacent connective tissue by a basement membrane. Note in *C* the terminal bars, which correspond in light microscopy to the zonula occludens and zonula adherens of the junctional complex.

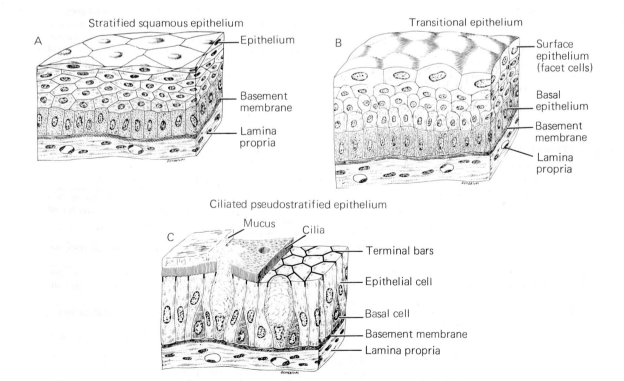

Figure 4–16. Diagrams of epithelial tissue. *A:* Stratified squamous epithelium. *B:* Transitional epithelium. *C:* Ciliated pseudostratified epithelium. The goblet cells secrete mucus that forms a continuous mucous layer over the ciliary layer.

Simple epithelium can, according to cell shape, be **squamous, cuboidal,** or **columnar.** The endothelium lining blood vessels and the mesothelium lining certain body cavities are examples of simple squamous epithelium (Fig 4–15A). Although endothelial and mesothelial cells present the same appearance in the light microscope, they should not be considered as one cell type differently localized. It is known that they differ not only in their embryologic origin and ultrastructural morphology but also in their pathologic responses. Thus, they react differently to several types of insults and even produce different types of tumors. An example of cuboidal epithelium is the surface epithelium of the ovary (Fig 4–15B), and an example of columnar epithelium is the lining of the small intestine (Fig 4–1A).

Stratified epithelium is classified according to the cell shape of its superficial layer. These include **squamous, cuboidal, columnar,** and **transitional** epithelium. Pseudostratified epithelium forms a separate group.

Stratified squamous keratinized epithelium is found mainly in the skin. Its cells form many layers; the cells closer to the underlying tissue are usually cuboidal or columnar. Toward the surface, the cells become irregular in shape and flatten progressively as they get closer to the surface, where they are thin and squamous (Fig 4–16A). (For details, see Chapter 19.)

Stratified squamous nonkeratinized epithelium lines wet cavities (eg, mouth, esophagus, vagina), in contrast to the skin, whose surface is dry. Stratified squamous nonkeratinized epithelium is characterized by a flattened layer of cells at the surface that retain their nuclei and are living cells. This is not the case in the keratinized variety of this epithelium, where the surface cells are dead and their nuclei are not discernible.

Stratified columnar epithelium is rare; it is present in the human body only in small areas such as the ocular conjunctiva and the ducts of large glands.

Transitional epithelium, which lines the urinary bladder, the ureter, and the upper part of the urethra, is characterized by the presence on its surface of dome-like cells that are neither squamous nor columnar (Fig 4–16B). The form of these cells changes according to the degree of distention of the bladder. It is not unusual for these cells to be binucleate. This type of epithelium is discussed in detail in Chapter 20.

Pseudostratified epithelium is so called because, although nuclei appear to lie in various layers, all cells are attached to the basal lamina, but some do not reach the surface. The best-known example of this tissue is the ciliated pseudostratified columnar epithelium present in the respiratory passages (Fig 4–16C).

Two other types of epithelium warrant brief mention. **Neuroepithelial cells** are cells of epithelial origin with specialized sensory functions (eg, cells of taste buds). **Myoepithelial cells** specialize in contraction (eg, in the sweat, mammary, and salivary glands).

Glandular Epithelia

Glandular epithelial tissues are those formed by cells specialized in producing a fluid secretion that differs in composition from blood or intercellular fluid. This process is usually accompanied by the intracellular synthesis of macromolecules. These compounds are generally stored in the cells in small membrane-bound vesicles called secretory granules.

The chemical nature of these macromolecules is variable. Glandular epithelial cells may synthesize, store, and secrete proteins (eg, pancreas), lipids (eg, adrenal and sebaceous glands), or complexes of carbohydrate and proteins (eg, salivary glands). In the mammary glands, all 3 substances—proteins, lipids, and carbohydrates—are secreted. Less common are the cells of glands which have low synthetic activity (eg, sweat glands) and in which secretion is mostly composed of substances transferred from the blood to the lumen of the gland.

In some cases, a gland may contain active synthesizing cells in association with cells specializing in ion transport. This occurs in most major mammalian salivary glands where secretory acini coexist with ion-transporting structures called **striated ducts** (see Chapter 17).

All gland cells produce and expel to an extracellular compartment products that are not used by the cell itself but are of importance to other parts of the organism.

Types of Glandular Epithelia

The epithelia that form the glands of the body can be classified according to various criteria; eg, unicellular glands consist of isolated glandular cells, and multicellular glands are composed of clusters of cells. An example of a unicellular gland is the goblet cell of the lining of the small intestine or of the respiratory tract. However, most glands are multicellular.

Glands always derive from covering epithelia by means of cell proliferation and invasion of subjacent connective tissue, subsequently followed by further differentiation. Fig 4–17 shows how this occurs. **Exocrine glands** are glands that retain their connection with the surface epithelium from which they originated. This connection takes the form of tubular ducts lined with epithelial cells through which the glandular secretions pass to reach the surface. **Endocrine glands** are glands whose connection with the surface from which they originated was obliterated during development. These glands are therefore ductless, and their secretions are picked up and transported to their site of action by the bloodstream rather than by a duct system.

Two types of endocrine glands can be differentiated according to cell grouping. In the first type, the agglomerated cells form anastomosing cords interspersed between dilated blood capillaries (eg, adrenal gland, parathyroid, anterior lobe of the pituitary) (Fig 4–17). In the second **(follicular)** type, the cells line a vesicle or follicle filled with noncellular material (eg, the thyroid gland) (Fig 4–17).

Exocrine glands have a **secretory portion,** which contains the cells responsible for the secretory process; and the **ducts,** which transport the secretion to the exterior of the gland (Fig 4–17). **Simple glands** have only one unbranched duct. **Compound glands** have ducts that branch repeatedly. The cellular organization within the secretory portion of the gland further classifies the glands. The simple glands can be tubular, coiled tubular, branched tubular, or acinar. The compound glands can be tubular, acinar, or tubuloacinar. Fig 4–18 illustrates these types of glands schematically. Some organs have both endocrine and exocrine functions, and one cell type may function both ways—eg, in the liver, where cells that secrete bile into the duct system also secrete some of their products into the bloodstream. In other organs, some cells are specialized in exocrine secretion whereas others are concerned exclusively with endocrine secretion, eg, in the pancreas, where the acinar cells secrete digestive enzymes into the intestinal lumen while the islet cells secrete insulin and glucagon into the blood.

According to the way the secretory products leave the cell, glands may be classified as **merocrine** or **holocrine.** In merocrine glands (eg, in the pancreas), the secretory granules leave the cell by exocytosis with no loss of other cellular material. In holocrine glands (eg, sebaceous glands), the product of secretion is shed with the whole cell—a process that involves destruction of the secretion-filled cells. In an intermediate type—the **apocrine** gland—the secretory product is discharged together with parts of the apical cytoplasm. This type of secretion is observed in mammary glands.

Multicellular glands are not merely collections of cells but complete organs with a definite and orderly architecture. They usually have a surrounding capsule of connective tissue and septa that divide the gland into lobules. These lobules then subdivide, and in this

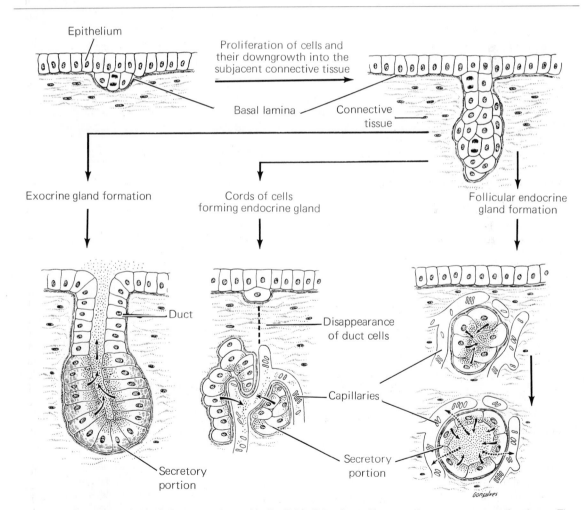

Figure 4–17. Formation of glands from covering epithelia. Epithelial cells proliferate and penetrate connective tissue. They may or may not maintain contact with the surface. When contact is maintained, exocrine glands are formed; when contact is not maintained, endocrine glands are formed. The cells of these glands can be arranged in cords or follicles. The lumens of follicles accumulate large quantities of secretion; cells of the cords store only small quantities in their cytoplasm. (Redrawn and reproduced, with permission, from Ham AW: *Histology,* 6th ed. Lippincott, 1969.)

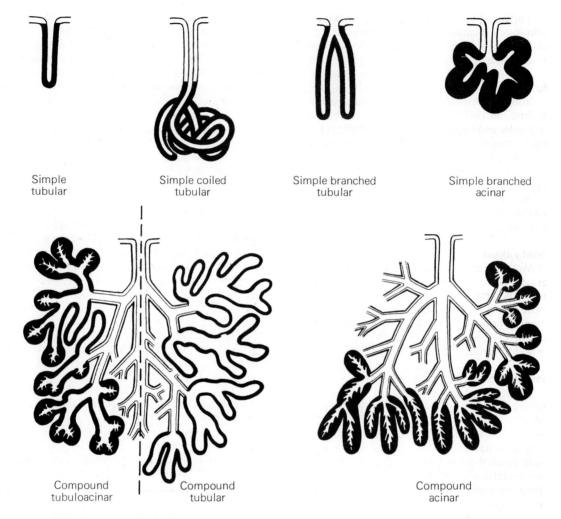

Simple tubular

Simple coiled tubular

Simple branched tubular

Simple branched acinar

Compound tubuloacinar

Compound tubular

Compound acinar

Figure 4–18. Principal types of exocrine glands. The part of the gland formed by secretory cells is shown in black; the remainder shows the ducts. The compound glands have ramified ducts.

way the connective tissue separates and binds together the glandular components. Blood vessels and nerves also penetrate and subdivide in the gland.

GENERAL BIOLOGY OF EPITHELIAL TISSUES

Underlying covering epithelial tissues is a layer of connective tissue called **lamina propria,** which is bound to the epithelium by the basal lamina. The lamina propria not only serves to support the epithelium but also binds it to neighboring structures. The contact between epithelium and lamina propria is increased by irregularities in the surface in the form of evaginations called **papillae.** These occur most frequently in epithelial tissues subject to stress, such as the skin and the tongue.

Polarity

An important feature of epithelia is their polarity; ie, they have a free, or apical, surface and a basal surface resting on a basal lamina. Since blood vessels do not normally penetrate an epithelium, all nutrients must pass out of capillaries in the underlying lamina propria. These nutrients and precursors of products of the epithelial cells then diffuse across the basal lamina and are taken up through the basolateral surface of the epithelial cell, usually by an energy-dependent process. Receptors for chemical messengers that influence the activity of epithelial cells (hormones, neurotransmitters) are localized in the basolateral membranes. In absorptive epithelial cells, the apical cell membrane contains, as integral membrane proteins, enzymes such as disaccharidases and peptidases, which complete the digestion of molecules to be absorbed. It is thought that tight junctions help prevent the intermingling of the integral membrane proteins of the various cell membrane regions, which might be expected to occur based on a simplified view of the fluid mosaic model of membrane structure.

Nutrition

Normally, blood vessels do not penetrate the epithelium, so that there is no direct contact between these cells and blood vessels. Epithelial nutrition depends, therefore, on the diffusion of metabolites through the basal lamina and, frequently, through parts of the lamina propria as well. The diffusion process is probably enhanced by the papillae, which increase the area of contact between epithelium and lamina propria, and it probably limits the thickness of the epithelium.

Innervation

Most epithelial tissues receive a rich supply of sensory nerve endings from nerve plexuses in the lamina propria. Everyone is aware of the exquisite sensitivity of the cornea, the epithelium covering the anterior surface of the eye. This is due to the great number of sensory nerve fibers that ramify between corneal epithelial cells.

Renewal of Epithelial Cells

Epithelial tissues are labile structures whose cells are renewed continuously by means of mitotic activity. This renewal rate is variable. It can be fast in such tissues as the intestinal epithelium, which is replaced every 2–5 days; or slow, as in the pancreas, where tissue renewal takes about 50 days. In stratified and pseudostratified epithelial tissues, mitosis occurs within the germinal layer, those cells closest to the basal lamina.

Metaplasia

Under certain physiologic or pathologic conditions, one type of epithelial tissue may undergo transformation into another epithelial type. This process is called metaplasia. It is reversible, and the following examples illustrate this process. (1) In heavy cigarette smokers, the pseudostratified epithelium lining the bronchi can be transformed into stratified squamous epithelium. (2) In individuals with chronic vitamin A deficiency, epithelial tissues of the type found in the bronchi and urinary bladder are gradually replaced by stratified squamous epithelium. Metaplasia is not restricted to epithelial tissue; it may also occur in connective tissue.

Control of Glandular Activity

The activity of a gland depends on 2 types of mechanisms: The first is genetic and depends on the expression of one or more genes that provide for the synthesis and secretion of specific compounds or products. During the differentiation of a glandular cell, the selection and expression of the genes that control secretion is determined.

The second type of mechanism is related to exogenous or environmental controls. The nervous and endocrine systems are the main participants in its control. Most glands are sensitive to both nervous and endocrine control, but one is frequently more important than the other. Thus, exocrine secretion in the pancreas depends mainly on stimulation by the hormones secretin and cholecystokinin. The salivary glands, on the other hand, are essentially under nervous control.

The nervous and endocrine control of glands occurs through the action of chemical substances called **chemical messengers.** Neurotransmitters are those messengers produced by nerve cells, while hormones are the controlling factors produced by endocrine glands.

Chemical messengers may act by either of 2 mechanisms. In the first case, the messenger enters the cell, reacts with intracellular receptors, and activates one or more genes, initiating the production of specific

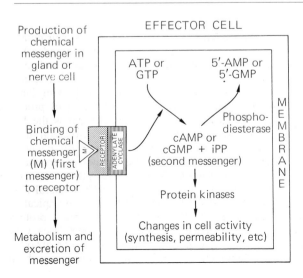

Figure 4–19 (at left). cAMP or cGMP is produced from ATP or GTP, respectively, owing to the activation of adenylate cyclase by the first messenger. Adenylate cyclase is located in the cell membrane, and a specific first messenger receptor is associated with this enzyme. These second messengers are produced inside the cell, while the first messenger remains outside. The actions of many neurotransmitters and hormones are mediated by cAMP or cGMP. The specificity of the first messengers on different cell types depends on the presence of specific receptors associated with adenylate cyclase. cGMP is usually found in lower concentrations than cAMP, but it also mediates a variety of cellular activities. In some cells, both cAMP and cGMP are known to interact, one stimulating and the other inhibiting a specific cellular activity. (Based on Sutherland EW: Studies on the mechanism of hormone action. *Science* 1972;**177**:401. Copyright © 1972 by the American Association for the Advancement of Science.)

proteins. Some steroid hormones, which are capable of easily crossing the cell membrane owing to their lipid structure, exhibit this type of action. The antibiotic dactinomycin blocks the synthesis of messenger RNA and is known to inhibit this type of messenger activity.

A second mechanism is related to the interaction of a chemical messenger with a receptor located in the outer surface of the cell membrane. This chemical substance, referred to as the **first messenger,** acts by inducing the synthesis of yet another messenger, called the **second messenger,** that initiates a series of events which ultimately promotes a specific cell activity. Fig 4–19 summarizes this concept. Protein or polypeptide hormones and neurotransmitters that do not readily cross the cell membrane are known to act via this second messenger mechanism.

BIOLOGY OF THE MAIN TYPES OF EPITHELIAL CELLS

As cells differentiate, they gradually acquire morphologic and physiologic characteristics related to the various functions they assume. Since these differentiated cells frequently have the same functions in different tissues and organs, descriptions of the basic epithelial cell types will be given.

Cells That Transport Ions

All cells have the ability to transport certain ions against a concentration and electrical potential gradient, utilizing ATP as an energy source. This is called **active transport** to distinguish it from passive diffusion down a concentration gradient. In mammals, the sodium ion (Na^+) concentration in the extracellular fluid is 140 mmol/L, while the intracellular concentration is 5–15 mmol/L. In addition, the interior of

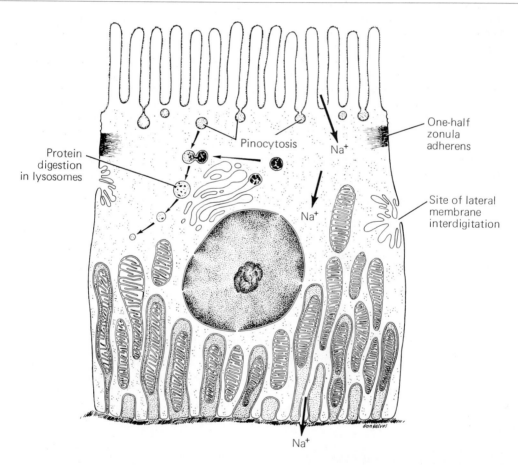

Figure 4–20. Ultrastructure of a proximal convoluted tubule cell of the kidney. Invagination of the basal cell membrane outlines regions filled with elongated mitochondria. This typical disposition is present in ion-transporting cells. Interdigitations from neighboring cells (stippled structures) interlock with those of this cell. Protein absorbed by pinocytosis and being digested by lysosomes is shown in the upper left portion of the diagram. Sodium ions diffuse passively through the apical membranes of renal epithelial cells. These ions are then actively transported out of the cells by Na^+/K^+-ATPase located in the basolateral membranes of the cells. Energy for this sodium "pump" is supplied by nearby mitochondria. This is an example of a cell with more than one function, since it transports ions in addition to providing for protein digestion.

the cells is electrically negative with respect to the extracellular environment. Under these conditions, the positively charged sodium ion would tend to diffuse down both an electrical and a concentration gradient. The cell uses the energy stored in ATP to actively extrude Na^+ by means of an Mg^{2+}-activated Na^+/K^+-ATPase (sodium pump), thereby maintaining the required low intracellular sodium concentration.

Some epithelial cells (eg, proximal and distal renal tubules, striated ducts of salivary glands) exploit this mechanism to transfer sodium across the epithelium, from the apex to the base—**transcellular transport.** The apical surface of the proximal renal tubule cell is freely permeable to Na^+. To maintain electrical and osmotic balance, equimolar amounts of Cl^- and water follow the Na^+ ion into the cell. The basal surfaces of these cells are elaborately folded; many long invaginations of the basal plasma membrane are seen in electron micrographs (Figs 4–20 and 20–14). In addition, there is elaborate interdigitation of basal processes between adjacent cells. It has been shown that Mg^{2+}-activated Na^+/K^+-ATPase (sodium pump) is preferentially localized in these invaginations of the basal plasma membrane but is also present in the lateral membranes. Located between the invaginations are vertically oriented mitochondria that supply the energy (ATP) for the active extrusion of Na^+ from the base of the cell. Chloride and water again follow passively. Thus, sodium is returned to the circulation and not lost in massive amounts in the urine.

Tight junctions play an important role in this process. Because of their relative impermeability to ions, water, and larger molecules, they prevent back-diffusion of materials already transported across the epithelium. Otherwise, a great deal of energy would be wasted.

Ion transport and the consequent flow of fluid may occur in opposite directions (ie, apical → basal, basal → apical) in different epithelial tissues. In the intestine, proximal convoluted tubules of the kidney, striated ducts of the salivary glands, gallbladder, etc, the flow is from the apex of the cell to its basal region. Flow is in the opposite direction in other epithelial sheets such as in the choroid plexus and ciliary body (Fig 4–21). In both cases, the tight junctions seal the apical portions of the cells and provide for inner and outer tissue compartments.

Cells That Transport by Pinocytosis

In various cells of the body, pinocytotic vesicles that form abundantly on plasmalemma surfaces permit the transport of macromolecules across the plasma membrane. This activity is clearly observed in the simple squamous epithelium lining the blood vessels (endothelia) or the body cavities (mesothelia). These cells have few organelles other than the abundant pinocytotic vesicles found on the cell surfaces and in the cytoplasm (Fig 4–22). These observations, in conjunction with results obtained by injection of electron-dense colloidal particles (eg, ferritin, colloidal gold, thorium) followed by observation with the electron microscope, indicate that the vesicles transporting the injected materials flow in both directions through the cells (Fig 4–22).

Calculations based on these studies suggest that a pinocytotic vesicle can cross these cells in 2–3 min-

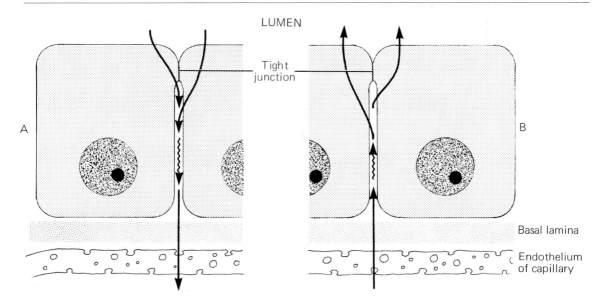

Figure 4–21. Ion and fluid transport can occur in different directions depending on which tissue is involved. *A:* The direction of transport is from the lumen to the blood vessel, as occurs in the gallbladder and intestine. This process is called absorption. *B:* Transport is in the opposite direction, as occurs in the choroid plexus, ciliary body, and sweat gland. This process is called secretion. Note the use of the intercellular space in the transport process and that the presence of occluding junctions is necessary to maintain compartmentalization and consequently control over ion distribution.

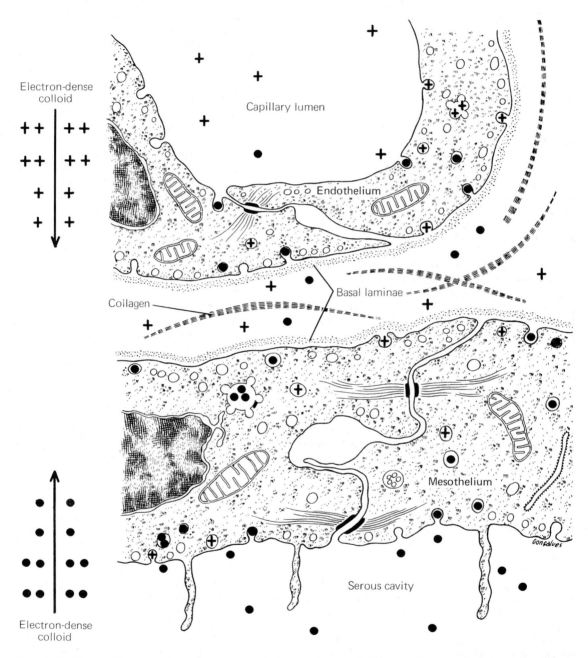

Electron-dense colloid

Capillary lumen

Endothelium

Basal laminae

Collagen

Mesothelium

Serous cavity

Electron-dense colloid

Gonçalves

Figure 4–22. Diagram illustrating how the transport of electron-dense colloids through the mesothelial and endothelial cells was studied. Simultaneous injections of colloids that differ morphologically were made, one intravenously and the other in a serous cavity (eg, the mesentery or pericardial cavity) lined by the cells. After short periods of time (minutes), fragments of the serous membranes were fixed and studied in the electron microscope. It was observed that the transport of colloid occurred in both directions. These particles are engulfed by pinocytosis and are transported across the cells in vesicles. (Redrawn and reproduced, with permission, from Staubesand J: Zur Histophysiologie des Herzbeutels. *Z Zellforsch Mikrosk Anat* 1963;**58**:915.)

utes. Since the frequency of vesicle formation and vesicle volume can be measured, it has been possible to calculate the quantity of the transferred fluid through the walls of capillaries. In the case of muscle tissue, the amount transported has been estimated to be 2 – 3 mL/h/kg of tissue.

Chemical Messenger–Producing Cells

The vertebrate body has many cell types whose main function is the production of messenger substances of a varied chemical nature that may influence the activities of other cells. These cells can be classified in 3 groups according to the mode of delivery of the messenger:

(1) Neurocrine cells release chemical messages at interfaces where cytoplasmic extensions of the messenger cell approach the surface of the target cells. Neurons are an example of this type of messenger-producing cell, and the site where its extension makes contact with the effector cell is called a **synapse** (see Chapter 9).

(2) Paracrine cells secrete a message that diffuses into the surrounding extracellular fluid and acts upon neighboring target cells. The mast cell, an example of this type of messenger-producing cell, secretes histamine that acts upon nearby capillary endothelial cells (see Chapter 12).

(3) Endocrine cells secrete their messenger substances into the blood, which carries them directly to the target cells. Most endocrine cells produce steroid or protein messenger compounds. However, some endocrine cells produce biologically active amines.

Chemical messenger–producing cells are derived from each of the 3 embryologic germ layers and subsequently reside in a variety of tissues within the body. For example, neurocrine cells derive from ectoderm; mast cells derive from mesoderm; and thyroid follicular cells, which produce thyroid hormone, derive from endoderm.

Protein-Synthesizing Cells

All cells continuously synthesize small amounts of protein in order to replace cytoplasmic subunits utilized or lost through the normal turnover of cellular components. Some cells, however, synthesize large amounts of protein as a consequence of their differentiated function. These cells can be divided into 2 classes based on the final distribution of their protein products. In one group, where the protein remains free within the cytoplasm, protein synthesis primarily occurs on free or unbound polyribosomes. Examples of cells within this group include embryonic cells and erythroblasts (Fig 14 – 6).

In the second group, synthesized proteins are segregated from other cytoplasmic components as a result of their injection into the rough endoplasmic reticulum. This group can be further subdivided in regard to whether the synthesized proteins are accumulated within or exported from the cell. Some leukocytes (eg, neutrophils and eosinophils) and macrophages synthesize lytic enzymes stored in membrane-bound

granules that are usually retained within the cytoplasm and subsequently utilized for intracellular digestion (see Chapter 5 and Fig 5 – 16). However, many protein synthesizers segregate their protein products and eventually release them into the extracellular space in a process called **secretion.** Examples of protein secretors include fibroblasts, plasma cells, and pancreatic acinar cells. Within these cells, proteins are synthesized on membrane-bound polyribosomes, and the newly synthesized polypeptides are injected directly into cisternae of the rough endoplasmic reticulum.

Some cells **synthesize, segregate,** and **release** proteins without first accumulating them within the cytoplasm. In such cells (eg, the **plasma cell** [Fig 5 – 23]), proteins are transferred from the endoplasmic reticulum to the Golgi complex. Small vesicles bud off the Golgi complex, migrate to the cell surface, and release their contents by exocytosis.

In other cell types, proteins are **synthesized, segregated,** and **accumulated** in the apex of the cell, and then they are **released** in response to specific stimuli. The acinar cells of the pancreas and parotid glands are typical examples of this cell type. They are polyhedral or pyramidal, with central, rounded nuclei and well-defined polarity. In the basal infranuclear region, these cells exhibit an intense basophilia, which results from local accumulation of rough endoplasmic reticulum in the form of parallel arrays of flattened cisternae studded with abundant ribosomes (Fig 4 – 23).

Filamentous mitochondria are frequently interspersed among endoplasmic reticulum cisternae. The position of the nucleus and the presence of an evident basal basophilic region in these cells are characteristics of protein-synthesizing cells and are criteria used to distinguish them from cells secreting mucus.

In the apical region just above the nucleus lies a well-developed Golgi complex. The rest of the cytoplasm is filled with rounded, protein-rich, membrane-bound **secretory granules.** In cells that produce digestive enzymes (eg, pancreatic acinar cells), these structures containing enzymes are called **zymogen granules** (Figs 4 – 23 and 4 – 24).

Enough evidence has been presented from biochemical and cytologic studies to define the secretory process in these cells as follows (see also Chapter 3):

(1) Amino acids from the bloodstream pass through the capillary walls and their basal lamina, through the secretory cell basal lamina and plasma membrane, and into the cytoplasm. The entry of amino acids through the membrane is greatly accelerated by an active transport mechanism.

(2) Within the cell, the amino acids become associated with transfer RNA (tRNA). Free ribosomes associated with a strand of messenger RNA (mRNA) initiate protein synthesis by utilizing the tRNA-associated amino acids to translate the message encoded in the mRNA. The mRNA code for segregated proteins includes a code for an additional N-terminal sequence of hydrophobic amino acids called a **signal peptide.** As the newly assembled peptide extends from

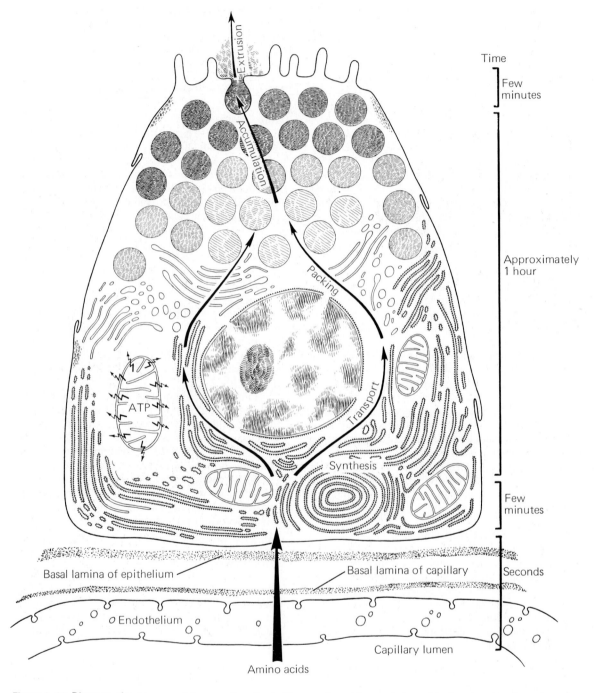

Figure 4–23. Diagram of a serous cell (pancreatic acinar). Observe its evident polarity, with abundant basal rough endoplasmic reticulum (ergastoplasm). The Golgi complex and secretory granules are in the supranuclear region. The secretory process is described in the text. To the right is a time scale indicating the approximate amount of time necessary for each step.

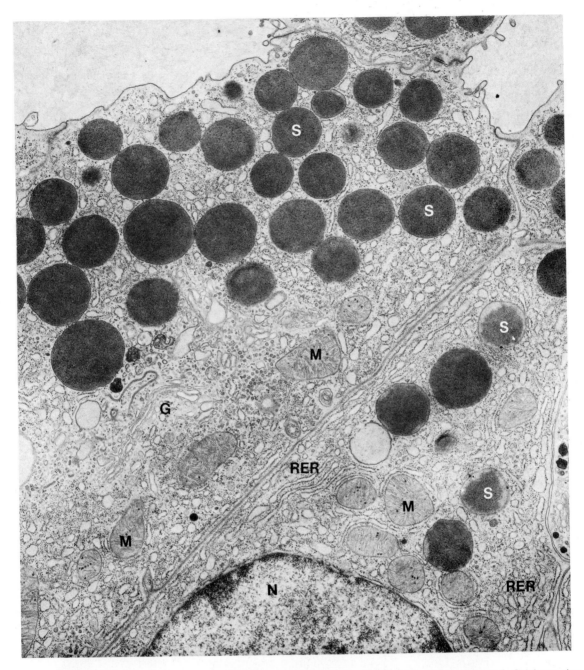

Figure 4–24. Electron micrograph of 2 frog pancreatic cells. Observe the nucleus (N), mitochondria (M), Golgi complex (G), secretory granules (S) in various stages of condensation, and rough endoplasmic reticulum (RER). × 13,000. (Courtesy of KR Porter.)

the central core of the ribosome (Fig 3–7), the hydrophobic signal peptide penetrates the endoplasmic reticulum membrane. As the protein chain is assembled and injected into the endoplasmic reticulum cisterna, additional ribosomes are simultaneously attached to both the mRNA and the endoplasmic reticulum membrane, which results in the formation of a membrane-bound polyribosome. The hydrophobic signal peptide is enzymatically clipped off after the assembled protein enters the endoplasmic reticulum cisterna. At this stage, the proteins are segregated within an extracytoplasmic space—the interior of the rough endoplasmic reticulum cisternae. This separation is significant in that it avoids direct contact of the secretory product, often digestive enzymes (eg, ribonuclease and protease), with cytoplasmic components.

(3) The proteins thus segregated are transported from the endoplasmic reticulum to the Golgi complex. The mechanism by which they reach the interior of the Golgi cisternae is still in question, but evidence shows that in several cell types this occurs by formation of small, protein-containing **transfer,** or **shuttle, vesicles** that bud from the endoplasmic reticulum, migrate to, and fuse with the convex surface of Golgi cisternae.

(4) This material is then accumulated in the Golgi cisternae. On the mature (concave) face of the Golgi, bulges form along the surface and lateral margins of the innermost cisterna. These bulges pinch off to form large membrane-bound **condensing vacuoles** or immature secretory granules (Fig 4–25).

(5) The newly formed granules in turn migrate to the cell apex and in doing so become more dense as water is removed from the protein. These have been designated **mature granules,** in contrast to the less dense, recently formed granules. Granules accumulate until they are mobilized. Accumulation occurs for periods of time that vary with the type of gland and its activity.

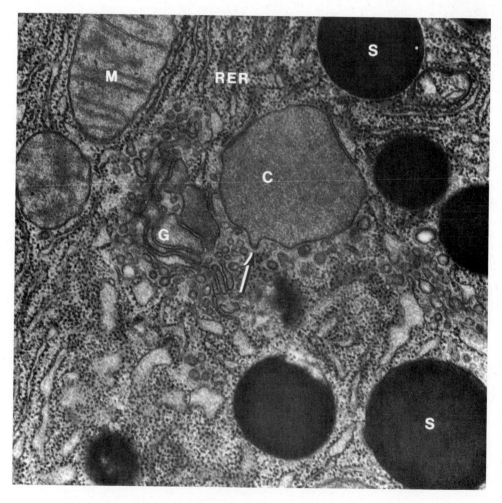

Figure 4–25. Electron micrograph of a part of a rat pancreatic acinar cell showing a condensing vacuole (C), which is presumed to be receiving a small quantity of secretory product (arrow) from the Golgi complex (G). M, mitochondrion; RER, rough endoplasmic reticulum; S, mature secretory (zymogen) granule. × 40,000.

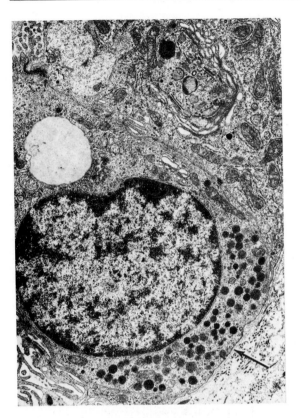

Figure 4–26. Electron micrograph of a somatostatin D cell from human gastrointestinal tract. Note the accumulation of secretory granules in the basal region of the cell. The arrow indicates the basal lamina. × 13,500. (Courtesy of AGE Pearse.)

(6) When the cells release their secretory products, the membranes of the secretory granules fuse to the cell membrane and the granule contents spill out of the cell in a process called **exocytosis.** The energy for these processes is known to be furnished by oxidative phosphorylation at the mitochondrial level.

Polypeptide-Secreting Cells

It is now well established that a class of cells having the capacity to synthesize and release low-molecular-weight polypeptides or proteins with hormonal activity also have some morphologic and histochemical characteristics in common. These cells are found in epithelia of the gastrointestinal and respiratory tracts and in the pancreas and thyroid gland. They have the ability to concentrate in their cytoplasm either ready-made biogenic amines, such as epinephrine, norepinephrine, or 5-hydroxytryptamine (serotonin), or precursors from which they can synthesize these amines. They also possess a high level of amino acid decarboxylase activity—an enzyme necessary for the synthesis of biogenic amines. These characteristics explain the designation **APUD** (*a*mine *p*recursor *up*take and *d*ecarboxylation) given to these cells. Some APUD cells also stain with silver salts, which resulted in the older terms ''argentaffin'' or ''argyrophil'' cells.

APUD cells fall into 2 broad classes: (1) the **open** type, in which the apex of the cell, with a few microvilli, contacts the lumen of the organ, and (2) the **closed** type, in which the apex is covered by epithelial cells characteristic of the organ where the APUD cell is found. APUD cells generally have small amounts of rough endoplasmic reticulum, a supranuclear Golgi complex, and numerous membrane-limited secretory granules near the basal pole of the cell (Fig 4–26). The granules are of distinctive size (100–400 nm in diameter), shape, and electron density in each of the 20 or more types of APUD cells now recognized.

Some APUD cells release their secretory product into blood or lymphatic vessels, and this product (**hormone**) is carried to a distant site where the hormone has its **endocrine** effect. The secretory products of other APUD cells regulate the functions of adjacent cells without having to pass through the vascular system, an effect termed **paracrine.**

The embryologic origin of APUD cells is the subject of continuing controversy. One view is that all APUD cells are derived from the neural crest. The experimental evidence obtained so far indicates that only a few APUD cells have this origin. APUD cells of the gastrointestinal tract appear to arise in situ from endodermal cells.

The characterization of polypeptides or proteins produced by these cells has been achieved mainly by the immunocytochemical methods described in Chapter 2. Using these methods, it has been possible to localize several types of APUD cells in humans (Table 4–2). The morphology and histochemistry of these cells vary with the species studied. At present, several polypeptides with biologic activity whose corresponding APUD cells have not thus far been located, as well as several cells with APUD morphology but of undetermined function, are known to exist.

Several tumors derived from APUD cells have been described. Tumors of the non-B islet cells of the pancreas that produce gastrin are responsible for Zollinger-Ellison syndrome; another example is the calcitonin-producing tumor of the thyroid. These tumors are called **apudomas.**

Table 4–2. Some of the better known APUD cells present in humans.

Cell Name	Location*	Polypeptide Produced
A	P	Glucagon
B	P	Insulin
C	T	Calcitonin
D	S, SI, P	Somatostatin
D1	S, SI, LI, P	Vasoactive intestinal polypeptide
EC	S, SI, LI, P	Motilin, Substance P
G	S, SI, P	Gastrin
I	SI	Cholecystokinin
K	SI	Gastric inhibitory polypeptide
N	SI	Neurotensin
S	SI	Secretin

*P, pancreas; S, stomach; SI, small intestine; LI, large intestine; T, thyroid.

Mucus-Secreting Cells

The most thoroughly studied example of a mucus-secreting cell is the **goblet cell** of the intestines. This cell is characterized by the presence of numerous large, lightly staining granules containing glycoproteins called **mucins** or **mucinogens.** Secretory granules fill the extensive apical pole of the cell. The nucleus is usually flattened vertically and is localized in the cell base. This region is rich in rough endoplasmic reticulum (Figs 4–27 and 4–28). The Golgi complex, located just above the nucleus, is exceptionally well developed, indicative of its important function in this cell. Data obtained by radioautography suggest that, in this cell, proteins are synthesized from amino acids

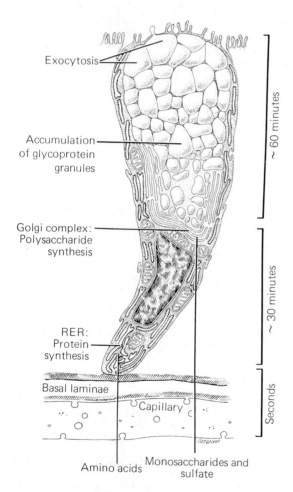

Figure 4–27. Diagram of a mucus-secreting intestinal goblet cell. Its constricted base, where the mitochondria and rough endoplasmic reticulum (RER) are located, is typical. Synthesis of the protein part of the glycoprotein complex occurs in the endoplasmic reticulum. A well-developed Golgi complex is present in the supranuclear region. In cells that secrete sulfated polysaccharides, the process of sulfation occurs in the Golgi complex. (Redrawn after Gordon and reproduced, with permission, from Ham AW: *Histology,* 6th ed. Lippincott, 1969.)

at the level of the rough endoplasmic reticulum present in the cell base. Monosaccharides are added to the core protein by enzymes termed **glycosyltransferases** located in Golgi membranes. The innermost monosaccharide is linked to the hydroxyl group of certain threonine or serine residues of the core protein (O-linked oligosaccharides). This is in contrast to the high-mannose oligosaccharides of other glycoproteins, which are N-linked to asparagine residues of the core protein (see Chapter 3). In cells that produce sulfated glycoproteins, sulfation of sugars also occurs in the Golgi complex.

Although not completely characterized, mucins consist of several glycoprotein subunits, each with a molecular weight of about 500,000 and containing numerous (> 600) complex oligosaccharide chains constituting about 80% of the mass. Each oligosaccharide chain, consisting of up to 20 monosaccharides, can be linear or branched, and sulfated or neutral. The subunits are linked together by disulfide bridges to form macromolecules with molecular weights in excess of 2 million. When mucins are released from the cell, they become highly hydrated and form a viscous, elastic gel now called **mucus.**

The goblet cell of the intestines is only one of several types of cells that synthesize mucin glycoproteins. Others are found in the stomach, salivary glands, respiratory tract, and genital tract. These show great variability in the chemistry of their secretion and have somewhat different morphologic characteristics, as described elsewhere in the text.

Serous & Mucous Cells

Pancreatic acinar cells and goblet cells are typical examples of cells called serous and mucous cells, respectively, because of the molecular nature and consistency of their products of secretion. Mucous cells are characterized by the presence of large, translucent secretory granules that occupy most of the cell and a flattened nucleus containing condensed chromatin at the cell base. Serous cells present a rounded euchromatic nucleus surrounded by rough endoplasmic reticulum in the basal third of the cell, in addition to clearly visible and easily stained secretory granules at the cell apex (Figs 4–29 and 17–1).

Differences between these 2 types of cells are not always clear, and in mammalian organisms various cell types have been described that produce variable proportions of polysaccharides and proteins. This occurs, for example, in the parotid and submandibular salivary glands. Close analysis of these cell types shows that there is an almost continuous gradient from serous to mucous cells, which consequently makes it impossible to classify certain cell types as either mucous or serous. In doubtful instances, an intermediate classification of **seromucous cells** has been proposed.

Myoepithelial Cells

Several glands (eg, sweat, lacrimal, salivary, and mammary glands) contain stellate or spindle-shaped myoepithelial cells. These cells embrace gland acini

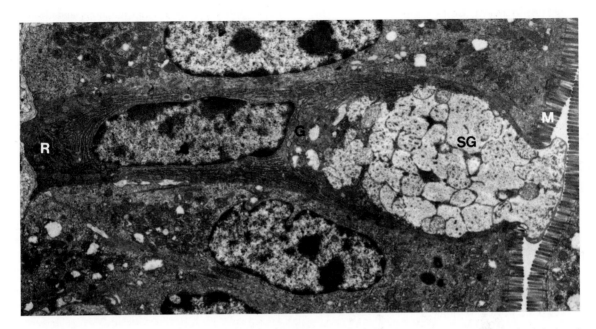

Figure 4–28. Electron micrograph of a typical goblet cell from the small intestine. The rough endoplasmic reticulum is present mainly in the basal portion of the cell (R), while the cell apex is filled with dense secretory granules (SG). The Golgi complex (G) lies just above the nucleus. Typical columnar absorptive cells with microvillar borders (M) lie adjacent to the goblet cell. × 7000. (Reproduced, with permission, from Junqueira LCU, Salles LMM: *Ultra-Estrutura e Função Celular*. Edgard Blücher, 1975).

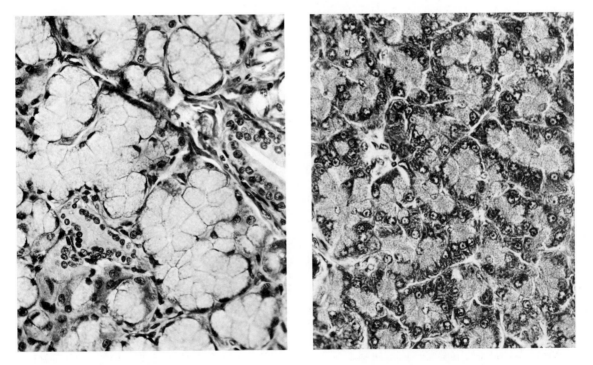

Figure 4–29. Two photomicrographs illustrating the differences between mucous cells (sublingual gland), *left,* and serous cells (pancreas), *right.* × 300.

as an octopus might embrace a rounded boulder. They are more longitudinally arranged along ducts. Myoepithelial cells are located between the basal lamina and the basal pole of secretory or ductal cells. The nucleus is usually located in the region where the lateral surfaces of 2 overlying epithelial cells meet. Myoepithelial cells are connected to each other and to the epithelial cells by gap junctions and desmosomes. The cytoplasm contains numerous microfilaments (actin), as well as tropomyosin and myosin. Myoepithelial cells also contain intermediate filaments (7–11 nm in diameter) belonging to the cytokeratin (prekeratin) family, thus confirming their epithelial origin. The function of myoepithelial cells

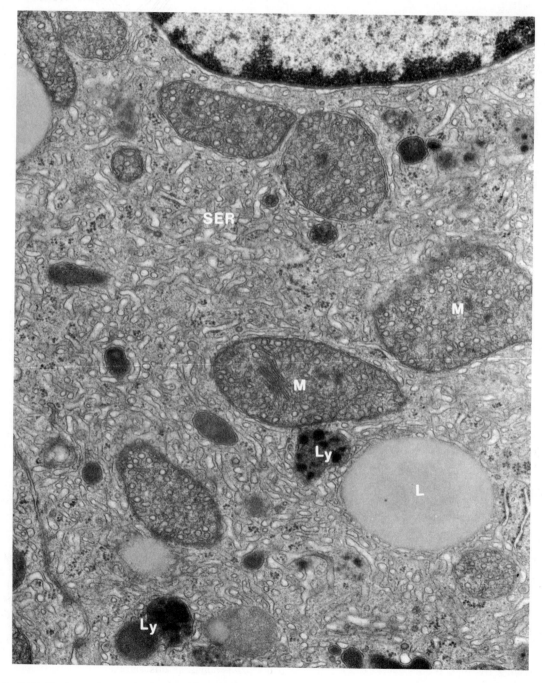

Figure 4–30. Electron micrograph of a steroid-producing cell from the human adrenal cortex. Note the mitochondria (M) with tubular cristae, the lipid droplets (L), the abundant smooth endoplasmic reticulum (SER), and the lysosomes (Ly). × 25,400.

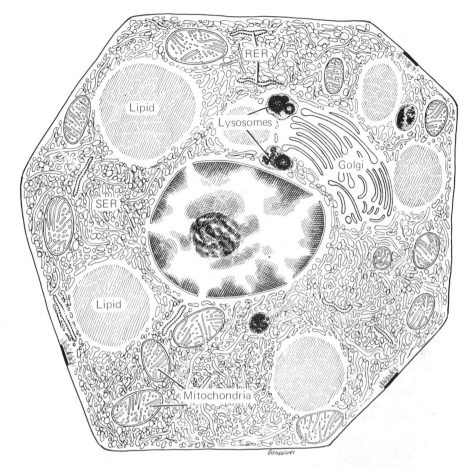

Figure 4–31. Diagram of the ultrastructure of a hypothetic steroid-secreting cell. Observe the abundance of the smooth endoplasmic reticulum (SER), lipid droplets, Golgi complex, and lysosomes. The numerous mitochondria have tubular cristae. They not only produce the energy necessary for activity of the cell but are also involved in steroid hormone synthesis. RER, rough endoplasmic reticulum.

is to contract around the secretory or conducting portion of the gland, thus helping to propel secretory products toward the exterior.

Steroid-Secreting Cells

Cells secreting steroids are found in various organs of the body (eg, testes, ovaries, adrenals). They are endocrine cells specialized for synthesizing and secreting steroids with hormonal activity. They have the following characteristics (Figs 4–30 and 4–31):

(1) They are polyhedral or rounded acidophilic cells with a central nucleus and a cytoplasm that is usually but not invariably rich in lipid droplets.

(2) The cytoplasm of steroid-secreting cells contains an exceptionally rich smooth endoplasmic reticulum, which takes the form of anastomosing tubules. Smooth endoplasmic reticulum contains the necessary enzymes to synthesize cholesterol from acetate and other substrates and to transform the pregnenolone produced in the mitochondria into androgens, estrogens, and progestogens.

(3) The spherical or elongated mitochondria that are present usually contain tubular rather than lamellar or shelflike cristae, which are common in mitochondria of other epithelial cells. Besides being the main site of energy production for cell function, these organelles have the necessary enzymatic equipment not only to cleave the cholesterol side chain and produce pregnenolone but also to participate in subsequent reactions that result in steroid hormones. The process of steroid synthesis results, therefore, from close collaboration between smooth endoplasmic reticulum and mitochondria, a striking example of cooperation between intracellular organelles. It also explains the close proximity observed between these 2 organelles in steroid-secreting cells.

REFERENCES

Alberts B et al: *Molecular Biology of the Cell*. Garland, 1983.

Bennett G, Leblond CP, Haddad A: Migration of glycoproteins from the Golgi apparatus to the surface of various cell types as shown by radioautography after labelled fucose injection into rats. *J Cell Biol* 1974;**60:**258.

Berridge MJ, Oschman JL: *Transporting Epithelia*. Academic Press, 1972.

Blöbel G: Mechanism for the intracellular compartmentalization of newly synthesized proteins. In: *FEBS Symposium*. Vol 43. Pergamon Press, 1977.

Bretscher MS: Some general principles of membrane structure. Page 17 in: *The Cell Surface in Development*. Moscona AA (editor). Wiley, 1974.

Claude P: Morphological factors influencing transepithelial permeability: A model for the resistance of the zonula occludens. *J Membr Biol* 1978;**39:**219.

Farquhar MG, Palade GE: Junctional complexes in various epithelia. *J Cell Biol* 1963;**17:**375.

Fawcett D: *The Cell,* 2nd ed. Saunders, 1981.

Hall PF: Cellular organization for steroidogenesis. *Int Rev Cytol* 1984;**86:**53.

Hanover JA, Lennarz WJ: Transmembrane assembly of membrane and secretory glycoproteins. *Arch Biochem Biophys* 1981;**211:**1.

Hertzberg EL, Lawrence TS, Gilula NB: Gap junctional communication. *Annu Rev Physiol* 1981;**43:**479.

Hull BE, Staehelin LA: The terminal web: A reevaluation of its structure and function. *J Cell Biol* 1979;**81:**67.

Jamieson JD, Palade GE: Intracellular transport of secretory protein in the pancreatic exocrine cell. 4. Metabolic requirements. *J Cell Biol* 1968;**39:**589.

Junqueira LCU: Control of cell secretion. In: *Secretory Mechanisms of Salivary Glands*. Schneyer LH, Schneyer CA (editors). Academic Press, 1967.

Junqueira LCU, Hirch GC: Cell secretion: A study of pancreas and salivary glands. *Int Rev Cytol* 1956;**5:**323.

Junqueira LCU et al: Evidence for collagen molecular orientation in basement membranes. *Histochem J* 1983;**15:**785.

Kefalides NA: *Biology and Chemistry of Basement Membranes*. Academic Press, 1978.

Krstić RV: *Ultrastructure of the Mammalian Cell*. Springer-Verlag, 1979.

Leader DP: Protein synthesis on membrane-bound ribosomes. *Trans Int Biol Soc* 1979;**4:**205.

Mooseker MS: Actin-binding proteins of the brush border. *Cell* 1983;**35:**11.

Mooseker MS: Organization, chemistry, and assembly of the cytoskeletal apparatus of the intestinal brush border. *Annu Rev Cell Biol* 1985;**1:**209.

Neutra M, Leblond CP: Radioautographic comparison of the uptake of galactose-H^3 and glucose ^3H in the Golgi region of various cells secreting glycoproteins or mucopolysaccharides. *J Cell Biol* 1966;**30:**137.

Pearse AGE: The cytochemistry and ultrastructure of polypeptide hormone-producing cells of the APUD series and the embryologic, physiologic and pathologic implications of the concept. *J Histochem Cytochem* 1969;**17:**303.

Pearse AGE, Polak JM: Endocrine tumours of neural crest origin: Neurolophomas, apudomas and the APUD concept. *Med Biol* 1974;**52:**3.

Rambourg A, Leblond CP: Electron microscope observations on the carbohydrate-rich cell coat present at the surface of cells in the rat. *J Cell Biol* 1967;**32:**27.

Revel JP, Karnovsky MJ: Hexagonal array of subunits in intercellular junctions of the mouse heart and liver. *J Cell Biol* 1967;**33:**C7.

Simons K, Fuller SD: Cell surface polarity in epithelia. *Annu Rev Cell Biol* 1985;**1:**243.

Staehelin LA, Hull B: Junctions between living cells. *Sci Am* (May) 1978;**238:**141.

Connective Tissue

5

The connective tissues are responsible for providing and maintaining form in the body. Functioning in a mechanical role, they provide a matrix that serves to connect and bind the cells and organs and ultimately give support to the body. Unlike the other tissue types (epithelium, muscle, and nerve) formed mainly by cells, the major constituent of connective tissue is its **extracellular matrix,** composed of protein **fibers,** an amorphous **ground substance,** and **tissue fluid,** the latter consisting primarily of bound water of solvation. Embedded within the extracellular matrix are the **connective tissue cells.**

In terms of structural composition, connective tissue can be subdivided into 3 classes of components: **cells, fibers,** and **ground substance.** The wide variety of connective tissue types in the body represents modulations in the degree of expression of these 3 components.

Connective tissue serves a variety of functions. Its most conspicuous function is structural. The capsules that surround the organs of the body and the internal architecture that supports their cells are composed of connective tissue. This tissue also makes up tendons, ligaments, and the areolar tissue that fills the spaces between organs. Bone and cartilage are specialized types of connective tissue that function to support the soft tissues of the body.

The role of connective tissue in defense of the organism is related to its content of phagocytic and immunocompetent cells and also cells that produce pharmacologically active substances important during inflammation. Phagocytic cells engulf inert particles and microorganisms that enter the body. Specific proteins called **antibodies** are produced by plasma cells in the connective tissue. These combine with foreign proteins of bacteria and viruses—or with the toxins produced by bacteria—and combat the biologic activity of these harmful agents. In addition, connective tissue matrix components provide a physical barrier, preventing the dispersion of microorganisms that pass through the epithelia.

The role of connective tissue in nutrition is due to its close association with blood vessels. The connective tissue matrix serves as the medium through which nutrients and metabolic wastes are exchanged between cells and their blood supply.

Most connective tissues develop from the middle layer of the embryo, the **mesoderm.** However, some of the connective tissues of the head derive from the neural crest, a derivative of the ectoderm. Mesodermal cells migrate from their site of origin, surrounding and penetrating developing organs. These cells are called **mesenchymal cells,** and the tissue they form is called **mesenchyme.** Mesenchymal cells are characterized by an oval nucleus with prominent nucleoli and fine chromatin. They have relatively little cytoplasm, which extends as multiple, thin processes away from the nucleus. The space between mesenchymal cells is occupied by a viscous ground substance containing few fibers. In addition to being the point of origin of all types of connective tissue cells, mesenchyme develops into other types of tissues such as blood cells and blood vessels. These structures may be considered very specialized types of connective tissue, but they are traditionally given separate consideration in histology texts.

GROUND SUBSTANCE

The amorphous intercellular ground substance is colorless, transparent, and homogeneous. It fills the space between cells and fibers of the connective tissue; it is viscous and acts as a lubricant and also as a barrier to the penetration of the tissues by foreign particles. Because of its high content of water and amorphous appearance, it is difficult to study in both fresh and fixed material. When fixed, its components aggregate and appear as a granular material in the electron microscope (Fig 5–1). The ground substance is formed mainly by 2 classes of components: **glycosaminoglycans** and **structural glycoproteins.**

Glycosaminoglycans are linear polysaccharides formed by characteristic repeating disaccharide units usually composed of a uronic acid and a hexosamine. The term **acid mucopolysaccharides** was used originally to designate hexosamine-rich acid polysaccharides extracted from connective tissue. In recent years, the term glycosaminoglycans has gained greater acceptance and is now used in place of mucopolysaccharides. The hexosamine can be **glucosamine** or **galactosamine,** and the uronic acid can be **glucuronic** or **iduronic acid.** With the exception of hyaluronic acid, these linear chains are bound covalently to a protein core (Fig 7–4), forming a **proteoglycan molecule.** In cartilage, these proteoglycan molecules have been shown to be bound to a hyaluronic acid chain, forming larger molecules—proteoglycan aggregates. Owing to the abundance of hydroxyl, carboxyl, and sulfate groups in the carbohydrate moiety of most proteoglycans, they are intensely hydrophilic and act as polyanions. Hyaluronic acid is the only nonsulfated

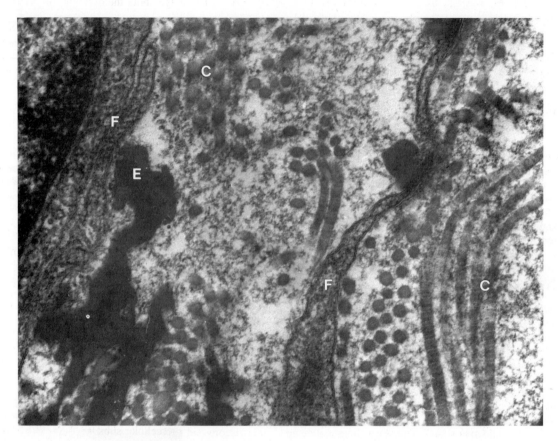

Figure 5–1. Electron micrograph showing the structural organization of the connective tissue matrix. The ground substance constitutes a fine granular material that fills the spaces between the collagen (C) and elastic (E) fibers, as well as surrounding fibroblast cells and processes (F). Ground substance granularity is an artifactual consequence of the glutaraldehyde –tannic acid fixation procedure. × 100,000.

Table 5–1. Composition and distribution of glycosaminoglycans in connective tissue and their interaction with collagen fibers.

| Glycosaminoglycan | Repeating Disaccharides | | Distribution | Electrostatic Interaction With Collagen |
	Hexuronic Acid	Hexosamine		
Hyaluronic acid	D-Glucuronic acid	D-Glucosamine	Umbilical cord, synovial fluid, vitreous humor, cartilage	. . .
Chrondroitin 4-sulfate	D-Glucuronic acid	D-Galactosamine	Cartilage, bone, cornea, skin, notochord, aorta	High levels of interaction, mainly with collagen type II
Chrondroitin 6-sulfate	D-Glucuronic acid	D-Galactosamine	Cartilage, umbilical cord, skin, aorta (media)	High levels of interaction, mainly with collagen type II
Dermatan sulfate	L-Iduronic acid or D-glucuronic acid	D-Galactosamine	Skin, tendon, aorta (adventitia)	Low levels of interaction, mainly with collagen type I
Heparan sulfate	D-Glucuronic acid or L-iduronic acid	D-Galactosamine	Aorta, lung, liver, basal laminae	Intermediate levels of interaction, mainly with collagen types III and IV
Keratan sulfate (cornea)	D-Galactose	D-Galactosamine	Cornea	. . .
Keratan sulfate (skeleton)	D-Galactose	D-Glucosamine	Cartilage, nucleus pulposus, annulus fibrosus	. . .

glycosaminoglycan. In proteoglycans, the carbohydrate portion is preponderant and constitutes 80–90% of the weight of this macromolecule. Because of the aforementioned characteristics, proteoglycans can bind to a great number of cations (usually sodium) by electrostatic (ionic) bonds, and they are intensely hydrated structures with a thick layer of solvation water surrounding the molecule. When fully hydrated, these molecules fill a much larger volume (domain) than in their anhydrous state.

The main proteoglycans are composed of a core protein associated with the glycosaminoglycans known as **dermatan sulfate, chondroitin sulfate, keratan sulfate,** and **heparan sulfate.** Table 5–1 shows the chemical composition and distribution of the glycosaminoglycans, as well as hyaluronic acid, in the tissues.

Dermatan sulfate is found mainly in dermis, tendons, ligaments, and fibrous cartilage, all structures that contain **collagen fibers** (collagen type I). Chondroitin sulfate predominates in hyaline and elastic cartilages, which are rich in collagen type II. Heparan sulfate seems to be associated with **reticular fibers,** which are composed of collagen type III. The various collagen types are discussed below. Proteoglycans bind to collagen owing to electrostatic interaction between their acidic groups and the basic amino acid residues of collagen.

The synthesis of proteoglycans begins in the rough endoplasmic reticulum with the synthesis of its protein moiety. Its glycosylation is initiated in the rough endoplasmic reticulum and completed in the Golgi complex where sulfation also occurs (see Chapter 3).

The degradation of proteoglycans is carried out by several cell types and depends on the presence of lysosomal enzymes. The turnover of these compounds is rapid—2–4 days for hyaluronic acid and 7–10 days for sulfated proteoglycans. Several disorders have been described in which, owing to a deficiency in lysosomal enzymes, glycosaminoglycan degradation is blocked, with a consequent accumulation of these compounds in tissues. Lack of specific hydrolases in the lysosomes has been found as the cause of several disorders in humans, including Hurler's syndrome, Hunter's syndrome, Sanfilippo syndrome, and Morquio's syndrome.

Glycosaminoglycans have a lubricating function in connective tissue, but their main function is probably structural, interacting with collagen fibrils to bind these structures together (Fig 7–4). Further information on the function of proteoglycans is presented in Chapter 7.

Structural glycoproteins are compounds containing a protein moiety to which carbohydrates are attached. In contrast to proteoglycans, the protein moiety usually predominates, and these molecules do not contain linear polysaccharides formed by disaccharides containing hexosamines. Rather, the carbohydrate moiety of glycoproteins is frequently a branched structure. Although the presence of glycoproteins in the ground substance has been known for

several years, recent studies have contributed to rapid progress in knowledge about the biologic importance of these compounds.

Several glycoproteins have been isolated from connective tissue, and evidence shows that they play an important role not only in the interaction between neighboring cells but also in the adhesion of cells to their substrate. **Fibronectin** (MW 220,000–240,000) is a glycoprotein synthesized by fibroblasts and some epithelial cells. This molecule has binding sites for cells, collagen, and glycosaminoglycans. These interactions help mediate normal cell adhesion and migration. Cancer cells do not synthesize fibronectin, and this may account for their increased capacity to invade other tissues. **Laminin** is a large glycoprotein composed of at least 2 polypeptide chains. It has been detected in basal laminae and is partially responsible for the adhesion of epithelial cells to the type IV collagen present in these structures. **Chondronectin** is present in cartilage, where it mediates the adhesion of chondrocytes to type II collagen.

In connective tissue, in addition to the amorphous substance, there is a very small quantity of fluid—called **tissue fluid**—that is similar to blood plasma in its content of ions and diffusible substances. Tissue fluid contains a small percentage of plasma proteins of low molecular weight that pass through the capillary walls as a consequence of the hydrostatic pressure of the blood. Under normal conditions, the quantity of tissue fluid is insignificant.

Edema

Water in the intercellular substance of connective tissue comes from the blood, passing through the capillary walls into the intercellular regions of the tissue. The capillary wall is only slightly permeable to macromolecules but permits the passage of water and small molecules, including low-molecular-weight proteins.

Blood brings to connective tissue the different nutrients required by the cells and carries metabolic waste products away to the detoxifying and excretory organs (liver, kidney, etc).

There are 2 forces acting on the water contained in the capillaries: (1) the hydrostatic pressure of the blood, a consequence of the pumping action of the heart, which forces water to pass through the capillary walls; and (2) the colloid osmotic pressure of the blood plasma, which draws water back into the capillaries (Fig 5–2). Osmotic pressure is due mainly to plasma proteins, because the ions and low-molecular-weight compounds that pass easily through the capillary walls have approximately the same concentration inside and outside these blood vessels. Therefore, osmotic pressures exerted by these substances are approximately equal on either side of the capillaries and cancel each other. However, the colloid osmotic pressure exerted by the blood protein macromolecules—that are unable to pass through the capillary walls—is not counterbalanced by outside pressure and therefore tends to bring water back into the blood vessel.

Normally, water passes through capillary walls to

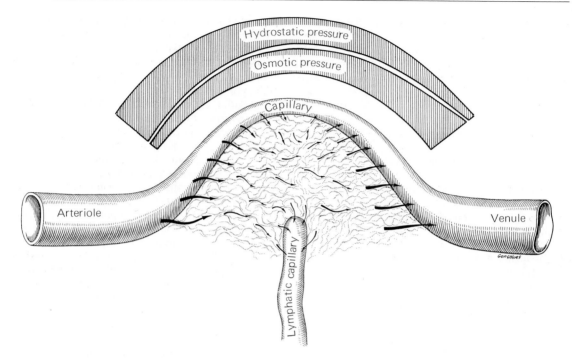

Figure 5–2. Movement of fluid through connective tissue. From the arterial to the venous ends of blood capillaries there is a decrease in hydrostatic pressure and an increase in osmotic pressure (upper part of drawing). Fluid leaves the capillary through its arterial end and repenetrates the blood at the venous end of the capillaries. Some fluid is drained by the lymphatic capillaries.

the surrounding tissues at the arterial end of a capillary. This occurs because the hydrostatic pressure here is greater than the colloid osmotic pressure. However, hydrostatic pressure decreases along the length of the capillary toward the venous end. As hydrostatic pressure falls, osmotic pressure rises because of the progressive increase in the concentration of proteins, which is caused by the passage of water from the capillaries. As a result of the increase in protein concentration and the fall in hydrostatic pressure, osmotic pressure becomes greater than hydrostatic pressure at the venous end of the capillary, and water is thus drawn back into the capillary (Fig 5–2).

The quantity of water drawn back is less than that which passes out through the capillaries. The water that remains in the connective tissue returns to the blood by the lymphatic vessels. The smallest lymphatic vessels are the lymphatic capillaries, which originate in connective tissue with blind ends. Lymphatic vessels drain into veins at the base of the neck (see Chapter 12).

There is, therefore, little free water in the tissue, because of the equilibrium that exists between the water entering and the water leaving the intercellular substance of connective tissue.

In several pathologic conditions, the quantity of tissue fluid may increase considerably, causing edema. Histologically, this condition is characterized by enlarged spaces between the components of the connective tissue caused by the increase in liquid. Macro-

scopically, edema can appear as an increase in volume that yields easily to localized pressure, which results in a depression that slowly disappears ("pitting edema").

Edema may result from venous obstruction or decrease in venous blood flow (eg, congestive heart failure). It may also be caused by starvation because the consequent protein deficiency results in lack of plasma proteins and a fall in colloid osmotic pressure. Water therefore accumulates in the connective tissue and is not drawn back into the capillaries.

Another possible cause of edema is increased permeability of the blood capillary endothelium due to mechanical injury or to some substance produced in the body (eg, histamine). Edema may be caused also by the obstruction of lymphatic vessels, eg, by plugs of parasites or tumor cells.

FIBERS

There are 3 main types of connective tissue fibers: **collagen fibers, reticular fibers,** and **elastic fibers.** Collagen and reticular fibers are known to be formed by the protein **collagen,** whereas the elastic fibers are composed mainly by the protein **elastin.** These fibers are distributed unequally among the different connective tissues. In many cases, the predominant fiber type is responsible for conferring specific properties on the tissue.

Brief Introduction to the Study of Collagen

During the process of evolution, a group of structural proteins developed that were modified to varying degrees of rigidity, elasticity, and strength depending upon environmental influences and the functional requirements of the animal organism. These proteins are known collectively as **collagen,** and the chief examples among its various types are the collagen from skin, bone, cartilage, smooth muscle, and basal lamina.

Collagen is the most abundant protein of the human body, representing 30% of its dry weight. Improvements in methodology have shown that the collagens of vertebrates are a family of proteins, produced by several cell types, that are distinguishable by their chemical composition and by their different morphologic and pathologic features, distribution in tissues, and functions (Table 5–2). Although many different types of collagen have been described, the most common, most important, and best studied are the collagen types I, II, III, IV, and V.

Collagen type I is the most abundant and has a widespread distribution. It occurs in tissues as structures classically designated as **collagen fibers** that form bones, dentin, tendons, organ capsules, dermis, etc.

Collagen type II is present mainly in hyaline and elastic cartilage. Only very thin fibrils are formed.

Collagen type III is usually associated with collagen type I in the tissues and is the collagenous component of **reticular fibers.**

Collagen type IV is present in the basal lamina (see Chapter 4). This type of collagen does not form fibrils or fibers.

Collagen type V is present in fetal membranes, in blood vessels, and in small amounts in other tissues. Its structure and function are still a subject of controversy and intensive investigation.

Recent studies on collagen biology have shown that collagen synthesis, an activity thought originally to be restricted to fibroblasts, chondroblasts, osteoblasts, and odontoblasts, is actually very widespread and many cell types produce this protein (Table 5–2). The principal amino acids composing collagen are glycine (33.5%), proline (12%), and hydroxyproline (10%). The amount of collagen in a tissue can thus be determined by measurement of its hydroxyproline content. Collagen contains 2 amino acids that are characteristic of this protein—**hydroxyproline** and **hydroxylysine.** These amino acids are not incorporated as such in the protein molecule but result from the hydroxylation of proline and lysine of nascent collagen polypeptides in the rough endoplasmic reticulum during collagen synthesis.

The protein unit that polymerizes to form collagen fibrils is the elongated molecule called **tropocollagen,**

Table 5–2. Main characteristics of the different collagen types.

Collagen Type	Molecular Formula	Tissue Distribution	Optical Microscopy	Ultrastructure	Site of Synthesis	Interaction With Glycosaminoglycans	Function
I	$[\alpha1(I)]_2\alpha2(I)$	Dermis, bone, tendon, dentin, fascias, sclera, organ capsules, fibrous cartilage.	Closely packed, thick, nonargyrophilic, strongly birefringent yellow or red fibers. Collagen fibers.	Densely packed, thick fibrils with marked variation in diameter.	Fibroblast, osteoblast, odontoblast, chondroblast.	Low level of interaction, mainly with dermatan sulfate.	Resistance to tension.
II	$[\alpha1(II)]_3$	Hyaline and elastic cartilages.	Loose, collagenous network visible only with picro-Sirius stain and polarization microscopy.	No fibers; very thin fibrils embedded in abundant ground substance.	Chondroblast.	High level of interaction, mainly with chondroitin sulfates.	Resistance to intermittent pressure.
III	$[\alpha1(III)]_3$	Smooth muscle, endoneurium, arteries, uterus, liver, spleen, kidney, lung.	Loose network of thin, argyrophilic, weakly birefringent greenish fibers. Reticular fibers.	Loosely packed thin fibrils with more uniform diameters.	Smooth muscle, fibroblast, reticular cells, Schwann cells, hepatocyte.	Intermediate level of interaction, mainly with heparan sulfate.	Structural maintenance in expansible organs.
IV	$[pro\alpha1(IV)]_2 pro\alpha2(IV)$	Epithelial and endothelial basal laminae and basement membranes.	Thin, amorphous, weakly birefringent membrane.	Neither fibers nor fibrils are detected.	Endothelial and epithelial cells, muscle cells, and Schwann cells.	Interacts with heparan sulfate.	Support and filtration.
V	$[\alpha1(V)]_2\alpha2(V)$	Placental basement membranes.	Insufficient data.	Insufficient data.	Insufficient data.	Insufficient data.	Insufficient data.

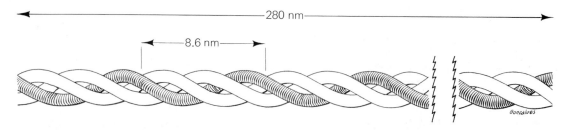

Figure 5–3. In the most abundant form of collagen, known as type I, each molecule (tropocollagen) is composed of two alpha 1 and one alpha 2 (shaded) peptide chains, each with a molecular weight of approximately 100,000, intertwined in a right-handed helix and held together by hydrogen bonds and hydrophobic interactions. Each complete turn of the helix spans a distance of 8.6 nm. The length of each tropocollagen molecule is 280 nm, and its width is 1.5 nm.

which measures 280 nm in length and 1.5 nm in width. Tropocollagen consists of 3 subunit polypeptide chains intertwined in a triple helix (Fig 5–3). Differences in chemical structure of these polypeptide chains are responsible for the different types of collagen. Molecular formulas of the several types of collagen are given in Table 5–2.

In collagen types I, II, and III, tropocollagen molecules aggregate into microfibrillar subunits that are packed together to form **fibrils.** Hydrogen bonds and hydrophobic interactions are important in the aggregation and packing of these units. In a subsequent step, this structure is reinforced by the formation of

covalent cross-links, a process catalyzed by the activity of the enzyme lysyl oxidase.

Collagen fibrils are thin, elongated structures with a variable diameter (ranging from 20 to 90 nm) that have a transverse striation with a characteristic periodicity of 64 nm (Fig 5–4). The transverse striation of the collagen fibrils is determined by the overlapping arrangement of the subunit tropocollagen molecules (Fig 5–5). The dark bands retain more of the stain used in electron microscopic studies because they have more free chemical groups that react more intensely with the lead solution used as a "stain" than the light bands. In collagen types I and III, these fibrils as-

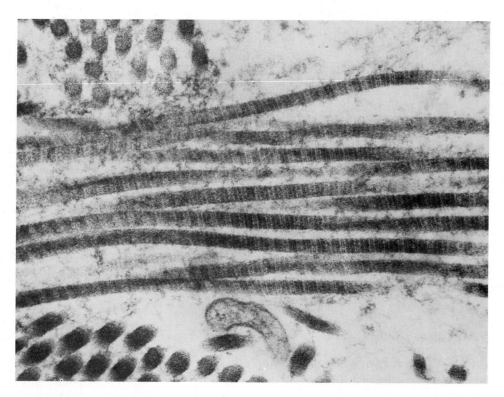

Figure 5–4. Electron micrograph of human collagen fibrils in cross and longitudinal sections. Each fibril consists of regular alternating dark and light bands, which are further divided by cross-striations. Amorphous ground substance completely surrounds the fibrils. × 100,000.

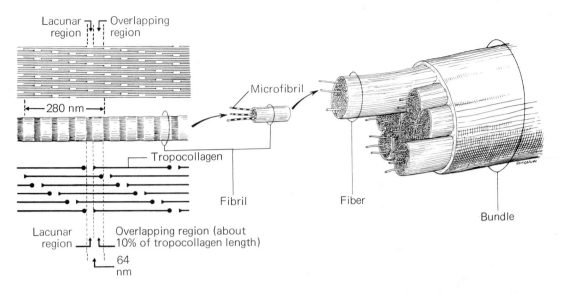

Lacunar region
Overlapping region
←280 nm→
Microfibril
Tropocollagen
Fibril
Fiber
Bundle
Lacunar region
Overlapping region (about 10% of tropocollagen length)
64 nm

Figure 5–5. Schematic drawing of collagen fibrils, fibers, and bundles. Under the electron microscope, the fibrils show periodicity of dark and light bands. This 64-nm periodicity is explained by the overlapping arrangement of rodlike tropocollagen subunits, each measuring 280 nm. Tropocollagen molecules are organized in a step-wise arrangement that produces lacunar and overlapping regions.

sociate to form fibers. In collagen type I, fibers can associate to form bundles (Fig 5–5). Collagen type II (present in cartilage) occurs as fibrils but does not form fibers (Fig 5–6). Collagen type IV, present in basal laminae, does not form fibrils or fibers and probably occurs as unpolymerized or scarcely polymerized procollagen molecules. Collagen types I, II, and III form fibrils and are often referred to as **interstitial** collagens to distinguish them, as a group, from collagen types IV and V, which do not form fibrils.

Collagen Biosynthesis

The synthesis of collagen proceeds through the following steps, which are summarized in Fig 5–7:

(1) Polypeptide alpha chains are assembled on polyribosomes bound to rough endoplasmic reticulum membranes and injected into the cisternae.

(2) Hydroxylation of proline and lysine occurs after these amino acids are incorporated into polypeptide chains. Hydroxylation begins after the peptide chain has reached a certain minimum length and is still

Figure 5–6 (at right). Electron micrograph of hyaline cartilage matrix showing the fine collagen fibrils of collagen type II interspersed with abundant amorphous ground substance. Fibril transverse striations are barely visible because of the interaction of collagen with chondroitin sulfate. In the center is a portion of a chondrocyte. Compare the appearance of these fibrils with those of fibrocartilage (Fig 7–9). × 14,000.

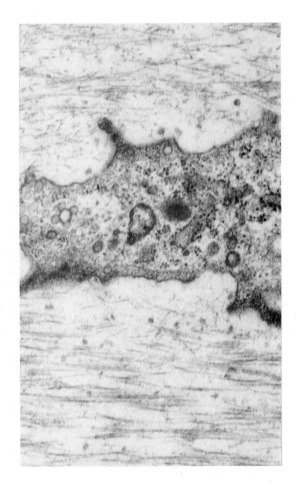

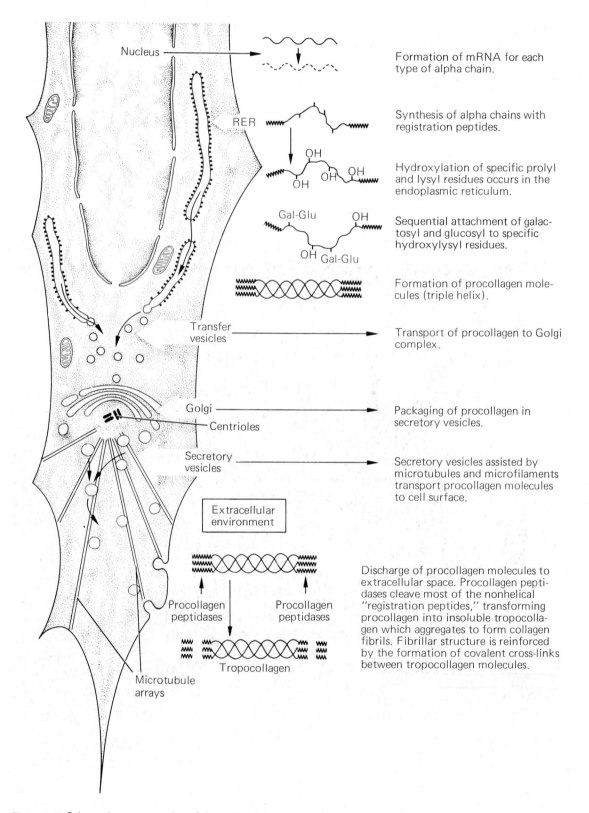

Figure 5–7. Schematic representation of the molecular events and organellar participation in the synthesis of collagen.

bound to the ribosomes. The 2 enzymes involved are (a) peptidyl proline hydroxylase and (b) peptidyl lysine hydroxylase.

(3) Glycosylation of hydroxylysine occurs after its hydroxylation. Different collagen types have variable amounts of carbohydrate in the form of galactose or glycosylgalactose linked to hydroxylysine.

(4) Each alpha chain is synthesized with an extra length of peptides on both NH₂- and COOH-terminal ends called **registration peptides.** Registration peptides probably ensure that the appropriate alpha chains (ie, α1, α2) assemble in the correct position. In addition, the extra peptides make the resulting **procollagen molecule** soluble and prevent its premature intracellular assembly and precipitation as collagen fibrils. Procollagen is transported as such out of the cell to the extracellular environment.

(5) Outside the cell, specific proteases called **procollagen peptidases** remove the registration peptides. This altered protein is known as **tropocollagen,** which is capable of assembling into polymeric collagen fibrils. The hydroxyproline residues contribute to the stability of the tropocollagen triple helix, forming hydrogen bonds between its polypeptide chains.

(6) In collagen types I and III, fibrils aggregate

Table 5–3. Examples of some disorders due to defects in collagen synthesis.

Disorder	Defect	Symptoms
Ehlers-Danlos type IV	Faulty transcription or translation of type III	Aortic and/or intestinal rupture
Ehlers-Danlos type VI	Faulty lysine hydroxylation	Augmented skin elasticity, rupture of eyeball
Ehlers-Danlos type VII	Decrease in procollagen peptidase activity	Increased articular mobility, frequent luxation
Scurvy	Lack of vitamin C, cofactor for proline hydroxylase	Ulceration of gums and hemorrhages

spontaneously to form fibers. Proteoglycans and structural glycoproteins very probably play an important role in the aggregation of tropocollagen to form fibrils and in the formation of fibers from fibrils.

(7) Fibrillar structure is reinforced by the formation of covalent cross-links between tropocollagen molecules. This process is catalyzed by the action of the enzyme **lysyl oxidase** that acts in the extracellular space.

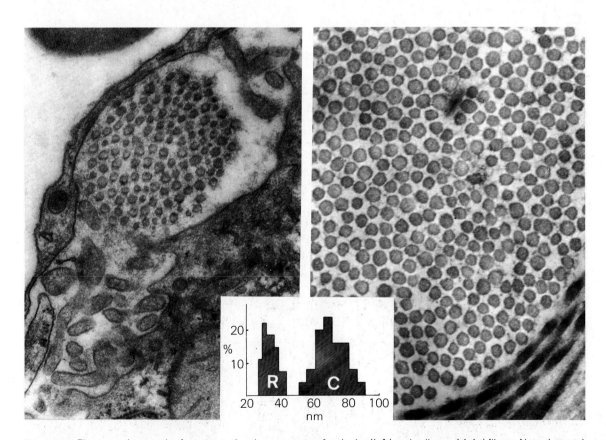

Figure 5–8. Electron micrograph of cross-sectional appearance of reticular *(left)* and collagen *(right)* fibers. Note that each fiber type is composed of numerous smaller collagen fibrils. Reticular fibers are composed of fibrils of significantly narrower diameter (see histogram inset), and in addition, the constituent fibrils reveal an abundant surface-associated granularity not present on regular collagen fibrils *(right).* × 70,000.

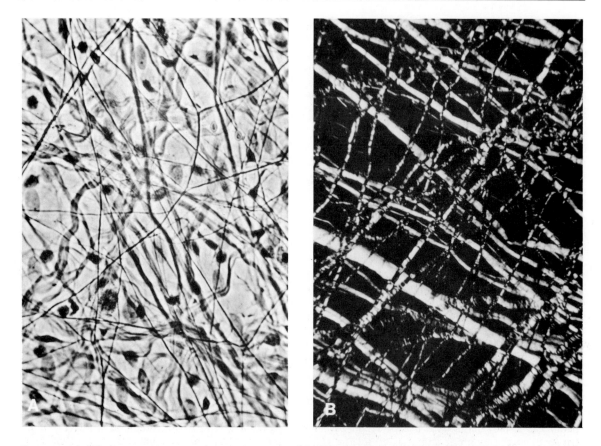

Figure 5–9. *A:* Whole mesentery spread on a microscope slide. The preparation was stained by the Weigert method for elastic fibers and photographed under the phase contrast microscope. The thin, taut filaments are elastic fibers that branch and form a woven network. Collagen fibers are the thick and wavy structures. × 200. *B:* A similar preparation stained with Sirius red and observed with polarization microscopy. Collagenous fibers are the only structures revealed. The birefringence of collagen is due to the tight packing and paracrystalline assembly of its tropocollagen subunits. × 300.

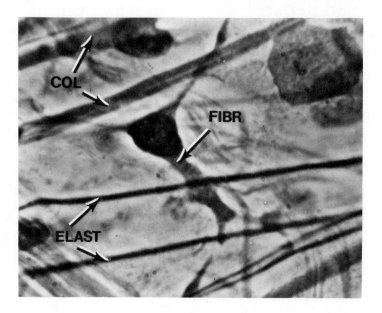

Figure 5–10. Phase contrast photomicrograph of a piece of mesentery spread on a glass slide. Shown are a fibroblast (FIBR), collagen fibers (COL), and elastic fibers (ELAST). H&E stain, × 800.

The synthesis of collagen involves a cascade of unique posttranslational biochemical modifications of the original procollagen polypeptide. All of these modifications are crucial to the structure and function of normal, mature collagen. These modifications are carried out by a series of different enzymes and cofactors, each of which is specifically designed for a particular role in the construction of the final product. Because there are so many steps in collagen biosynthesis, there are many points at which the process may be interrupted or changed by faulty enzymes or by disease processes. Thus, it should not be surprising that a large number of pathologic conditions have been described which are directly attributable to insufficient or abnormal collagen synthesis. Table 5–3 lists examples of the many disorders due to failure of collagen biosynthesis.

Collagen Fibers

Collagen fibers are the most numerous fibers in connective tissue. Fresh collagen fibers are colorless strands, but when present in great numbers they cause the tissues in which they lie to be white—for example, in tendons and aponeuroses.

Owing to the oriented disposition of the elongated tropocollagen molecules in these fibers, these structures are birefringent. When fibers containing collagen are stained with an acidic dye composed of elongated molecules (eg, Sirius red) that binds to collagen in a parallel array to its molecules, collagen's normal birefringency increases considerably. This increase in birefringency occurs only in oriented collagen structures and is used as a specific method for their detection (Fig 5–9).

Collagen fibers are inelastic and, because of their molecular configuration, have a greater tensile strength than steel. Consequently, collagen imparts a unique combination of flexibility and strength to the tissues in which it lies.

Collagen fibers consist of closely packed thick fibrils with an average diameter of 75 nm (Fig 5–8) in mammals. The diameter of the fibers depends on the number of fibrils they contain. In many parts of the body, collagen fibers are organized in a parallel array, forming **collagen bundles** (Fig 5–5).

Because of their long and tortuous course, the morphologic characteristics of collagen fibers are better studied in spread preparations than in histologic sections. Mesentery is frequently used for this purpose, for when spread on a slide, it is sufficiently thin to be stained and examined under the microscope. Mesentery is composed of a central portion of connective tissue lined on both surfaces by a simple squamous epithelium, the mesothelium. The collagen fibers in a spread preparation appear as elongated and tortuous cylindric structures of indefinite length and with a diameter that varies from 1 to 20 μm (Figs 5–9 and 5–10).

Seen in the light microscope, collagen fibers are acidophilic; they stain pink with eosin, blue with Mallory's trichrome stain, green with Masson's trichrome stain, and red with Sirius red.

Reticular Fibers

Reticular fibers are extremely thin, with a diameter between 0.5 and 2 μm. They form an extensive network in certain organs. They are not visible in hematoxylin and eosin preparations but can be easily stained black by impregnation with silver salts. Owing to their affinity for silver salts, they are called **argyrophilic fibers** (Fig 5–11).

Reticular fibers are also PAS-positive. Both PAS-

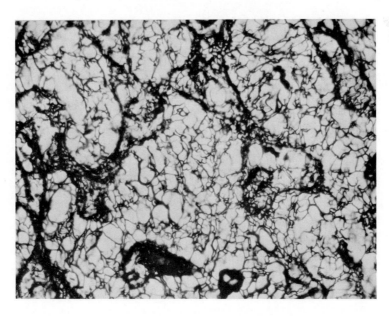

Figure 5–11. Section from a lymph node stained with silver. Note the thin black lines representing the argyrophilic reticular fibers. × 200.

positivity and argyrophilia are considered to be due to the high content of glycoproteins characteristic of these fibers. Reticular fibers have 6–12% hexoses as opposed to 1% in collagen fibers. Immunocytochemical and histochemical evidence reveals that reticular fibers, in contrast to collagen fibers, which consist of collagen type I, are composed mainly of collagen type III in association with glycoproteins and proteoglycans. They are formed by loosely packed, thin (average, 45 nm) fibrils bound together by abundant small interfibrillar bridges probably composed of proteoglycans and glycoproteins (Fig 5–8). Owing to their small diameter, reticular fibers have a weak birefringency when stained with Sirius red and observed by means of polarizing microscopy.

Reticular fibers are particularly abundant in smooth muscle, endoneurium, and the framework of hematopoietic organs (eg, spleen, lymph nodes, red bone marrow) and constitute a network around the cells of parenchymal organs (eg, liver, kidney, and endocrine glands). During embryogenesis, inflammatory processes, and wound healing, most connective tissues have an abundance of reticular fibers, but these are subsequently replaced by regular collagen fibers.

The small diameter and the loose disposition of reticular fibers create a flexible network in organs that are subjected to changes in form or volume such as the arteries, spleen, liver, uterus, and intestinal muscle layers.

Reticular fibers, considered until recently to be immature collagen fibers, are separate entities with characteristic biochemical, morphologic, functional, and pathologic features.

Elastic Fibers

Elastic fibers are easily distinguished from the collagen fibers in stretched connective tissue preparations, because they are thinner and tauter than collagen fibers, which are present as broad, wavy, diffusely stained bundles. Elastic fibers branch and unite with one another, forming an irregular network (Fig 5–9). When they are fresh and present in great quantity, elastic fibers have a characteristic yellow color. Elastic fibers predominate in elastic tissue and are known as yellow fibers of connective tissue, while collagen fibers are known as white fibers. Elastic fibers, capable of stretching to one and one-half times their length, yield easily to very small traction forces but return to their original shape when these forces are relaxed. The presence of elastic fibers in blood vessels contributes to the efficiency of blood circulation and has contributed to the successful evolution of vertebrates.

Elastic fibers may stain weakly and irregularly with hematoxylin and eosin, but they usually appear unstained with this method. Selective methods to demonstrate elastic fibers, although they are devoid of histochemical specificity, include resorcin-fuchsin, aldehyde-fuchsin, and orcein, resulting in purple, black, or dark-blue staining of these fibers.

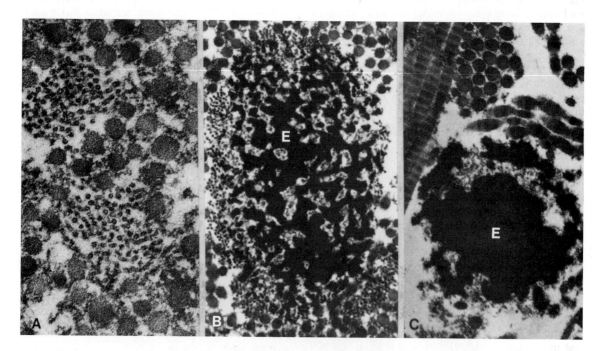

Figure 5–12. Electron microscopic observations of developing elastic fibers. **A:** In early stages of formation, developing fibers consist of numerous small glycoprotein microfibrils. The larger round structures are cross sections of collagen fibrils. **B:** With further development, amorphous elastin molecules (E) are found among the microfibrils. **C:** The amorphous elastin (E) accumulates, ultimately occupying the center of an elastic fiber delineated by microfibrils. Note the collagen fibrils, seen in cross and longitudinal section, at upper left. A × 75,000; B and C × 35,000. (Courtesy of G Cotta-Pereira.)

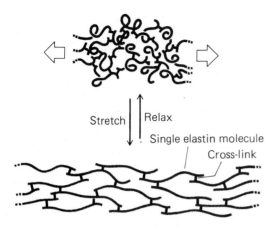

Stretch | Relax

Single elastin molecule

Cross-link

Figure 5–13. Elastin molecules are joined together by covalent bonds to generate an extensive cross-linked network. Because each elastin molecule in the network can expand and contract as a random coil, the entire network can stretch and recoil like a rubber band. (Reproduced, with permission, from Alberts B et al: *Molecular Biology of the Cell.* Garland, 1983.)

Electron microscopic observations reveal that elastic fibers consist of 2 components: an amorphous central region containing **elastin** surrounded by a sheath of 14-nm tubular **microfibrils.** In elastic fiber development, the microfibrils appear first, creating a matrix within which small amounts of elastin are deposited (Fig 5– 12). The amorphous elastin component gradually accumulates until it occupies the center of a fiber delineated by a tubular sheath of microfibrils. The microfibrils are composed of a structural glycoprotein as judged by biochemical, immunochemical, and electron microscopic techniques. Elastin is secreted as proelastin, a globular molecule of MW 70,000 that polymerizes, producing the amorphous rubberlike glycoprotein called elastin that predominates in the mature fibers (Fig 5– 12). Elastin is a significantly "younger" protein in terms of evolution than collagen and much more resistant to extraction procedures. It is produced by fibroblasts in skin and tendon and by smooth muscle cells in the large blood vessels with elastic tissue. Elastin is resistant to boiling and extraction with dilute acids and alkalis and is not digested by trypsin. All of this is apparently due to its tertiary and quaternary structure, stabilized by hydrophobic interactions between the nonpolar peptide chains. This probably also explains the affinity of elastin for lipids. Pepsin at pH 2.0 acts slowly upon elastin, but elastin is easily hydrolyzed by the pancreatic enzyme **elastase.**

The amino acid composition of elastin resembles that of collagen in that elastin is rich in glycine and proline. Differences include greater quantities of valine and alanine along with small amounts of hydroxyproline and no hydroxylysine. Elastin contains 2 unusual amino acids, **desmosine** and **isodesmosine,** formed by covalent reactions among 4 lysine residues.

This effectively cross-links elastin and is thought to account for the rubberlike qualities of this protein (Fig 5– 13).

Elastin also occurs in a nonfibrillar form as **fenestrated membranes** (elastic laminae) present in the walls of some blood vessels.

CELLS

Some cells of connective tissue such as fibroblasts and adipose cells are produced and remain locally, while others such as leukocytes come from other territories and can be transient inhabitants of connective tissue. These cells have various functions that are summarized in Table 5– 4.

Cells of the connective tissue interact, creating complex mechanisms that help defend the organism from invasion. Thus, macrophages can influence antibody production by lymphocyte-derived plasma cells, and lymphocytes and mast cells can produce substances that attract eosinophils.

Fibroblasts

The fibroblast is the cell most commonly found in connective tissue. It is responsible for the synthesis of fibers and amorphous intercellular substance. There are 2 quite different morphologic types of fibroblasts and several with intermediate characteristics. The young cell with intense synthetic activity is morphologically distinct from the quiescent fibroblast that is found scattered within the matrix it has already synthesized. Some histologists reserve the term fibroblast to denote the young cell and call the mature cell a **fibrocyte.**

The young fibroblast has an abundant and irregularly branched cytoplasm. Its nucleus is ovoid, large,

Table 5–4. Functions of connective tissue cells.

Cell Type	Main Product or Activity	Main Function
Fibroblast, chondroblast, osteoblast, odontoblast	Fibers and ground substance production	Structural
Plasma cell, lymphocyte, eosinophilic leukocyte	Production of antibodies (humoral immunity) and of immunocompetent cells (cell-mediated immunity), phagocytosis of antigen-antibody complex	Immunologic
Macrophages, neutrophilic leukocyte	Phagocytosis of foreign substances, phagocytosis of bacteria	Defense
Mast cells, basophilic leukocyte	Liberation of pharmacologically active substances (eg, histamine)	Release of pharmacologically active substances
Adipose cell	Storage of neutral fats, heat production	Energy reservoir

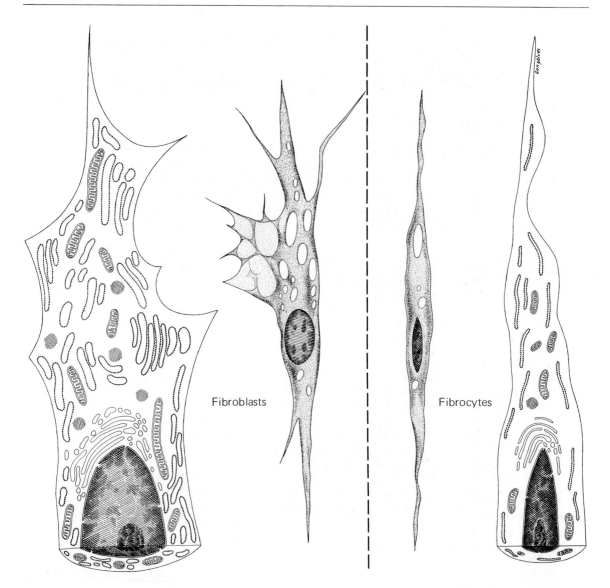

Fibroblasts

Fibrocytes

Figure 5–14. Immature *(left)* and mature *(right)* fibroblasts. External morphology and ultrastructure of each cell are shown. Synthetically active immature or young fibroblasts are richer in mitochondria, lipid droplets, Golgi complex, and rough endoplasmic reticulum than mature fibroblasts, often called fibrocytes.

and pale-staining, with fine chromatin and a prominent nucleolus. The cytoplasm is rich in rough endoplasmic reticulum, and the Golgi complex is well developed (Figs 5–14 and 5–15).

The fibrocyte is a smaller cell than the fibroblast. It tends to be spindle-shaped and has fewer processes than the young fibroblast. It has a smaller, darker, elongated nucleus and an acidophilic cytoplasm (Fig 5–10).

The electron microscope shows that the fibrocyte has a less well developed rough endoplasmic reticulum and Golgi complex than the young fibroblast. When it is adequately stimulated, the fibrocyte may revert

to the fibroblast state, and its synthetic activities are reactivated. This occurs during wound healing, and in such instances the cell reassumes the form and appearance of a young fibroblast.

The functions of the fibroblasts have been studied in light and electron microscopic radioautographs. These cells synthesize collagen, reticular and elastic fibers, and the glycosaminoglycans and glycoproteins of the amorphous intercellular substance.

Radioautographic techniques reveal that procollagen synthesized by the rough endoplasmic reticulum accumulates in the cisternae of this structure. It is subsequently encountered in the Golgi complex and

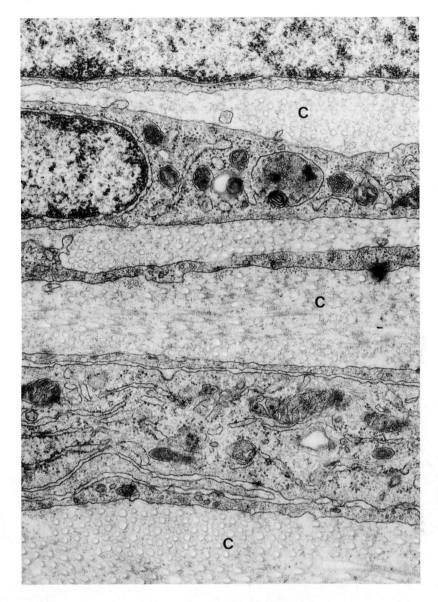

Figure 5–15. Electron micrograph revealing portions of several flattened <u>fibroblasts</u> in dense connective tissue. Abundant mitochondria, rough endoplasmic reticulum, and vesicles distinguish these cells from the less active fibrocytes. Multiple strata of collagen fibrils (C) lie among the fibroblasts. × 30,000.

is then transported to the outside of the cell via small vesicles. Collagen, therefore, follows the same path as other secreted proteins (Fig 5–7).

The synthesis of glycosaminoglycans has been studied mainly by radioautography after the administration of sulfate labeled with ^{35}S, since most connective tissue glycosaminoglycans are sulfated. Fibroblasts synthesize collagen and glycosaminoglycans simultaneously, although some cell culture experiments indicate that a cell which produces collagen in substantial amounts produces little glycosaminoglycan and vice versa. The rate of secretion of different molecules of connective tissue by the same cell may vary with the age of the individual or in response to hormonal influences.

In adults, fibroblasts in connective tissue rarely undergo division. Mitoses are observed only when the organism requires additional fibroblasts, ie, when connective tissue is damaged.

Macrophages

These are cells discovered and initially characterized by their phagocytic capacity. When a vital dye such as trypan blue or India ink is injected in an animal, these cells engulf and accumulate it in their cytoplasm in the form of granules or vacuoles visible

Table 5–5. Cells of the mononuclear phagocyte system.

Name	Location
Histiocytes	Connective tissue
Kupffer cells	Liver
Alveolar macrophages	Lung
Macrophages	Lymph nodes
Macrophages	Spleen
Pleural and peritoneal macrophages	Serous cavities
Osteoclasts	Bone
Microglial cells	Central nervous system

in the light microscope. Macrophages derive mainly from precursor cells from the bone marrow that divide, producing **monocytes.** These cells circulate in the blood and in a second step migrate into the connective tissue where they mature and are called macrophages. Tissue macrophages can proliferate locally, producing more of these cells.

Macrophages are present in most organs and constitute the **mononuclear phagocyte system.** The spe-

cial names given to macrophages in different organs are listed in Table 5 – 5. To be classified as components of this system, phagocytes must be derived from bone marrow stem cells, have a characteristic morphology, and exhibit relatively intense phagocytic activity mediated by immunoglobulins or serum complement. Previously, most of the body's macrophages were considered to be constituents of what was referred to as the **reticuloendothelial system.** Certain components of the reticuloendothelial system are excluded from the mononuclear phagocyte system, notably the reticular cells of lymphoid organs. Conversely, a few cell types not originally considered as components of the reticuloendothelial system (eg, alveolar macrophages of the lung) are included in the mononuclear phagocyte system.

Although mononuclear phagocytes have a wide spectrum of morphologic features according to their state of functional activity and to the tissue they inhabit, they are characterized by an irregular surface with pleats, protrusions, and indentations—a morphologic expression of their active pinocytotic and

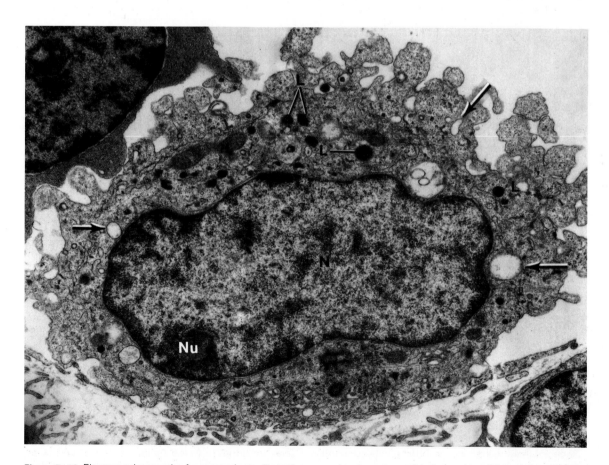

Figure 5–16. Electron micrograph of a macrophage. Note the secondary lysosomes (L), the nucleus (N), and the nucleolus (Nu). The arrows point to phagocytic vacuoles.

phagocytic activities. They generally have a well-developed Golgi complex, many lysosomes, and a prominent rough endoplasmic reticulum (Fig 5–16). In the process of monocyte-to-macrophage transformation, there is an increase in protein synthesis and cell size. An increase in the Golgi complex as well as in the number of lysosomes, microtubules, and microfilaments is also apparent. Macrophages measure between 10 and 30 μm and usually have an oval or kidney-shaped nucleus located eccentrically. Macrophages are long-living cells and may survive for months in the tissues. When adequately stimulated, these cells may increase in size, forming **epithelioid cells,** or several may fuse to form **multinuclear giant cells**—cell types usually found only in pathologic conditions (Fig 5–17).

The major function of macrophages is the ingestion of particles and their digestion by the lysosomes. Ingestion is performed by surrounding the particle with thin extensions of the cell surface that ultimately fuse. The particle is thus isolated within a phagocytic vacuole. Next, lysosomes fuse with the phagocytic vacuole and digest the contents. A working hypothesis of the mechanism of phagocytosis is summarized in Fig 5–18. In addition to this function, macrophages participate in the immune system of the body; there is evidence that these cells influence activation of the immune response. They also participate in cell-mediated resistance to infection by bacteria, viruses, protozoa, fungi, and metazoa (such as parasitic worms) and in cell-mediated resistance to tumors.

The diversity of macrophage morphology extends

to its metabolism, which also varies according to this cell's functional activity and environment. Thus, lung macrophages exhibit a high level of aerobic glycolysis (probably related to the high oxygen tension available locally), whereas peritoneal macrophages have a high level of anaerobic glycolysis.

When macrophages are stimulated (by injection of foreign substances or by infection), they change

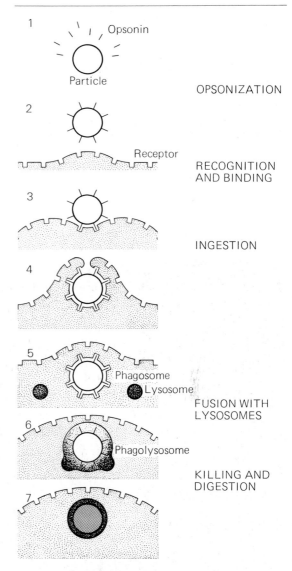

Figure 5–18. Phagocytosis of foreign particles. (1) Coating of a foreign particle by substances such as immunoglobulins (opsonins) for which the phagocyte has receptors. (2) Binding of opsonized particle to phagocyte. (3 and 4) Uptake of the opsonized particle involves sequential interaction of phagocyte membrane receptors with the particle ("zippering"). Subsequent events include fusion of the phagocytic vacuole with lysosomes and killing and digestion of the foreign particle (5, 6, and 7). (Redrawn and reproduced, with permission, from Stites DP et al: *Basic & Clinical Immunology,* 5th ed. Lange, 1984.)

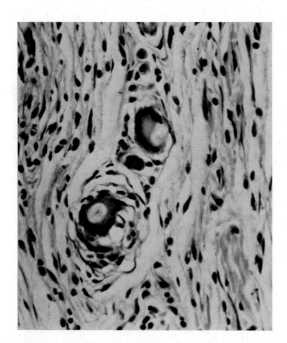

Figure 5–17. Photomicrograph of 2 foreign body giant cells. Both cells contain, in their cytoplasm, phagocytized material that appears lightly stained. At the periphery of these cells, many nuclei can be seen. H&E stain, × 320.

their morphology and metabolism. Under these conditions, they are called **activated macrophages** and acquire characteristics not present in their nonactivated state. Thus activated, macrophages, in addition to showing an increase in their capacity for phagocytosis and intracellular digestion, exhibit enhanced metabolic and lysosomal enzyme activity. Activated macrophages can also produce and secrete collagenase and exhibit increased tumor cell–killing capacity.

Cells of Regeneration

Some believe that in adults there are cells that persist with the same potential as embryonic mesenchymal cells—ie, the ability to give rise to any kind of connective tissue cells. It is also believed that they have the capacity to give rise to smooth muscle cells. This occurs when an injured blood vessel grows and new muscle cells, derived from the multiplication and differentiation of mesenchymal cells, appear in its wall. Sometimes these cells are called **adventitial cells,** because they are usually found in the periphery of blood capillaries.

Morphologically, adventitial cells are similar to fibroblasts, which makes their identification difficult in some cases. They are usually smaller than fibroblasts and possess elongated nuclei with coarse chromatin.

The opposing view is that new connective tissue arises from existing cells such as fibroblasts, smooth muscle cells, etc, which retain their capacity to divide following certain stimuli.

Mast Cells

Mast cells are oval to round connective tissue cells, 20–30 μm in diameter, whose cytoplasm is filled with basophilic granules. The nucleus is rather small, spherical, and centrally situated; it is frequently obscured by the cytoplasmic granules (Fig 5–19).

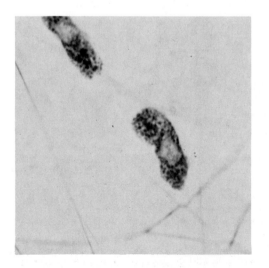

Figure 5–19. Whole mount of spread mesentery. Two mast cells appear stained by Gomori's aldehyde-fuchsin. × 400.

"Mast" is from a German word meaning to stuff or fatten. Erhlich called these cells "mast" cells because he wrongly believed they formed their granules by taking up extracellular materials.

The electron microscope reveals a few small spherical mitochondria, short cisternae of rough endoplasmic reticulum, and a well-developed Golgi complex. The secretory granules are 0.3–0.5 μm in diameter and are limited by a membrane. Their interior is heterogeneous in appearance, with a prominent scroll-like substructure (Fig 5–20).

Mast cell granules are metachromatic because of their content of glycosaminoglycans. **Metachromasia** is a property of certain basic aniline dyes (such as toluidine blue) in which the stained material takes on a different color (purple-red) from that of the applied dye (blue). Other constituents of mast cell granules are histamine, neutral proteases, and eosinophil chemotactic factor of anaphylaxis (ECF-A). Mast cells also release leukotrienes (SRS-A), but these substances are not stored in the cell. Rather, they are synthesized from membrane phospholipids and immediately released upon appropriate stimulation.

An important new finding is that there are at least 2 populations of mast cells in connective tissues. One type is called the connective tissue mast cell. In these cells, the proteoglycan in the granules is heparin. In the second type, termed mucosal mast cells, the granules contain chondroitin sulfate instead of heparin. In addition, the 2 types react differently to pharmacologic agents.

Mast cells were formerly considered to be resident cells of connective tissues because they were thought to arise locally. It is now known that mast cells originate from stem cells in the bone marrow. Although mast cells are, in many respects, similar to basophilic leukocytes, they have a separate stem cell and are not basophils found in connective tissue. Likewise, basophils are not circulating mast cells.

The surface of mast cells contains specific receptors for IgE, a type of immunoglobulin produced by plasma cells. Most IgE molecules are fixed on the surface of mast cells and blood basophils, while very few remain in the plasma.

Release of the chemical mediators stored in mast cells promotes the allergic reactions known as "immediate hypersensitivity reactions" because they occur within a few minutes after penetration by antigen of an individual previously sensitized to the same or a very similar antigen. There are many examples of immediate hypersensitivity reaction; a dramatic one is **anaphylactic shock,** a potentially fatal condition. It may occur when a person is injected with tetanus antitoxin months after having had one or several injections of it. The process of anaphylaxis consists of the following sequential events: The first exposure to an antigen (allergen), such as tetanus antitoxin or bee venom, results in production of the IgE class of immunoglobulins (antibodies) by plasma cells. IgE is avidly bound to the surfaces of mast cells. A second exposure to the antigen results in binding of the antigen

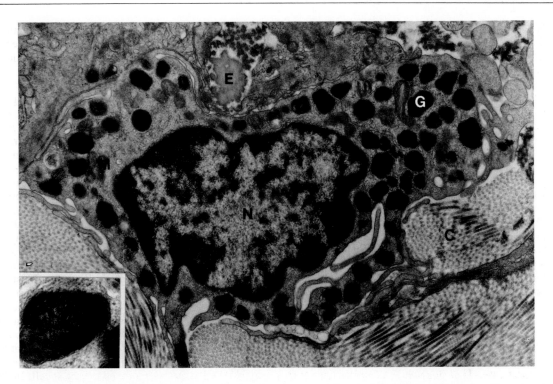

Figure 5–20. Electron micrograph of a human mast cell. The granules (G) contain heparin and histamine. Note the characteristic scroll-like structures within the granules. M, mitochondrion; N, nucleus; C, collagen fibrils; E, elastic fibril. *Inset:* Higher magnification view of a mast cell granule. (Courtesy of MC Williams.) × 14,700. Inset × 44,600.

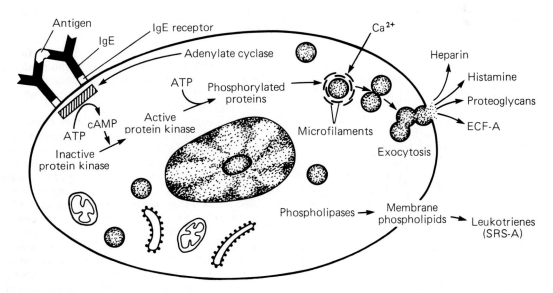

Figure 5–21. Mast cell secretion. After a second exposure to an antigen (eg, bee venom), IgE molecules bound to surface receptors are cross-linked by the antigen. This activates adenylate cyclase and results in the phosphorylation of certain proteins. At the same time, Ca^{2+} enters the cell. These events lead to exocytosis of mast cell granules. In addition, phospholipases act on membrane phospholipids to produce leukotrienes.

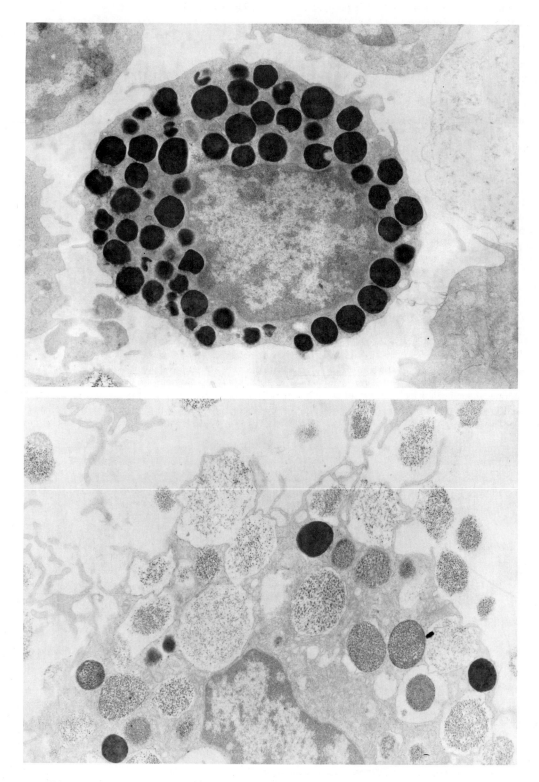

Figure 5–22. This pair of electron micrographs illustrates the liberation of granules by mast cells. *Top:* A resting mast cell with its numerous cytoplasmic granules. *Bottom:* A similar cell after injection of protamine, which stimulates liberation of the granules. The cell surface is irregular, and the granular content is dissolving out. Magnification is the same for both cells: × 20,000. (Courtesy of I Vugman and RM Hofmeister.)

to IgE on mast cells. This event triggers release of mast cell granules, liberating histamine, heparin, leukotrienes, and ECF-A (Figs 5–21 and 5–22).

Histamine causes contraction of smooth muscle (mainly the bronchioles), dilates blood capillaries, and increases their permeability. Leukotrienes produce slow contractions in smooth muscle, and ECF-A attracts blood eosinophils. Heparin is a blood anticoagulant, but in humans blood clotting remains normal during anaphylactic shock. Any liberated histamine is inactivated immediately after release.

Extrusion of mast cell granules is an active, energy-consuming process that may be easily observed with the light microscope. Electron microscopic studies show that the membranes of peripheral granules fuse with the cell membrane to discharge their contents (Fig 5–22). Simultaneously, peripheral granules fuse with granules located deep inside the mast cell, creating channels that facilitate a rapid passage of material to the cell exterior. The process of extrusion does not damage the mast cell, which remains viable and synthesizes new granules. Extrusion is inhibited by cytochalasin, a compound which inhibits the activity of microfilaments, suggesting that microfilaments participate in the release of mast cell granules.

Mast cells are widespread in the human body but are particularly abundant in the dermis and digestive and respiratory tracts. Mast cells are typical of cells that liberate pharmacologically active substances which act locally and therefore are classified as **paracrine cells** (defined in Chapter 4).

Plasma Cells

Plasma cells are few in number in connective tissue in most areas of the body. They are numerous in sites subject to penetration by bacteria and foreign proteins (eg, intestinal mucosa) and in areas where there is chronic inflammation.

Plasma cells are large, ovoid cells that have a basophilic cytoplasm owing to their richness in rough endoplasmic reticulum (Figs 5–23 and 5–24). The juxtanuclear Golgi complex and the centrioles occupy a region that appears pale in regular histologic preparations.

The nucleus of the plasma cell is spherical and eccentrically placed, containing compact, coarse heterochromatin alternating with lighter areas of approximately equal size. This configuration resembles the face of a clock with the heterochromatin clumps corresponding to the numerals. Thus, the nucleus of a plasma cell is commonly described as having a clock-face appearance (Fig 5–25).

Plasma cells are responsible for the synthesis of the antibodies found in the bloodstream. Antibodies are specific globulins produced by the organism in response to penetration by antigens. Each antibody is specific for the one antigen that gave rise to its production and reacts specifically with it, although it is possible for an antibody to cross-react with antigens possessing similar molecular configurations. The results of the antibody-antigen reaction are variable. Its capacity to neutralize harmful effects caused by antigens is important. When an antigen is a toxin (eg,

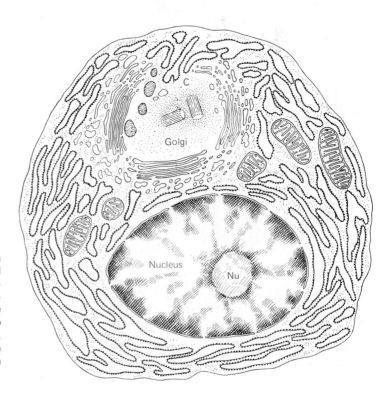

Figure 5–23. Ultrastructure of a plasma cell. The cell contains a well-developed rough endoplasmic reticulum, with dilated cisternae containing gamma globulins (antibodies). In plasma cells, the secreted proteins do not aggregate into secretory granules. Nu, nucleolus; C, centriole. (Redrawn and reproduced, with permission, from Ham AW: *Histology,* 6th ed. Lippincott, 1969.)

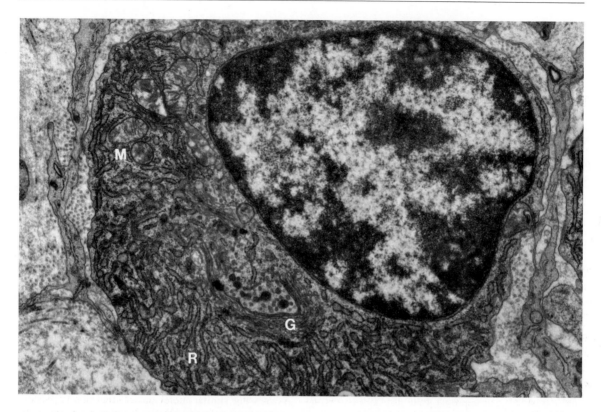

Figure 5–24. A plasma cell seen under the electron microscope. The micrograph shows the abundance of rough endoplasmic reticulum (R). Observe that many cisternae are dilated. M, mitochondria; G, Golgi complex. × 18,000.

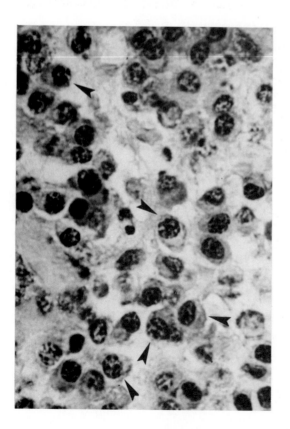

tetanus, diphtheria), it may lose its capacity to do harm when it combines with its respective antibody.

By means of immunofluorescence and cytochemical techniques, it has been demonstrated that after injection of an antigen, the corresponding antibody appears first in the cytoplasm of the plasma cell. Electron microscopic studies have shown that the first intracellular site in which antibodies appear is the cisternae of the rough endoplasmic reticulum.

Many of the antibodies synthesized by the plasma cells are specific for bacterial antigens and thus protect the body against these microorganisms. Since bacteria are never found inside plasma cells but rather are engulfed by the macrophages, it was thought that there was a mechanism by which the plasma cell ''learned'' about the nature of the bacterial antigens present in the macrophage. Although the process by which this information is transmitted has not been completely elucidated, electron microscopic studies have shown that cellular contact occurs between macrophages and

Figure 5–25 (at left). Photomicrograph of plasma cells (arrowheads). Observe the coarse chromatin and light juxtanuclear area corresponding to the region of the Golgi complex and centriole. Compare with Fig 5–23. × 600.

presumed precursor plasma cells (see Chapters 14 and 15). This suggests a transfer of information-bearing substances. It has also been demonstrated that extracts of macrophages which have phagocytized certain antigens are able to induce the appearance of plasma cells that form antibodies against these antigens (Fig 5–26).

Some antigens must establish contact with macrophages in order to stimulate the production of antibody-forming plasma cells. Other antigens act directly on plasma cell precursors (B lymphocytes). In such instances, the resulting plasma cells synthesize antibodies without assistance from macrophages.

Adipose Cells

Adipose cells (adipocytes) are connective tissue cells that have become specialized for storage of neutral fats or heat production. They are discussed in Chapter 6.

Leukocytes

Leukocytes, or white blood corpuscles, are frequently found in connective tissue. In general, they migrate across capillary and venule walls from the blood. There is a continuous movement of leukocytes from blood to connective tissue, and this process (diapedesis) increases greatly during inflammation. After having resided in connective tissue, these cells do not move back into the blood. In addition to the neutrophils, eosinophils, basophils, and lymphocytes are leukocytes frequently encountered in normal connective tissue.

A. Eosinophils: The main morphologic characteristics of eosinophils are the eosinophilic granules in their cytoplasm (lysosomes). Electron microscopic examination shows that these granules are membrane-bound and, in their interior, possess a flat crystalloid embedded in a granular substance. The nucleus of these cells usually has 2 lobes (Fig 5–27).

The number of eosinophils increases during the course of allergic and parasitic diseases as well as other types of disease.

The injection of antigenic protein causes an increase in the number of eosinophils in the injected area. This attraction is due to the complex formed by the reaction of the injected protein and its antibody. The antigen-antibody complex is promptly phagocytosed by eosinophils, although these cells are not very active in the phagocytosis of bacteria and foreign particles.

Substances secreted by eosinophils are involved in allergic reactions. Both mast cells and basophils release **eosinophil chemotactic factors** (ECF-A and ECF-C) that attract these cells to allergic inflammatory areas. Under these conditions, eosinophils release the enzymes **arylsulfatase** and **histaminase** (probably from their granules), which cleave 2 of the main mediators involved in the allergic reaction, ie, leukotriene C (formerly SRS-A) and histamine. Eosinophils thus can exert a negative feedback control in allergic processes not only by removing the antigen-antibody complexes through phagocytosis but also by hydrolyzing mediators.

B. Basophils: Basophils are a form of leukocyte

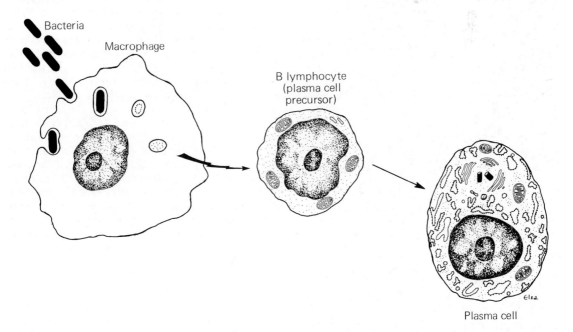

Figure 5–26. Possible relationships between macrophages and plasma cells. It has been shown that some kind of information passes from macrophages to plasma cell precursors.

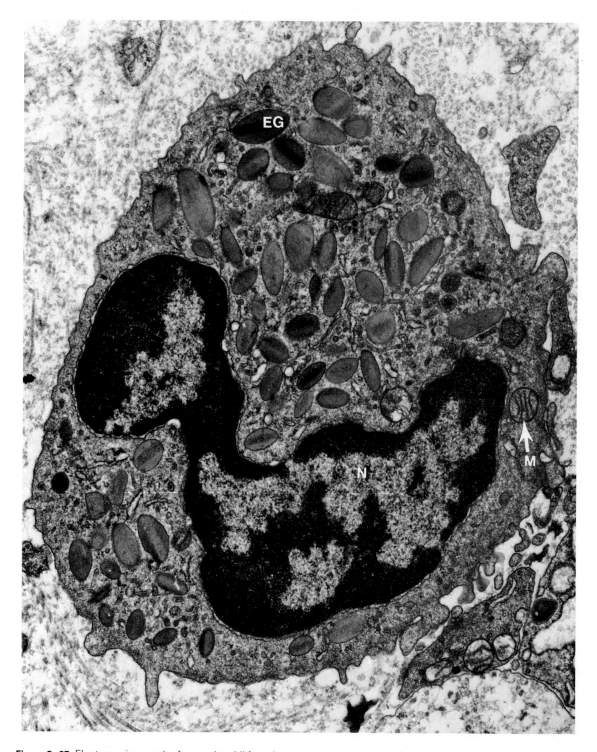

Figure 5–27. Electron micrograph of an eosinophil from human connective tissue. Typical eosinophilic granules are clearly seen. Each granule has a disk-shaped crystal that is electron-dense and appears surrounded by a matrix which is enveloped by a unit membrane. EG, eosinophil granule; N, nucleus; M, mitochondria. × 20,000.

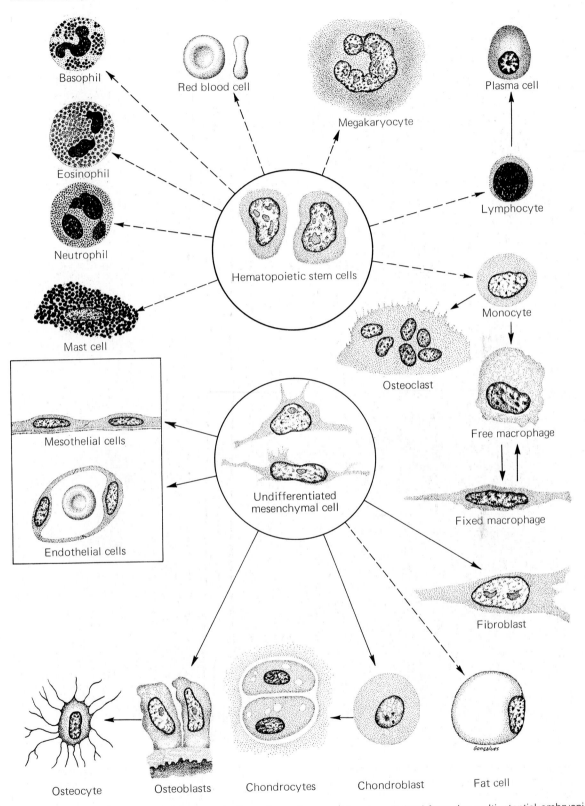

Basophil

Red blood cell

Megakaryocyte

Plasma cell

Eosinophil

Lymphocyte

Neutrophil

Hematopoietic stem cells

Monocyte

Mast cell

Osteoclast

Free macrophage

Mesothelial cells

Undifferentiated
mesenchymal cell

Fixed macrophage

Endothelial cells

Fibroblast

Osteocyte Osteoblasts Chondrocytes Chondroblast Fat cell

Figure 5–28. Simplified representation of the connective tissue cell lineages derived from the <u>multipotential embryonic mesenchyme cell.</u> Dotted arrows indicate that intermediate cell types exist between illustrated examples. The 2 cells in the rectangle are epithelial derivatives that still maintain some mesenchymal characteristics. Cells are not drawn in proportion to actual sizes (eg, adipocyte, megakaryocyte, and osteoclast cells are significantly larger than other illustrated cells).

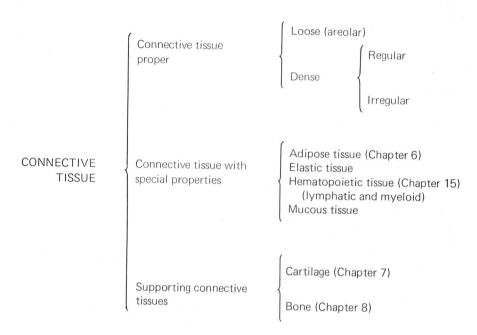

Figure 5–29. Simplified scheme classifying the principal types of connective tissue.

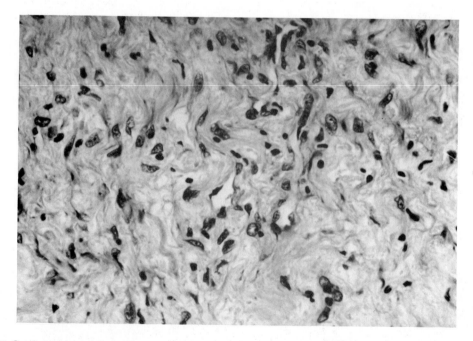

Figure 5–30. Section of loose connective tissue. Note the abundance of cells, most of which are fibroblasts, but macrophages and other types are also present. × 400.

that contains granules similar in composition and function to those of mast cells. Basophils are the only source of histamine in blood, and these cells also play a role in allergic phenomena. Blood from allergic individuals releases histamine when placed in contact with allergens.

C. Lymphocytes: Connective tissue lymphocytes have a diameter of 6–8 μm (small lymphocytes). They have a small amount of slightly basophilic cytoplasm and a large, dark nucleus with condensed chromatin that sometimes shows an indentation. The nucleolus is not visible under the light microscope.

The lymphocytes of connective tissue represent a heterogeneous population. Some have a long life span (many months to several years), whereas others live for only a short time (a few days or weeks). At least 2 functional types have been recognized: (1) the **T lymphocytes,** which are responsible for initiating cell-mediated immune responses and have a long life; and (2) the **B lymphocytes,** which, when stimulated by an antigen, divide several times and generate plasma cells that in turn secrete antibodies specific to the antigen. Plasma cells seldom divide, and they live for only 2–3 days.

The relationships among cells found in different types of connective tissue are shown in Fig 5–28. For further discussions of lymphocytes, see Chapters 13, 14, and 15.

TYPES OF CONNECTIVE TISSUE

There are several types of connective tissue that consist of the basic components already described—fibers, cells, and ground substance. The names given to the different types denote either the component that predominates in the tissue or a structural characteristic of the tissue.

The classification shown in Fig 5–29 does not include all possible types of connective tissue.

Connective Tissue Proper

There are 2 classes of connective tissue proper: loose and dense.

A. Loose Connective Tissue: This tissue, also called **areolar** tissue, is the more abundant of the 2 types. It fills spaces between fibers and muscle sheaths, supports epithelial tissue, and forms a layer that ensheathes the lymphatic and blood vessels. Loose connective tissue is also found in the papillary layer of the dermis, in the hypodermis, in the serosal linings of peritoneal and pleural cavities, and in glands and mucous membranes (wet membranes that line the hollow organs) supporting the epithelial cells.

Loose connective tissue is composed of all the main components of connective tissue proper (Fig 5–30). The most numerous cells are fibroblasts and macrophages, but all of the other types of connective tissue cells are present also. Collagen, elastic, and reticular fibers also appear in this tissue, though the proportion of reticular fibers is small. A major constituent of loose connective tissue is the amorphous ground substance.

Loose connective tissue has a delicate consistency; it is flexible, not very resistant to stress, and very well vascularized.

B. Dense Connective Tissue: This type of tissue is composed of the same components found in loose

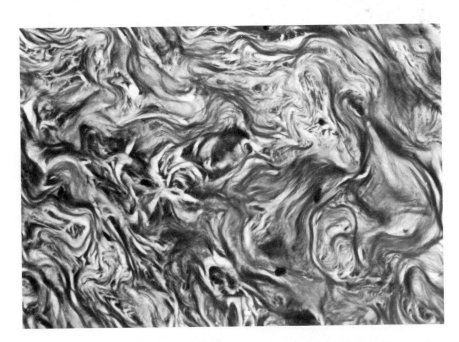

Figure 5–31. Dense irregular connective tissue. This tissue contains many randomly oriented large collagen fibers, sparse ground substance, and few cells. H&E stain, × 320.

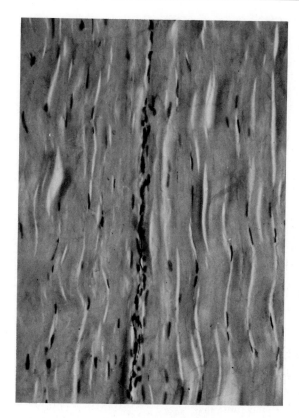

Figure 5–32. Dense regular connective tissue (longitudinal section through a tendon). There are numerous collagen bundles in parallel array. Fibrocyte nuclei are seen between the collagen bundles. H&E stain, × 320.

connective tissue, but there is a clear predominance of collagen fibers at the expense of the ground substance components. Histologic preparations reveal that this tissue has fewer cells than loose connective tissue. Fibroblasts are most common. Dense connective tissue is less flexible and far more resistant to stress. It is known as **dense irregular** connective tissue when the collagen fibers are arranged in bundles without a definite orientation. The collagen fibers form a 3-dimensional network in this tissue and provide resistance to stress from all directions (Fig 5–31). This type of tissue is encountered in the dermis of the skin, in the submucosa of the digestive tract, and in the connective tissue capsules around such organs as the spleen, lymph nodes, and liver.

The collagen bundles of **dense regular** connective tissue are arranged according to a definite pattern. The collagen fibers of this tissue are formed in response to prolonged stresses exerted in the same direction and consequently offer great resistance to traction forces.

Tendons are the most common example of dense regular connective tissue. They are elongated, cylindric structures that function to attach striated muscle to bone; they are white and inextensible by virtue of

their richness in collagen fibers. They have parallel, closely packed bundles of collagen separated by a small quantity of amorphous intercellular substance. Their fibrocytes contain elongated nuclei parallel to the fibers and a sparse cytoplasm that envelops portions of the collagen bundles. Their cytoplasm is rarely revealed in hematoxylin and eosin stains—not only because it is sparse but also because it stains the same color as the fibers (Figs 5–32 and 5–33).

The collagen bundles of the tendons (primary bundles) aggregate into larger bundles (secondary bundles) that are enveloped by loose connective tissue containing blood vessels and nerves. Externally, the tendon is surrounded by a sheath of dense connective tissue. In some tendons, this sheath is made up of 2 layers, both lined by squamous cells of mesenchymal origin. One layer is fixed to the tendon, and the other lines the neighboring structures. A cavity containing a viscous fluid (similar to synovial fluid) is formed between the 2 layers. This fluid, which contains water, proteins, glycosaminoglycans, and ions, is a lubricant that permits an easy sliding movement of the tendon within its sheath.

Elastic Tissue

Elastic tissue is composed of bundles of thick, parallel elastic fibers. Around each bundle there is a small amount of loose connective tissue, and flattened fibrocytes, similar to those of tendons, are found between the elastic fibers. The abundance of elastic fibers in this tissue confers on it a typical yellow color and great elasticity. Elastic tissue occurs infrequently. It is present in the yellow ligaments of the vertebral column and in the suspensory ligament of the penis.

Reticular Tissue

Reticular tissue is a specialized loose connective tissue variation that provides the architectural framework of the myeloid (bone marrow) and lymphoid (lymph nodules and nodes, spleen) hemopoietic organs. In this form of connective tissue, **reticular cells** elaborate a fine matrix of branched reticular fibers composed of type III collagen. Reticular cells are simply fibroblasts specialized for secreting the constituents of reticular fibers. The reticular cells are dispersed along this matrix and ensheathe the reticular fibers and ground substance with cytoplasmic processes (Fig 5–8). The resulting cell-lined trabecular system creates a spongelike matrix (Fig 5–34) within which cells and fluids of a given organ are readily mobile.

In addition to the reticular cells, cells of the mononuclear phagocyte system are also strategically dispersed along the trabeculae. These cells monitor the flow of materials through the sinuslike spaces and phagocytically remove antigens and other forms of cellular debris.

Mucous Tissue

Mucous tissue has an abundance of amorphous ground substance composed chiefly of hyaluronic acid.

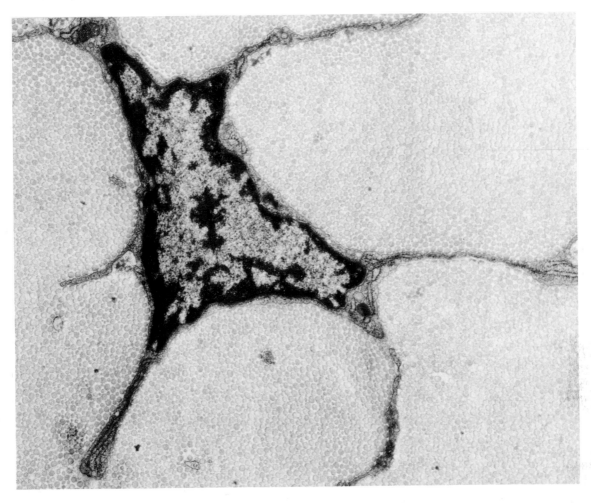

Figure 5–33. The cytoplasm of fibrocytes in dense regular connective tissue is rarely visualized. As this electron micrograph reveals, the sparse cytoplasm of the fibrocyte is subdivided into numerous thin cytoplasmic processes that interdigitate among the coarse collagen fibers. Note that the thick collagen fibers are composed of smaller, parallel collagen fibrils of variable diameter. × 25,000.

It is a jellylike tissue containing collagen fibers and a few elastic or reticular fibers. The cells in this tissue are mainly fibroblasts. Mucous tissue is the principal component of the umbilical cord, where it is referred to as Wharton's jelly. It is also found in the pulp of young teeth.

HISTOPHYSIOLOGY

Connective tissues have the functions of support, packing, storage, transport, defense, and repair. The functions of support and packing are obvious—epithelial, muscular, and nerve tissues are associated with connective tissue that supports and fills the tissue spaces between their cells. The support function is carried out mainly by connective tissue fibers.

Fibers, predominantly composed of collagen, constitute tendons, aponeuroses, capsules of organs, and membranes that envelop the central nervous system (meninges). They also make up the trabeculae and walls inside several organs, forming the most resistant component of the stroma (support tissue) of these organs.

Storage

Lipids, which are important nutritional reserves, are stored in adipose tissue (see Chapter 6). In addition, because of its richness in glycosaminoglycans, loose connective tissue stores water and electrolytes. The most abundant electrolyte is sodium. Although only a small percentage of connective tissue consists of plasma proteins, because of its wide distribution it is estimated that as much as one-third of the plasma proteins of the body are stored in the intercellular connective tissue matrix.

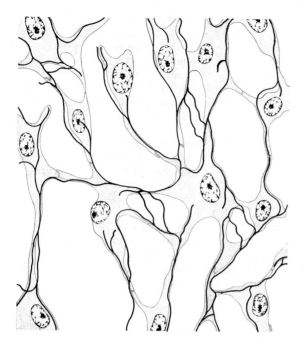

Figure 5–34. Schematic drawing of reticular connective tissue showing only the fixed cells and the fibers. Free cells are not represented. Reticular fibers are enveloped by the cytoplasm of reticular cells; however, the fibers are extracellular, being separated from the cytoplasm by the cell membrane. Within the sinuslike spaces, cells and tissue fluids of the organ are freely mobile.

Defense

Several defense mechanisms depend upon the cells and intercellular components of connective tissue. This tissue contains phagocytic cells (macrophages) and plasma cells, which synthesize antibodies. In addition, because of its viscosity, the intercellular substance acts as a barrier to penetration by bacteria and inert particles. Bacteria that produce **hyaluronidase** have great invasive power, for this enzyme hydrolyzes hyaluronic acid and other glycosaminoglycans of the connective tissue, thus reducing the viscosity of the intercellular substance and facilitating their invasion.

The diverse mechanisms that constitute the reaction known as **inflammation** take place principally in connective tissue. Inflammation is a vascular and cellular defensive reaction against foreign bodies. In most cases, it is a reaction against pathogenic bacteria or irritating chemical substances. The classic signs of inflammation were first enunciated by Celsus (first century AD) as redness and swelling with heat and pain *(rubor et tumor cum calore et dolore)*. Much later, disturbed function *(functio laesa)* was added as the fifth cardinal sign. Increased blood flow and capillary permeability due to the liberation of histamine by mast cells result in these signs. Edema is produced in this way, and an increase in the volume of bound water results in swelling of the inflamed area. This, in turn, causes pressure on nerves, resulting in pain and loss of function.

As a consequence of their motile behavior, leukocytes cross the walls of venules and capillaries, invading the inflamed area. This migration is called **diapedesis.**

During the initial or acute phase of inflammation, the neutrophils predominate; when the inflammation persists and enters the **chronic phase,** the cell population changes. The main types of cells in the chronic phase are lymphocytes and monocytes, which come from the blood, and plasma cells, which originate from B lymphocytes. Macrophages in the area of inflammation represent wandering connective tissue cells that have migrated to that site, or they may differentiate from monocytes that arrive via the circulation.

The cells in the inflamed area engulf the remains of cells and fibers altered by this process and participate in the production of antibodies against invading microorganisms. If the bacteria are not destroyed, surrounding connective tissue forms a retaining fibrous wall, or capsule, around the inflammation.

Repair

Connective tissue has great regenerative capacity, and the areas destroyed by inflammation or traumatic injury are easily repaired. The spaces left by injuries to tissues whose cells do not divide (eg, cardiac muscle) are filled by connective tissue, which forms a scar. The healing of surgical incisions depends on the reparative capacity of connective tissue.

Transport

There is a close association between blood capillaries, lymphatic capillaries, and connective tissue. These vessels, except in nerve tissue, are always ensheathed by connective tissue. Consequently, the connective tissue carries nutrients from the blood to various tissues in the body and moves metabolic wastes from the cells to the blood.

Hormonal Effects

Different hormones influence the metabolism of connective tissue. An example is the hormone **cortisol (hydrocortisone),** produced by the cortical layer of the adrenal gland, which inhibits the synthesis of fibers by connective tissue cells. **Adrenocorticotropic hormone (ACTH),** elaborated by the pituitary, which stimulates the production of cortisol, has the same effect. Injection of either cortisol or ACTH has a detrimental effect on wound healing. These hormones also suppress or attenuate the inflammatory process. Their action is also directed against the cells of the connective tissue (lymphocytes, plasma cells, etc).

Hypothyroidism causes an accumulation of glycosaminoglycans in connective tissues. Adult hypothyroidism is called **myxedema (mucous edema)** and is associated with an excess of glycosaminoglycans in the connective tissue.

Nutritional Factors

Vitamin C (ascorbic acid) deficiency leads to **scurvy,** a disease characterized by generalized degeneration of connective tissue. In the absence of this vitamin, fibroblasts synthesize defective collagen and the defective fibers are not replaced. Ascorbic acid is a cofactor for proline hydroxylase, which is essential for the normal synthesis of collagen. In this step of hydroxylation, iron, molecular oxygen, and α-ketoglutarate are also necessary. Changes in the concentration of these substances within the cell also influence the rate of collagen biosynthesis. The roles of vitamins A, C, and D in connective tissue are also discussed in Chapter 8.

Renewal of Collagen

Collagen is a stable protein, and its renewal is very slow. Its **turnover rate** is different in different anatomic structures. The collagen of tendons is renewed very slowly or not at all, whereas the collagen of loose connective tissue is renewed more rapidly.

In vitamin C deficiency, once collagen fibers are destroyed they are not replaced. This leads to a generalized degeneration of connective tissue that becomes more pronounced in areas where collagen renewal takes place at a faster rate. The periodontal ligament that holds teeth in their sockets exhibits a relatively high collagen turnover; consequently, this ligament is markedly affected by scurvy, which leads to a loss of teeth.

The physiologic degradation of collagen is initiated by collagenase, an enzyme produced by macrophages and neutrophils. This enzyme affects only collagen and not other proteins. It is active at the normal pH of the connective tissue (about 7.0). The existence of collagenase in mammals has recently been confirmed, although the fact of collagen removal has been known for some time. Some bacteria of the genus *Clostridium* that cause gas gangrene produce collagenase, which greatly increases the invasive power of these microorganisms.

REFERENCES

Cleary EG, Gibson MA: Elastin-associated microfibrils and microfibrillar proteins. *Int Rev Connect Tissue Res* 1983;**10**:97.

Cotta-Pereira G, Guerra Rodrigo F: Elastic system fibers and basement lamina. In: *Biology and Chemistry of Basement Membranes.* Kefalides N (editor). Academic Press, 1978.

Deyl Z, Adam M: *Connective Tissue Research: Chemistry, Biology and Physiology.* Riss, 1981.

Eyre DR: Collagen: Molecular diversity in the body's protein scaffold. *Science* 1980;**207**:1315.

Gay S, Miller EJ: *Collagen in the Physiology and Pathology of Connective Tissue.* Gustav Fischer, 1978.

Gray WR et al: Molecular model for elastin structure and function. *Nature* 1973;**246**:461.

Hay ED: Extracellular matrix. *J Cell Biol* 1981;**91**:205s.

Hay ED (editor): *Cell Biology of Extracellular Matrix.* Plenum, 1982.

Heathcote JG, Grant ME: The molecular organization of basement membranes. *Int Rev Connect Tissue Res* 1981;**9**:191.

Junqueira LCU, Montes GS: Biology of collagen proteoglycan interaction. *Arch Histol Jpn* 1983;**46**:589.

Kefalides NA, Alper R, Clark CC: Biochemistry and metabolism of basement membranes. *Int Rev Cytol* 1979;**61**:167.

Kitamura YK et al: Spleen colony-forming cells as common precursors for tissue mast cells and granulocytes. *Nature* 1981;**291**:159.

Kleinman HK, Klebe RJ, Martin GR: Role of collagenous matrices in the adhesion and growth of cells. *J Cell Biol* 1981; **88**:473.

Lagunoff D: Membrane fusion during mast cell secretion. *J Cell Biol* 1973;**57**:252.

Lindhal U, Hook M: Glycosaminoglycans and their binding to biological macromolecules. *Annu Rev Biochem* 1978;**47**:385.

Mathews MB: *Connective Tissue, Macromolecular Structure and Evolution.* Springer-Verlag, 1975.

Montes GS et al: Collagen distribution in tissues. In: *Ultrastructure of the Connective Tissue Matrix.* Ruggieri A, Motta PM (editors). Martinus Nijhoff, 1984.

Montes GS et al: Histochemical and morphological characterization of reticular fibers. *Histochemistry* 1980;**65**:131.

Page RC, Davies P, Allison AC: The macrophage as a secretory cell. *Int Rev Cytol* 1978;**52**:119.

Porter R (editor): Basement membranes and cell movement. Ciba Foundation Symposium No. 108. Pitman, 1984.

Prockop DJ et al: The biosynthesis of collagen and its disorders. *N Engl J Med* 1979;**301**:13.

Ruoslahti E et al: Fibronectin: Current concepts of its structure and functions. *Collagen Res* 1981;**1**:95.

Sandberg LB et al: Elastin structure, biosynthesis, and relation to disease state. *N Engl J Med* 1981;**304**:556.

Stanley JR et al: Structure and function of basement membrane. *J Invest Dermatol* 1982;**79**:69s.

Vander Rhee HJ et al: The differentiation of monocytes into macrophages, epithelioid cells and multinucleated giant cells in subcutaneous granulomas. 1. Fine structure. *Cell Tissue Res* 1979;**197**:355.

Van Furth R (editor): *Mononuclear Phagocytes: Functional Aspects.* 2 vols. Martinus Nijhoff, 1980.

Von der Mark K: Localization of collagen types in tissues. *Int Rev Connect Tissue Res* 1981;**9**:265.

6

Adipose Tissue

Adipose tissue is a special type of connective tissue in which adipose cells (**adipocytes**) predominate. These cells may be found either isolated or in small groups within connective tissue itself, but most are found in large aggregates making up the adipose tissue spread throughout the body. Adipose tissue is, in a sense, one of the largest organs in the body. In men of normal weight, adipose tissue represents 15–20% of the body weight; in women of normal weight, 20–25% of body weight.

Adipose tissue is the largest repository of energy (in the form of triglycerides) in the body. The other organs that store energy (in the form of glycogen) are the liver and skeletal muscle. Since eating is a periodic activity and the supply of glycogen is limited, there must be a large store of calories that can be mobilized between meals. Because triglycerides are of lower density than glycogen and have a higher caloric value (9.3 kcal/g for triglycerides versus 4.1 kcal/g for carbohydrates), adipose tissue is a very efficient storage tissue. It is in a state of continuous turnover and is sensitive to nervous and hormonal stimuli. Subcutaneous layers of adipose tissue help to shape the surface of the body, while deposits in the form of pads act as shock absorbers, chiefly in the soles and palms. Since fat is a poor heat conductor, it contributes to the thermal insulation of the body. Adipose tissue also fills up spaces between other tissues and helps to keep some organs in position.

Two types of adipose tissue are known to exist, characterized by the structure of their cells, localization, and color. **Common, yellow,** or **unilocular adipose tissue** is composed of cells which, when completely developed, contain one large central droplet of fat in their cytoplasm. **Brown,** or **multilocular, adipose tissue** is composed of cells containing numerous lipid droplets and mitochondria. Both types of adipose tissue have a rich blood supply.

UNILOCULAR ADIPOSE TISSUE

The color of unilocular adipose tissue varies from white to dark yellow, depending on the diet, and is mainly due to the presence of carotenoids dissolved in fat droplets of the cells. Almost all adipose tissue in adults is of this type. It is found throughout the human body except for the eyelids, the penis and scrotum, and all of the auricle of the external ear except the lobule. The distribution and density of adipose deposits are determined by age and sex.

In the newborn, unilocular adipose tissue has a uniform thickness throughout the body; with age, it tends to disappear from some parts of the body and increase in others, since its distribution is partly regulated by sex hormones and adrenocortical hormones, which control the accumulation of fat and are largely responsible for male or female body contour.

Histologic Structure of Unilocular Adipose Tissue

Unilocular adipose cells are spherical when isolated but are polyhedral in adipose tissue, where they are closely packed. Each cell is between 50 and 150 μm in diameter. Since lipid droplets are removed by the alcohol and xylol used in routine histologic techniques, in standard microscope preparations each cell appears as a thin ring of cytoplasm surrounding the vacuole left by the dissolved lipid droplet—the **signet ring cell.** Consequently, these cells have eccentric

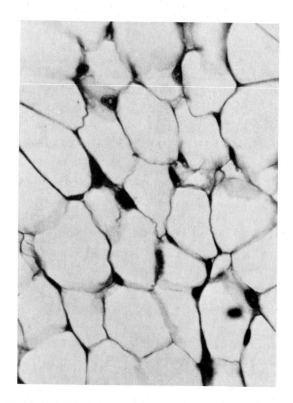

Figure 6–1. Photomicrograph of unilocular adipose tissue. H&E stain, × 320.

124

and flattened nuclei (Fig 6– 1). The rim of cytoplasm that remains after removal of the stored triglycerides (neutral fats) may rupture and collapse, distorting the tissue structure.

The thickest portion of the cytoplasm surrounds the nucleus of these cells and contains a Golgi complex, mitochondria of the filamentous and ovoid variety, poorly developed cisternae of rough endoplasmic reticulum, and free ribosomes. The rim of cytoplasm surrounding the lipid droplet contains vesicles of smooth endoplasmic reticulum, occasional microtubules, and numerous pinocytotic vesicles. Electron microscopic studies reveal that each adipose cell usually possesses minute lipid droplets other than the single large one seen with the light microscope. Lipid droplets are not surrounded by a membrane. Each adipose cell is surrounded by a basal lamina.

Unilocular adipose tissue is subdivided into incomplete lobules by a partition of connective tissue containing a rich vascular bed and network of nerves. Reticular fibers form a fine interwoven network that supports individual fat cells and binds them together.

Although blood vessels are not always apparent, adipose tissue is richly vascularized. Considering the amount of cytoplasm that exists in fat cells, the ratio of blood volume to volume of cytoplasm is greater in adipose tissue than in striated muscle.

Histophysiology of Unilocular Adipose Tissue

The lipids stored in adipose cells are chiefly triglycerides—ie, esters of fatty acids and glycerol. Fatty acids stored by these cells have their origin (1) in dietary fats that are brought to adipose tissue cells in the form of chylomicron triglycerides; (2) in triglycerides synthesized in the liver and transported to adipose tissue in the form of very low density lipoproteins (VLDL); and (3) by synthesis of free fatty acids and glycerol from glucose to form triglycerides in adipose cells.

Chylomicrons are particles up to 3 μm in diameter formed in intestinal epithelial cells and transported in blood plasma and mesenteric lymph. They consist of a central core composed mainly of triglycerides and

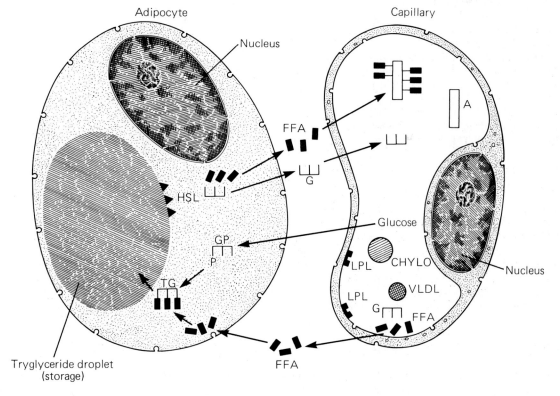

Figure 6–2. The process of lipid storage and release by the adipocyte. Triglycerides (TG) are transported in blood from the intestine and liver by lipoproteins known as chylomicrons (CHYLO) and very low density lipoproteins (VLDL). In adipose tissue capillaries, these lipoproteins are partially broken down by lipoprotein lipase (LPL), releasing free fatty acids (FFA) and glycerol (G). The free fatty acids diffuse from the capillary into the adipocyte, where they are reesterified to glycerol phosphate (GP). The resulting triglycerides are stored in droplets until needed. Norepinephrine activates hormone-sensitive lipase (HSL), which hydrolyzes stored triglycerides to free fatty acids and glycerol. These substances diffuse into the capillary, where free fatty acids are bound to albumin (A) for transport to distant sites for utilization as an energy source.

a small amount of cholesteryl esters surrounded by a stabilizing monolayer consisting of apolipoproteins, cholesterol, and phospholipids. **Very low density lipoproteins (VLDL)** have proportionately more lipid in their surface layer because they are smaller (greater surface-to-volume ratio), have different apolipoproteins at the surface, and contain a higher proportion of cholesteryl esters to triglycerides when compared with chylomicrons. Chylomicrons and VLDL are hydrolyzed at the luminal surfaces of blood capillaries of adipose tissue by lipoprotein lipase, an enzyme synthesized by the adipocyte and transferred to the capillary cell membrane. Free fatty acids enter the adipocyte by mechanisms that are not completely understood. An active transport system as well as free diffusion seems to be involved. It is probable that the numerous pinocytotic vesicles seen at the surfaces of adipocytes are not involved. Thus, the fatty acids cross the following layers in passing from the endothelium into the adipose cell: (1) capillary endothelium, (2) capillary basal lamina, (3) connective tissue ground substance, (4) adipocyte basal lamina, and (5) adipocyte plasma membrane. The movement of fatty acids across the cytoplasm into the lipid droplet is incompletely understood but may utilize specific carrier proteins (Fig 6–2). Within the adipocyte, the fatty acids combine with an intermediate product of glucose metabolism, glycerol phosphate, to form triglyceride molecules. These are then deposited in the triglyceride droplets. Mitochondria and smooth endoplasmic reticulum are organelles that are very active in the process of uptake and storage of lipids.

Adipose cells can synthesize fatty acids from glucose, a process accelerated by insulin. Insulin also stimulates the uptake of glucose into the adipose cells through an increase in the synthesis of lipoprotein lipase.

Stored lipids are mobilized by humoral and neurogenic mechanisms, resulting in the liberation of fatty acids and glycerol into the blood. An enzyme known as **hormone-sensitive lipase** (triglyceride lipase) is activated by adenylate cyclase when the tissue is stimulated by norepinephrine. Norepinephrine is liberated at the endings of the postganglionic sympathetic nerves present in adipose tissue. The activated enzyme breaks down triglyceride molecules located mainly at the surface of the lipid droplets. The relatively insoluble fatty acids are transported in association with serum albumin to other tissues of the body, while the more soluble glycerol remains free and is taken up by the liver.

Growth hormone, glucocorticoids, prolactin, corticotropin, insulin, and thyroid hormone also have roles in different steps in the metabolism of adipose tissue.

Under circumstances of bodily need, mobilization of lipids does not occur in uniform proportion in all parts of the body. Subcutaneous, mesenteric, and retroperitoneal deposits are the first to be mobilized, while adipose tissue in the hands, feet, and retroorbital fat pads resists long periods of starvation. After such periods, unilocular adipose tissue loses nearly all of its fat and becomes a tissue containing polyhedral or spindle-shaped cells with very few lipid droplets. These cells remain as quiescent adipocytes and do not modulate into fibroblasts or other types of connective tissue cells.

Both the brown and white types of adipose tissue are richly innervated by the sympathetic division of the autonomic nervous system. In white adipose tissue, nerve endings are found only in the walls of blood vessels; adipocytes are not directly innervated. Brown fat cells do receive direct sympathetic innervation. Release of the neurotransmitter (norepinephrine) activates the hormone-sensitive lipase described above. This innervation plays an important role in the mobilization of fats when the body is subjected to long periods of fasting or severe cold.

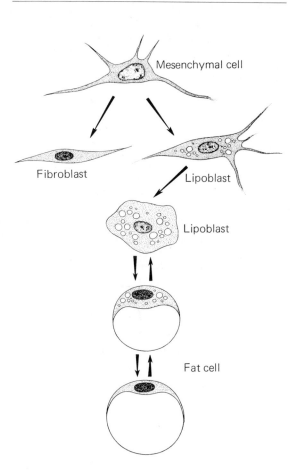

Figure 6–3. Development of unilocular fat cells. Undifferentiated mesenchymal cells are transformed into lipoblasts that accumulate fat and thus give rise to mature fat cells. When a large amount of lipids is mobilized by the body, mature fat cells return to the lipoblast stage. Undifferentiated mesenchymal cells also give rise to a variety of other cell types, including fibroblasts. The mature fat cell is in reality larger than shown here when compared with the other cell types of this illustration.

Histogenesis of Unilocular Adipose Tissue

Adipose cells develop from mesenchymally derived lipoblasts. These cells have the appearance of fibroblasts but are able to accumulate fat in their cytoplasm. The lipid droplets appear initially at one pole of the cell and then at the opposite pole. Lipid accumulations are at first isolated from one another but soon fuse to form the single larger droplet that is characteristic of unilocular tissue cells (Fig 6–3). When lipoblasts or adipose cells contain more than one lipid droplet, they are said to be in the multilocular stage.

The human being is one of the few mammals born with fat stores; they begin to accumulate at the 30th week of gestation. After birth, the development of new adipose cells is common mainly around small blood vessels, where undifferentiated mesenchymal cells are usually found.

It is now possible to estimate the size and number of adipose cells in the body by lipid analysis of a sample of adipose tissue (obtained by needle biopsy) for which a count of adipocytes has also been made. When these data are combined with a measure of total body fat, it is possible to estimate the total number of fat cells in the body as well as to determine the average lipid content per cell, which is a measure of its size. With these techniques, it has been determined that cells of adults of normal weight contain an average of 0.6 μg of lipid and that the average number of cells is 25×10^9. It is believed that during a finite postnatal period, nutritional and other influences can cause an increase in the number of adipocytes, but after that period the cells do not increase in number but only accumulate more lipid under conditions of excess caloric intake. This early increase in the number of adipocytes may predispose an individual to increased adiposity in later life.

MULTILOCULAR ADIPOSE TISSUE

Multilocular adipose tissue is also called **brown fat** because of its color, which is due to both the large number of blood capillaries in this tissue and the numerous mitochondria (containing colored cytochromes) in the cells. Unlike unilocular tissue, which is present throughout the body, brown adipose tissue has a more limited distribution. It is common in hibernating animals and is improperly called the hibernating gland.

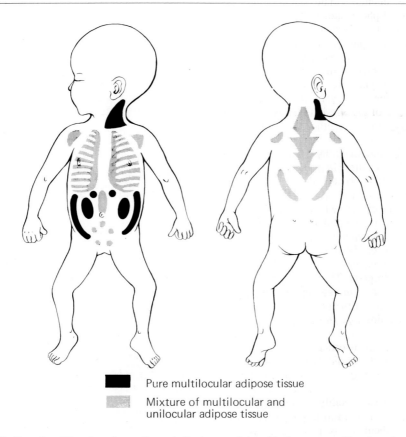

■ Pure multilocular adipose tissue

▨ Mixture of multilocular and unilocular adipose tissue

Figure 6–4. Distribution of multilocular adipose tissue in the human fetus. Black areas: multilocular adipose tissue. Shaded areas: mixture of multilocular and unilocular adipose tissue. (Modified, redrawn, and reproduced, with permission, from Merklin RJ: Growth and distribution of human fetal brown fat. *Anat Rec* 1974;**178**:637.)

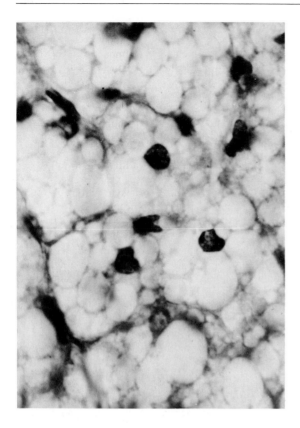

Figure 6–5. Photomicrograph of multilocular adipose tissue with its characteristic cells containing central spherical nuclei and multiple lipid droplets. × 1000.

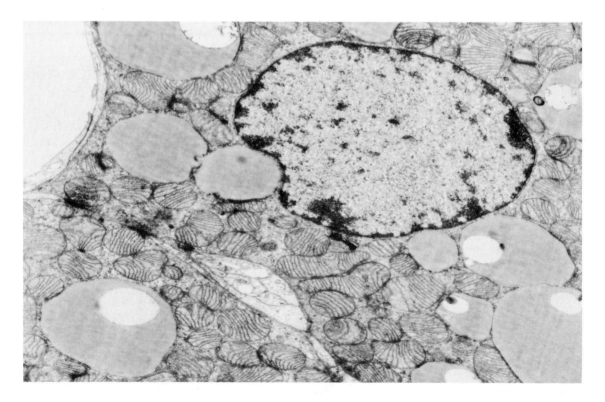

Figure 6–6. Electron micrograph of multilocular adipose tissue. Observe the central nucleus, multiple fat droplets, and abundant mitochondria. × 10,000.

In rats and several other mammals, this tissue is found mainly about the shoulder girdle. In the human embryo and the newborn, multilocular adipose tissue is encountered in several areas and remains restricted to these locations after birth (Fig 6–4). It is greatly reduced in adulthood. The function of this tissue in humans appears to be of importance mainly in the first months of postnatal life, when it produces heat and thus protects the newborn against cold.

Histologic Structure of Multilocular Adipose Tissue

Multilocular tissue cells are polygonal and smaller than cells of unilocular adipose tissue. Their cytoplasm contains a great number of lipid droplets of different sizes (Figs 6–5 and 6–6), a spherical and central nucleus, and numerous mitochondria with abundant long cristae. Endoplasmic reticulum is not abundant.

Brown adipose tissue resembles an endocrine gland in that its cells assume an almost epithelial arrangement of closely packed masses associated with blood capillaries. This tissue is subdivided by partitions of connective tissue into lobules that are better delineated than in unilocular adipose tissue lobules.

Histophysiology of Multilocular Adipose Tissue

The physiology of multilocular adipose tissue is understood best in the study of hibernating species.

In animals ending their hibernation period, or when newborn mammals (including humans) are exposed to a cold environment, nerve impulses liberate norepinephrine into the tissue. This neurotransmitter activates the hormone-sensitive lipase present in adipose cells, promoting hydrolysis of triglycerides to fatty acids and glycerol. Oxygen consumption and liberation of heat are increased, elevating the temperature of the tissue and warming the blood passing through it. Heat production is increased, because when stimulated, the mitochondria of multilocular adipose cells can uncouple their process of oxidative phosphorylation; consequently, no ATP is synthesized and all of the chemical energy liberated from the electron transport chain is dissipated as heat. Under unstimulated conditions, these mitochondria can recouple their oxidative phosphorylation and function normally. Warmed blood circulates throughout, heating the body and carrying fatty acids not metabolized in the adipose tissue, which will be utilized by other organs.

Histogenesis of Multilocular Adipose Tissue

Multilocular adipose tissue develops differently from unilocular tissue. The mesenchymal cells that constitute the brown tissue resemble epithelium, suggesting an endocrine gland, before they accumulate fat. Apparently there is no formation of brown adipose tissue after birth, nor is one type of adipose tissue transformed into another.

REFERENCES

Angel A, Hollenberg CH, Roncari DAK (editors): *The Adipocyte and Obesity: Cellular and Molecular Mechanisms*. Raven Press, 1983.

Bonnet FP (editor): *Adipose Tissue in Childhood*. CRC Press, 1981.

Hull D: The structure and function of brown adipose tissue. *Br Med Bull* 1965;**22:**92.

Imaizumi M: On the fine structure of the surface of lipid droplets in adipose cells. *Arch Histol Jpn* 1969;**30:**353.

Lindberg O: *Brown Adipose Tissue*. American Elsevier, 1970.

Lindberg O et al: Studies of the mitochondrial energy transfer system of brown adipose tissue. *J Cell Biol* 1967;**34:**293.

Napolitano L: The differentiation of white adipose cells: An electron microscope study. *J Cell Biol* 1963;**18:**663.

Nedergaard J, Lindberg O: The brown fat cell. *Int Rev Cytol* 1982;**74:**310.

Renold AE, Cahill GF Jr (editors): *Handbook of Physiology*. Section 5: *Adipose Tissue*. American Physiological Society, 1965.

Slavin BG: The cytophysiology of mammalian adipose cells. *Int Rev Cytol* 1972;**33:**297.

Smith RE, Horwitz BA: Brown fat and thermogenesis. *Physiol Rev* 1969;**49:**330.

7

Cartilage

Cartilage is a specialized form of connective tissue in which the extracellular matrix has a firm consistency. This matrix endows cartilage with the resilience that allows the tissue to bear mechanical stresses without distortion. The main functions of cartilage are to support soft tissues and, by virtue of its smooth surface, to provide a sliding area for joints, thus facilitating bone movements. Cartilage is also essential for the development and growth of long bones both before and after birth (see Chapter 8).

As is characteristic of other connective tissues, cartilage consists of cells **(chondrocytes)** and an extensive **extracellular matrix** composed of fibers and ground substance. Chondrocytes synthesize and secrete the extracellular matrix and become surrounded by its components. Cartilage cells occupy a potential space, or **lacuna**, which can be observed only upon the death or shrinkage of the cell. Collagen, hyaluronic acid, proteoglycans, and small amounts of several glycoproteins are the principal macromolecules present in all types of cartilage matrix. Elastic cartilage, characterized by its great pliability, contains significant amounts of elastin in the matrix.

Since collagen and elastin are flexible, the firm, gel-like consistency of cartilage depends upon (1) electrostatic bonds that occur between collagen fibers and the glycosaminoglycan side chains of matrix proteoglycans, and (2) binding of water (solvation water) to negatively charged glycosaminoglycan chains that extend from the proteoglycan core proteins. An example of the importance of matrix proteoglycans is observed after intravenous injection of papain in rabbits. Within hours after the injection of this protease, the cartilages supporting the ears of these animals lose their turgidity and the ears droop (Fig 7–1, inset). The loss of turgidity is due to digestion of proteoglycan

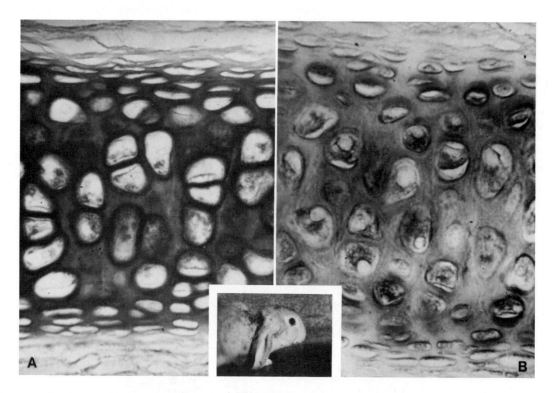

Figure 7–1. Sections of rabbit ear cartilage with its proteoglycan stained by alcian blue. *A* presents a section from a control animal, whereas *B* is from an animal previously injected intravenously with papain, an enzyme that hydrolyzes the proteoglycan moiety of the cartilage matrix. Observe the decrease of proteoglycan content in the cartilage of the injected animal (less intense staining by alcian blue). The inset shows the collapsed ear of the papain-injected animal. This experiment dramatically illustrates the functional role of proteoglycans in cartilage matrix. × 600.

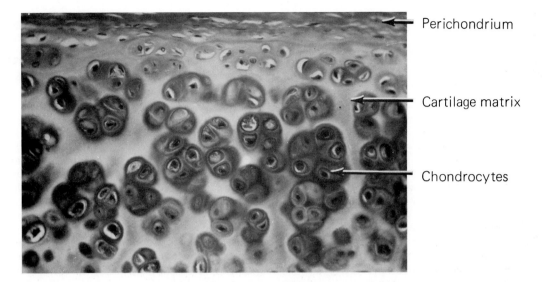

Perichondrium

Cartilage matrix

Chondrocytes

Figure 7–2. Photomicrograph of hyaline cartilage. Most chondrocytes are organized in isogenous groups. An enriched concentration of glycosaminoglycans in the matrix—the capsular, or territorial, matrix—is present around the chondrocytes. The upper part of the figure shows the perichondrium where fibroblasts may differentiate into chondrocytes during cartilage growth. H&E stain, × 300.

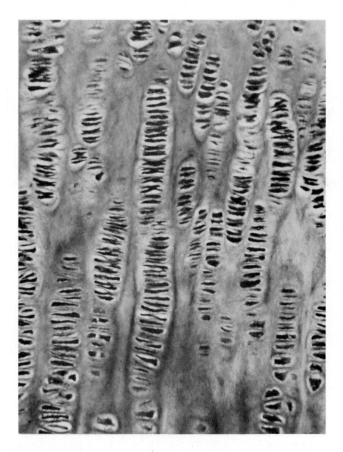

Figure 7–3. Photomicrograph of a portion of the epiphyseal plate cartilage. As illustrated, large numbers of chondrocytes in the proliferative zone of this cartilage are arranged side by side in parallel columns. H&E stain, × 320.

core proteins and the consequent dissolution of glycosaminoglycan side chains (Fig 7–1).

As a consequence of different functional requirements, 3 forms of cartilage have evolved, each exhibiting variations in matrix composition. **Hyaline cartilage,** the most common form, possesses a matrix containing collagen type II as the principal collagen type. The more pliable and distensible **elastic cartilage** possesses, in addition to collagen type II, an abundance of elastic fibers within its matrix. **Fibrocartilage,** present in regions of the body subject to great stress or the demands of weight bearing, is characterized by a matrix containing a dense network of coarse collagen type I fibers.

In all 3 types, cartilage is avascular and is nourished by diffusion of nutrients from capillaries in adjacent connective tissue (perichondrium) or by means of synovial fluid from joint cavities. In some instances, blood vessels traverse a cartilage to nourish other tissues, but these vessels do not supply nutrients to the cartilage. As might be expected of cells in an avascular tissue, chondrocytes exhibit low metabolic activity. Cartilage has no lymphatic vessels or nerves.

The **perichondrium** (Figs 7–2 and 7–5) is a capsulelike sheath of dense connective tissue that surrounds cartilage in most places, forming an interface between the cartilage and the tissue the cartilage serves to support. The perichondrium harbors the vascular supply for the avascular cartilage. Articular cartilage, which covers the surfaces of the bones of movable joints, is notably devoid of perichondrium and is sustained by the diffusion of oxygen and nutrients from the synovial fluid.

HYALINE CARTILAGE

Hyaline cartilage (Fig 7–2) is the most common and best studied of the 3 types. Most experimental data on cartilage have been obtained from studies of hyaline cartilage, but the findings are most likely applicable to the other types as well.

Fresh hyaline cartilage is bluish-white and translucent. In the embryo, it serves as a temporary skeleton until it is replaced gradually by bone. Between the diaphysis and the epiphysis of growing long bones, the **epiphyseal plate,** composed of hyaline cartilage, is responsible for the longitudinal growth of bone (Fig 7–3).

In adult mammals, hyaline cartilage is located in the articular surfaces of movable joints; the walls of larger respiratory passages (nose, larynx, trachea, bronchi); and the ventral ends of ribs, where they articulate with the sternum.

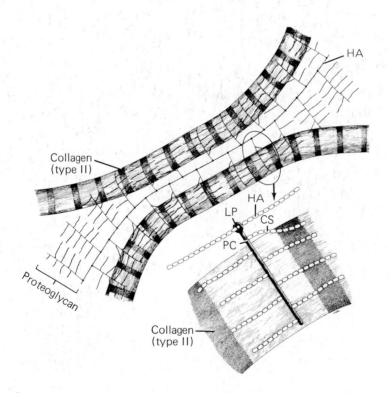

Collagen (type II)

Proteoglycan

HA

HA
LP
CS
PC

Collagen (type II)

Figure 7–4. Schematic representation of proposed molecular organization in cartilage matrix. Linking proteins (LP) covalently bind the protein core (PC) of proteoglycans to the linear hyaluronic acid (HA) molecules. The chondroitin sulfate (CS) side chains of the proteoglycan electrostatically bind to the collagen fibrils, forming a cross-linked matrix. The oval outlines an area enlarged in the lower part of the figure.

Matrix

Forty percent of the dry weight of hyaline cartilage consists of collagen embedded in an amorphous intercellular substance. In routine histologic preparations, the collagen is indiscernible from the amorphous substance for 2 reasons: (1) the collagen is in the form of fibrils, which have submicroscopic dimensions; and (2) the refractive index of the fibrils is almost the same as that of the ground substance in which they are embedded.

Electron micrographs show that collagen fibrils, finer than those in other forms of connective tissue, are the dominant component of the matrix. These fibrils have a 64-nm periodicity similar to that of typical connective tissue collagen. Although hyaline cartilage fibrils have a 64-nm periodicity, this is not clearly seen in most fibrils from routine sections, for it is masked by its interaction with the proteoglycans (Fig 7–4). Variations in the assembly and appearance of cartilage collagen reflect its chemical composition. Hyaline cartilage contains primarily type II collagen consisting of 3 alpha 1 type II chains ([α1(II)]$_3$). This type of collagen differs from type I collagen in that

Table 7–1. Approximate composition of cartilage proteoglycans (average molecular weight = 2.5×10^6).*

Component	Number of Chains	Molecular Weight	Percent of Dry Weight
Core protein	1	200,000–350,000	7–12
Chondroitin sulfates	100	20,000	85
Keratan sulfate	50	5000	7

*Modified and reproduced, with permission, from Hardingham TE: Structure and associations of proteoglycans in cartilage. In: Arnott S, Rees DA, Morris ER: *Molecular Biophysics of the Extracellular Matrix.* Humana Press, 1984.

it possesses higher levels of hydroxylysine, increasing the hydrophilia of its matrix.

In cartilage, proteoglycans are composed of chondroitin 4-sulfate, chondroitin 6-sulfate, and keratan sulfate, covalently linked to core proteins (Table 7–1). Up to 200 of these proteoglycans are noncovalently associated with long molecules of hyaluronic acid, forming **proteoglycan aggregates** that interact with collagen (Fig 7–4). Structurally, proteoglycans re-

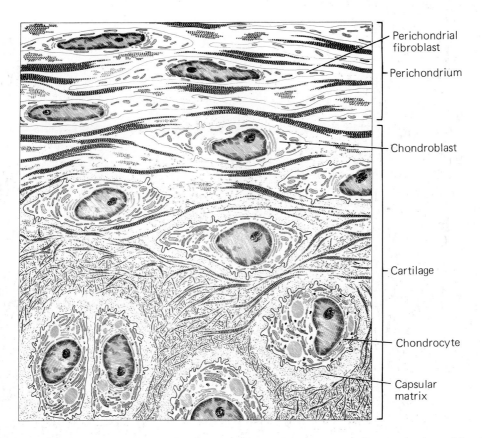

Figure 7–5. Diagram of the area of transition between the perichondrium and hyaline cartilage. As perichondrial cells differentiate into chondrocytes, they become round, with an irregular surface. Cartilage matrix contains numerous fine collagen fibrils except around the periphery of the chondrocytes, where the matrix primarily consists of glycosaminoglycans; this region is called the capsular, or territorial, matrix.

semble bottle brushes, the protein core being the backbone and the radiating glycosaminoglycan chains the bristles. The aggregates may be up to 4 μm in length and have a mass of 350×10^6 daltons.

The relative proportions of collagen, hyaluronic acid, and sulfated proteoglycans and the disposition of collagen fibrils in the matrix vary with anatomic site and age. The high content of solvation water bound to the negative charges of glycosaminoglycans acts as a shock absorber or biomechanical spring that is of great functional importance, especially in articular cartilages.

Within the cartilage matrix, immediately surrounding each chondrocyte, is a zone of glycosaminoglycan-rich, collagen-poor matrix. This peripheral

zone, called the **capsular,** or **territorial, matrix,** histochemically exhibits an intense basophilia, metachromasia, and greater PAS positivity than other portions of the **interterritorial matrix** (Figs 7–2 and 7–5).

Perichondrium

Except in articular cartilage of joints, all hyaline cartilage is covered by a layer of dense connective tissue, the perichondrium, which is essential for the growth and maintenance of cartilage (Figs 7–2 and 7–5). It is rich in collagen (type I) fibers and contains numerous fibroblasts. Some of the cells in the inner layer of the perichondrium resemble fibroblasts, but they have the capacity to differentiate into chondro-

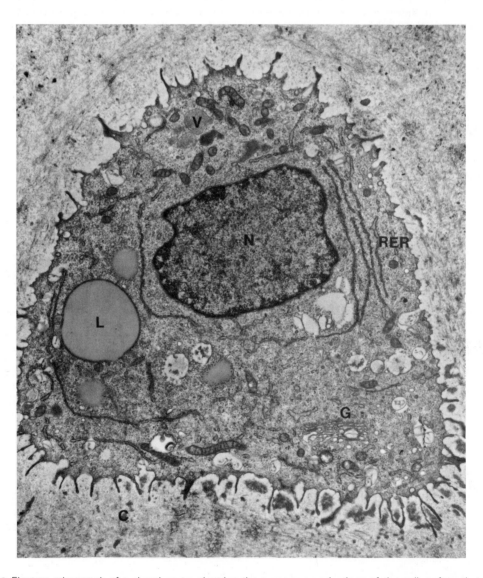

Figure 7–6. Electron micrograph of a chondrocyte, showing the numerous projections of the cell surface that facilitate metabolic exchanges. The large vacuoles (V) contain procollagen and glycosaminoglycans that will be released into the extracellular matrix. Note the long cisternae of rough endoplasmic reticulum (RER) and the Golgi complex (G), characteristic features of glycoprotein secreting cells. L, lipid droplet; N, nucleus. × 10,710. (Courtesy of C Basbaum.)

blasts. For this reason, the inner cells are better thought of as undifferentiated mesenchymal cells.

Chondrocytes

At the periphery of hyaline cartilage, young chondrocytes have an elliptic shape, with the long axis parallel to the surface. Farther in, they are round, 10–30 μm in diameter, and may appear in groups (Fig 7–2) of up to 8 cells originating from mitotic divisions of a single chondrocyte. These groups are designated **isogenous groups.** In epiphyseal plate cartilage, the proliferating chondrocytes are accumulated in rows (Fig 7–3).

Cartilage cells and the matrix shrink during histologic preparation, causing the irregular shape of the chondrocytes and their retraction from the capsule. In living tissue, the chondrocytes or groups of chondrocytes fill the lacunae completely. Upon examination with the light microscope, their surface appears smooth, but the electron microscope reveals indentations and protrusions, larger and more frequent in young chondrocytes (Fig 7–6). These structural characteristics increase their surface area, facilitating exchange with the extracellular medium; this has an important function in maintaining nutrition of these cells, since they are located at a distance from the bloodstream.

Mature chondrocytes have organelles typical of protein secretory cells—an elaborate rough endoplasmic reticulum and well-developed Golgi complex (Figs 7–6 and 7–9). Large accumulations of glycogen and lipid vesicles are characteristic of mature chondrocytes and reflect their metabolic activity as influenced by their long distance from the nourishing bloodstream. The chondrocyte is a cell that synthesizes large amounts of glycosaminoglycans and type II collagen (α1[II])$_3$.

In growing cartilage, studies using injection of ^{35}S in the form of sulfate, which is incorporated into the sulfated glycosaminoglycans, revealed that radioactivity appeared first in the cytoplasm of the chondrocytes and afterward in the intercellular substance. Synthesis and sulfation of the glycosaminoglycans take place in the Golgi complex. Additionally, the core protein synthesized in the rough endoplasmic reticulum combines here with the repeated units of glycosaminoglycans to form the proteoglycans. Radioautographic studies of collagen synthesis with the electron microscope after ^{3}H-proline administration demonstrated that radioactivity appeared first in the rough endoplasmic reticulum, then in the Golgi complex, and finally in the intercellular substance. In other words, there is evidence that chondrocytes can synthesize all of the macromolecular components of cartilage matrix. One cell apparently can simultaneously synthesize proteoglycans and collagen.

Histophysiology

Since cartilage is devoid of blood capillaries, chondrocytes respire under low oxygen tension. Hya-

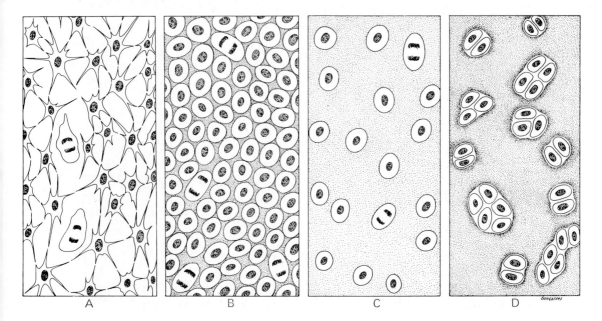

Figure 7–7. Histogenesis of hyaline cartilage. *A:* The mesenchyme, which is the precursor tissue of all types of cartilage. *B:* Mitotic proliferation of mesenchymal cell gives rise to a very cellular tissue. *C:* Rounded cells are separated from one another by the formation of a great amount of matrix. *D:* Multiplication of cartilage cells gives rise to isogenous groups that are surrounded by a condensation of the matrix (capsule).

line cartilage cells metabolize glucose mainly by anaerobic glycolysis to produce lactic acid as the end product. Nutrients from the blood diffuse from the perichondrium to the more deeply placed chondrocytes. Because of this, the maximum width of the cartilage is limited. The nutrients diffuse through the solvation water of the matrix. There is almost no free water in cartilage matrix.

Chondrocyte function depends on a proper hormonal balance. The synthesis of sulfated glycosaminoglycans is accelerated by growth hormone, thyroxine, and testosterone. It is retarded by cortisone, hydrocortisone, and estradiol.

Histogenesis

Cartilage derives from the mesenchyme (Fig 7–7). The first modification observed is the rounding up of the mesenchymal cells, which retract their protoplasmic extensions, multiply rapidly, and form mesenchymal condensations. The cells formed by this direct differentiation of mesenchymal cells, now called **chondroblasts,** have a ribosome-rich basophilic cytoplasm. Synthesis and deposition of the matrix then begin to separate the chondroblasts from one another. The differentiation of cartilage takes place from the center outward; therefore, the more central cells have characteristics of chondrocytes while the peripheral cells are typical chondroblasts. The superficial mesenchyme develops into fibroblasts of the perichondrium.

Growth

The growth of cartilage is attributable to 2 processes: **interstitial growth,** due to mitotic division of preexisting chondrocytes; and **appositional growth,** due to the differentiation of perichondrial cells. In both cases, newly formed chondrocytes synthesize collagen fibrils and ground substance. Real growth is thus much greater than that due to the simple increase in the number of cells. Interstitial growth is the less important of the 2 processes and occurs only during the early phases of cartilage formation when it increases tissue mass by expanding the cartilage matrix from within. Interstitial growth also occurs in the epiphyseal plates of long bones and within articular cartilage. In the epiphyseal plates, interstitial growth is important in increasing the length of long bones and in providing a cartilage model for endochondral bone formation (see Chapter 8). In articular cartilage, as cells and matrix near the articulating surface are gradually worn away, the cartilage must be replaced from within, since there is no perichondrium here to add cells by apposition. In cartilage found elsewhere in the body, as the matrix becomes increasingly rigid because of cross-linking of matrix components, interstitial growth becomes less pronounced. Cartilage then grows in girth only by apposition. Cells of the perichondrium adjacent to the cartilage multiply and differentiate into chondroblasts, which become chondrocytes once they have surrounded themselves with cartilaginous matrix and are incorporated into the existing cartilage (Figs 7–2 and 7–5).

Regressive Changes

In contrast to other tissues, hyaline cartilage is frequently subjected to degenerative processes. The most common is calcification of the matrix, and this is preceded by an increase in the size and volume of the cells followed by their death. Although calcification is a regressive alteration, it occurs normally in certain cartilages, providing a model for bone development. (See Endochondral Ossification, Chapter 8.)

Regeneration

Except in young children, damaged cartilage regenerates with difficulty and often incompletely. In adults, regeneration occurs because of the activity of the perichondrium. When cartilage fractures, cells from the perichondrium invade the fractured area and generate new cartilage. In extensively damaged areas (and occasionally in small areas), the perichondrium, instead of forming new cartilage, generates a scar of dense connective tissue.

ELASTIC CARTILAGE

Elastic cartilage is found in the auricle of the ear, in the walls of the external auditory canals, in the auditory (eustachian) tubes and epiglottis, and in the cuneiform cartilage in the larynx.

Basically, elastic cartilage is identical to hyaline cartilage except that in addition to collagen type II

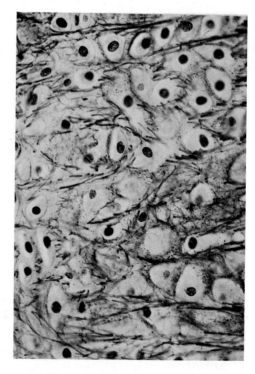

Figure 7–8. Photomicrograph of elastic cartilage. Weigert staining method for elastic fibers. × 350.

fibrils, it contains an abundant network of fine elastic fibers. Fresh elastic cartilage has a yellowish color caused by the presence of elastin in the elastic fibers, which may be demonstrated by standard elastin stains (eg, orcein) (Fig 7–8).

Elastic cartilage may be present by itself or in combination with hyaline cartilage. Because the chondrocytes of elastic and hyaline cartilage tissues are very similar, elastic cartilage is frequently found to be gradually continuous with hyaline cartilage. As with hyaline cartilage, elastic cartilage possesses a less susceptible to degenerative processes than hyaline cartilage.

FIBROCARTILAGE

Fibrocartilage is a tissue with characteristics intermediate between those of dense connective tissue and hyaline cartilage. It is found in intervertebral disks, in attachments of certain ligaments to bones, and in the symphysis pubica. Fibrocartilage is always associated with dense connective tissue, and the border areas between these 2 tissues are not clear-cut but show a gradual transition.

Fibrocartilage contains chondrocytes similar to those of hyaline cartilage, either singly or in isogenous groups (Fig 7–9). Very often, the chondrocytes are arranged in long columns. Fibrocartilage matrix is acidophilic because it contains a great number of coarse type I collagen fibers, which are easily seen under the light microscope (Fig 7–10). The amorphous matrix is less abundant in this type of cartilage and contains equal amounts of chondroitin sulfate and dermatan sulfate.

In fibrocartilage, the numerous collagenous fibers either form irregular bundles between the groups of chondrocytes or are aligned in a parallel arrangement along the columns of chondrocytes (Fig 7–10). This orientation depends upon the stresses acting on fibrocartilage, since the collagenous bundles take up a direction parallel to those stresses. There is no identifiable perichondrium in fibrocartilage.

Fibrocartilage develops from dense connective tissue by means of differentiation of fibroblasts into chondrocytes.

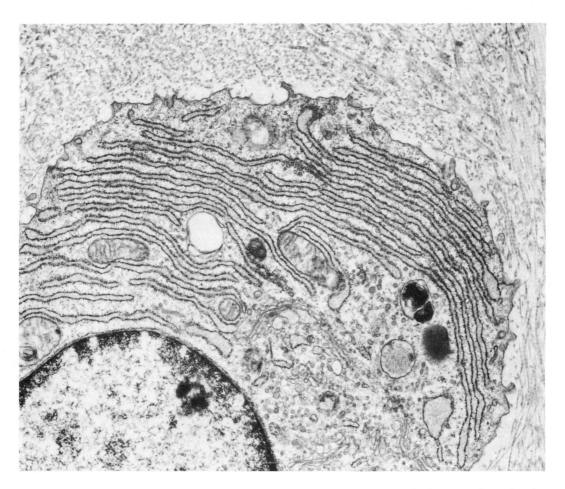

Figure 7–9. Electron micrograph of fibrocartilage. Observe the densely packed collagen fibrils surrounding a chondrocyte. × 20,000.

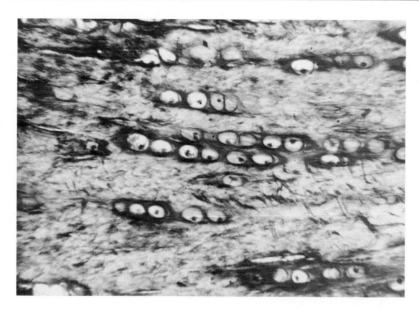

Figure 7–10. Photomicrograph of fibrocartilage. Observe columns of chondrocytes separated by collagen fibers. Picro-Sirius–hematoxylin, × 500.

INTERVERTEBRAL DISKS

Each intervertebral disk is situated between 2 vertebrae and held to them by means of ligaments. The disks have 2 components: the cartilaginous annulus fibrosus and the liquid nucleus pulposus.

The **annulus fibrosus** has an external layer of dense connective tissue, but it is mainly composed of overlapping laminae of fibrocartilage in which collagenous bundles are orthogonally arranged in adjacent layers. The multiple lamellae, with the 90-degree registration of collagen fibers in adjacent layers, provide the disk with an unusual resilience that enables it to withstand the pressures generated by impinging vertebrae. In tangential section, the disk presents a characteristic herringbone pattern as a result of the orthogonal alignment of collagen in alternating lamellae.

The **nucleus pulposus** is situated in the center of the annulus fibrosus. It is derived from the notochord and consists of a few rounded cells embedded in an amorphous viscous fluid rich in hyaluronic acid. In children, the nucleus pulposus is large, but with age it gradually becomes smaller and is partially replaced by fibrocartilage.

Herniation of the Intervertebral Disk

The intervertebral disk acts as a lubricated cushion that prevents adjacent vertebrae from being eroded by abrasive forces during movement of the spinal column. The liquid nucleus pulposus serves as a shock absorber to cushion the impact between adjacent vertebrae. Rupture of the annulus fibrosus, which most frequently occurs in the posterior region where there are fewer collagenous bundles, results in expulsion of the liquid nucleus pulposus and a concomitant flattening of the disk. As a consequence, the disk frequently dislocates or "slips" from its position between the vertebrae. If it moves toward the spinal cord, it can compress the nerves and result in severe pain and neurologic disturbances. The pain accompanying a slipped disk may be perceived in areas innervated by the compressed nerve fibers—usually the lower lumbar region.

REFERENCES

Anderson DR: The ultrastructure of elastic and hyaline cartilage in the rat. *Am J Anat* 1964;**114**:403.

Chakrabarti B, Park JW: Glycosaminoglycans: Structure and interaction. *CRC Crit Rev Biochem* 1980;**8**:225.

Eyre DR, Muir H: The distribution of different molecular species of collagen in fibrous, elastic and hyaline cartilages of the pig. *Biochem J* 1975;**151**:595.

Godman GC, Lane N: On the site of sulfation in the chondrocyte. *J Cell Biol* 1964;**21**:353.

Hall BK (editor): *Cartilage*. Vol 1: *Structure, Function, and Biochemistry*. Academic Press, 1983.

Junqueira LCU et al: Quantitation of collagen-proteoglycan interaction in tissue sections. *Connect Tissue Res* 1980;**7**:91.

Lindahl U, Höök M: Glycosaminoglycans and their binding to biological macromolecules. *Annu Rev Biochem* 1978;**47**:385.

Minns RJ, Stevens FS: The collagen fibril organization in human articular cartilage. *J Anat* 1977;**123**:437.

Revel JP, Hay ED: An autoradiographic and electron microscopic study of collagen synthesis in differentiating cartilage. *Z Zellforsch Mikrosk Anat* 1963;**61**:110.

Roden L: Structure and metabolism of connective tissue proteoglycans. In: *The Biochemistry of Glycoproteins and Proteoglycans*. Lennarz WJ (editor). Plenum, 1980.

Salpeter MM: ^{3}H-proline incorporation into cartilage: Electron microscope autoradiographic observations. *J Morphol* 1968;**124**:387.

Searls RL: Newer knowledge of chondrogenesis. *Clin Orthop* 1973;**96**:327.

Smith PH: Autoradiographic evidence for the concurrent synthesis of collagen and chondroitin sulfates by chick sternal chondrocytes. *Connect Tissue Res* 1972;**1**:181.

Stockwell RA: *Biology of Cartilage Cells*. Cambridge Univ Press, 1979.

Thomas L: Reversible collapse of rabbit ears after intravenous papain, and prevention of recovery by cortisone. *J Exp Med* 1956;**104**:245.

Zambrano NZ et al: Collagen arrangement in cartilages. *Acta Anat* 1982;**113**:26.

8

Bone

Bone is one of the hardest tissues of the human body and second only to cartilage in its ability to withstand stress. As the main constituent of the adult skeleton, it supports fleshy structures, protects vital organs such as those contained in the cranial and thoracic cavities, and harbors the bone marrow, where blood cells are formed. Bone also serves as a reservoir of calcium, phosphate, and other ions that can be released or stored in a controlled fashion to maintain constant concentrations of these important ions in body fluids.

Besides these functions, bones form a system of levers that multiply the forces generated during skeletal muscle contraction, transforming them into bodily movements.

Bone is a specialized connective tissue composed of intercellular calcified material, the **bone matrix** (Fig 8–1); and 3 different cell types: **osteocytes,** which are found in cavities **(lacunae)** within the matrix; **osteoblasts,** which synthesize the organic components of the matrix; and **osteoclasts,** which are multinucleated giant cells involved in the resorption and remodeling of bone tissue.

Since metabolites are unable to diffuse through the calcified matrix of bone, the exchanges between osteocytes and blood capillaries depend on cellular communication through the **canaliculi,** which perforate the matrix. These canaliculi permit the osteocytes to communicate via filopodial processes with their neighbors, with the internal and external surfaces of the bone, and with the blood vessels traversing the matrix.

All bones are lined on both internal and external surfaces by layers of connective tissue called **endosteum** and **periosteum,** respectively.

Because of its hardness, bone is difficult to section with the microtome; therefore, special techniques must be used for its study. One of these consists of grinding slices of bone with abrasives until they are thin enough to be translucent. The preparation thus obtained is referred to as a ground section. This technique does not preserve the cells but does permit detailed study of the matrix, its lacunae, and its canaliculi. Owing to differences in refractive index between lacunae and canaliculi (which are both filled with air in these preparations) and the medium used in mounting, light rays striking the lacunae and canaliculi are deflected and do not penetrate the objective lens of the microscope. Lacunae and canaliculi consequently appear black in ground sections (Fig 8–2).

Another frequently used technique that permits the observation of the cells and organic matrix is based on the decalcification of bone preserved by standard fixatives. The mineral is removed by immersion in a dilute acid solution (eg, 5% nitric acid) or in a solution containing a calcium-chelating substance (eg, ethylenediamine-tetraacetic acid, EDTA). The decalcified tissue is then embedded, sectioned, and stained by routine techniques.

BONE CELLS

Osteoblasts

Osteoblasts are responsible for the synthesis of the organic components of bone matrix (type I collagen,

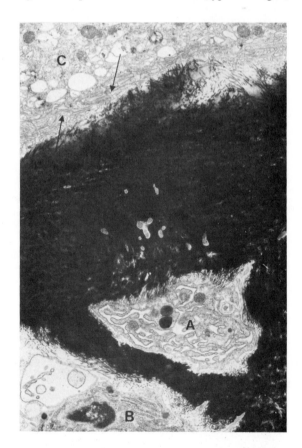

Figure 8–1. A portion of calcified bone (in black). Inside the calcified matrix there is a portion of the cytoplasm of an osteocyte (A). On the periphery there is a portion of an osteoblast (B) and of an osteoclast (C). The ruffled border (arrows) of the osteoclast is in contact with the matrix. × 7100. (Courtesy of E Katchburian.)

proteoglycans, and glycoproteins). Deposition of the inorganic components of bone is dependent on the presence of viable osteoblasts. They are exclusively located at the surfaces of bone tissue, side by side, in a way resembling simple epithelium (Fig 8–3). When they are actively engaged in matrix synthesis, osteoblasts have a cuboidal to columnar shape, basophilic cytoplasm, and high alkaline phosphatase activity. When their synthesizing activity declines, they flatten, and cytoplasmic basophilia declines, as does alkaline phosphatase activity.

Osteoblasts have cytoplasmic processes that bring them into contact with neighboring osteoblasts. The processes are more evident when the cell begins to surround itself with matrix. Once surrounded by newly synthesized matrix, the osteoblast is referred to as an **osteocyte.** Lacunae and canaliculi appear, because the matrix is formed around a cell and its cytoplasmic extensions.

During matrix synthesis, osteoblasts have the ultrastructure of cells synthesizing proteins for export, eg, well-developed rough endoplasmic reticulum (Fig 8–4) and Golgi complex. In the light microscope, a pale-staining area is often seen between the nucleus and the bone surface. This represents the location of

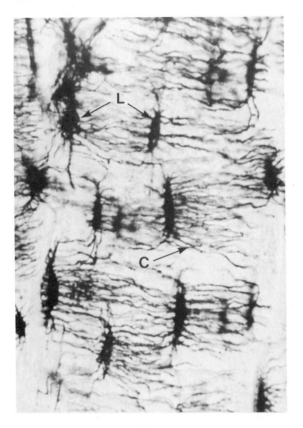

Figure 8–2 (at left). Photomicrograph of ground section of bone. Lacunae (L) and canaliculi (C) appear black. × 900.

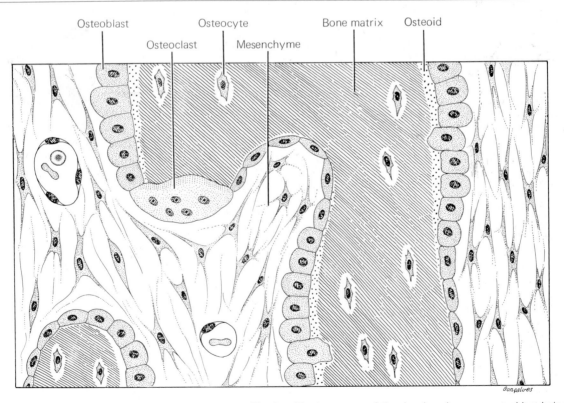

Figure 8–3. Advanced stage of intramembranous ossification. The lower part of the drawing shows an osteoblast being entrapped in the newly formed bone matrix.

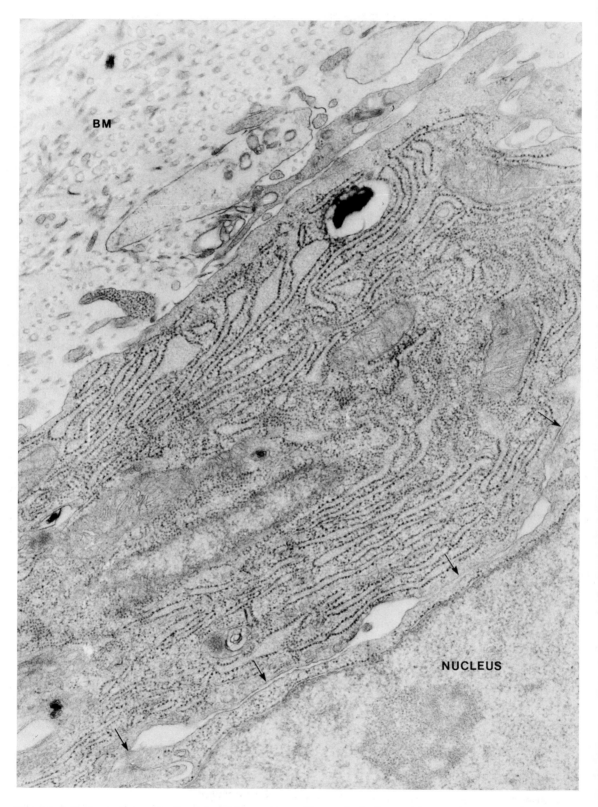

Figure 8–4. Electron micrograph of portions of 2 osteoblasts. The one in the lower right part of the figure shows mainly the nucleus. The border between the 2 cells is indicated by arrows. In the upper left corner there is a small amount of bone matrix (BM) with sectioned collagen fibers. Observe the abundant rough endoplasmic reticulum. × 25,000.

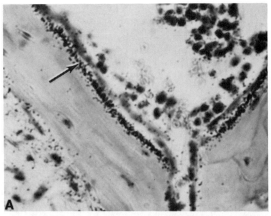

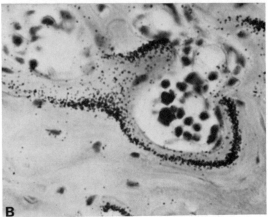

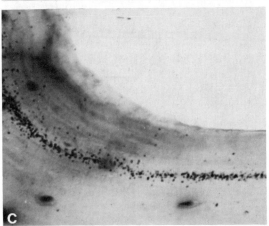

Figure 8–5. Radioautographs of bone tissue from mice injected with ³H-glycine and sacrificed at different intervals after the injection. *A:* From a mouse killed 4 hours after injection. At this time, osteoid is strongly radioactive (arrow). It contains ³H-glycine–labeled collagen synthesized by the osteoblasts. There is some radioactivity remaining in the osteoblasts. Bone marrow cells (upper right) are also radioactive. *B:* From a mouse killed 7 days after injection. The radioactive band is deeper into the calcified matrix because of the subsequent accumulation of the nonradioactive collagen formed after utilization of all labeled glycine. *C:* From a mouse killed 45 days after injection. The radioactive band is more deeply situated in comparison with the sections from previous intervals. H&E stain. × 300.

the Golgi complex. Osteoblasts are polarized cells; extrusion of the synthesized molecules takes place at the cell surface in contact with bone matrix. The large, round nucleus contains finely dispersed chromatin and is found at the side of the cell away from the matrix.

The newly synthesized, not yet calcified matrix adjacent to osteoblasts is termed the organic component, or **osteoid.** In active osteoblasts, PAS-positive cytoplasmic granules have been found that are probably precursors of the glycosaminoglycans of the matrix.

The role of osteoblasts in secreting bone collagen has been studied by radioautography in animals injected with ³H-glycine (an amino acid constituting one-third of the residues in collagen). Thirty minutes after ³H-glycine administration, the label was found mainly in osteoblasts; 4 hours later, it was located in osteoid (Fig 8–5A); and after 35 hours, a radioactive band was observed in the calcified matrix. The extracellular label appeared as a radioactive band that was displaced from the proximity of the osteoblasts by the nonradioactive matrix formed after utilization of the injected, labeled glycine. By the seventh (Fig 8–5B) and especially by the 45th day (Fig 8–5C) after the labeling injection, radioactivity was found deep in the matrix. The unlabeled matrix between the radioactive matrix and the osteoblast layer indicates the amount of bone formed in the interval between the injection of ³H-glycine and the termination of the experiment.

Osteocytes

Osteocytes are simply osteoblasts that have surrounded themselves with bone matrix (Figs 8–6 and 8–7). They lie in spaces (lacunae) situated between lamellae of matrix. Only one osteocyte is found in each lacuna. Thin, cylindric spaces in the matrix, called canaliculi, house osteocyte filopodial processes. Processes of adjacent cells make contact via gap junctions. This coupling provides for the intercellular flow of ions and small molecules (eg, hormones controlling bone growth and development). Filopodial contact between encapsulated osteocytes provides a mechanism wherein nutrients and metabolites can be passed between blood vessels and distant osteocytes. This ''bucket brigade'' phenomenon can provide support for a chain of about 15 cells.

When compared to osteoblasts, the flat, almond-shaped osteocytes exhibit a significantly reduced rough endoplasmic reticulum (Fig 8–7) and Golgi complex and more condensed nuclear chromatin. Although these are signs of reduced synthetic activity, these cells are actively involved with the maintenance of the bony matrix. Death of the osteocytes is followed by resorption of this matrix.

Osteoclasts

Osteoclasts are very large, extensively branched motile cells. Dilated portions of the cell body (Fig 8–8) contain from 2 to 50 or more nuclei. The branches of the cell are quite irregular and vary in both thickness and shape. Since sections reveal only a limited aspect of the osteoclast, the true morphology of the cell has only recently been described through the use of the scanning electron microscope. In areas of bone undergoing resorption, portions of the giant osteoclasts are found to lie within enzymatically etched depressions in the matrix known as **Howship's lacunae.** Frequently, some portions of the osteoclast will be actively resorbing bone while other branches of the same cell will appear quiescent.

It was formerly thought that osteoclasts were derived from osteoprogenitor cells and that they could revert back to those stem cells by having individual nuclei bud off of the multinucleated osteoclasts and form mononucleated osteoblasts. However, this hypothesis is currently in question, since more recent evidence strongly indicates that osteoclasts are derived from the fusion of blood-derived monocytes.

Osteoclasts usually have acidophilic cytoplasm. The cells possess numerous lysosomes and consequently give a positive histochemical reaction for acid phosphatase. Electron micrographs show that the active osteoclast surface facing bone matrix is folded into irregular, often subdivided projections, forming

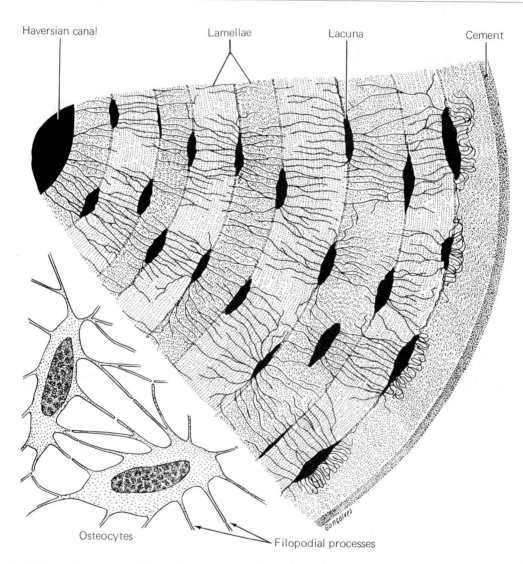

Haversian canal   Lamellae   Lacuna   Cement

Osteocytes   Filopodial processes

Figure 8–6. Schematic drawings of 2 osteocytes and part of a haversian system. Collagen fibers of contiguous lamellae are sectioned at different angles. Observe the numerous canaliculi which form intercommunications of the lacunae with each other and with the haversian canals. Although it is not apparent in this simplified diagram, each indicated lamella actually consists of multiple lamellae in which the parallel arrays of collagen fibers in adjacent lamellae are oriented in different directions. The presence of large numbers of lamellae with different fiber orientations provides the bone with great strength despite its light weight. (Redrawn and reproduced, with permission, from Leeson TS, Leeson CR: *Histology*, 2nd ed. Saunders, 1970.)

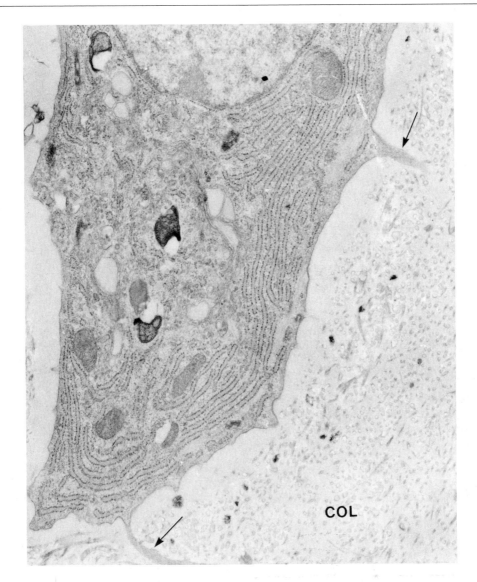

Figure 8–7. Electron micrograph of a young osteocyte. The section shows 2 cell processes (arrows) and the collagen fibers (COL) of bone matrix. × 6000.

a ruffled border. Besides establishing a device whereby small particles may be easily trapped and subjected to enzymatic activity, this arrangement considerably increases the active resorptive area. Numerous free polysomes, some rough endoplasmic reticulum, abundant mitochondria, and a well-developed Golgi complex are found in addition to the great number of lysosomes that are present within the cell.

Crystals containing calcium have been observed in the spaces between the folds as well as in cytoplasmic vacuoles probably derived from the surface membrane of the osteoclasts. Disintegrating collagen fibers have also been reported in the extracellular space close to the folds of the osteoclast, but they never occur within the cytoplasm.

The precise role of osteoclasts in bone resorption is not yet clear. They secrete acid, collagenase, and other proteolytic enzymes that attack the bone matrix and liberate the calcified ground substance. The cells are actively engaged in elimination of debris formed during bone resorption.

BONE MATRIX

Inorganic matter represents about 50% of the dry weight of bone matrix. Calcium and phosphorus are especially abundant, but bicarbonate, citrate, magnesium, potassium, and sodium are also found. X-ray diffraction studies have shown that calcium and phos-

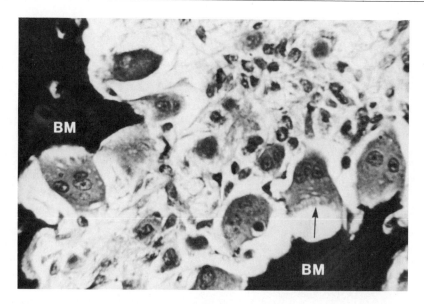

Figure 8–8. Photomicrograph of a bone section showing several osteoclasts. Observe the ruffled border (arrow). Bone matrix (BM) appears dark. The separation between some osteoclasts and the bone matrix is an artifact. Sirius red and hematoxylin, × 800.

phorus form hydroxyapatite crystals with the composition $Ca_{10}(PO_4)_6(OH)_2$. Significant quantities of amorphous (noncrystalline) calcium phosphate are also present. In electron micrographs, hydroxyapatite crystals of bone appear as plates measuring $40 \times 25 \times 3$ nm. They lie alongside the collagen fibrils but are surrounded by an amorphous ground substance. The surface ions of hydroxyapatite are hydrated, and a layer of water and ions forms around the crystal. This layer, the **hydration shell,** facilitates the exchange of ions between the crystal and the body fluids.

The organic matter is composed of collagen fibers (95%) (collagen type I) and the amorphous ground substance, which contains glycosaminoglycans associated with proteins. Several specific glycoproteins have been isolated from bone. Bone sialoprotein and osteocalcin (containing several γ-carboxyglutamic acid residues) both bind calcium avidly and may be responsible for promoting calcification of bone matrix. Other tissues containing type I collagen are not normally calcified and do not contain these glycoproteins. Among the glycosaminoglycans of bone are chondroitin 4-sulfate, chondroitin 6-sulfate, and keratan sulfate.

Because of its high collagen content, decalcified bone matrix binds selective stains for collagen fibers. It is also stained by the PAS technique, in which case the color intensity is proportionate to the quantity of galactose, fucose, and other carbohydrates present in glycoproteins.

The association of hydroxyapatite with collagen fibers is responsible for the hardness and resistance that are characteristic of bone. After a bone is decalcified, its shape is preserved, but it becomes as flexible as a tendon. Removal of the organic part of the matrix—which is mainly collagenous in nature—also leaves the bone with its original shape; however, it becomes fragile and breaks easily when handled.

PERIOSTEUM & ENDOSTEUM

External and internal surfaces of bone are covered by layers of bone-forming cells and connective tissue called periosteum and endosteum.

The **periosteum** consists of an outer layer of collagen fibers and fibroblasts (Fig 8–10). Periosteal collagen fibers that penetrate the bone matrix, binding the periosteum to bone, are called **Sharpey's fibers.** The inner, more cellular layer of the periosteum is composed of flattened cells with the potential to divide by mitosis and differentiate into osteoblasts. These **osteoprogenitor cells** are characterized by their location, their spindle shape, a small amount of rough endoplasmic reticulum, and their poorly developed Golgi complex. Autoradiographic studies demonstrate that these cells take up ^{3}H-thymidine, which is subsequently encountered in osteoblasts. These cells play a prominent role in bone growth and repair.

The **endosteum** (Fig 8–10) lines all internal surfaces of bone and is composed of osteoprogenitor cells and a very small amount of connective tissue. Thus, the endosteum is considerably thinner than the periosteum.

The principal functions of periosteum and endosteum are nutrition of osseous tissue and provision of a continuous supply of new osteoblasts for repair or growth of bone. For these reasons, precautions are taken to preserve the periosteum and endosteum during bone surgery.

TYPES OF BONE TISSUE

Gross observation of bone in cross section shows dense areas without cavities—corresponding to **compact bone**—and areas with numerous interconnecting cavities—corresponding to **spongy bone** (Fig 8–9). Under the microscope, however, both compact bone and the trabeculae separating the cavities of spongy bone have the same basic histologic structure.

In long bones, the bulbous ends—called **epiphyses**—are composed of spongy bone covered by a thin layer of compact bone. The cylindric part—**diaphysis**—is almost totally composed of compact bone, with a small component of spongy bone on its inner surface around the bone marrow cavity (Fig 8–16). Short bones usually have a core of spongy bone completely surrounded by compact bone. The flat bones that form the calvaria have 2 layers of compact bone

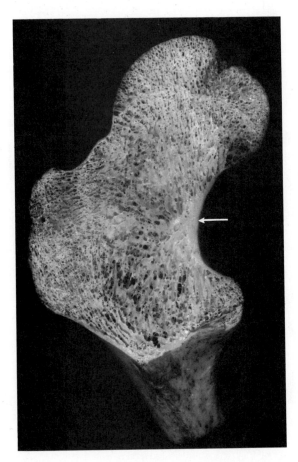

Figure 8–9. Section through the head of the femur. This dry bone shows the complex trabeculae of spongy (cancellous) bone. The arrow indicates compact bone. (Courtesy of E Katchburian.)

called **plates** (tables), separated by a layer of spongy bone called the **diploë.**

The cavities of spongy bone and the marrow cavity in the diaphyses of long bones contain **bone marrow,** of which there are 2 kinds: **red bone marrow,** in which blood cells are forming; and **yellow bone marrow,** composed mainly of fat cells.

Histologically, there are 2 varieties of bone tissue: **immature, primary,** or **woven bone;** and **mature, secondary,** or **lamellar bone.** Both varieties contain the same structural components, but in immature bone collagen bundles are randomly placed while in mature bone these bundles are organized into **bone lamellae.**

Primary Bone Tissue

In the formation of each bone, as well as in the repair process, the first bone tissue to appear is immature, or woven, bone. It is temporary and is replaced in adults by secondary bone tissue except in a very few places in the body, eg, near the sutures of the flat bones of the skull, in tooth sockets, and in the insertions of some tendons.

Besides the irregular array of collagen fibers, other characteristics of primary bone tissue are a smaller content of minerals (it is more easily penetrated by x-rays) and a higher proportion of osteocytes than in secondary bone tissue.

Secondary Bone Tissue

Secondary bone is the variety usually found in adults. Characteristically, it shows collagen fibers arranged in lamellae (3–7 μm thick) that are parallel to each other (**cancellous,** or spongy, bone) or concentrically organized around a vascular canal (**compact,** or dense, bone). The whole complex of concentric lamellae of bone surrounding a canal containing blood vessels, nerves, and loose connective tissue is called a **haversian system** or **osteon** (Figs 8–6 and 8–10). Lacunae containing osteocytes are found between and occasionally within the lamellae. In each lamella, collagen fibers are parallel to each other. Surrounding each haversian system is a deposit of amorphous material called the **cementing substance** that consists of mineralized matrix with few collagen fibers.

In compact bone (eg, the diaphysis of long bones), the lamellae exhibit a typical organization consisting of haversian systems, outer circumferential lamellae, inner circumferential lamellae, and interstitial lamellae. The 4 types of lamellar bone are easily identified in cross section (Fig 8–10). Since the principal function of haversian systems is to bring nutrients to compact bone, it is not surprising to find that haversian systems are absent in the thin spicules of cancellous bone. Here, nutrients can diffuse into the bony tissue from surrounding blood capillaries.

Each haversian system is a long, often bifurcated cylinder parallel to the long axis of the diaphysis. It consists of a central canal surrounded by 4–20 concentric lamellae. Each endosteum-lined canal contains blood vessels, nerves, and loose connective tissue.

The haversian canals communicate with the marrow cavity, with the periosteum, and with each other through transverse or oblique Volkmann's canals (Fig 8–10). Volkmann's canals do not have concentric lamellae. Instead, they perforate the lamellae (Fig 8–10). All vascular canals found in bone tissue come into existence when matrix is laid down around preexisting blood vessels.

Examination of haversian systems with polarized light shows bright anisotropic layers alternating with dark isotropic layers (Fig 8–11). When observed under polarized light at right angles to their length, collagen fibers are birefringent (anisotropic). The alternating bright and dark layers are due to the orientation of collagen fibers in the lamellae. In each lamella, fibers are parallel to each other and follow a helical course. The pitch of the helix is, however, different for different lamellae, so that at any given point fibers from adjacent lamellae intersect at approximately right angles (Fig 8–10). Cross sections of a haversian system show transverse sections of collagen fibers in one lamella and oblique, almost longitudinal sections of

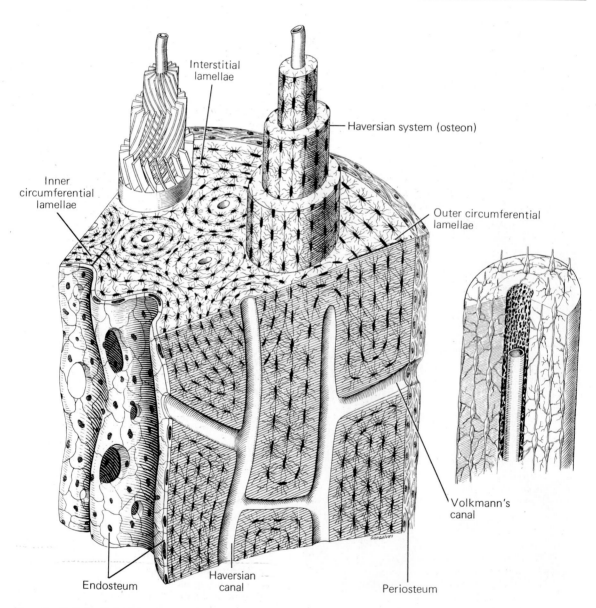

Figure 8–10. Schematic drawing of the wall of a long bone diaphysis. Observe the 4 types of lamellar bone: haversian system, outer and inner circumferential lamellae, and interstitial lamellae. The protruding haversian system on the left shows the orientation of collagen fibers in each lamella. At the right is a haversian system showing lamellae, a central blood capillary, and many osteocytes with their processes.

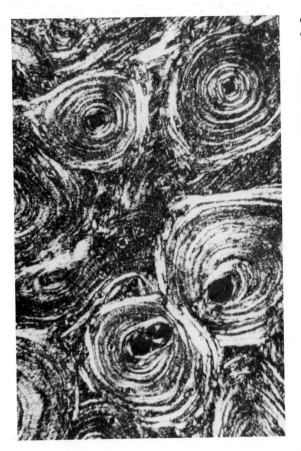

Figure 8–11. Transverse section of decalcified diaphysis; polarization microscopy showing the alternating light and dark bands that surround the haversian canal. The birefringence is due to the presence of collagen fibers disposed in different orientations in contiguous lamellae. × 150.

cavity as the center. There are more outer than inner circumferential lamellae (Fig 8–10).

Between the 2 circumferential systems there are numerous haversian systems, and among the latter are triangular or irregularly shaped groups of parallel lamellae called **interstitial** (or intermediate) **lamellae.** These structures represent lamellae left by haversian systems destroyed during growth and remodeling of bone (Fig 8–12).

HISTOGENESIS

Bone tissue arises either by intramembranous ossification, which occurs within a layer (membrane) of condensed mesenchymal tissue, or by endochondral ossification, which takes place within a cartilaginous model. The model is gradually destroyed and replaced by bone formed by incoming cells from surrounding periosteal connective tissues.

In both processes, the bone tissue that appears first is primary or immature. Primary bone is a temporary tissue and is soon replaced by the definitive, lamellar variety of bone, referred to as secondary bone. During bone growth, areas of primary bone, areas of resorption, and areas of lamellar bone appear side by side. This combination of bone synthesis and removal (remodeling) occurs not only in growing bones but also throughout adult life, though its rate of change then is considerably slower.

Intramembranous Ossification

Intramembranous ossification, the source of most of the flat bones, is so called because it takes place within condensations of mesenchymal tissue. The frontal and parietal bones of the skull—as well as parts of the occipital and temporal bones and the mandible and maxilla—are formed by intramembranous ossification. Intramembranous ossification also contributes to the growth of short bones and the thickening of long bones.

In the mesenchymal condensation layer, the starting point for ossification is called a **primary ossification center.** The process begins when groups of cells differentiate into osteoblasts. Osteoid synthesis and calcification follow (Fig 8–13), resulting in the encapsulation of some osteoblasts which then become osteocytes (Fig 8–14). These islands of developing bone are known as **spicules.** Several such groups arise almost simultaneously at the ossification center, so that the fusion of the spicules gives the bone a spongy structure (Fig 8–15). The connective tissue that remains among the bone spicules is penetrated by growing blood vessels and additional undifferentiated mesenchymal cells, which give rise to the bone marrow cells.

Cells of the mesenchymal tissue condensation divide, giving rise to more osteoblasts, which are responsible for the continued growth of the ossification center. The several ossification centers of a bone grow radially and finally fuse together, replacing the orig-

collagen fibers in the adjacent lamella. The structure of haversian systems as shown in the light microscope is compatible with this interpretation. In one lamella, the collagen fibers are sectioned transversely and appear granular; in the next, the fibers are sectioned obliquely and have an elongated appearance (Fig 8–6).

There is great variability in the diameter of haversian canals. Each system is formed by successive deposition of lamellae, starting from the periphery, so that younger systems have larger canals. Thus in mature haversian systems, the most recently formed lamella is the one closest to the central canal.

During growth—and even in adult bone—there is continuous destruction and rebuilding of haversian systems, so that one often sees systems with only a few lamellae and a large central canal.

Inner and outer circumferential lamellae are, as their names indicate, located around the marrow cavity and immediately beneath the periosteum. Their lamellae have a circular distribution, with the marrow

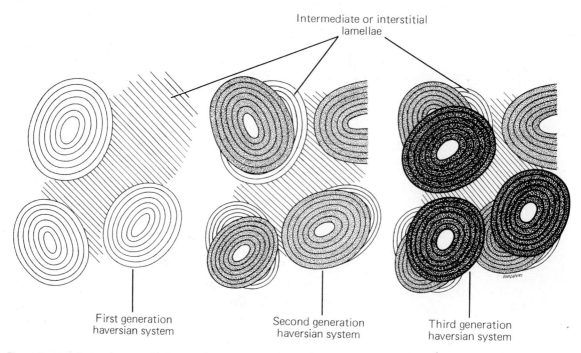

Intermediate or interstitial lamellae

First generation haversian system

Second generation haversian system

Third generation haversian system

Figure 8–12. Schematic view of diaphyseal bone remodeling. Three generations of haversian systems are shown. At right, the contribution of first and second generation haversian systems to the formation of intermediate or interstitial lamellae can be seen.

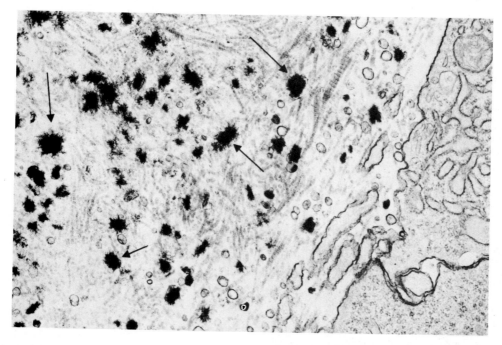

Figure 8–13. Calvarium in the early stage of mineral deposition. In the collagen-rich matrix, there are numerous foci of mineralization (arrows), presumably originating within matrix vesicles. × 18,000. (Courtesy of E Katchburian.)

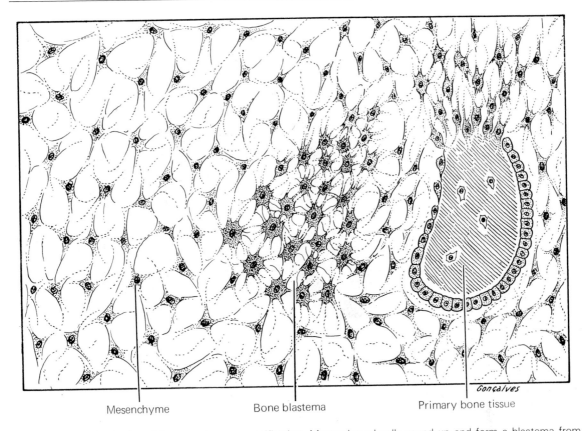

Mesenchyme   Bone blastema   Primary bone tissue

Figure 8–14. The beginning of intramembranous ossification. Mesenchymal cells round up and form a blastema from which osteoblasts differentiate.

Bone
spicule   Osteo-
blast   Osteo-
clast

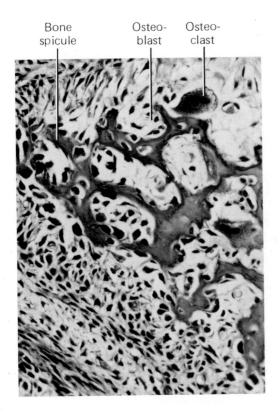

Figure 8–15 (at left). Photomicrograph of intramembranous ossification from the head of a young rat. Bone tissue shows osteocytes in lacunae. Around the newly formed bone tissue there are numerous osteoblasts and an osteoclast. Mallory's azan stain, × 350.

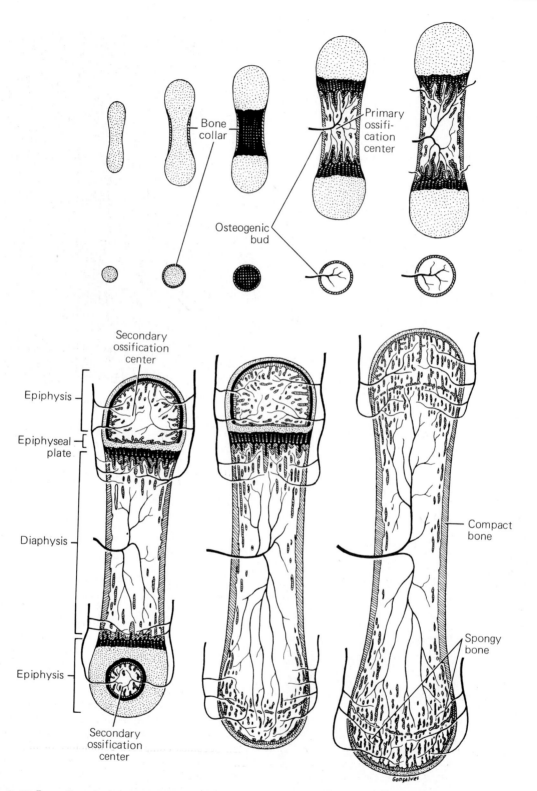

Figure 8–16. Formation of a long bone on a model made of cartilage. Hyaline cartilage is stippled; calcified cartilage is black; and bone tissue is indicated by oblique lines. The 5 small drawings in the middle row represent cross sections through the mid regions of the figures shown in the upper row. (For details, see text.) (Redrawn and reproduced, with permission, from Bloom W, Fawcett DW: *A Textbook of Histology,* 9th ed. Saunders, 1968.)

inal connective tissue. In newborn infants, the fontanelles are soft areas in the skull that correspond to parts of the connective tissue not yet ossified.

In cranial flat bones, especially after birth, there is a marked predominance of bone formation over bone resorption at both the internal and the external surfaces. Thus, 2 layers of compact bone (internal and external plates) arise, whereas the central portion (diploë) maintains its spongy nature.

That portion of the connective tissue layer which does not undergo ossification gives rise to the endosteum and the periosteum of intramembranous bone.

Endochondral Ossification

Endochondral ossification takes place within a piece of hyaline cartilage whose shape resembles a small version or model of the bone to be formed. This type of ossification is principally responsible for the formation of short and long bones (Fig 8–16).

Basically, endochondral ossification consists of 2 phases. The first phase is hypertrophy and destruction of the chondrocytes of the model of the bone, leaving expanded lacunae separated by septa of calcified cartilage matrix. In the second phase, an **osteogenic bud** consisting of osteoprogenitor cells and blood capillaries penetrates the spaces left by the degenerating chondrocytes. The osteoprogenitor cells give rise to osteoblasts, which form an osseous matrix on the remnants of the calcified cartilage matrix. In this way, bone tissue appears at the site where there was cartilage, and there is no transformation of the cartilage into bone tissue. The septa of calcified cartilage tissue serve as supports for the beginning of ossification (Fig 8–16).

Long bones are formed from cartilaginous models with dilatations (epiphyses) at each end of a cylindric shaft (diaphysis). The first bone tissue to be formed appears by means of intramembranous ossification within the perichondrium surrounding the diaphysis (Fig 8–16). Thus, a hollow bone cylinder, the **bone collar,** is produced in the deep portions of the perichondrium surrounding the cartilage. The perichondrium is then called periosteum, because it covers the newly developed bone. Internal to the forming bone collar, chondrocytes of the cartilage model begin to degenerate, since the new osseous collar prevents the diffusion of nutrients into the cartilage matrix. As the chondrocytes begin to degenerate, they resorb their surrounding matrix, causing an enlargement of the lacunae. As the chondrocytes lose their ability to maintain the matrix, calcium deposits form and the cartilage becomes **calcified.**

Blood vessels of the osteogenic bud, coming from the periosteum through holes made by osteoclasts in the bone collar, penetrate the calcified cartilage matrix. Along with the blood vessels, osteoprogenitor cells also invade the area; they proliferate and give rise to osteoblasts. Osteoblasts form a continuous layer over the calcified cartilaginous matrix and start to synthesize bone matrix. Thus, primary bone synthesis takes place over the remnants of calcified cartilage

Remnants of cartilage matrix

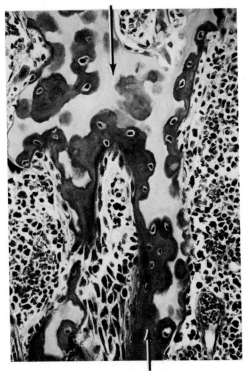

Bone tissue

Figure 8–17. Photomicrograph of endochondral ossification from the finger of a human fetus. Remnants of calcified cartilage matrix appear covered by primary bone tissue. Calcified cartilage matrix has no cells, while bone matrix contains many osteocytes. Mallory's trichrome stain, × 238.

(Fig 8–17). Bone marrow stem cells are circulating in the blood and are brought into the forming bone by the osteogenic bud.

In histologic sections, calcified cartilage can be distinguished as basophilic, whereas the bone tissue deposited over it is acidophilic. As the spongy bone matrix develops, calcified cartilage remnants are resorbed by the giant multinucleated **chondroclasts.** These cells are structurally and functionally equivalent to osteoclasts except that they break down cartilage rather than osseous matrix.

The ossification center described above, which appears in the diaphysis, is called the **primary ossification center** (Fig 8–16). Its rapid longitudinal growth ends by occupying the whole diaphysis, which then becomes composed completely of bone tissue. This expansion of the primary ossification center is accompanied by expansion of the periosteal bone collar, which also grows in the direction of the epiphyses. From the beginning of the formation of the ossification center, osteoclasts are active, and resorption of the bone occurs at the center, which results in formation of a hollow marrow cavity that grows toward the

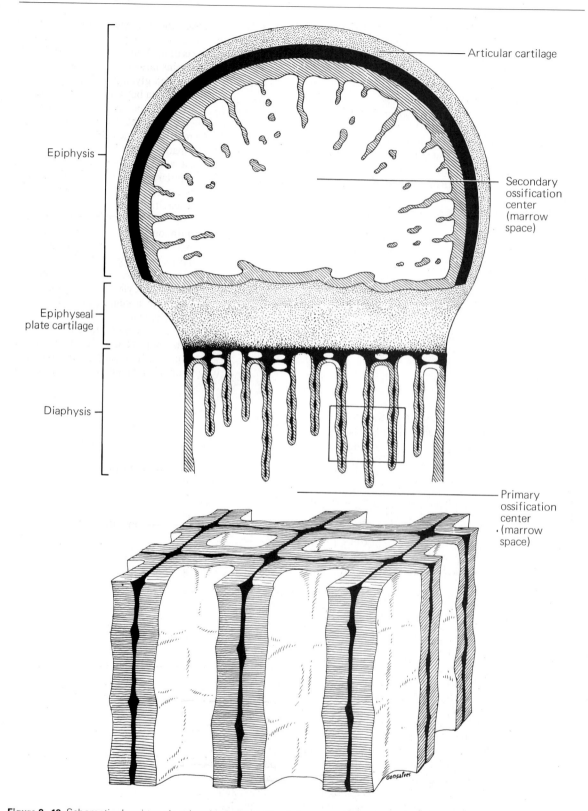

Figure 8–18. Schematic drawings showing the 3-dimensional shape of bone spicules in the epiphyseal plate area. Hyaline cartilage is stippled; calcified cartilage is black; and bone tissue is indicated by parallel lines. The upper drawing shows the region represented 3-dimensionally in the lower drawing. (Redrawn and reproduced, with permission, from Ham AW: *Histology,* 6th ed. Lippincott, 1969.)

epiphyses as ossification continues toward the ends of the finally complete bone model.

At later stages in embryonic development, a **secondary ossification center** (Fig 8–16) arises at the center of each epiphysis, although even within one bone, all centers do not develop simultaneously. The function of these centers is similar to that of the primary center, but their growth is radial instead of longitudinal. Furthermore, since the articular cartilage has no perichondrium, the equivalent of a bone collar is not formed here (Fig 8–16).

When bone tissue that originated at the secondary centers occupies the epiphysis, cartilage remains restricted to 2 places: articular cartilage, which persists throughout adult life and does not contribute to bone formation; and epiphyseal cartilage, or the epiphyseal plate, which connects epiphysis to diaphysis (Figs 8–18 and 8–19). As the cartilage of the epiphyseal plate grows, it is replaced continuously by newly formed bone matrix mainly from the diaphyseal center. No further longitudinal growth of the bone takes place after the growth of the epiphyseal plate ceases.

Epiphyseal cartilage is divided into 5 zones (Fig 8–19), starting from the epiphyseal side of cartilage: (1) The **resting zone** consists of hyaline cartilage without morphologic changes in the cells. (2) In the **proliferative zone,** chondrocytes divide rapidly and form columns (isogenous groups) of stacked cells parallel to the long axis of the bone. (3) The **hypertrophic cartilage zone** contains large chondrocytes whose cytoplasm has accumulated glycogen. The resorbed matrix is reduced to thin septa between the chondrocytes. (4) Simultaneously with the death of chondrocytes occurring in the **calcified cartilage zone,** the thin septa of cartilage matrix become calcified by the deposition of hydroxyapatite (Figs 8–18 and 8–19). (5) In the **ossification zone,** endochondral bone tissue appears. Blood capillaries and osteoprogenitor cells formed by mitosis of cells originating from the periosteum invade the cavities left by the chondrocytes. The osteoprogenitor cells form osteoblasts, which in turn form a discontinuous layer over the septa of calcified cartilage matrix. Over these septa, the osteoblasts deposit bone matrix (Fig 8–17).

The bone matrix calcifies, and some osteoblasts are transformed into osteocytes. In this way, **bone spicules** are formed with a central area of calcified cartilage and a superficial layer of primary bone tissue. The spicules are so called because of their appearance in histologic sections; they are sections of walls which delineate elongated cavities containing capillaries, bone marrow cells, and undifferentiated cells (Fig 8–18).

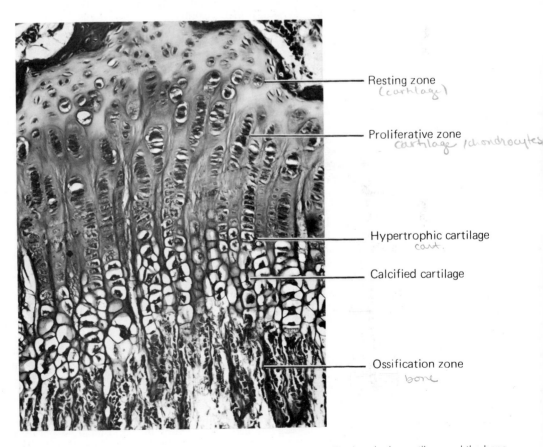

Figure 8–19. Photomicrograph of the epiphyseal plate, showing the changes that take place in the cartilage and the bone spicules formed. H&E stain, × 110.

In summary, growth in length of a long bone occurs by proliferation of chondrocytes in the epiphyseal plate adjacent to the epiphysis. At the same time, chondrocytes on the diaphyseal side of the plate hypertrophy; their matrix becomes calcified; and the cells die. Osteoblasts lay down a layer of primary bone on the calcified cartilage spicules. The rates of these 2 opposing events (proliferation and destruction) are approximately equal, and thus the epiphyseal plate does not change thickness. Instead, it is displaced away from the middle of the diaphysis, resulting in growth in length of the bone.

Mechanisms of Calcification

Normally, only certain regions of the body undergo ossification (bones) or calcification (some cartilages). Much research effort has been devoted to determining the factors that control selective deposition of calcium phosphate salts in these regions. No satisfactory mechanism can be presented at this time. Some of the prevalent hypotheses are outlined below.

The first theory was formulated by Robison in the 1920s. He noted that both calcium and phosphate ions are present in body fluids in concentrations less than that necessary to produce precipitation of the salt. Robison proposed that alkaline phosphatase activity, prominent in osteoblasts, could locally increase the phosphate ion concentration in calcifying tissues. The substrates for this enzyme were thought to be organic phosphates such as hexose phosphates or glycerophosphates. As a result of enzymatic activity, phosphate concentrations would be increased to the point at which precipitation of calcium phosphate would occur. This theory has fallen into disfavor.

Other workers proposed that nucleation sites, the ''lacunae'' (or ''holes'') in collagen fibrils (Fig 5–5), could induce calcium phosphate precipitation. This idea contends with the fact that type I collagen in other areas of the body does not calcify. The presence of calcium-binding glycoproteins, present only in bone (see p 146), has been invoked to overcome this objection.

A third group of theories revolves around a structure called the matrix vesicle, which is seen in calcifying cartilage, osteoid, and predentin. This is a membrane-limited vesicle, about 100 nm in diameter, thought to be pinched off from cells such as osteoblasts. Matrix vesicles can accumulate calcium phosphate by an active transport mechanism, and they contain alkaline phosphatase and pyrophosphatase. The latter enzyme cleaves pyrophosphates, which are known to be inhibitors of calcification, yielding inorganic phosphate. According to this mechanism of calcification, matrix vesicles would accumulate calcium phosphate and, after membrane rupture, the contents would act as nucleation sites for the addition of calcium, phosphate, and other ions, ultimately forming hydroxyapatite crystals in areas undergoing calcification.

GROWTH & REMODELING OF BONE

Bone growth is generally associated with partial resorption of preformed tissue and the simultaneous laying down of new bone. This permits the shape of the bone to be maintained while it grows.

Cranial bones grow mainly owing to formation of bone tissue by the periosteum located between the sutures and on the external bone surface. At the same time, resorption takes place on the internal surface. Since bone is an extremely plastic tissue, it responds to the growth of the brain and forms a skull of adequate size. The skull will be small if the brain does not develop completely and larger than normal in a person suffering from hydrocephalus, a disorder characterized by abnormal accumulation of spinal fluid and dilatation of the cerebral ventricles.

The growth of long bones is a complex process. The epiphyses increase in size owing to the radial growth of the cartilage, followed by endochondral ossification. In this way, the spongy part of the epiphysis increases.

The diaphysis (the bone formed between the 2 epiphyseal plates) consists initially of a bone cylinder. Because of the faster growth of the epiphyses, the extremities of the diaphysis soon become larger, forming 2 **diaphyseal funnels** separated by the **diaphyseal shaft.**

The diaphyseal shaft increases in length mainly as a result of the osteogenic activity of the epiphyseal plate; it increases in width as a result of the formation of bone by the periosteum on the external surface of the bone collar. At the same time, bone is removed from the internal surface, and in this way the bone marrow cavity increases in diameter.

In both diaphyseal funnels, owing to the osteogenic activity of the endosteum, deposition of bone occurs on the internal surface (Fig 8–20). At the same time, bone is resorbed from opposite areas on the external surface. The narrow parts of the diaphyseal funnels therefore become gradually cylindric, and this is due mainly to the osteogenic activity of the epiphyseal plate (Fig 8–21). As a result of this process, the cylindric diaphyseal shaft increases in length, and the 2 diaphyseal funnels grow farther apart as the bone lengthens. Gradually, osteogenic activity in the endosteum of the cylindric portion of the diaphyseal funnel ceases, permitting the bone marrow cavity to maintain or to increase its diameter slowly by resorption. As the central bone spicules become eroded to make room for the bone marrow cavity, the epiphyseal cartilage remains firmly attached to the diaphyseal funnel by means of the peripheral spicules (Figs 8–20 and 8–21).

In brief, it can be said that long bones become longer as a result of the activity of the epiphyseal plates and wider as a result of the apposition of bone formed by the periosteum. When the cartilage of the epiphyseal plate stops growing, it is replaced by bone tissue through the process of ossification. This closure of the epiphyses occurs around age 20. Afterward,

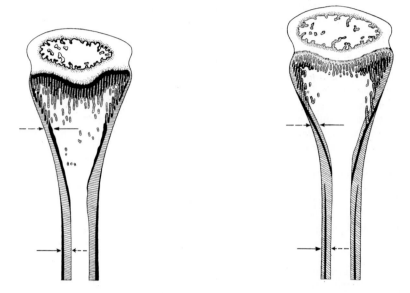

Figure 8 –20. Drawings based on radioautographs of animals injected with radioactive phosphate at several time intervals before being killed. Black areas indicate radioactive matrix, solid arrows indicate zones of bone deposition, and broken arrows indicate zones of bone resorption. In diaphyseal funnels, bone deposition occurs mainly at the internal surface. In the diaphysis, bone is laid down mainly on the outer surface. (Based on the work of CP Leblond et al. Redrawn and reproduced, with permission, from Greep RO, Weiss L: *Histology,* 3rd ed. McGraw-Hill, 1973.)

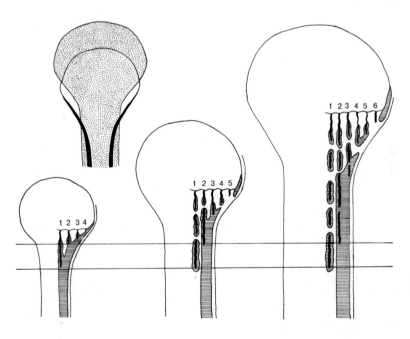

Figure 8 –21. *Upper left:* The importance of bone resorption in the external surface of the funnel for bone growth. *Lower drawings:* Bone growth taking place by diaphyseal displacement. (Use the 2 parallel lines as reference.) Observe also how epiphyseal bone spicules contribute to the diaphyseal development; eg, spicule 2 is being incorporated into the diaphysis. (Based on the work of CP Leblond et al.)

longitudinal growth of bones becomes impossible, although widening may still occur.

FRACTURE REPAIR

When a bone is fractured, the damaged blood vessels produce a localized hemorrhage with formation of a blood clot. Destruction of bone matrix and death of bone cells adjoining the fracture also occur.

During repair, the blood clot, the remaining cells, and the damaged bone matrix are removed by macrophages. The periosteum and the endosteum around the fracture respond with intense proliferation of osteoprogenitor cells, which form a cellular tissue surrounding the fracture and penetrating between the extremities of the fractured bone (Fig 8–22A and B).

Immature bone is then formed by endochondral ossification of small cartilage fragments that appear in the connective tissue of the fracture. Bone is also formed by means of intramembranous ossification. Therefore, areas of cartilage, intramembranous ossification, and endochondral ossification are simultaneously encountered in fractures. Repair progresses in such a way that irregularly formed trabeculae of immature bone temporarily unite the extremities of the fractured bone, forming a **bone callus** (Figs 8–22C and 8–23).

Normal stress imposed on the bone during repair and during the patient's gradual return to activity serves to remodel the bone callus. Since these stresses are identical to those that occurred during the growth of the bone, thus influencing its structure, remodeling of the callus reconstitutes the bone as it was prior to fracture. The primary bone tissue of the callus is therefore gradually reabsorbed and replaced by lamellar bone, resulting in restoration of the original bone structure (Fig 8–22D).

HISTOPHYSIOLOGY

Support & Protection

Bones form the skeleton, the function of which is to bear the weight of the body. Voluntary (skeletal) muscles are inserted onto the bones via intercalation of the tendons with the connective tissue of the periosteum. Long bones constitute a system of levers that increase the forces produced by muscular contractions. Bones protect the central nervous system (which is enclosed in the skull and the spinal canal), the bone marrow, and the thoracic contents.

Plasticity

In spite of its hardness, bone is capable of remodeling its internal structure according to the different stresses to which it is subjected. For example, the positions of the teeth in the jawbone may be modified by lateral pressures produced by orthodontic appliances. Bone formation takes place on the side where traction is applied and is reabsorbed where pressure is exerted (on the opposite side). In this way, teeth move within the jawbone while the alveolar bone is being remodeled. This capacity for reconstruction is a characteristic of all bones.

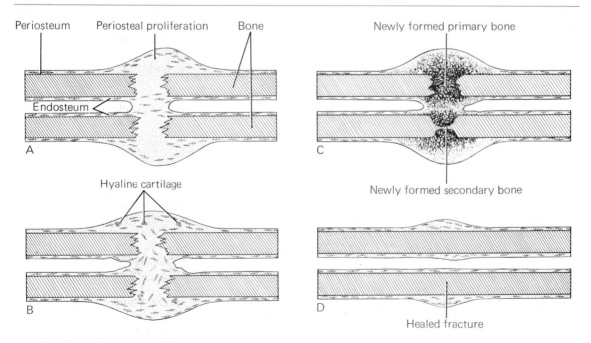

Figure 8–22. Repair of a fractured bone by formation of new bone tissue through proliferation of periosteal and endosteal cells.

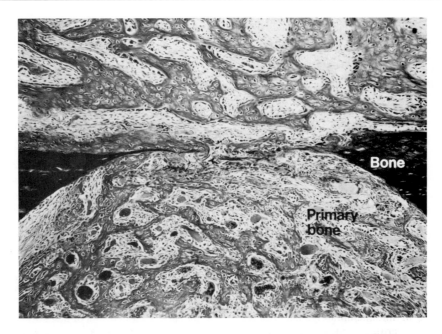

Figure 8–23. Photomicrograph of a mouse bone callus 7 days after fracture. The early callus contains mainly primary bone tissue made by cells originating in the periosteum. This is a micrograph corresponding to the central area in Fig 8–23C. Mallory's stain, × 118.

Calcium Reserve

The skeleton contains 99% of the total calcium of the body and acts as a calcium reservoir. The concentration of calcium in the blood and in tissues is quite stable. Calcium is important for the activity of several enzymatic systems, including those responsible for muscular contraction and transmission of nerve impulses. Calcium in the extracellular compartment is essential to several functions such as coagulation of the blood and cell adhesion.

There is a continuous interchange between blood calcium and bone calcium. The calcium absorbed from a meal, which would otherwise increase the blood calcium level, is rapidly deposited in bones or excreted in the feces or urine. Calcium in bones is mobilized when the concentration in blood decreases.

Bone calcium is mobilized by 2 mechanisms, one rapid and the other slow. The first is the simple transference of ions from hydroxyapatite crystals to interstitial fluid—from which, in turn, calcium passes into the blood. This purely physical mechanism, which takes place mainly in spongy bone, is aided by the large surface area of the hydroxyapatite crystals. The younger, slightly calcified lamellae that exist even in adult bone because of continuous remodeling receive and lose calcium more readily. These lamellae are more important for the maintenance of calcium concentration in the blood than the older, greatly calcified lamellae, whose role is mainly that of support and protection.

The second mechanism for mobilizing calcium depends on the action of hormones on bone. **Para-thyroid hormone** activates and increases the number of cells promoting resorption (osteoclasts) of the bone matrix, with the consequent liberation of calcium.

Another hormone, **calcitonin,** which is synthesized by the clear (C) cells of the thyroid gland, inhibits matrix resorption by increasing matrix formation and calcium deposition. Its effect on bone, therefore, is opposite to that of parathyroid hormone.

Since the concentration of calcium in tissues and blood must be kept constant, nutritional deficiency of calcium results in decalcification of bones; they then are more liable to fracture and are more transparent to x-rays. Decalcification of bone may also be caused by excessive production of parathyroid hormone (hyperparathyroidism), which results in intense resorption of bone, elevation of blood calcium, and abnormal deposits of calcium in several organs, mainly the kidneys and arterial walls.

Nutrition

Especially during growth, bone is sensitive to several nutritional factors. Insufficient dietary protein causes a deficiency of amino acids and leads to reduced synthesis of collagen by osteoblasts. Deficiency of calcium leads to incomplete calcification of the organic bone matrix; it may be due either to the lack of calcium in the diet or to the lack of vitamin D, which is important for the absorption of calcium by the small intestine.

Calcium deficiency in children causes **rickets,** a disease in which the bone matrix does not calcify normally and the bone spicules formed by the epiphyseal plate become distorted when subjected to the normal strains of body weight and muscular activity. Consequently, ossification processes at this level are hindered and the bones not only grow more slowly but also become deformed.

Calcium deficiency in adults gives rise to **osteomalacia,** characterized by deficient calcification of recently formed bone and partial decalcification of already calcified matrix. However, since adults have no epiphyseal cartilage, the deformation of long bones and retardation of growth that is characteristic of rickets in children does not occur, and of course growth is not affected. Osteomalacia may be aggravated during pregnancy, since the developing fetus requires a great deal of calcium.

Osteomalacia should not be confused with **osteoporosis,** a condition not related to nutrition. In the former, there is a decrease in the amount of calcium per unit of bone matrix. Osteoporosis, frequently expressed in immobilized patients and postmenopausal women, is a decrease in bone mass caused by either decreased bone formation or increased bone resorption or both. In osteoporosis, the ratio of mineral to matrix is normal.

Besides the aforementioned effect on intestinal absorption, vitamin D has a direct effect on ossification, as has been demonstrated with in vitro ex-

periments. Bone tissue cultivated in a medium rich in calcium but deficient in vitamin D does not calcify properly. Excessive amounts of vitamin D are toxic and give rise to bone resorption.

Vitamin A, also related to the distribution and activity of the osteoblasts and osteoclasts, affects the balance between production and resorption of bone. This vitamin is essential to normal growth in response to mechanical factors acting on bones, an effect that becomes evident when, as a result of vitamin A deficiency, the bones of the skull do not develop fast enough to respond to the pressure exerted by the growing brain, resulting in damage to the central nervous system. This does not occur in laboratory control animals receiving adequate doses of vitamin A, for the skull then grows to the exact size necessary to contain the brain.

In vitamin A deficiency, the osteoblasts do not synthesize the bone matrix normally, and the individual therefore does not reach normal stature. Vitamin A excess accelerates ossification of the epiphyseal plates without a concomitant effect on the growth of cartilage in these plates. Consequently, epiphyseal cartilage is rapidly replaced by bone, and body growth ceases. For these reasons, either vitamin A deficiency or administration of toxic doses of vitamin A may cause small stature.

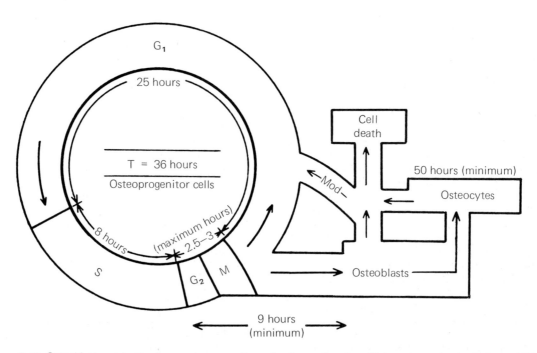

Figure 8–24. Osteoblasts originating from osteoprogenitor cells. Generation time (T) is estimated to be 36 hours (tibia of young rats). The period of DNA synthesis (S) is 8 hours; G$_1$ consumes 25 hours of the cycle, whereas G$_2$ and mitosis (M) take 2.5–3 hours. The minimum time for an osteoprogenitor cell to be transformed into an osteoblast is 9 hours. Once formed, osteocytes remain as such for at least 50 hours or, very often, longer. Osteoblasts and osteocytes can modulate (Mod) back to an osteoprogenitor cell. It has been demonstrated that osteoclasts are derived primarily from blood monocytes. (Slightly modified and reproduced, with permission, from Young RW: *J Cell Biol* 1962;**14**:357.)

Another vitamin that acts directly on bone is vitamin C (ascorbic acid), which is essential for collagen synthesis by both osteoblasts and osteocytes. Vitamin C deficiency interferes with bone growth and hinders repair of fractures by altering collagen deposition.

Hormonal Factors

In addition to parathyroid hormone and calcitonin, several other hormones act on bone.

The anterior lobe of the pituitary synthesizes growth hormone, which stimulates overall growth but especially that of epiphyseal cartilage. Consequently, lack of growth hormone during the growing years causes pituitary dwarfism, and growth hormone excess causes gigantism owing to excessive growth of long bones. Adult bones cannot increase in length when stimulated by an excess of growth hormone because of the lack of epiphyseal cartilage, but they do increase in width by periosteal growth. In adults, an increase in growth hormone causes **acromegaly,** a disease in which the bones—mainly the long ones—become very thick.

The sex hormones, both male (androgen) and female (estrogens), have a complex effect on bones and are, in a general way, stimulators of bone formation. They influence the time of appearance and the development of ossification centers. Thus, precocious sexual maturity due to sex hormone–producing tumors or to the administration of sex hormones retards bodily growth, since the epiphyseal cartilage is quickly replaced by bone. In hormone deficiencies due to abnormal development of the gonads or castration, epiphyseal cartilage remains functional for a longer period of time, resulting in tall stature.

Interrelationships Between the Cells of Bone

Radioautographic studies performed after the administration of ³H-thymidine to young animals—whose bone cells proliferate rapidly—reveal that osteoblasts and osteocytes do not divide after having been formed from the **osteoprogenitor cell,** which is a slightly differentiated mesenchymal cell. The osteoprogenitor cell has a "generation time" of about 36 hours; this means that during this interval its number doubles. Some of the new cells thus formed differentiate, giving rise to osteoblasts (Fig 8–24).

A. Fate of the Osteoblasts: Most of the osteoblasts give rise to osteocytes; others remain as osteoblasts for long periods of time; and some return to the state of the osteoprogenitor cell.

B. Fate of the Osteocytes: When destruction of the matrix occurs during the process of remodeling, it appears that some of the osteocytes die, but most of these cells probably return to the state of the osteoprogenitor cell. As a result of the extensive remodeling of bone that takes place in the epiphyseal disk, many of the osteocytes remain as osteocytes for a short period (minimum of 50 hours). In other sites (eg, in the haversian system), the cells may persist as osteocytes for a long time.

JOINTS

Bones are joined to one another to form the skeleton by means of connective tissue structures called joints. Joints may be classified as **diarthroses,** which permit free bone movement, and **synarthroses,** in which very limited or no movement occurs. There are 3 types of synarthrosis: synostosis, synchondrosis, and syndesmosis.

Synostosis

In joints of this type, bones are united by bone tissue. No movement takes place. In elderly people, this type of synarthrosis unites the skull bones. In children and young adults, these bones are united by dense connective tissue.

Synchondrosis

Synchondroses are articulations in which the bones are joined by hyaline cartilage. Limited movement may take place. The ribs are attached to the sternum in this way; the epiphyseal plate is another example.

Syndesmosis

As is the case with synchondroses, a syndesmosis permits a certain amount of movement. The bones are joined by an interosseous ligament (eg, the inferior tibiofibular articulation).

Diarthrosis

Diarthroses are joints that generally unite long bones and have great mobility. In a diarthrosis, a

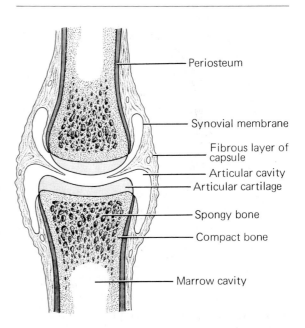

Figure 8–25. Schematic drawing of a diarthrosis. The capsule is formed by 2 parts, not clearly delimited: the external **fibrous layer** and the **synovial layer** (synovial membrane) that lines the articular cavity except the cartilaginous areas.

Periosteum

Synovial membrane

Fibrous layer of capsule

Articular cavity

Articular cartilage

Spongy bone

Compact bone

Marrow cavity

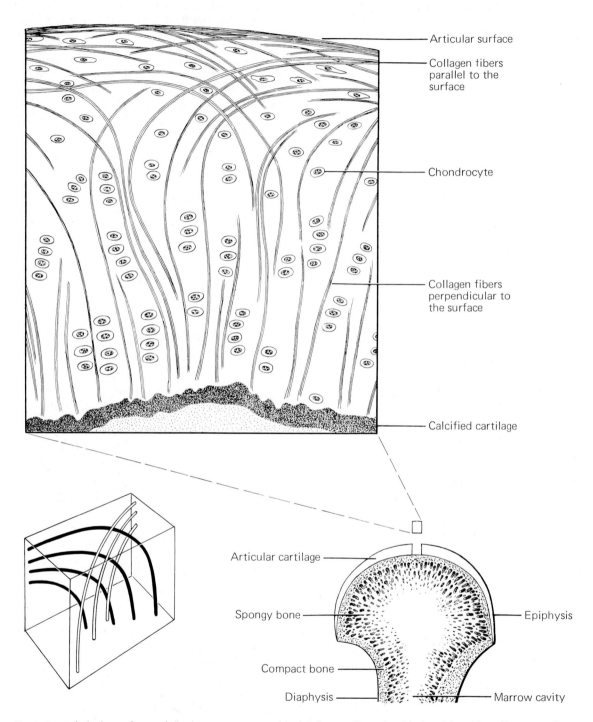

Figure 8–26. Articular surfaces of diarthroses are covered by hyaline cartilage devoid of perichondrium. The upper figure shows that in this cartilage collagen fibers are first perpendicular and then parallel to the cartilage surface. Deeply located chondrocytes are globular and are arranged in vertical rows. Superficially placed chondrocytes are flattened and are not organized in groups. The lower left drawing shows the organization of collagen fibers in articular cartilage in 3 dimensions.

capsule joins the extremities of the bones and encloses a sealed **articular cavity** that contains a colorless, transparent, viscous fluid, rich in hyaluronic acid, called **synovial fluid.** The sliding of articular surfaces covered by hyaline cartilage and having no perichondrium is facilitated by the lubricating synovial fluid, which also supplies nutrients and oxygen to the avascular articular cartilage (Figs 8–25 and 8–26).

The capsules of diarthroses (Fig 8–25) vary in structure according to the joint. Generally, however, this capsule is composed of 2 layers, one external **(fibrous layer)** and one internal **(synovial layer).**

The fluid encountered in the articular cavity is formed by the synovial layer, which is arranged in folds that occasionally penetrate deep into the interior of the articular cavity. The internal surface of the synovial membrane is usually lined by a layer of squamous or cuboidal cells. Underneath these cells is a layer of loose or dense connective tissue with areas of adipose tissue. The lining cells of the synovial membrane originate in the mesenchyme. They are separated from each other by a small amount of connective tissue ground substance (Figs 8–27 and 8–28).

Observations made with the electron microscope have shown 2 cell types lining the synovial membrane (Fig 8–28). Some of these cells are intensely phagocytic and are called **A cells.** They have a large Golgi complex and many lysosomes but only a small amount of rough endoplasmic reticulum. The other cell type is called the **B cell.** Cells of this type have a well-developed rough endoplasmic reticulum and are more electron-dense than A cells. A cells and B cells probably represent different functional stages of the same cell type.

Radioautographs analyzed under the light microscope show that the A cells synthesize hyaluronic acid, which is secreted into the synovial fluid. Much of the protein in synovial fluid derives from blood plasma,

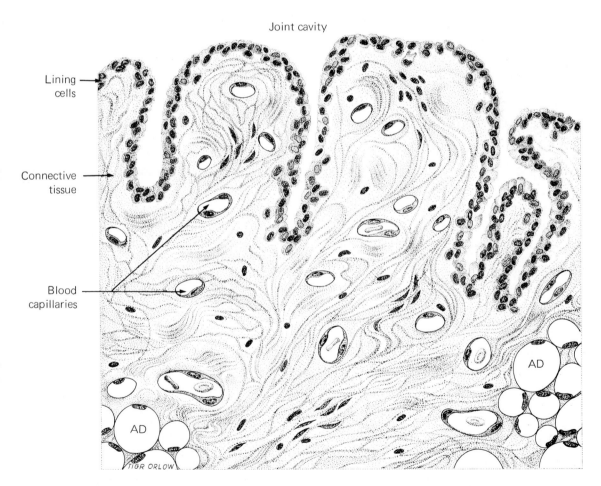

Figure 8–27. Histologic structure of the synovial membrane, with its lining cells in epitheloid arrangement. There is no basal lamina between the lining cells and the underlying connective tissue. This tissue is rich in blood capillaries and contains a variable amount of adipose cells (AD). (Reproduced, with permission, from Cossermelli W: *Reumatologia Básica.* Sarvier, 1971.)

but it is possible that the B cells make some contribution. Both A and B cells are phagocytic, but A cells are more active in this respect.

The fibrous layer is made of dense connective tissue that is better developed in parts subject to great strain. This layer envelops the ligaments of the joint and some of the tendons inserted into the bone near the joint.

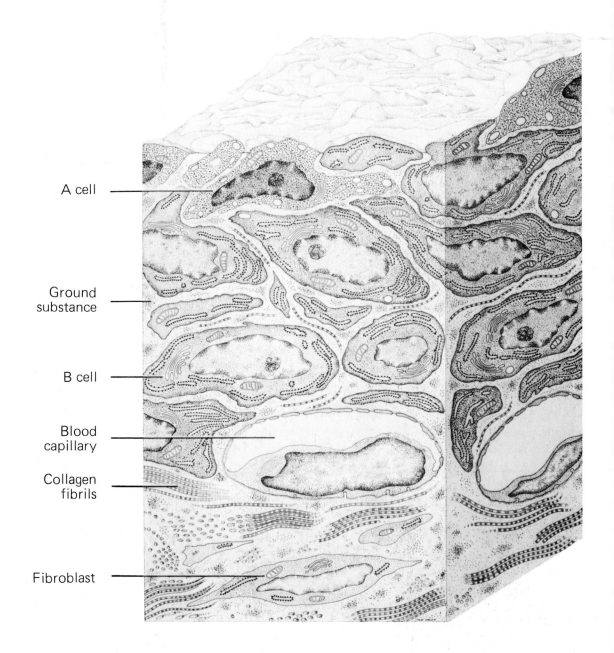

A cell

Ground substance

B cell

Blood capillary

Collagen fibrils

Fibroblast

Figure 8–28. Schematic representation of the ultrastructure of a synovial membrane. B and A cell types are separated by a small amount of connective tissue ground substance. No basal lamina is seen separating the lining cells from the connective tissue. Blood capillaries are of the fenestrated type, which facilitates exchange of substances between blood and synovial fluid.

REFERENCES

Anderson HC: Introduction to the second conference on matrix vesicle calcification. *Metab Bone Dis Relat Res* 1978;**1**:83.

Barland P, Novikoff AB, Hamerman D: Electron microscopy of the human synovial membrane. *J Cell Biol* 1962;**14**:207.

Barland P, Smith C, Hamerman D: Localization of hyaluronic acid in synovial cells by radioautography. *J Cell Biol* 1968;**37**:13.

Bourne GH (editor): *The Biochemistry and Physiology of Bone*, 2nd ed. 4 vols. Academic Press, 1971–1976.

Carneiro J, Leblond CP: Role of osteoblasts and odontoblasts in secreting the collagen of bone and dentin, as shown by radioautography in mice given tritium-labelled glycine. *Exp Cell Res* 1959;**18**:291.

Carneiro J, Leblond CP: Suitability of collagenase treatment for the radioautographic identification of newly-formed collagen labeled with ^{3}H-glycine or ^{3}H-proline. *J Histochem Cytochem* 1966;**14**:334.

Ghadially FN: *Fine Structure of Synovial Joints*. Butterworth, 1983.

Gothlin G, Ericsson JLE: The osteoclast: Review of ultrastructure, origin and structure-function relationship. *Clin Orthop* 1976;**120**:201.

Ham AW, Harris WR: Repair and transplantation of bone. In: *The Biochemistry and Physiology of Bone*, 2nd ed. Vol 3. Bourne GH (editor). Academic Press, 1976.

Hancox NM: *Biology of Bone*. Cambridge Univ Press, 1972.

Holtrop ME: The ultrastructure of bone. *Ann Clin Lab Sci* 1975;**5**:264.

Howell DS: Calcification mechanisms. *Isr J Med Sci* 1976;**12**:91.

Jones SJ, Boyde A: The migration of osteoblasts. *Cell Tissue Res* 1977;**184**:179.

Jones SJ, Boyde A: Some morphologic observations on osteoclasts. *Cell Tissue Res* 1977;**185**:387.

Jotereau FV, LeDouarin NM: The developmental relationship between osteocytes and osteoclasts: A study using the quail-chick nuclear marker in endochondral ossification. *Dev Biol* 1978;**63**:253.

Katchburian E: Initiation of mineral deposition in dentine. *Calcif Tissue Res* 1977;**22(Suppl).**

Katchburian E: Membrane-bound bodies as initiators of mineralization of dentine. *J Anat* 1973;**116**:285.

Owen M: Cellular dynamics of bone. In: *The Physiology and Biochemistry of Bone*. Vol 3. Bourne GH (editor). Academic Press, 1971.

Owen M: Histogenesis of bone cells. *Calcif Tissue Res* 1978;**25**:205.

Taylor AN, Wasserman RH: Immunofluorescent localization of vitamin D−dependent calcium-binding protein. *J Histochem Cytochem* 1970;**18**:107.

Termine JD et al: Osteonectin, a bone-specific protein linking mineral to collagen. *Cell* 1981;**26**:99.

Urist MR: Biochemistry of calcification. In: *The Biochemistry and Physiology of Bone*, 2nd ed. Vol 4. Bourne GH (editor). Academic Press, 1976.

Vaughan JM: *The Physiology of Bone*, 3rd ed. Clarendon Press, 1981.

Nerve Tissue

The human nervous system contains at least 10 billion neurons. These basic building blocks of the nervous system have evolved from primitive neuro-effector cells that respond to various stimuli by contracting. In higher animals, contraction became the specialized function of muscle cells, while transmission of nerve impulses became the specialized function of neurons.

Nerve tissue is distributed throughout the body as an integrated communications network. Anatomically, the nervous system is divided into the **central nervous system,** consisting of the brain and the spinal cord; and the **peripheral nervous system,** composed of nerve fibers and small aggregates of nerve cells called **nerve ganglia.**

Structurally, nerve tissue consists of 2 classes of cell types: **nerve cells,** or **neurons,** which usually show numerous long processes; and several types of **glial cells,** or **neuroglia,** which support and protect neurons and participate in neural activity, neural nutrition, and the defense processes of the central nervous system.

In the central nervous system, nerve cell bodies are concentrated in groups **(nuclei)** located at some distance from the tips of their processes. The brain and spinal cord are composed of **gray matter** and **white matter.** The former contains mainly nerve cell bodies and neuroglia but also a complicated network of nerve cell processes. White matter does not contain nerve cell bodies; it consists of neuronal processes and neuroglia. It takes its name from the presence of a whitish material called **myelin** that envelops most of the neuronal processes. The brain stem exhibits zones containing both nerve cells and myelinated fibers—an area where gray matter is mixed with white matter.

Neurons respond to environmental changes **(stimuli)** by altering electrical potential differences that exist between the inner and the outer surfaces of their membranes. Cells with this property (eg, neurons, muscle cells, some gland cells) are called "excitable" or "irritable." Neurons react promptly to stimuli, and modification of electrical potential may be restricted to the place that received the stimulus or may be spread (propagated) throughout the neuron by the membrane. This propagation, called the **action potential** or **nerve impulse,** transmits information to other neurons, muscles, and glands.

The 2 fundamental functions of the nervous system are (1) to detect, analyze, integrate, and transmit all information generated by sensory stimuli (such as heat and light) and by mechanical and chemical changes that take place in the internal and external milieu; and (2) to organize and coordinate, directly or indirectly, most functions of the body, especially the motor, visceral, endocrine, and mental activities.

DEVELOPMENT OF NERVE TISSUE

Nerve tissues develop from embryonic ectoderm that is induced to differentiate in this direction by the underlying notochord. First, a neural plate forms; then the edges of the plate thicken, forming the neural groove. The edges of the groove grow toward each other and ultimately fuse, forming the neural tube. This structure gives rise to the entire central nervous system, including neurons, glial cells, ependymal cells, and epithelial cells of the choroid plexus.

Some cells lateral to the neural groove, comprising the **neural crest,** undergo extensive migrations and give rise to most of the peripheral nervous system, as well as a number of other structures. The following is a list of neural crest derivatives: (1) chromaffin cells of the adrenal medulla (see Chapter 22); (2) melanocytes of skin and subcutaneous tissues (see Chapter 19); (3) odontoblasts (see Chapter 16); (4) cells of the pia mater and the arachnoid; (5) sensory neurons of cranial and spinal sensory ganglia; (6) postganglionic neurons of sympathetic and parasympathetic ganglia; (7) Schwann cells of peripheral axons; (8) satellite cells of peripheral ganglia.

NEURONS

Nerve cells, or neurons, are independent anatomic and functional units with complex morphologic characteristics. Most neurons consist of 3 parts: the **dendrites,** which are multiple elongated processes specialized in receiving stimuli from the environment, from sensory epithelial cells, or from other neurons; the **cell body,** or **perikaryon,** which represents the trophic center for the whole nerve cell and is also receptive to stimuli; and the **axon,** which is a single process specialized in generating or conducting nerve impulses to other cells (nerve, muscle, and gland cells). The distal portion of the axon is usually branched and constitutes the **terminal arborization.** Each branch of this arborization terminates on the next cell in dilatations called **end bulbs** (boutons), which form a

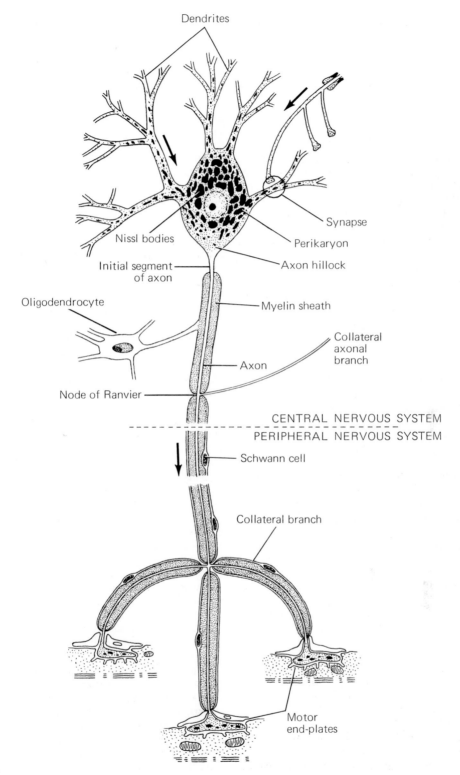

Figure 9–1. Schematic drawing of a Nissl-stained motor neuron. The myelin sheath is produced by oligodendrocytes in the central nervous system and by Schwann cells in the peripheral nervous system. The neuronal cell body has an unusually large, euchromatic nucleus with a well-developed nucleolus. The perikaryon contains Nissl bodies, which are also found in large dendrites. An axon from another neuron is shown at upper right. It has 3 end bulbs, one of which synapses with the neuron. Note also 3 motor end-plates, which transmit the nerve impulse to striated skeletal muscle fibers. Arrows show the direction of the nerve impulse.

part of the **synapse.** Synapses transmit information to the next cell in the chain (Fig 9–1).

Neurons usually receive information through dendrites and cell bodies, where it is integrated, and then transmit this information onward via the axons. This sequence, termed **dynamic polarization** by Cajal, constitutes a general mechanism in neuronal function, although several exceptions exist.

Neurons and their processes are extremely variable in size and shape (Fig 9–2). Perikaryons can be spherical, ovoid, or angular in contour; some are very large, measuring up to 150 μm in diameter—large enough to be visible to the naked eye. Other nerve cells are among the smallest cells in the body; for example, the perikaryons of granular cells of the cerebellum are only 4–5 μm in diameter.

According to the size and shape of their processes, most neurons can be placed in one of the following categories: **multipolar neurons,** which have more than 2 cell processes, one being the axon and the others dendrites; **bipolar neurons,** with one dendrite and one axon; and **pseudounipolar neurons,** which have a single process close to the perikaryon but which divides into 2 branches, forming a T shape, one branch extending to a peripheral ending and the other toward the central nervous system (Fig 9–2).

In the embryo, a pseudounipolar neuron starts as a bipolar cell with a dendrite and an axon, each arising from opposite ends of the perikaryon. During later development, the 2 processes come together on one side of the cell and fuse for a certain distance close to the perikaryon. Certain cells, like the amacrine cells of the retina, do not have axons in the ordinary sense, and their processes appear to be both axonic and dendritic. In typical pseudounipolar neurons, both branches are axons on both structural and electrophysiologic grounds. In pseudounipolar neurons, the arborizations of the peripheral branches receive stimuli and are functional dendrites. The significance of this type of neuron is that stimuli picked up by the dendrites travel directly to the axon terminal without passing through the perikaryon.

Most neurons of the body are multipolar. Bipolar neurons are found in the cochlear and vestibular ganglia as well as in the retina and the olfactory mucosa. Pseudounipolar neurons are found in the spinal ganglia, which are sensory ganglia located in the dorsal roots of the spinal nerves, and they are also found in most cranial ganglia.

Neurons can also be classified according to their functional roles. **Motor neurons** control effector organs such as muscle fibers and exocrine and endocrine glands. **Sensory neurons** are involved in the reception of sensory stimuli from the environment and from within the body. **Interneurons** establish interrelationships among other neurons, forming complex functional chains or circuits.

During mammalian evolution there has been a great increase in the number and complexity of interneurons. Highly developed functions of the nervous system cannot be ascribed to simple neuron circuits; rather, they depend on complex interactions established by the integrated functions of many neurons.

In the central nervous system, nerve cell bodies are present only in the gray matter. White matter contains neuronal processes but no perikaryons. In the peripheral nervous system, perikaryons are found in ganglia and in some sensory regions (eg, retina, olfactory mucosa).

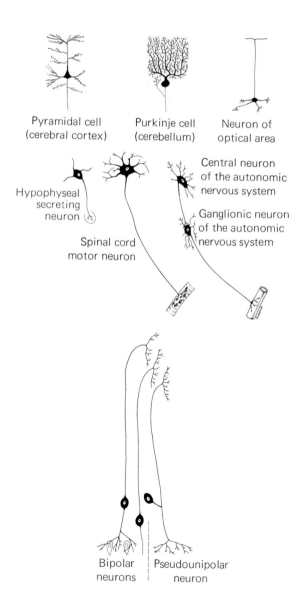

Pyramidal cell (cerebral cortex)

Purkinje cell (cerebellum)

Neuron of optical area

Hypophyseal secreting neuron

Central neuron of the autonomic nervous system

Ganglionic neuron of the autonomic nervous system

Spinal cord motor neuron

Bipolar neurons

Pseudounipolar neuron

Figure 9–2 (at left). Diagrams of several types of neurons. Neurons have a very complex morphology. Except for the bipolar and pseudounipolar neurons, which are not very numerous in nerve tissue, all others shown here are of the common multipolar variety.

PERIKARYON, OR SOMA

The perikaryon is the part of the neuron that contains the nucleus and surrounding cytoplasm exclusive of the cell processes. It is primarily a trophic center, but it also has receptive capabilities. The perikaryon of most neurons receives a great number of nerve endings that convey excitatory or inhibitory stimuli generated in other nerve cells (Fig 9–3).

Nucleus

Most nerve cells have a spherical, unusually large, euchromatic (pale-staining) nucleus with a prominent nucleolus. The nucleus is most often located in the center of the cell body except in the nerve cells of Clarke's column of the spinal column and in some sympathetic ganglia, where it is situated eccentrically. Binuclear nerve cells are seen in sympathetic and sensory ganglia. The chromatin is finely dispersed,

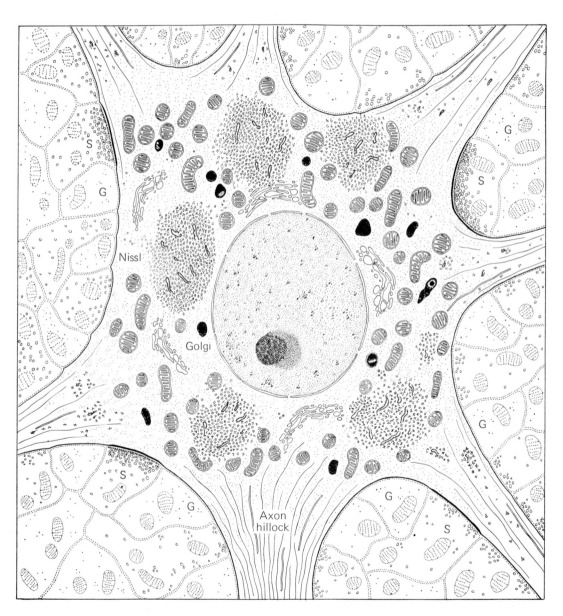

Figure 9–3. Ultrastructure of a neuron. The neuronal surface is completely covered either by synaptic endings of other neurons (S) or by processes of glial cells (G). At synapses, the neuronal membrane is thicker and is called the postsynaptic membrane. The neuronal process devoid of ribosomes (lower part of figure) is the axon hillock. The other processes of this cell are dendrites.

reflecting the intense synthetic activity of these cells. In females, between the large nucleolus and the nuclear membrane, a special chromatin clump (**Barr body**) is found in neurons. This is the sex chromatin, first discovered in nerve cells from female cats and later located in other cells of the body of females. This chromatin represents the inactivated X chromosome that remains condensed during interphase.

Rough Endoplasmic Reticulum

Perikaryons contain a highly developed rough endoplasmic reticulum organized into aggregates of parallel cisternae. In the cytoplasm between the cisternae, there are numerous polysomes, which usually form rosettes; these cells synthesize both structural proteins and proteins for transport. When appropriate stains are used, rough endoplasmic reticulum and free ribosomes appear under the light microscope as basophilic granular areas called **Nissl bodies** (Figs 9–1 and 9–4).

The number of Nissl bodies varies according to neuronal type and functional state. They are particularly abundant in large nerve cells such as the motor neurons (Fig 9–4).

Injury to axons or neuron exhaustion resulting from strong or prolonged stimuli causes a reduction in the number of Nissl bodies. This alteration is called **chromatolysis** and occurs simultaneously with nuclear migration to the periphery of the perikaryon. However, moderate stimuli may increase the amount of RNA in the perikaryon.

Golgi Complex

The Golgi complex is located only in the perikaryon and consists of multiple parallel arrays of smooth cisternae arranged around the periphery of the nucleus. There are also a number of smaller, spherical vesicles that likely represent both transfer and secretory vesicles (Fig 9–3). With the use of osmic acid or silver impregnation techniques, the Golgi complex takes on the appearance of a network of irregular filaments. Some profiles of smooth endoplasmic reticulum are seen near the Golgi area.

Mitochondria

Mitochondria are found in neurons and are especially abundant in the axon terminals. They are scattered throughout the cytoplasm of the perikaryon.

Neurofilaments & Microtubules

Intermediate filaments with a diameter of 10 nm, called neurofilaments, are abundant in perikaryons and cell processes. Neurofilaments agglutinate as a result of the action of certain fixatives. When impregnated with silver, they form **neurofibrils** that are visible with the light microscope. In tissue cultures under certain conditions, it is possible to see neurofibrillike structures in living neurons. The neurofilaments can probably be seen because they are often aligned as closely packed, parallel bundles of filaments, though they are actually below the limit of resolution of the light microscope. Crisscrossing arrays of neurofilaments cut through the agglomerations of rough endoplasmic reticulum and free polysomes and, as a consequence, carve up this basophilic material into the discrete clusters recognized, after appropriate staining, as Nissl bodies. The perikaryon also contains microtubules with a diameter of 24 nm identical to those found in many other cells (Fig 9–5).

Inclusions

In certain areas of the central nervous system, the perikaryons contain dark brown or black granules. Areas where this pigmentation is seen are the dorsal motor nucleus of the vagus nerve, the spinal and sympathetic ganglia, the substantia nigra of the midbrain, and the locus ceruleus in the floor of the fourth ventricle. The functional role of this **melanin** pigment in nerve cells is obscure. Another pigment sometimes found in nerve cell bodies is **lipofuscin**. This is a light brown lipid-containing pigment that accumulates in increasing amounts with age. It probably represents a residue of material undigested by lysosomes. Lipid droplets may occur in nerve cell bodies.

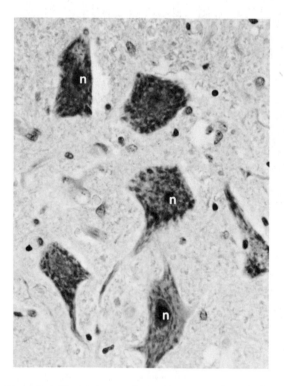

Figure 9–4. Photomicrograph of motor neurons from the human spinal cord. The cytoplasm contains a great number of Nissl bodies, making it difficult to see the cell nucleus (n). Although their cellular boundaries are not evident, nuclei of numerous glial and endothelial cells are present around the neurons. H&E stain, × 360.

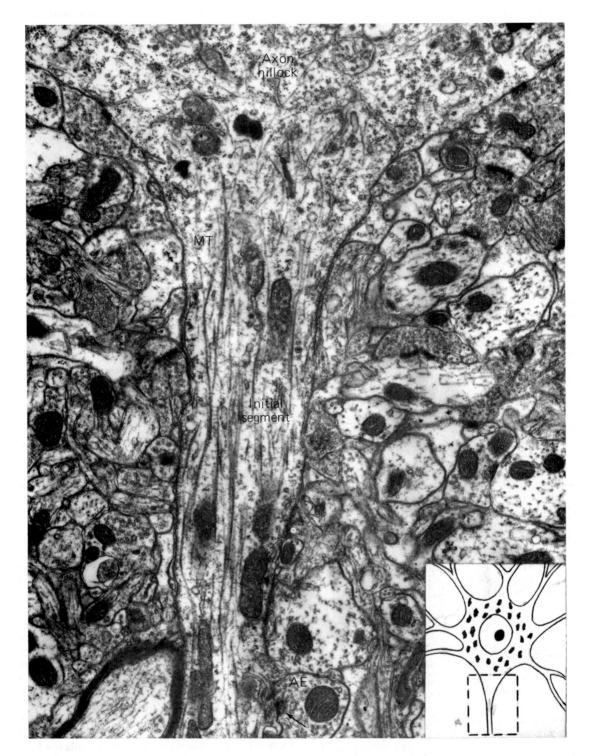

Figure 9–5. Electron micrograph of the axon hillock and the axon's first segment. (Position in relation to the neuron is indicated in the inset.) The axon hillock lacks ribosomes and endoplasmic reticulum. The parallel arrangement of microtubules (MT) in bundles is initiated in the axon hillock and becomes more pronounced in the initial segment of the axon. An axon ending (AE—arrow) synapses with the initial segment in the lower portion of the micrograph. Note that there is virtually no intercellular material in nerve tissue. (See also Fig 9–3.) × 26,000. (Courtesy of A Peters.)

DENDRITES

Most nerve cells have numerous dendrites, which increase considerably the receptive area of the cell. Dendrite arborization makes it possible for one neuron to receive and integrate a great number of axon terminals from other nerve cells. It has been estimated that up to 200,000 axonal terminations establish functional contact with the dendrites of the Purkinje cell found in the cerebellum (Fig 9–2). In other nerve cells, that number may be even higher. Neurons with only one dendrite (bipolar neurons) are uncommon and are found only in special sites. In contrast to axons, which maintain a constant diameter from one end to the other, dendrites become thinner as they subdivide into branches.

The composition of dendritic cytoplasm is very similar to that of the perikaryon; however, dendrites are devoid of Golgi complexes. Nissl bodies and mitochondria are present except in very thin dendrites. Neurofilaments (10 nm) and microtubules (about 24 nm), also found in axons, are more numerous in dendrites. Dendrites are usually short and divide like the branches of a tree (arborization). In some instances, however, they assume other forms—for example, the characteristic dendrites of the cerebellar Purkinje cells branch in one plane only, assuming the shape of a fan (Fig 9–2) and increasing the surface area of each Purkinje cell from 250 μm² in early development to 27,000 μm² in the mature cell. Dendrites are usually covered by a large number of thorny spines or gemmules, which are small dendritic projections representing sites of synaptic contact.

AXONS

Most neurons have only one axon; a very few do not have an axon at all. An axon is a cylindric process that varies in length and diameter according to the type of neuron. Although some neurons have short axons, axons are usually very long processes. For example, axons of the motor cells of the spinal cord that innervate the foot muscles may have a length of up to 100 cm (about 40 inches).

All axons originate from a short pyramid-shaped region called the **axon hillock** that usually arises from the perikaryon (Fig 9–3) but in a few cases originates from the stem of a major dendrite. The axon hillock can be differentiated from dendrites by distinctive cytologic features. (1) The rough endoplasmic reticulum and ribosomes found in perikaryons and dendrites do not extend into the axon hillock. (2) In the axon hillock, the microtubules are arranged in fascicles or bundles (Figs 9–3 and 9–5). The plasma membrane of the axon is called the **axolemma** and its contents **axoplasm.**

In neurons that give rise to a myelinated axon, the portion of the axon between the axon hillock and the point at which myelination begins is named the **initial segment.** The initial segment of the axon is the site where various excitatory and inhibitory stimuli impinging on the neuron are algebraically summed, resulting in the "decision" to propagate an action potential or not. It is known that several types of ion channels are localized in the initial segment and that these channels are important in generating the propagating electrical potential change that constitutes the action potential, or nerve impulse. The initial segment of the axon is characterized by a thin layer of electron-dense material beneath the plasma membrane called **dense undercoating.** Microtubules and neurofilaments continue in fascicles from the axon hillock into the initial segment.

In contrast to dendrites, axons have a constant diameter and do not branch profusely. Occasionally, the axon, shortly after its departure from the cell body, gives rise to a branch that returns to the area of the nerve cell body. These branches are known as **collaterals** (Fig 9–1).

Axonal cytoplasm (axoplasm) possesses a few mitochondria, microtubules, and neurofilaments and some cisternae of smooth endoplasmic reticulum. The absence of organelles involved in protein synthesis emphasizes the dependence of the axon on the perikaryon for its maintenance. If an axon is severed, its peripheral parts degenerate and die.

SYNAPSES

When axons are artificially stimulated, they conduct the nerve impulse in both directions from the stimulation point. The impulse directed to the cell body, however, does not excite other neurons, and only the impulse reaching the final arborization of the axon, the axon terminal, can excite the next cell in the chain, be it neuron, muscle, or gland cell.

This dynamic polarization of the transmission of the nerve impulse depends on highly specialized structures called synapses, which are classically defined as the contact of one axon with the dendrites or perikaryon and, very rarely, with the axon of another neuron. Synaptic contact also is established between neurons and muscle and gland cells. Most central nervous system synapses are between an axon and a dendrite (axodendritic) or between an axon and a cell body (axosomatic). But there are also synapses between dendrites (dendrodendritic) and between axons (axoaxonic). Synapses function by altering the membrane potential of neurons and other effector cells. The influence of a particular synapse on a neuron is related to its distance from the initial segment of the axon. Consequently, the influence of incoming information on neuronal activity is intimately related to the distribution and location, as well as number, of synapses on the dendritic tree and cell body.

Morphologically, several types of synapses can be identified. The axon terminal may form bulbous expansions, basketlike structures, or club-shaped terminations (Fig 9–6). These synaptic end bulbs are often called **boutons terminaux.** More often the axon are firmly bound together at the synaptic region, and in some instances dense filaments form bridges between them. The plasma membranes of the 2 neurons appear to be thicker at the presynaptic and postsynaptic areas of the synapse than elsewhere. This apparent increase in membrane thickness is due to the accumulation of dense-staining cytoplasmic proteins beneath the membranes forming the synapse. This accumulation may be more abundant on the postsynaptic side of the synapse (asymmetric, or type I, synapse) or equally distributed on both sides (symmetric, or type II, synapse). Cytoplasmic filaments resembling those found in desmosomes are anchored to the inside of each of these membranes.

The cytoplasm in the endings of the terminal typically contains numerous **synaptic vesicles** (Figs 9–7 and 9–23) with a diameter of 20–65 nm, although some vesicles as large as 160 nm have been observed.

Synaptic vesicle shape and content have been correlated with the function of the synapse. Thus, round, clear vesicles are associated with acetylcholine-mediated excitatory transmission at the neuromuscular junction and at other sites in the central nervous system. Flattened, 20- × 50-nm vesicles are often (but not universally) seen in neuron endings whose effect is inhibitory on the postsynaptic neuron. The pre- and postsynaptic densities are more symmetric at these inhibitory junctions (type II synapse). Norepinephrine-secreting axons display vesicles with an overall diameter of 40–60 nm and a dense-staining core with a diameter of 15–25 nm. Larger vesicles (80–90 nm in diameter, 50-nm core) have been observed in many synaptic endings, but their content has not been identified, and thus their significance is unknown. Neurosecretory axons (eg, axons of the paraventricular and supraoptic nuclei of the hypothalamus that contain oxytocin, vasopressin, and their associated neurophysins) have larger secretory granules, 120–150 nm in diameter. Electron-dense material fills these granules with no intervening clear space.

Neurofilaments are infrequent, but mitochondria are numerous. The synaptic vesicles contain substances called **neurotransmitters** that are responsible for the transmission of the nerve impulse across the synapse. These mediators are liberated at the presynaptic membrane by exocytosis and act on the postsynaptic membrane to initiate an excitatory or inhibitory response. The membranes of synaptic vesicles that are incorporated into the presynaptic membranes undergo endocytosis and are reused to form new synaptic vesicles (see new vesicle formation in Fig 9–25).

Besides the chemical synapses described above, in which a chemical substance mediates the transmission of the nerve impulse, there are also the electrical synapses. Here the nerve cells are linked through a gap junction (see Chapter 4), which permits the passage of ions from one cell to another, thus providing for their electrical coupling. Electrical synapses are less numerous than chemical synapses, but they are being observed with increasing frequency owing to technical improvements in electron microscopy.

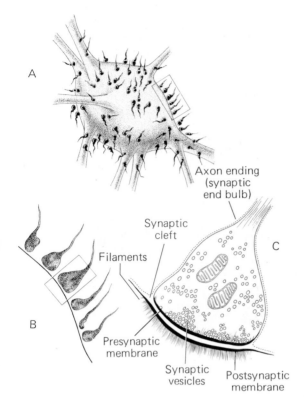

Figure 9–6. *A:* External morphology of a neuron and some of its processes. Axon endings from other neurons are shown in black. The area outlined by a rectangle appears enlarged at *B. B:* At synaptic junctions, the 2 cell membranes are separated by a slender space—the synaptic cleft. *C:* Ultrastructure of the synapse outlined in *B.* Presynaptic and postsynaptic membranes appear to be thicker than the neuronal membrane elsewhere. This is due to the accumulation of cytoplasmic proteins adjacent to these membranes. The axon ending shows 2 mitochondria as well as numerous synaptic vesicles that contain neurotransmitters. Liberation of the mediator substance transmits the nerve impulse from the presynaptic to the postsynaptic membrane. (Redrawn and reproduced, with permission, from De Robertis, Novinsky, and Saez: *Biologia Celular,* 8th ed. El Ateneo [Buenos Aires], 1970.)

establishes several synapses along its course. In this case, there are enlargements along the axon, called **boutons en passage.** The analysis of a synapse under the electron microscope shows that it is actually a specialized, localized region of a contact between 2 cells (Figs 9–6 and 9–23). It is composed of a terminal membrane (presynaptic membrane), a region of extracellular space (the **synaptic cleft**), and a postsynaptic membrane belonging to a dendrite, perikaryon, axon of another neuron, or membrane of a muscle or gland cell. At a synapse, the plasma membranes of the 2 neurons are usually separated by a distance of 20–30 nm (the synaptic cleft). These membranes

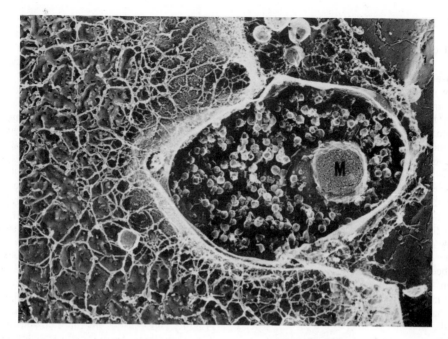

Figure 9–7. View of a rotary-replicated freeze-etched synapse. Synaptic vesicles surround a mitochondrion (M) in the axon terminal. × 25,000. (Reproduced, with permission, from Heuser JE, Salpeter SR: Organization of acetylcholine receptors in quick-frozen, deep-etched, and rotary-replicated Torpedo postsynaptic membrane. *J Cell Biol* 1979;**82**:150.)

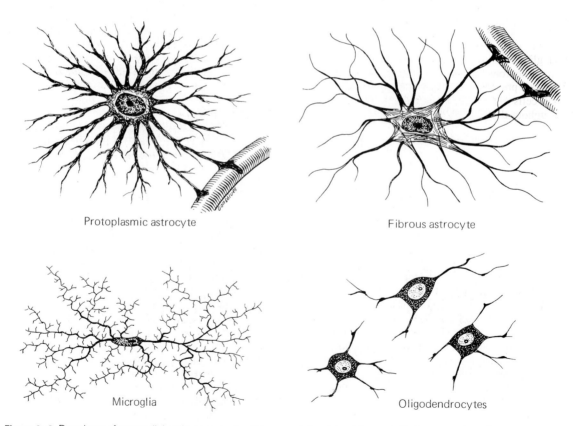

Protoplasmic astrocyte

Fibrous astrocyte

Microglia

Oligodendrocytes

Figure 9–8. Drawings of neuroglial cells as seen in slides specially stained by metallic impregnation. Observe that only astrocytes exhibit vascular end-feet, which cover the walls of blood capillaries.

NEUROGLIA

Several cell types found in the central nervous system in association with the neurons are classified as **neuroglia,** or **glial cells.** The several types of neuroglia show morphologic and functional differences (Figs 9–8 and 9–9).

Routine hematoxylin and eosin preparations are not adequate to study neuroglia, since with this staining technique only their small nuclei (3–10 μm in diameter) can be seen among the larger nuclei of nerve cells (Fig 9–4). The cytoplasm and processes of the neuroglia are not identifiable, for it is impossible to distinguish them from the processes of the neurons. The neuroglia play an important role in the normal function of the nervous system. For the study of the morphology of neuroglia, special procedures involving silver or gold impregnation techniques are used.

It has been estimated that in the central nervous system there are 10 glial cells for each neuron. However, since neuroglia are much smaller, they occupy only about half of the total volume of nervous tissue.

Neuroglia include several varieties: astrocytes, oligodendrocytes, microglia, and ependymal cells. Astrocytes and oligodendrocytes are referred to as the **macroglia.**

Neuroglial cells are not thought to generate action potentials, and they do not form synapses with other cells. Oligodendroglial cells form the myelin sheaths of axons in the central nervous system and are probably necessary for the maintenance and viability of neurons. This latter possibility is supported by the fact that glial cells are necessary for tissue culturing of normal neurons, which cannot be grown unless neuroglia are present in the culture. In contrast to neurons, glial cells retain their ability to undergo mitosis throughout the life of the organism.

1. ASTROCYTES

Astrocytes are the largest of the neuroglia, possessing numerous long processes. They have spherical, centrally located nuclei that stain lightly (Fig 9–8). Many of their processes have expanded pedicles at their ends that attach to the walls of blood capillaries. These pedicles, called the "vascular feet" of the neuroglia, completely surround and ensheathe all vessels of the nourishing vascular network. Processes of astrocytes are also present at the periphery of the brain and spinal cord, forming a layer under the pia mater. This layer, which also contains processes of other neuroglia, separates the connective tissue of the pia mater from the nerve cells. Astrocytes provide some structural support for nervous tissue. In certain regions, astrocyte processes appear to isolate groups of synaptic endings from adjacent endings. This may limit "cross talk" between neighboring communication channels. There are 2 types of astrocytes: protoplasmic, which are found in the gray matter of the brain and spinal cord; and fibrous, which are found chiefly in the white matter. In electron micrographs, astrocytes are identified by their light-staining, relatively organelle-free cytoplasm. Intermediate filaments, which are 8 nm in diameter and composed of glial fibrillar acidic protein, are abundant.

Protoplasmic Astrocytes

Protoplasmic astrocytes have abundant granular cytoplasm. Their processes have many branches, are shorter than those of fibrous astrocytes, and are relatively thick (Figs 9–8 and 9–9). Their processes envelop the surface of nerve cells, the synaptic areas, and blood vessels.

Fibrous Astrocytes

Fibrous astrocytes have long, slender, smooth processes that branch infrequently. In special silver-stained preparations, their cytoplasm shows fibrillar material

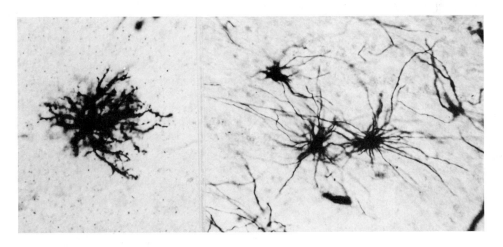

Figure 9–9. Photomicrographs of cerebrum sections silver-stained to show glial cells. *Left:* One protoplasmic astrocyte. *Right:* Several fibrous astrocytes. × 500.

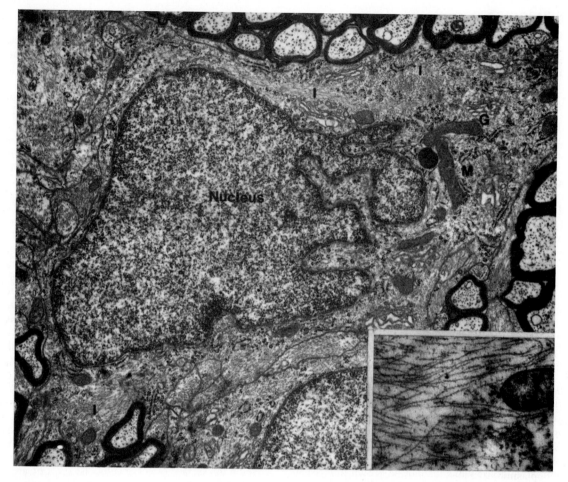

Figure 9–10. Electron micrograph of a fibrous astrocyte. G, Golgi complex; M, mitochondrion; I, intermediate (8-nm) filaments. × 12,000. In the inset, the magnification is × 42,000 and shows the abundant filaments in the cytoplasm. (Courtesy of A Peters.)

that is probably formed by the aggregation of 10-nm intermediate filaments (see Chapter 3) abundant in the cell bodies and processes of fibrous astrocytes (Figs 9–9 and 9–10).

2. OLIGODENDROCYTES

Oligodendrocytes are much smaller than astrocytes, and their processes are less numerous and shorter than those present in other neuroglia (Fig 9–8). Their nuclei are smaller and more intensely stained than nuclei of astrocytes. Oligodendrocytes are found both in gray and in white matter. In gray matter, they are mainly localized close to perikaryons.

The number of oligodendrocytes increases with increasing complexity of the nervous system in different species. Human nerve tissue has the highest number of oligodendrocytes per nerve cell.

In white matter, oligodendrocytes appear in rows among the myelinated nerve fibers. Study of fetal

nerve tissue with the electron microscope shows that the myelin sheath of central nervous system tissue is produced by the processes of oligodendrocytes. In this aspect of their function, the oligodendrocytes are analogous to the Schwann cells of peripheral nerves (Fig 9–12). Unlike Schwann cells, oligodendroglial cells can participate in the myelination of more than one axon (Fig 9–12).

The cytoplasm of oligodendrocytes is electron-dense and contains many mitochondria, a large Golgi complex, cisternae of rough endoplasmic reticulum, and numerous microtubules. These characteristics permit their identification in electron micrographs.

3. MICROGLIA

The cell bodies of microglia are small, dense, and elongated. Their nuclei show highly condensed chromatin and an elongated shape along the axis of the cell body. The shape of the nuclei of microglia permits their identification in hematoxylin and eosin preparations, for other neuroglia have spherical nuclei. Microglia have short processes covered by numerous small expansions, giving them a thorny appearance (Fig 9–8). Microglia are not numerous, but they are found in both white and gray matter.

Although many microglia might be evident using special silver-stained light microscope preparations, very few microglial cells are observed in electron microscopic studies. It appears that many of the so-called microglial cells seen in the light microscope actually represent oligodendroglia or immature **glioblasts.** However, there are some phagocytic microglial cells that apparently arise from blood-borne monocytes and represent the mononuclear phagocyte system in nervous tissue.

4. EPENDYMAL CELLS

Ependymal cells derive from the internal lining of the neural tube and retain their epithelial arrangement, whereas the other cells from the neural tube develop processes and give rise to neurons or to neuroglia. Ependymal cells line the cavities of the brain and spinal cord and are bathed by the cerebrospinal fluid, which fills these cavities. Most ependymal cells possess motile cilia that serve to produce movement of the cerebrospinal fluid. Regional differences do occur; eg, the lower wall of the third ventricle is almost devoid of cilia.

Ependymal cells possess an abundance of mitochondria, an apical Golgi complex, and a sparse rough endoplasmic reticulum. The lateral surfaces of some ependymal cells exhibit gap junctions and zonulae adherentes, but in most areas of the brain, tight junctions (zonulae occludentes) are absent. Thus, substances in the cerebrospinal fluid can come in contact with cells deep within the thick neuroepithelium.

The contour of the basal surface of the ependymal cell varies with its position in the brain or spinal cord. Most ependymal cells have a flattened base, but some have a long process that extends deep into the subjacent neural tissue. This latter type of cell is called a **tanycyte** and is conspicuous in the floor of the third ventricle. Here, the tanycyte may play a role in transferring chemical signals from cerebrospinal fluid to the primary capillary plexus of the hypophyseal-pituitary portal system (see Chapter 21).

HISTOPHYSIOLOGY OF NEUROGLIA

In the central nervous system, connective tissue layers form the enveloping protective and vascular coats (meninges) of the organ. The very small amount of connective tissue which extends into the nerve tissue is restricted to sheaths that are present around the larger blood vessels. In the central nervous system, the supporting function of connective tissue is assumed by neuroglia. Because of their number and their long processes, astrocytes seem to be the most important supporting elements.

Glial cells, especially astrocytes, participate in the repair process following injury to the central nervous system. Repair consists of proliferation of glial cells that fill the defect left by the degeneration of neurons and their processes. Astrocytes may also participate in the formation of the blood-brain barrier, although it is now generally believed that tight junctions between endothelial cells have the major role in preventing indiscriminate access of circulating molecules to neural tissue.

The idea that astrocytes can selectively take up and transfer materials to neurons, thereby serving a trophic function, is now generally discounted. The intercellular space between neurons and glial cells seems adequate for this function.

Oligodendroglial cells are frequently found adjacent to neurons, and this association has given rise to the concept that oligodendroglial cells have a symbiotic relation with neurons. Cytochemical studies performed on neurons and satellite cells isolated by microsurgery have shown a metabolic dependency between them. Any stimulus that alters the chemical composition of the nerve cell is also reflected in the satellite cell. Electron microscopic examination has revealed processes of astrocytes between the neuron in question and its supposedly symbiotic oligodendroglial cell. The concept is thus called into question, and further research is needed. It is known that, in tissue cultures, neurons do not survive unless they are associated with their satellite cells.

NERVE FIBERS

Nerve fibers consist of axons enveloped by special sheaths. The axon sheaths are of ectodermal origin. Groups of nerve fibers constitute the tracts of the brain, spinal cord, and peripheral nerves. Nerve fibers exhibit differences in their enveloping sheaths related to whether the fibers are part of the central or peripheral nervous system.

Most axons in adult nerve tissue are ensheathed by single or multiple folds of a sheath cell. In peripheral nerve fibers, the sheath cell is the **Schwann cell,** and in central nerve fibers it is the oligodendrocyte. Axons of small diameter are usually **unmyelinated nerve fibers** (Figs 9–11 and 9–16). Progressively thicker axons are generally ensheathed by increasingly numerous concentric wrappings of the enveloping cell. When enveloped by **myelin sheaths,** the fibers are known as **myelinated nerves** (Figs 9–12 and 9–14). Axonal conduction of the nerve impulse is faster in axons with larger diameters and thicker myelin sheaths. Fresh myelinated fibers appear as white, homogeneous, glistening cylinders.

Myelinated Fibers

In these fibers, the plasmalemma of the covering Schwann cell winds around and enwraps the axon. In

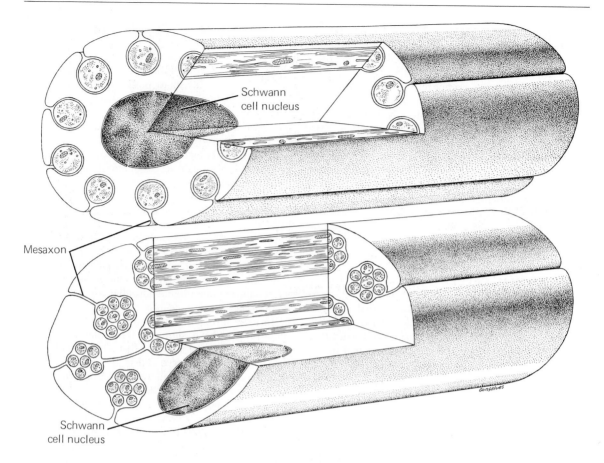

Schwann
cell nucleus

Mesaxon

Schwann
cell nucleus

Figure 9–11. *Above:* The most frequent type of unmyelinated nerve fiber, in which isolated axons are surrounded by a Schwann cell and each axon has its own mesaxon. *Below:* Many very thin axons are sometimes found together surrounded by the Schwann cell. In such cases, there is one mesaxon for several axons.

this process, the layers of membranes of the sheath cell unite and form a lipoprotein complex called **mye-lin,** which can be partly removed (the lipid component) by standard histologic procedures. Its presence can be demonstrated by osmium tetroxide, which preserves myelin and stains it black (Fig 9–14).

Each axon is surrounded by myelin formed by a series of Schwann cells. The myelin sheath shows gaps along its path called the **nodes of Ranvier** (Fig 9–15), which represent the spaces between adjacent Schwann cells along the length of the axon. At the node of Ranvier, the membrane of the axon (axolemma) shows an inner layer of electron-dense material forming a dense undercoat. Interdigitating processes of Schwann cells partially cover the node (Fig 9–16). The distance between 2 nodes is called an **internode** and consists of one Schwann cell (Figs 9–1, 9–15, and 9–16). The length of the internode varies between 1 and 2 mm, depending on the diameter of the axon (Figs 9–15 and 9–16). The thickness of the myelin sheath varies according to the axonal diameter, but it is constant along the extent of a particular axon. Under the light microscope, the myelin

sheath shows cone-shaped clefts called **clefts** or **incisures of Schmidt-Lanterman** that are actually helical cytoplasmic tunnels from the outside of the sheath to the inside. They represent distentions within the myelin cell layers due to the localized presence of Schwann cell cytoplasm. This cytoplasm and, consequently, the clefts move up and down the sheath. Their apexes do not always point in the same direction (Fig 9–15).

Myelin consists of many layers of modified cell membranes. These membranes have a higher proportion of lipids than other cell membranes. Central nervous system myelin contains 2 major proteins called myelin basic protein and proteolipid protein. Several human demyelinating diseases are due to the deficiency or lack of one or both of these proteins. Embryologic studies have shown that the first step in myelin formation is axon penetration of an existing groove of the Schwann cell cytoplasm. The edges of the groove come together to form a mesaxon, so that the plasma membranes of the 2 edges fuse together on their outer surface. Next, through a process not yet fully understood, the mesaxon wraps itself around

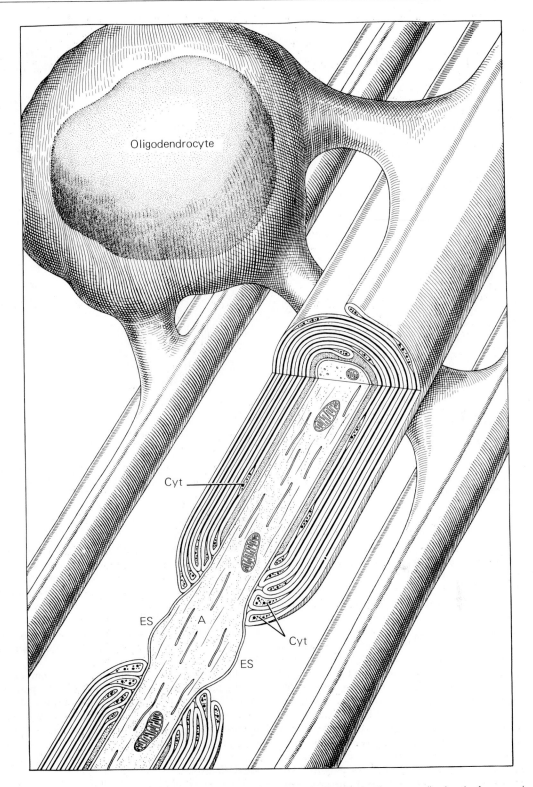

Figure 9–12. Myelin sheath of the central nervous system. The same oligodendrocyte forms myelin sheaths for several nerve fibers (3–50). In the central nervous system, the nodes of Ranvier are covered sometimes by processes of other cells or there is at that point considerable extracellular space (ES). The axolemma shows a thickening where the cell membrane of the oligodendrocyte comes into contact with it, thus limiting diffusion of materials into the periaxonal space between the axon and the myelin sheath. At upper left is a surface view of the cell body of an oligodendrocyte. Cyt, cytoplasm of glial cell; A, axon. (Redrawn and reproduced, with permission, from Bunge et al: *J Biophys Biochem Cytol* 1961;**10**:67.)

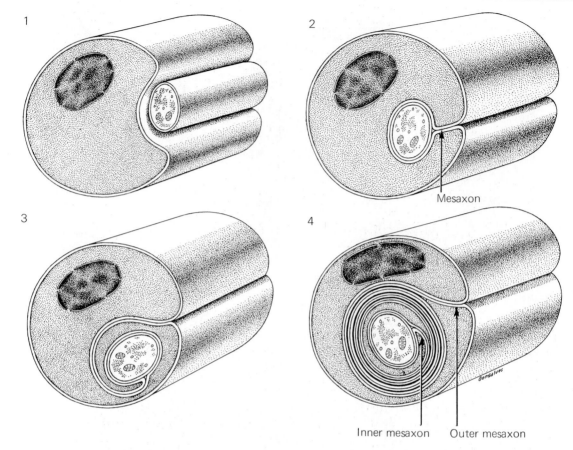

Figure 9–13. Four consecutive phases of myelin formation in peripheral nerve fibers.

the axon several times, the number of turns determining the thickness of the myelin layer. Close examination of Fig 9–14 (bottom) reveals continuous dark lines alternating with more diffuse lines. The regular dark lines are called **major dense lines** and represent the line of fusion of *cytoplasmic* surfaces of Schwann cell membranes. The less regular lines are called **intraperiod lines** and are sites of close contact, but not fusion, of the *extracellular* surfaces of adjacent layers of Schwann cell membrane (Figs 9–12 and 9–13). After this process, an internal and an external mesaxon can be seen (Figs 9–13 and 9–14). The clefts of Schmidt-Lanterman are areas in which the cytoplasm of the Schwann cells is present within the myelin layer. These cytoplasmic areas were left behind during the winding process of the cytoplasm around the axon (Figs 9–15 and 9–16).

There are no Schwann cells in the central nervous system; here, the myelin sheath is formed by the processes of the oligodendrocytes. Oligodendrocytes differ from Schwann cells in that different branches of one cell can envelop segments of several axons (Fig 9–12). The nodes of Ranvier may be uncovered in the central nervous system; Schmidt-Lanterman clefts are absent.

Unmyelinated Fibers

In both the central and peripheral nervous systems, not all axons are ensheathed in myelin. In the peripheral system, all **unmyelinated axons** are enveloped within simple clefts of the Schwann cells (Fig 9–11). Unlike their associations with individual myelinated axons, each Schwann cell can ensheathe many unmyelinated axons. Unmyelinated nerve fibers do not have nodes of Ranvier, since abutting Schwann cells are longitudinally united to form a continuous sheath.

The central nervous system is rich in unmyelinated axons, but these axons, unlike those in the peripheral system, are not ensheathed. In the brain and spinal cord, unmyelinated axonal processes run free among the other neuronal and glial processes.

NERVES

In the peripheral nervous system, the nerve fibers are grouped in bundles to form the nerves. Except for a few very thin nerves made up of unmyelinated fibers, nerves have a whitish appearance because of their myelin content.

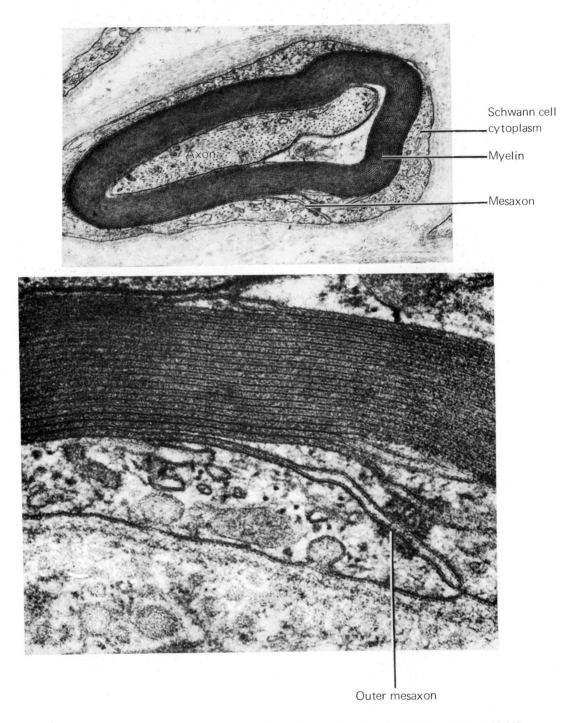

Schwann cell
cytoplasm

Myelin

Mesaxon

Axon

Outer mesaxon

Figure 9–14. Electron micrographs of a myelinated nerve fiber. Top, × 20,000; bottom, × 80,000.

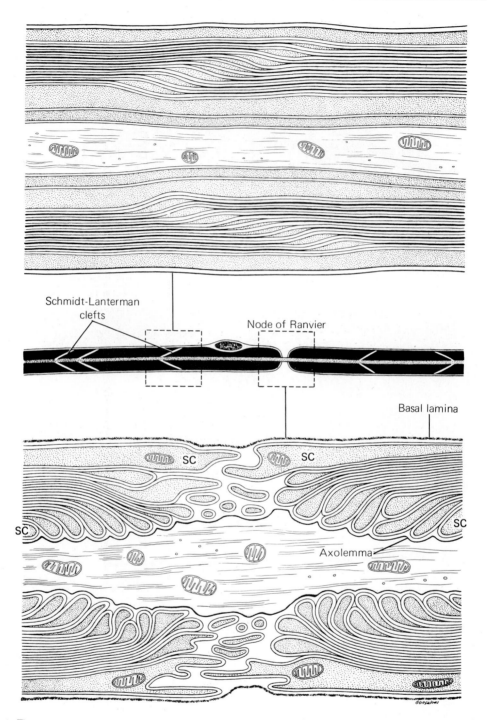

Schmidt-Lanterman clefts

Node of Ranvier

Basal lamina

SC

SC

SC

SC

Axolemma

Figure 9–15. The center drawing shows a myelinated peripheral nerve fiber as seen under the light microscope. The stippled process is the axon enveloped by the myelin sheath (in black) and by the cytoplasm of Schwann cells. A Schwann cell nucleus is seen, as well as the Schmidt-Lanterman clefts and a node of Ranvier. The upper drawing shows the ultrastructure of the Schmidt-Lanterman cleft. This cleft is formed by Schwann cell cytoplasm that is not displaced to the periphery during myelin formation. The lower drawing shows the ultrastructure of a node of Ranvier. Note the appearance of loose interdigitating processes of the outer leaf of the cytoplasm of the Schwann cells (SC) and that a close contact of the inner leaf of the cytoplasm with the axolemma exists, thus acting as a sort of barrier to the movement of materials in and out of the space between the axolemma and the membrane of the Schwann cell. This space is called periaxonal space. The basal lamina around the Schwann cell is continuous. Covering the nerve fiber is a connective tissue layer—mainly reticular fibers—which forms the endoneurial sheath of the peripheral nerve fibers.

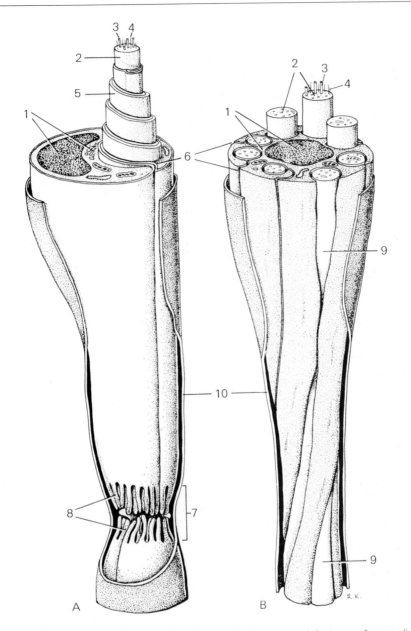

Figure 9–16. Schematic tridimensional drawings showing several ultrastructural features of a myelinated *(A)* and an unmyelinated *(B)* nerve fiber. 1, nucleus and cytoplasm of Schwann cell; 2, axon; 3, microtubule; 4, neurofilament; 5, myelin sheath; 6, mesaxon; 7, node of Ranvier; 8, interdigitating processes of Schwann cells at the node of Ranvier; 9, side view of an unmyelinated axon; 10, basal lamina. (Slightly modified and reproduced, with permission, from Krstić RV: *Ultrastructure of the Mammalian Cell.* Springer-Verlag, 1979.)

Nerves have an external fibrous coat of dense connective tissue called **epineurium,** which also fills the space between the bundles of nerve fibers. Each bundle is surrounded by the **perineurium,** a sleeve formed by layers of flattened epitheliumlike cells. These cells of each layer of the perineural sleeve are joined at their edges by tight junctions, an arrangement that makes the perineurium a barrier to the passage of most macromolecules. Within the perineurial sheath run the Schwann cell–ensheathed axons and their en-

veloping connective tissue, called the **endoneurium.** The endoneurium consists of a thin layer of reticular fibers (Figs 9–17, 9–18, and 9–19). Endoneurial reticular fibers are probably produced by Schwann cells.

The nerves establish communication between brain and spinal cord centers and the sense organs and effectors (muscles, glands, etc). They possess afferent and efferent fibers in relation to the central nervous system. The afferent fibers carry the information ob-

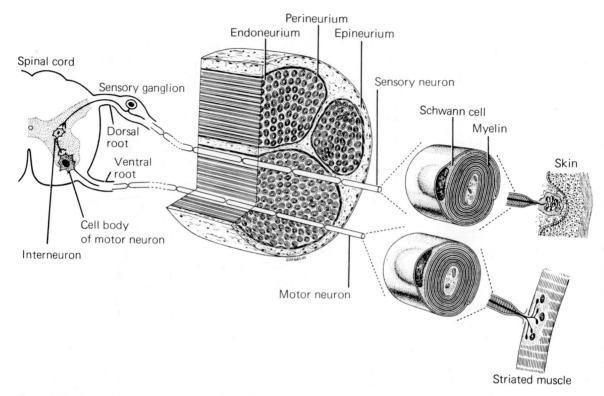

Figure 9–17. Schematic representation of a nerve and a reflex arc. In this example, the sensory stimulus starts in the skin and passes to the spinal cord via the dorsal root ganglion. The sensory stimulus then activates a motor fiber innervating skeletal muscle. Examples of the operation of this reflex are withdrawal of the finger from a hot surface and the knee-jerk reflex. (Slightly modified, redrawn, and reproduced, with permission, from Ham AW: *Histology,* 6th ed. Lippincott, 1969.)

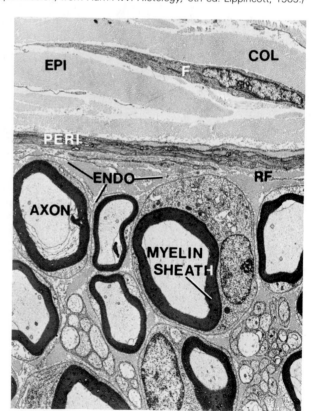

Figure 9–18 (at right). Electron micrograph of a cross section through a nerve, showing the epineurium (EPI), the perineurium (PERI), and the endoneurium (ENDO). The epineurium is a dense connective tissue rich in collagen fibers (COL) and fibroblasts (F). The perineurium is made up of several layers of flat cells tightly joined together to form a barrier to the penetration of the nerve by macromolecules. The endoneurium is composed mainly of reticular fibers (RF) synthesized by Schwann cells (SC). × 1200.

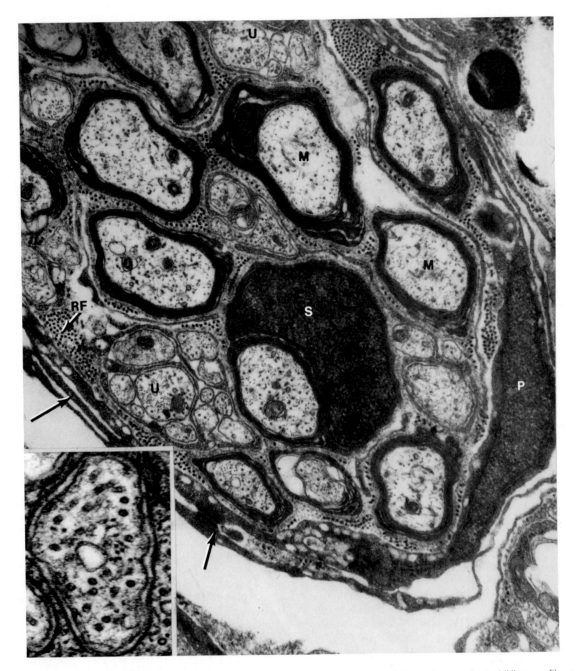

Figure 9–19. Electron micrograph of a peripheral nerve containing both myelinated (M) and unmyelinated (U) nerve fibers. The reticular fibers (RF) seen in cross section belong to the endoneurium. Near the center of the figure there is a Schwann cell nucleus (S). The perineurial cells (P and arrows) form a barrier that controls access of materials to nerve tissue. × 30,000. The inset shows part of an axon, where numerous neurofilaments and microtubules are seen in cross section. × 60,000.

tained from the interior of the body and the environment to the central nervous system. The efferent fibers carry impulses from the central nervous system to the effector organs commanded by these centers. Nerves possessing only sensory fibers (afferent) are called **sensory nerves;** those composed only of fibers carrying impulses to the effectors are called **motor nerves.** Most nerves have both sensory and motor fibers and are called **mixed nerves** (Fig 9–17); these nerves have both myelinated and unmyelinated axons (Fig 9–19).

AUTONOMIC NERVOUS SYSTEM

The autonomic nervous system is related to the control of smooth muscle, the secretion of some glands, and the modulation of cardiac rhythm. Its function is to make adjustments in certain activities of the body in order to maintain a constant internal environment (homeostasis). Although the autonomic nervous system is by definition a motor system, fibers that receive sensation originating in the interior of the organism accompany the motor fibers of the autonomic system.

Although the term autonomic implies that this part of the nervous system functions independently, this is not the case; its functions are constantly subject to the influences of conscious activity.

The concept of the autonomic nervous system is mainly functional. Anatomically, it is composed of collections of nerve cells located in the central nervous system; of fibers that leave the central nervous system through cranial or spinal nerves; and of nerve ganglia situated in the paths of these fibers. The term "autonomic" covers all the neural elements concerned with visceral function.

The first neuron of the autonomic chain is located in the central nervous system. Its axon forms a synapse with the second multipolar neuron in the chain, located in a ganglion of the peripheral autonomic system. The nerve fibers (axons) of the first neuron are called preganglionic fibers; the axons of the second neuron to the effectors—muscle or gland—are called postganglionic fibers. The chemical mediator present in the synaptic vesicles of all preganglionic endings and at anatomically parasympathetic postganglionic endings is acetylcholine. It is released from the terminals by nerve impulses.

The adrenal medulla is the only organ that receives preganglionic fibers, because the majority of the cells, after migration into the gland, do not differentiate into ganglion cells but into secretory cells. Consequently, its innervation is still preganglionic.

The autonomic nervous system is composed of 2 parts that differ both anatomically and functionally: the sympathetic system and the parasympathetic system (Fig 9–20).

Sympathetic System

The nuclei (nerve cell bodies) of the sympathetic system are located in the thoracic and lumbar segments of the spinal cord. The sympathetic system is also called the thoracolumbar division of the autonomic nervous system. The axons of these neurons—preganglionic fibers—leave the central nervous system by the ventral roots and white communicating rami of the thoracic and lumbar nerves. The ganglia of the sympathetic system form the paravertebral chain and plexuses situated near the viscera. The chemical mediator of the postganglionic fibers of the sympathetic system is **norepinephrine,** which is also produced by the medulla of the adrenal.

Parasympathetic System

The parasympathetic system has its nuclei in the medulla and midbrain and in the sacral portion of the spinal cord. The preganglionic fibers of these neurons leave through 4 of the cranial nerves (III, VII, IX, and X) and also through the second, third, and fourth sacral spinal nerves. The parasympathetic system is therefore also called the craniosacral division of the autonomic system.

The second neuron of the parasympathetic series is found in ganglia smaller than those of the sympathetic system; it is always located near or within the effector organs. These neurons are usually located in the walls of organs (eg, stomach, intestines), in which case the preganglionic fibers enter the organs and synapse there with the second neuron in the series.

The chemical mediator released by the pre- and postganglionic nerve endings of the parasympathetic system is **acetylcholine.** Acetylcholine is readily inactivated by acetylcholinesterase—one of the reasons parasympathetic stimulation has both a more discrete and a more localized action than sympathetic stimulation.

Distribution

Most of the organs innervated by the autonomic nervous system receive both sympathetic and parasympathetic fibers (Fig 9–20). Generally, in organs where the sympathetic system is the stimulator, the parasympathetic system has an inhibitory action, and vice versa. For example, stimulation of the sympathetic system accelerates cardiac rhythm, whereas stimulation of parasympathetic fibers slows it down. In some instances, the activity of these 2 components is complementary and not antagonistic. This is true in the case of some salivary glands, whose secretion is greater when stimulated by both systems than when stimulated by either one separately.

HISTOPHYSIOLOGY OF NERVE TISSUE

The integrative function of nerve tissue depends on the generation and conduction of nerve impulses and on the production of neurohormones by special nerve cells. (The neurohormones are discussed in Chapter 21.)

Axonal conduction of nerve impulses (action potentials) is one of the basic and better understood

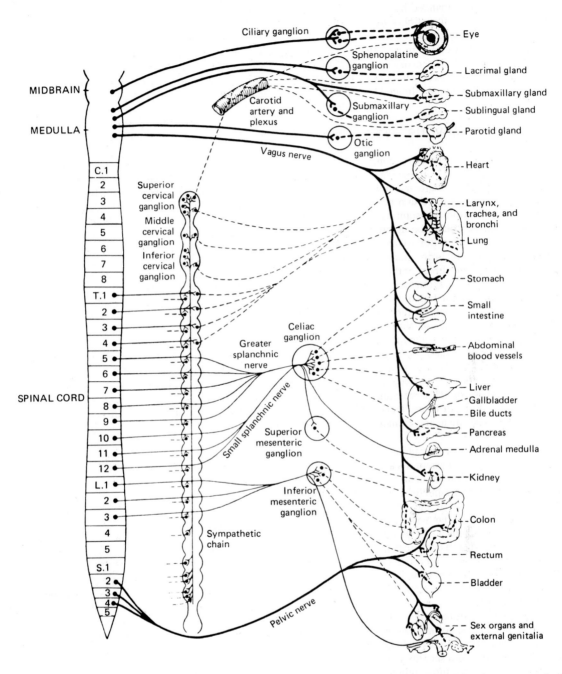

Figure 9–20. Diagram of the efferent autonomic pathways. Preganglionic neurons are shown as solid lines, postganglionic neurons as dotted lines. The heavy lines are parasympathetic fibers; the light lines are sympathetic. (Slightly modified and reproduced, with permission, from Youmans W: *Fundamentals of Human Physiology,* 2nd ed. Year Book, 1962.)

functions of nerve tissue. It is now well established that the key role in impulse conduction is played by the cell membrane. In the following discussion, the basis for the resting potential, how an action potential is generated, and how the action potential is conducted along an axon will be established.

Resting Potential

Intracellular ionic concentrations differ greatly from those found in extracellular fluids. The K^+ concentration inside a neuron is about 20 times greater than the concentration of this ion in the extracellular fluid. Conversely, Na^+ ions are about 10 times more concentrated outside the cell than inside. The cell membrane is much more permeable to K^+ than it is to any of the other ions. Potassium therefore tends to diffuse outward, down its concentration gradient. As a consequence, positive charges accumulate at the outer surface of the membrane and are balanced by the negative charge provided by impermeable macromolecules within the cell. This process continues until the diffusion force, provided by the concentration gradient, is just balanced by the increasing difficulty of moving a positive charge into an already positively charged region. At this point, there is no *net* movement of potassium ions. This separation of charge across the cell membrane is the **resting membrane potential.** Conventionally, the external medium (extracellular fluid) is considered to be at ground potential (0 volts); the interior of the cell is from 40 to 100 mV negative with respect to the exterior.

The concentration differences are maintained by a group of "pumps" that utilize the energy in ATP to actively transport ions. The best known is the Na^+/K^+-ATPase, which exchanges internal Na^+ ions for external K^+ ions.

Action Potential

Plasma membranes of neurons and muscle cells (and some other cells) contain integral membrane proteins that function as ion-selective channels. At any one time, these channels can be in one of 3 states—open, closed, or inactivated. The transition from the closed to the open state is governed by the membrane potential, and the channels are therefore termed **voltage-gated channels.**

In the resting neuron, the membrane potential is about −90 mV, as indicated in Fig 9–21 (left electrode pair), and most of the sodium and potassium channels are in the closed state. One result of excitatory synaptic input on the postsynaptic cell is partial depolarization of the cell; ie, the membrane potential is displaced toward 0 volts. When this depolarization reaches a critical level, called the **threshold** (eg, −70 mV in our example), sodium channels open, allowing sodium ions to enter. This has the effect of further depolarizing the cell and causing more sodium channels to open, resulting in reversal of the membrane potential at this site (right electrode pair in Fig 9–21). This explains the upward swing of the curve in the lower half of Fig 9–21. Sodium channels now undergo

spontaneous inactivation and remain in this state for 1–2 milliseconds.

Also as a result of membrane potential changes, potassium channels open but more slowly and for more prolonged periods of time. This has the effect of bringing the membrane potential back to its original level and even below it (**hyperpolarization**) (Fig 9–21). This sequence of events is called the **action potential.** This is an all-or-nothing event, since only stimuli above threshold will evoke it and the action potential is of constant amplitude and duration. After 1–2 milliseconds (the **refractory period**), the channels return to their original states and the membrane can again respond to a stimulus. Axons can generate action potentials up to 1000 times per second.

The explanation of the propagation of an action potential down an axon (away from the cell body) may now be given.

The sodium ions that enter the cell at a particular site not only serve to depolarize that site, but they can also diffuse longitudinally and depolarize adjacent sites. Diffusion toward the cell body (**antidromic spread**) has no effect, because the sodium channels are inactivated. However, diffusion of sodium ions toward the synaptic end of the axon (**orthodromic spread**) does depolarize the adjacent region of the membrane, leading to the generation of an action potential at this new site. This leads to a rapid, constant amplitude signal being propagated down the axon, with frequency being the only information encoded.

Myelinated axons are structurally adapted for rapid conduction of the action potential (Fig 9–22). Since most of their surface is encased in an insulating layer of myelin, only the nodes of Ranvier are exposed to the extracellular environment and thus available to

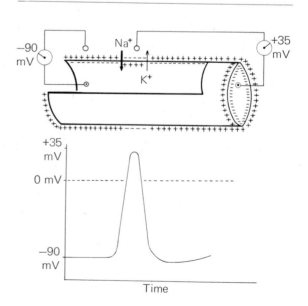

Figure 9–21. Diagrammatic representation of resting and action potentials in an axon.

Figure 9–22 (at right). Saltatory conduction in a myelinated nerve fiber. When a node of Ranvier becomes depolarized (2), the sodium current travels along the axon in both directions. The current can leave the axon only at nodes of Ranvier because of the good electrical insulating properties of myelin. When this current leaves the fiber at node 3, another action potential is developed that leads to the rapid leaping of the stimulus down the axon. After its stimulation, a node of Ranvier is refractory to further stimulation for a short time (1). For this reason, even though ionic currents spread in both directions from a stimulated node, action potentials move in one direction only (solid arrow in center of fiber).

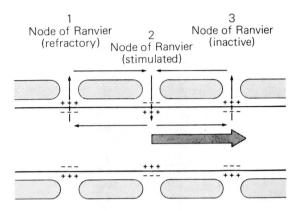

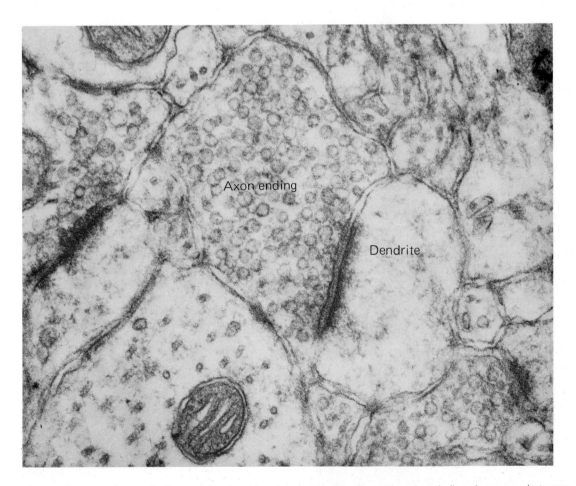

Figure 9–23. Electron micrograph of cerebral cortex. Near the center of the figure there is a cholinergic synapse between one axon ending and a dendrite. The postsynaptic (dendritic) membrane shows a greater accumulation of electron-dense material than the presynaptic (axonal) membrane. This is an asymmetric, or type I, synapse. The axon ending contains numerous synaptic vesicles. × 90,000. (Courtesy of A Peters.)

complete the ionic circuits necessary for the generation of action potentials. In addition, sodium and potassium channels are concentrated at the nodes, with very few channels being found in the internodal axonal membranes. Therefore, the depolarization required for an action potential is conducted quickly from one node to the next **(saltatory conduction)**. As a result of myelination, an action potential is conducted much more rapidly over a myelinated axon (1–100 m/s) than it is over unmyelinated axons (0.6–2 m/s). In addition, less energy is required by the pumps to reestablish the ionic gradients, although the changes in ionic concentration due to the propagation of an action potential are very small.

The energy used in the conduction of the impulse is restored by an increase in axonal metabolism, with enhanced oxygen consumption and heat production.

Nerve impulse conduction can be blocked by cold, heat, or pressure on the nerve fiber. More complete blocking is obtained by application of local anesthetics.

According to their conduction velocities, nerve fibers may be divided into 3 classes: A, B, and C. Type A fibers are myelinated, have large diameters and long internodes, and conduct impulses with high velocity (15–100 m/s). Type B fibers have smaller diameters, shorter internodes, and medium velocity of conduction (3–14 m/s). Type C fibers are thin and unmyelinated, with slow conduction velocity (0.5–2 m/s).

Nerve impulses are transmitted from one neuron to another or to an effector cell by the neurotransmitters liberated at synapses (Figs 9–23 and 9–24). When an action potential invades an axonal terminus, or ending, calcium ions are allowed to enter the ending. Ca^{2+} ions facilitate the fusion of synaptic vesicles containing a neurotransmitter (eg, acetylcholine) with the presynaptic membrane. The transmitter (about 10,000 molecules of acetylcholine per vesicle) is released by exocytosis into the synaptic cleft. It diffuses across the cleft and binds to receptors on the postsynaptic membrane, leading to increased ionic permeability of this membrane, its depolarization, and generation of an action potential in the postsynaptic cell.

After performing its function, the excess neurotransmitter (eg, acetylcholine) is removed by the degradative action of the enzyme acetylcholinesterase. This enzyme is secreted from cells and is bound to the basal lamina in the synaptic cleft. Other mechanisms of disposal exist for other neurotransmitters (Figs 9–25 and 9–26). The entire process is very rapid and can occur, for brief periods of time, over 1000 times a second.

The neurotransmitter in postganglionic endings of the sympathetic system is norepinephrine. Synaptic vesicles containing norepinephrine are usually larger than those containing acetylcholine, and they usually have an electron-dense core separated from its limiting membrane by a light zone (Fig 9–24).

Other neurotransmitters exist besides acetylcholine and norepinephrine. This function has been demonstrated for gamma-aminobutyric acid (GABA), glutamic acid, dopamine, serotonin (5-hydroxytryptamine, 5-HT), and glycine.

In mammals, gamma-aminobutyric acid is localized exclusively in the central nervous system. There is evidence suggesting that it may function as an inhibitory chemical transmitter. Recent investigations have demonstrated the presence of a new class of peptide neurotransmitters that are potent inhibitors of pain receptors. Endorphins and enkephalins are natural brain peptides exhibiting morphinelike analgesic powers that may also regulate behavior. Several peptide hormones such as cholecystokinin, vasoactive intestinal polypeptide, and bombesin, originally described in the digestive tract where they are produced

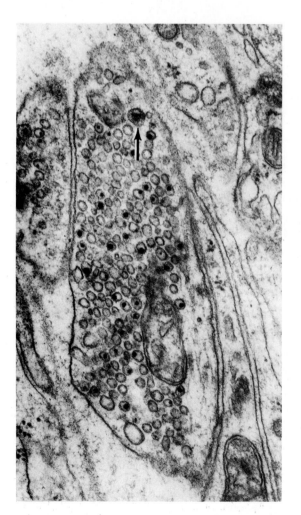

Figure 9–24 (at left). Norepinephrine nerve ending in the pineal gland. There are many vesicles with a diameter of 50 nm containing a dark, electron-dense core. There are also a few large, dense-core vesicles (arrow) whose function is not known. × 40,000. (Courtesy of A Machado.)

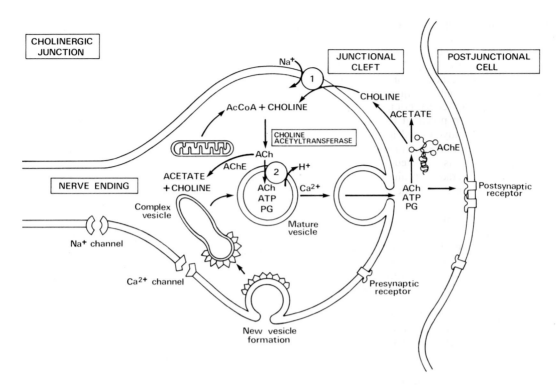

Figure 9–25. Schematic illustration of a generalized cholinergic junction (not to scale). Two cellular structures, the cholinergic nerve terminal (left) and the postjunctional cell (right), are separated by the junctional (synaptic) cleft. Choline is transported into the nerve terminal by a carrier (1) that cotransports sodium ion, using the sodium gradient for energy. This transport can be inhibited by hemicholinium. Inside the nerve terminal, choline combines with activated acetate (AcCoA), in a reaction catalyzed by choline acetyltransferase, to form acetylcholine (ACh). Formation of storage vesicles is initiated by the deposition of clathrin molecules on the inner surface of the terminal membrane (shown as the fencelike structure on the new vesicle). Upon being pinched off from the surface, a "complex vesicle" is formed that eventually gives rise to a mature storage vesicle. ACh is transported into the storage vesicle by the action of a carrier (2) that utilizes the outward flux of protons as its source of energy. ATP and proteoglycan (PG) are also stored in the vesicle. Release of transmitter occurs when an action potential, carried down the axon by the action of voltage-sensitive sodium channels, invades the nerve terminals. Voltage-sensitive calcium channels in the terminal membrane are opened, allowing an influx of calcium. The increase in intracellular calcium causes fusion of vesicles with the surface membrane, resulting in exocytotic expulsion of ACh, ATP, and proteoglycan into the junctional cleft. This step is blocked by botulin. ACh reaching prejunctional and postjunctional receptors modifies the function of the corresponding cell. (Note: Some cholinergic junctions appear to lack prejunctional receptors.) ACh also diffuses into contact with the enzyme acetylcholinesterase (AChE), a polymeric enzyme that splits ACh into choline and acetate. At some cholinergic junctions, a polypeptide cotransmitter, vasoactive intestinal polypeptide (VIP), is released along with ACh into the junctional cleft. (Reproduced, with permission, from Katzung BG [editor]: *Basic & Clinical Pharmacology,* 2nd ed. Lange, 1984.)

by APUD cells (see Chapter 4), have been localized in different areas of the central nervous system. Their function as neurotransmitters, however, has not yet been established. The present concepts of the production, liberation, and inactivation of the 2 best-known chemical mediators are summarized in Figs 9–25 and 9–26.

The abundance of RNA in the perikaryon suggests intense protein synthesis, which has been confirmed by radioautographic studies using ^{3}H-leucine and other labeled amino acids. Axons do not contain ribosomes, and thus all the proteins in these processes are synthesized in the perikaryon and moved down the axon by an energy-requiring mechanism known as **axonal**

transport. Newly synthesized and labeled protein molecules migrate down the axons (anterograde transport) at several speeds, but there are 2 main rates: a fast rate in the range of hundreds of millimeters per day and a slow rate in the range of several millimeters per day. The fast transport mechanism moves membranes, mitochondria, and synaptic vesicles, among other things, down the axon from their site of formation in the neuron cell body. Substances such as actin, tubulins, metabolic enzymes, and neurofilament proteins are transported at the slow rate. Agents that disrupt microfilaments and microtubules greatly slow both the fast and slow anterograde transport systems. Experimental evidence has been presented to show

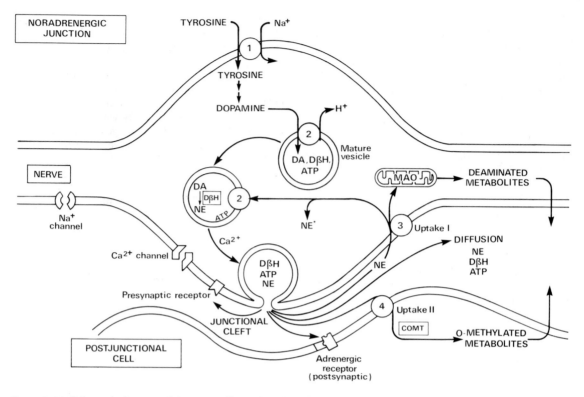

Figure 9–26. Schematic diagram of the neuroeffector junction of the peripheral sympathetic nervous system. The nerves terminate in complex networks with varicosities or enlargements that form synaptic junctions with effector cells. Some of the processes occurring in the noradrenergic varicosity are analogous to those in cholinergic terminals, eg, new vesicle formation in the varicosity. Tyrosine is transported into the noradrenergic varicosity by a carrier (1) that is linked to sodium uptake. Tyrosine is decarboxylated to dopa and then hydroxylated to form dopamine (DA) in the cytoplasm. Dopamine is transported into the vesicle by a carrier mechanism (2) that can be blocked by reserpine. The same carrier transports norepinephrine (NE) and several other amines into these granules. Dopamine is converted to norepinephrine through the catalytic action of dopamine β-hydroxylase (DβH). ATP is also present in high concentration in the vesicle. Release of 13transmitter occurs when an action potential is conducted to the varicosity by the action of voltage-sensitive sodium channels. Depolarization of the varicosity membrane opens voltage-sensitive calcium channels and results in an increase in intracellular calcium. The elevated calcium facilitates exocytotic fusion of vesicles with the surface membrane and expulsion of norepinephrine, ATP, and some of the dopamine β-hydroxylase. Release is blocked by drugs such as guanethidine and bretylium. Norepinephrine reaching either pre- or postsynaptic receptors modifies the function of the corresponding cells. Norpinephrine also diffuses out of the cleft, or it may be transported into the cytoplasm of the varicosity (uptake I [3], blocked by cocaine, tricyclic antidepressants) or into the postjunctional cell (uptake II [4]). The nonvesicular norepinephrine, shown schematically as NE*, can be released by tyramine and a variety of the other indirectly acting adrenergic agonists. (Reproduced, with permission, from Katzung BG [editor]: *Basic & Clinical Pharmacology,* 2nd ed. Lange, 1984.)

that transport of protein also occurs in a centripetal direction (retrograde transport) from the axon to the perikaryon. Thus, receptors and synaptic membrane proteins are removed from the periphery and shipped back to the cell body, where they may be reused. The use of enzymatic markers such as peroxidase that are captured by axon terminals and transported to the perikaryon has been used extensively to study the physiology and morphology of the nervous system.

A trophic function has been ascribed to the nervous system of mammals for the structures it innervates. It is known that denervation of organs such as glands and muscles can lead to their atrophy, with functional

and morphologic recuperation after reinnervation. Whether this atrophy is solely a consequence of disuse is an open question. In lower vertebrates, peripheral nerves have a trophic function that is not dependent on the nerve impulse.

DEGENERATION & REGENERATION OF NERVE TISSUE

Neurons do not divide; their degeneration represents a permanent loss. Neuronal processes in the central nervous system are, within very narrow limits, replaceable by growth through the synthetic activity of their perikaryons. Peripheral nerve fibers also can regenerate if their perikaryons are not destroyed.

Death of a nerve cell is limited to its perikaryon and processes. The neurons functionally connected to the dead neuron do not die, except for those neurons with only one link. In this latter instance, the isolated neuron undergoes **transneuronal degeneration.**

In contrast to nerve cells, neuroglia of the central nervous system and Schwann cells and ganglionic satellite cells of the peripheral nervous system are able to divide by mitosis. Spaces left in the central nervous system by nerve cells lost by disease or injury are invaded by neuroglia.

Since nerves are widely distributed throughout the body, they are often subjected to injury. When a nerve axon is transected, degenerative changes take place, followed by a reparative phase.

In a wounded nerve fiber, it is important to distinguish the changes occurring in the proximal segment from those in the distal segment. The proximal segment maintains its continuity with the trophic center (perikaryon) and frequently regenerates. The distal segment, separated from the nerve cell body, degenerates totally and is removed by tissue macrophages (Fig 9–27).

Axonal injury causes the following changes in the perikaryon: (1) chromatolysis, ie, dissolution of Nissl

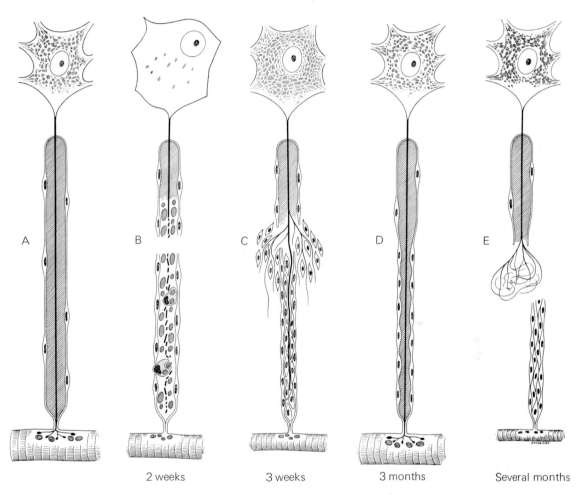

| A | B | C | D | E |
| | 2 weeks | 3 weeks | 3 months | Several months |

Figure 9–27. Main changes that take place in an injured nerve fiber. *A:* Normal nerve fiber, with its perikaryon and the effector cell (striated skeletal muscle). Note the position of the neuron nucleus and the amount and distribution of Nissl bodies. *B:* When the fiber is injured, the neuronal nucleus moves to the cell periphery and Nissl bodies become greatly reduced in number. The nerve fiber distal to the injury degenerates along with its myelin sheath. Debris is phagocytosed by macrophages. *C:* The muscle fiber shows a pronounced disuse atrophy. Schwann cells proliferate, forming a compact cord penetrated by the growing axon. The axon grows at a rate of 0.5–3 mm/d. *D:* In this example, the nerve fiber regeneration was successful. Note that the muscle fiber was also regenerated after receiving nerve stimuli. *E:* When the axon does not penetrate the cord of Schwann cells, its growth is not organized. (Redrawn and reproduced, with permission, from Willis RA, Willis AT: *The Principles of Pathology and Bacteriology,* 3rd ed. Butterworth, 1972.)

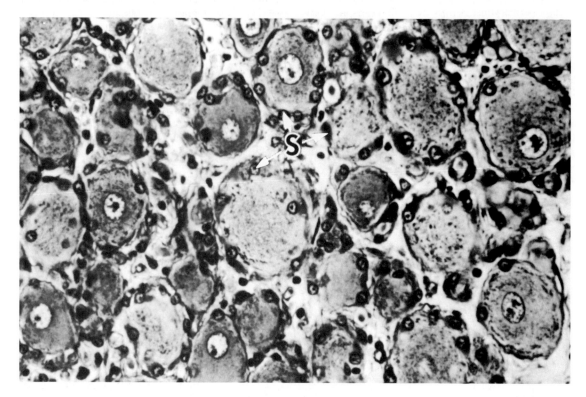

Figure 9–28. Photomicrograph of a spinal ganglion section, showing neurons and satellite cells (S). Azan stain, × 300. (Reproduced, with permission, from Junqueira LC, Carneiro J: *Histologie*. Schiebler TH, Peiper U [translators]. Springer-Verlag, 1984.)

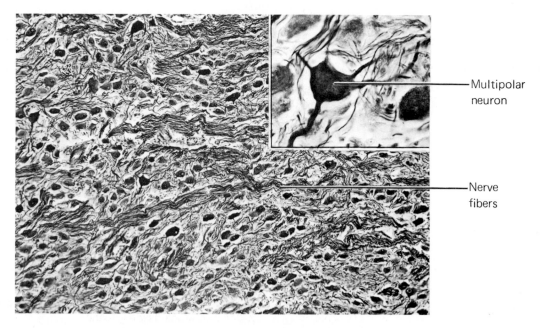

Multipolar
neuron

Nerve
fibers

Figure 9–29. Photomicrographs of silver-stained section from an autonomic nerve ganglion. Neurons and nerve fibers appear black. × 80. The inset shows a multipolar neuron. × 250.

substances with a consequent decrease in cytoplasmic basophilia; (2) increase in the volume of the perikaryon; and (3) migration of the nucleus to a peripheral position in the perikaryon. The proximal segment of the axon degenerates close to the wound for a short distance, but growth starts as soon as debris is removed by macrophages.

In the nerve stub distal to the injury, both the axon (now separated from its trophic center) and the myelin sheath degenerate completely, and their remnants, excluding their connective tissue and perineurial sheaths, are removed by macrophages (Fig 9–27B). While these regressive changes take place, Schwann cells proliferate within the remaining connective tissue sleeve, giving rise to solid cellular columns. These rows of Schwann cells serve as guides to the sprouting axons formed during the reparative phase.

After these regressive changes, the proximal segment of the axon grows and branches, forming several filaments that progress in the direction of the columns of Schwann cells (Fig 9–27C). Only those fibers that penetrate these Schwann cell columns will continue to grow and reach an effector organ (Fig 9–27D). When there is an extensive gap between the distal and proximal segments, or when the distal segment disappears altogether (as in the case of amputation of a limb), the newly grown nerve fibers may form a swelling or neuroma that can be the source of spontaneous pain (Fig 9–27E).

Regeneration is functionally efficient only when the fibers find the columns of Schwann cells directed to the correct place. This possibility is increased for the reason that each regenerating fiber gives origin to several processes and each column of Schwann cells receives processes from several regenerating fibers. In an injured mixed nerve, however, if regenerating sensory fibers grow into columns connected to motor end-plates that were occupied by motor fibers, the function of the muscle will not be reestablished.

GANGLIA

An aggregation of nerve cell bodies outside the central nervous system is called a **nerve ganglion.** Ganglia are usually ovoid structures encapsulated by dense connective tissue and associated with nerves.

Intramural ganglia are very small, consisting of only a few nerve cells, and are located within viscera, especially the walls of the digestive tract. All intramural ganglia belong to the parasympathetic system.

Two types of nerve ganglia can be distinguished on the basis of differing morphology and function: **craniospinal** or **dorsal root ganglia** (sensory), which occur at the dorsal (posterior) root of the spinal nerves and also in the path of some cranial nerves; and **autonomic ganglia,** which are associated with nerves of the autonomic system.

A capsule of connective tissue surrounding each ganglion is continuous with the connective tissue within it and with the perineurium and epineurium of the pre- and postganglionic nerves.

In ganglia, the body of each ganglion cell is enveloped by a layer of small cuboidal cells called **satellite cells.** A thin fibrous layer of connective tissue envelops each satellite cell–encapsulated perikaryon.

Craniospinal Ganglia

Craniospinal ganglia are located in the dorsal roots of the spinal nerves and in the paths of some cranial nerves. Their function is to carry to the central nervous system impulses generated by various sensory receptors.

Craniospinal ganglia have pseudounipolar neurons whose T-shaped process sends one branch to the periphery and the other to the central nervous system. The 2 branches of the single T-shaped process constitute one axon, and the peripheral branch has a dendritic arborization. In this instance, the dendrites are not expansions of the cell body but of an axon. The nerve impulse goes directly from the periphery to the central nervous system, bypassing the perikaryon. The perikaryons of pseudounipolar neurons therefore do not receive nerve impulses, and their function is exclusively trophic. The single axonal process of this cell makes several irregular turns around the cell body before its bifurcation, which occurs outside the capsule of satellite cells.

The ganglia from the acoustic nerve are the only cranial ganglia whose cells are bipolar. During the expansion of other craniospinal ganglia, the neurons, which are initially bipolar, fuse the initial segments of their axonal and dendritic processes, giving rise to the T-shaped process.

Craniospinal ganglia contain, side by side, small nerve cell bodies 15–30 μm in diameter and large ones about 120 μm in diameter. The cell bodies predominate in the periphery of the ganglion, where they form the cortical zone, which is poor in nerve fibers. The central part of the ganglion shows a great predominance of nerve fibers, forming an axial or medullary zone where only a few perikaryons occur in isolated groups.

In histologic sections, perikaryons of pseudounipolar neurons are round and surrounded by satellite cells. The site of emergence of the single process is rarely seen. These neurons usually show fine Nissl bodies and droplets of lipofuscin (Fig 9–28).

Autonomic Ganglia

Autonomic ganglia appear as bulbous dilatations in autonomic nerves. Some are located within certain organs, especially in the walls of the digestive tract, where they constitute the intramural ganglia. Intramural ganglia are devoid of connective tissue capsules, and their cells are supported by the stroma of the organ in which they are found.

In autonomic ganglia, the cell bodies do not show the peripheral localization seen in craniospinal ganglia; consequently, a cortical layer is not observed. Autonomic ganglia usually have multipolar neurons, which may appear star-shaped in histologic sections (Fig 9–29). As with craniospinal ganglia, autonomic ganglia have neuronal perikaryons with fine Nissl bodies.

The neurons of autonomic ganglia are frequently enveloped by a layer of satellite cells, which is usually incomplete. In intramural ganglia, only a few satellite cells are seen around each neuron.

GRAY MATTER & WHITE MATTER

The central nervous system is composed of white matter and gray matter. White matter contains myelinated and unmyelinated fibers, oligodendrocytes, fibrous astrocytes, and microglial cells. Gray matter contains perikaryons, unmyelinated and myelinated fibers (mostly the former), protoplasmic astrocytes, oligodendrocytes, and microglial cells. The characteristic color of the white matter is a clue to the predominance of myelinated nerve fibers.

In cross sections of the spinal cord, white matter appears peripherally and gray matter appears centrally, assuming the shape of an H (Fig 9–30). In the horizontal bar of this H is an opening, the central canal, which is a remnant of the lumen of the embryonic neural tube lined by ependymal cells. The gray matter of the ventral bars of the H forms the anterior horns, which contain motor neurons whose axons compose the ventral roots of the spinal nerves. Gray matter also forms the posterior horns, which receive sensory fibers from neurons in the spinal ganglia (dorsal roots).

Spinal cord neurons are large and multipolar, especially in the anterior horns, where large motor neurons are found (Fig 9–30).

The cerebellum has 2 hemispheres separated by the **vermis.** The surface of the cerebellum has many furrows (sulci) perpendicular to the vermis. These furrows divide the organ into lobules, each of which has a superficial layer of gray matter (cortex) and a core of white matter (Fig 9–31). In the interior of the white matter, deep in the cerebellum, isolated regions of gray matter (nuclei) also appear.

The cerebellar cortex has 3 layers: an outer molecular layer, a central layer of Purkinje cells, and an inner granular layer (Fig 9–32). The neurons of the granular layer are the smallest in the human body (5 μm in diameter) and have a typical structure. Each granular cell (cerebellar granule) has 3–6 dendrites and, as usual, one axon. The Purkinje cells are quite large. The dendrites of Purkinje cells divide repeatedly in one plane, forming a sort of fan (Fig 9–2). The most superficial layer of the cerebellum (the molecular layer) has few perikaryons and many unmyelinated nerve fibers.

Like the cerebellum, the cerebrum also has a cortex of gray matter and a central area of white matter in which are found nuclei of gray matter. The surface of the cerebrum is increased by many **gyri,** which are elevations separated by depressions named **sulci.** The cytology of the cerebral cortex varies according to the area. The majority of the cells of the cortex have perikaryons that are pyramidal, stellate, or spindle-shaped.

MENINGES

The central nervous system is protected by the skull and the vertebral column. It is also encased in membranes of connective tissue called the meninges.

Starting with the outermost layer, the meninges are named **dura mater, arachnoid,** and **pia mater.** Dura mater is also called **pachymeninx.** The arachnoid and the pia mater are linked together and are often considered as a single membrane called the **pia-arachnoid** or **leptomeninx** (Fig 9–33).

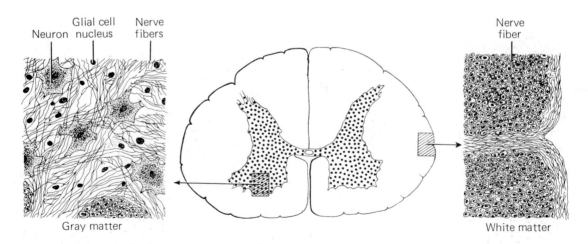

Glial cell   Nerve
Neuron   nucleus   fibers

Nerve
fiber

Gray matter

White matter

Figure 9–30. *Center:* Cross section through the spinal cord. *Left:* Gray matter. *Right:* White matter.

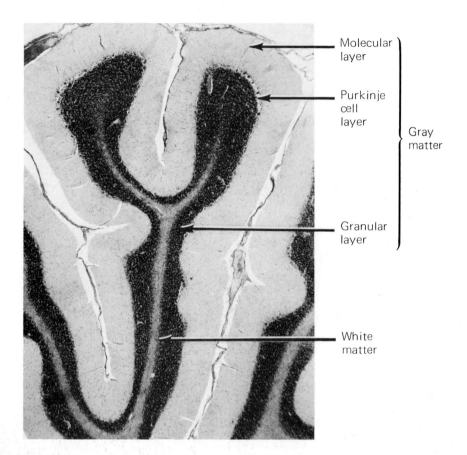

Molecular layer

Purkinje cell layer

Gray matter

Granular layer

White matter

Figure 9–31. Photomicrograph of a portion of cerebellum. Each lobule contains a core of white matter and 3 layers of gray matter: granular, Purkinje, and molecular layers. H&E stain, × 28.

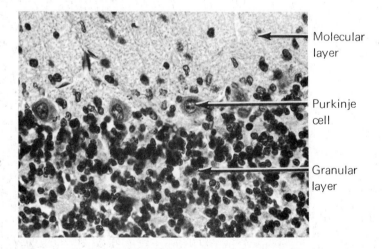

Molecular layer

Purkinje cell

Granular layer

Figure 9–32. Photomicrograph of cerebellar cortex. This staining procedure does not reveal the unusually large dendritic arborization of the Purkinje cell, which is diagrammatically illustrated in Fig 9–2. H&E stain, × 250.

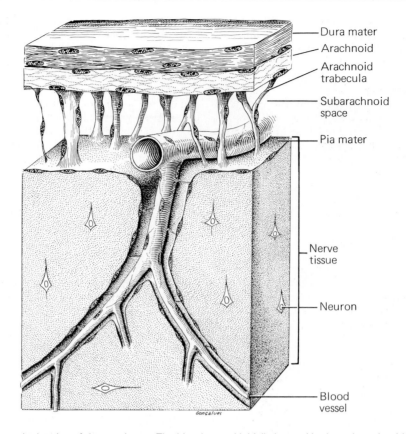

Figure 9–33. Schematic drawing of the meninges. The blood vessel initially located in the subarachnoid space penetrates the nerve tissue and is partly enveloped by the pia mater.

Dura Mater

The dura mater is the external meninx, composed of dense connective tissue continuous with the periosteum of the skull. The dura mater that envelops the spinal cord is separated from the periosteum of the vertebrae by the epidural space, which contains thin-walled veins, loose connective tissue, and adipose tissue.

The dura mater is always separated from the arachnoid by a thin space, the subdural space. The internal surface of all dura mater, as well as its external surface in the spinal cord, is covered by simple squamous epithelium of mesenchymal origin (Fig 9–33).

Arachnoid

The arachnoid has 2 components: a layer in contact with the dura mater and a system of trabeculae connecting that layer with the pia mater. The cavities between the trabeculae form the **subarachnoid space,** which is filled with cerebrospinal fluid and is completely separated from the subdural space. The subarachnoid space communicates with the ventricles of the brain via the unpaired median aperture and the paired lateral apertures.

The arachnoid is composed of connective tissue devoid of blood vessels. Its surfaces are covered by the same type of simple squamous epithelium that covers the dura mater. Since, in the spinal cord, the arachnoid has fewer trabeculae, it can be more clearly distinguished from pia mater.

In some areas, the arachnoid perforates the dura mater, forming protrusions that terminate in venous sinuses in the dura mater. These protrusions, which are covered by endothelial cells of the veins, are called **arachnoid villi.** Their function is to resorb cerebrospinal fluid into the blood of the venous sinuses.

Pia Mater

The pia mater is a loose connective tissue containing many blood vessels and is located quite close to the nerve tissue, but it is not in contact with nerve cells or fibers. Between the pia mater and the neural elements is a thin layer of neuroglial processes, firmly adherent to the pia mater.

The pia mater follows all the irregularities of the surface of the central nervous system and penetrates it to some extent along with the blood vessels. Pia mater is covered by squamous cells of mesenchymal origin.

Blood vessels penetrate the central nervous system through tunnels covered by pia mater and called the **perivascular spaces** (Fig 9–33). The pia mater disappears before the blood vessels are transformed into capillaries. In the central nervous system, the blood capillaries are completely covered by expansions of the neuroglial cell processes.

Blood-Brain Barrier

There is a barrier that prevents the passage of certain substances from the blood to nerve tissue. This functional barrier is termed the **blood-brain barrier.** For example, intravenously injected trypan blue appears in the intercellular spaces of all tissues except the central nervous system.

The blood-brain barrier results from the reduced permeability that is a property of blood capillaries of nerve tissue. Occluding junctions, which provide continuity between the endothelial cells of these capillaries, represent the main structural component of the barrier. The cytoplasm of these endothelial cells does not have the fenestrations found in many other locations, and very few pinocytotic vesicles are observed. It is also possible that expansions of neuroglial cell processes that envelop the capillaries are partly responsible for their low permeability.

THE CHOROID PLEXUS & THE CEREBROSPINAL FLUID

Choroid Plexus

The choroid plexus (tela choroidea) consists of invaginated folds of pia mater that penetrate the interior of the ventricles. It is found in the roofs of the third and fourth ventricles and in part in the walls of the lateral ventricles.

The choroid plexus is composed of loose connective tissue of the pia mater, covered by a simple cuboidal or low columnar epithelium that is continuous with the ependyma in other regions of the brain (Fig 9–34). The epithelial cells possess numerous irregular microvilli whose free ends are dilated. Their cytoplasm is rich in mitochondria, and there are junctional complexes near their free ends.

The connective tissue of the choroid plexus is quite cellular, containing many macrophages. The endothelium of its fenestrated capillaries has pores closed by thin diaphragms. The endothelial cells are held together by tight junctions. The epithelial and endothelial cells form the so-called blood–cerebrospinal fluid barrier that is responsible for the difference in composition between blood plasma and the cerebrospinal fluid.

The main function of the choroid plexus is to secrete cerebrospinal fluid, a thin watery fluid actively secreted by the epithelial cells covering the plexuses. Within the plexus are a few absorbing cells.

Cerebrospinal Fluid

The choroid plexus elaborates cerebrospinal fluid, which contains only a small amount of solids and completely fills the ventricles, central canal of the spinal cord, subarachnoid space, and perivascular space. It is important for the metabolism of the central nervous system and represents a protective device, forming a liquid layer in the subarachnoid space. This layer cushions the nerve tissue against trauma.

Adult humans have about 140 mL of cerebrospinal fluid in the cerebral ventricles and the subarachnoid space. The fluid is clear, has a low density (1.004–1.008

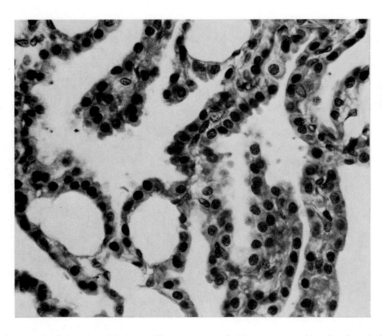

Figure 9–34. Photomicrograph of the choroid plexus. The numerous folds are covered by simple cuboidal epithelium. H&E stain, × 400.

g/mL), and is very low in protein content. A few desquamated cells and 2–5 lymphocytes per milliliter are also present. The ionic composition of cerebrospinal fluid is very close to that of plasma, ie, high sodium and chloride but low potassium concentrations. It is produced by ultrafiltration and diffusion from the blood as well as by active transport across epithelial cells of the choroid plexus. Between 600 and 700 mL of cerebrospinal fluid are produced each day.

Cerebrospinal fluid circulates through the ventricles, from which it passes into the subarachnoid space. Here, arachnoid villi provide the main pathway for reabsorption of cerebrospinal fluid into the venous circulation. Lymphatic vessels are not present in nervous tissue. If reabsorption is decreased or outflow from the ventricles is blocked, the condition known as **hydrocephalus** results.

REFERENCES

Akert K et al: The fine structure of the perineurial endothelium. *Cell Tissue Res* 1976;**165**:281.

Axelrod J: Neurotransmitters. *Sci Am* (June) 1974;**230**:58.

Bourne GH (editor): *The Structure and Function of Nervous Tissue.* Vol 1. Academic Press, 1968.

Brightman MW, Palay SL: The fine structure of ependyma in the brain of the rat. *J Cell Biol* 1963;**19**:415.

Brightman MW, Reese TS: Junctions between intimately apposed cell membranes in the vertebrate brain. *J Cell Biol* 1969;**40**:648.

Brightman MW et al: The blood-brain barrier to proteins under normal and pathological conditions. *J Neurol Sci* 1970;**10**:215.

Bunge MB et al: Comparison of nerve cell and nerve cell plus Schwann cell cultures, with particular emphasis on basal lamina and collagen formation. *J Cell Biol* 1980;**84**:184.

Bunge RP: Glial cells and the central myelin sheath. *Physiol Rev* 1968;**48**:197.

Cajal S: *Histologie du Système nerveux de l'Homme et des Vertébrés.* Vol 2. Librairie Maloine (Paris), 1911.

Davis R, Koelle GB: Electron microscopic localization of acetylcholinesterase at the neuromuscular junction by the gold-thiocholine and gold-thiolacetic acid methods. *J Cell Biol* 1967;**34**:157.

De Robertis EDP: Ultrastructure and cytochemistry of the synaptic region. *Science* 1967;**156**:907.

Droz B: Protein metabolism in nerve cells. *Int Rev Cytol* 1969;**25**:363.

Friede RL: Enzyme histochemistry of neuroglia. In: *Biology of Neuroglia.* De Robertis EDP, Correa R (editors). Elsevier, 1965.

Friede RL, Samorajski T: The clefts of Schmidt-Lanterman: A quantitative electron microscopic study of their structure in developing and adult sciatic nerves of the rat. *Anat Rec* 1969;**165**:89.

Friede RL, Samorajski T: Myelin formation in the sciatic nerve of the rat: A quantitative electron microscopic, histochemical, and radioautographic study. *J Neuropathol Exp Neurol* 1968;**27**:546.

Heuser JE, Reese TS: Evidence for recycling of synaptic vesicle membrane during transmitter release at the frog neuromuscular junction. *J Cell Biol* 1973;**57**:315.

Heuser JE, Reese TS: Structural changes after transmitter release at the frog neuromuscular junction. *J Cell Biol* 1981;**88**:564.

Hubbard JI (editor): *The Peripheral Nervous System.* Plenum Press, 1974.

Jacobson M, Hunt RK: The origins of nerve-cell specificity. *Sci Am* (Feb) 1973;**228**:26.

Junqueira LCU, Montes GS, Krisztán RM: The collagen of the vertebrate peripheral nervous system. *Cell Tissue Res* 1979; **202**:453.

Katz B: Elementary components of synaptic transmission. *Naturwissenschaften* 1979;**66**:606.

Keynes RD: Ion channels in the nerve-cell membrane. *Sci Am* (March) 1979;**240**:126.

Kreutzberg GW: Neuronal dynamics and axonal flow. 4. Blockage of intra-axonal enzyme transport by colchicine. *Proc Natl Acad Sci USA* 1969;**62**:722.

Krstić RV: Observations on the nodes of Ranvier of rat sciatic nerve fibers under the scanning and transmission electron microscope. *Period Biol* 1974;**76**:105.

Landon DN (editor): *The Peripheral Nerve.* Chapman & Hall, 1976.

Ling EA et al: Identification of glial cells in the brain of young rats. *J Comp Neurol* 1973;**149**:43.

Morales R, Duncan D: Specialized contacts of astrocytes with astrocytes and other cell types in the spinal cord of the cat. *Anat Rec* 1975;**182**:255.

Morell P, Norton WT: Myelin. *Sci Am* (May) 1980;**242**:88.

Palay SL, Chan-Palay V: *Cerebellar Cortex, Cytology and Organization.* Springer-Verlag, 1974.

Pappas GD, Waxman SG: Synaptic fine structure: Morphological correlates of chemical and electronic transmission. In: *Structure and Function of Synapses.* Pappas GD, Purpura DP (editors). Raven Press, 1972.

Peters A, Palay SL, Webster HF: *The Fine Structure of the Nervous System: The Neurons and Supporting Cells.* Saunders, 1976.

Reichardt LF, Kelly RB: A molecular description of nerve terminal function. *Annu Rev Biochem* 1983;**52**:871.

Schwartz JH: Axonal transport: Components, mechanisms, and specificity. *Annu Rev Neurosci* 1979;**2**:467.

Shepherd GM: Microcircuits in the nervous system. *Sci Am* (Feb) 1978;**238**:93.

Stevens CF: The Neuron. *Sci Am* (March) 1979;**241**:55.

Thomas PK, Olsson Y: Microscopic anatomy and function of the connective tissue components of peripheral nerve. In: *Peripheral Neuropathy.* Dyck PJ, Thomas PK, Lambert EH (editors). Saunders, 1975.

Wuerker RB, Kirkpatrick JB: Neuronal microtubules, neurofilaments, and microfilaments. *Int Rev Cytol* 1972;**33**:45.

The Sense Organs

10

Information about the external world is conveyed to the central nervous system by sensory units consisting of (1) a neuron with its cell body located in a dorsal (posterior) root ganglion or a cranial nucleus; (2) peripheral dendritic arborizations of the neuron; and (3) the central connections of this neuron to higher brain centers. The peripheral end of the afferent neuron or a nonneural secondary sensory cell acts as the receptor for one sensory modality, eg, touch, pain, smell, taste, vision, or hearing. This is called the **adequate stimulus** for the sensory cell. Most receptors can respond to excessive stimuli of any modality. For example, pressure on the eye can produce the sensation of light.

Three types of receptors are recognized based on the relationship of the sensory surface to the nervous system.

A **neuronal receptor** consists of an afferent nerve ending that acts as a biologic transducer to convert a specific stimulus to electrical events. This type of receptor is found in cutaneous sense organs and in many proprioceptors. The ending may be encapsulated or free. When the stimulus impinges on the nerve ending, graded changes in the membrane are produced (the **generator potential**) that will be summed, and if the generator potential reaches threshold, an action potential will be conducted to the central nervous system.

The second type consists of specialized **epithelial receptor cells** (eg, retinal photoreceptors, hair cells in the inner ear, sensory cells in taste buds) that detect the stimulus and respond by producing a **receptor potential** which causes the release of neurotransmitter molecules from the receptor cell. The transmitter may bring an associated sensory nerve fiber to threshold, with the result that one or more action potentials will be conducted centrally. Epithelial receptor cells are also called **secondary receptor cells** because they modulate the sensory stimulus before passing it along to the afferent (primary) neuron.

The only example of the third type of receptor in mammals is the sensory cell of the olfactory epithelium. Here, the cell body of the sensory neuron is peripherally located, where it serves as a **neuroepithelial receptor.**

An important generalization about sensory systems is the concept of a **receptive field.** This is the area in which an adequate stimulus (eg, touch) will evoke a response and is related to the extent of branching of the dendritic end of the afferent neuron. When many receptive endings are branches of one axon and are spread over a large area, the field is diffuse and spatial discrimination is poor.

Another general property of sensory receptors is their rate of adaptation. If a prolonged stimulus leads to a burst of action potentials that quickly subside, then we speak of a rapidly adapting receptor. This type of receptor can detect high-frequency stimuli. Conversely, slowly adapting receptors are more suited for detecting sustained stimuli such as the force of gravity.

The sensory systems described above detect information from the external world; there are also sensory systems that detect the internal status of the body. These include receptors for joint position, degree of muscle stretch, and O_2 and CO_2 concentrations.

Classification of Receptors

According to their functions, the principal receptors can be classified as follows:

(1) A system of receptors related to **somatic** and **visceral sensitivity.** These receptors are sensitive to pressure, vibration, temperature, and pain. In this group we include the mechanoreceptors responsible for relaying information on the degree of distention of hollow viscera, the digestive tract, the carotid sinus, etc.

(2) A **proprioceptor system,** which provides information on the position in space of different parts of the body. This system comprises the receptors of the vestibular part of the ear and receptors from the muscles, tendons, and joints.

(3) A **chemoreceptor system,** which participates in the gustatory and olfactory senses, including the receptors sensitive to CO_2 and O_2 present in the walls of blood vessels and those sensitive to food found in the digestive tract.

(4) A **photoreceptor system** responsible for vision.

(5) An **audioreceptor system** responsible for hearing.

RECEPTORS RELATED TO SUPERFICIAL & DEEP SENSATION

These receptors can be divided on morphologic grounds into free and encapsulated nerve terminals according to the absence or presence of a connective tissue capsule. The receptors consist of dendritic nerve endings or specialized, nonneuronal cells and are responsible for the senses discussed below.

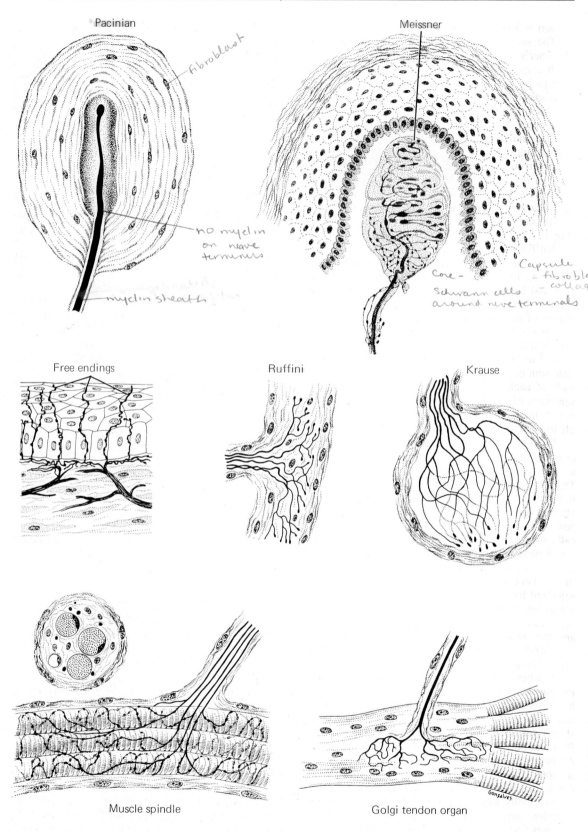

Pacinian

Meissner

fibroblast

no myelin
on nerve
terminus

myelin sheath

Core—

Capsule
— fibrobla
— collage

Schwann cells
around nerve terminals

Free endings

Ruffini

Krause

Muscle spindle

Golgi tendon organ

Gonsalves

Figure 10–1. Various types of sensory endings of nerves (not drawn to the same scale). (Based partially on a drawing in Ham AW: *Histology,* 6th ed. Lippincott, 1969.)

Touch & Pressure

The sense of touch and pressure is detected by Meissner's corpuscles, Ruffini's endings, Merkel's touch corpuscles, sensory endings around hairs, and perhaps by free nerve endings.

Meissner's corpuscles are most abundant in hairless (glabrous) skin of the palms and soles, their digits, the nipples, and the lips. They are found in dermal papillae and are about 150 μm long $\times$ 50 μm wide. The capsule consists of fibroblasts and thick collagen fibers surrounding an inner core of Schwann cells and nerve terminals. The characteristic appearance of Meissner's corpuscles in histologic sections is due to the horizontal arrangement of Schwann cells that enfold the nerve terminals as they wind their way upward (Fig 10–1).

Ruffini's endings are spindle-shaped encapsulated endings, ranging from 0.5 to 2 mm in length and lying in the dermis of both glabrous and hairy skin and in joints. A thin capsule surrounds a myelinated fiber that branches repeatedly to form a dense cluster of endings (Fig 10–1).

Hair follicles have a circumferential and a longitudinal array, or "palisade," of unmyelinated fibers around most of the length of the follicle. Sheets of Schwann cell cytoplasm encircle all but the extreme ends of each nerve fiber. When a hair is bent, the sensation of touch is elicited, but the receptive field is very large, since one parent axon may receive stimuli from several hundred hair follicles.

Merkel's touch corpuscles of the skin are an example of secondary sensory cells as transducers of a sensory stimulus—in this case, the sensation of touch. The receptor potential causes release of a neurotransmitter that may elicit an action potential in the primary afferent (sensory) nerve fiber. The corpuscle is composed of specialized epithelial cells, called **Merkel cells,** that are in close contact with unmyelinated fibers which penetrate the basal lamina of the epidermis and form large, flattened disks (**Merkel's disks**) beneath the Merkel cell. This specialized epithelial cell is characterized by a lobulated nucleus and the presence of numerous dense-core granules in the cytoplasm adjacent to the nerve ending. Many synapselike junctions are seen between the Merkel cell and the dendritic nerve ending. The neurotransmitter has not been identified, but it is not a catecholamine.

The best-studied mechanoreceptor is the **pacinian corpuscle.** It consists of many (20–70) layers of fibroblasts alternating with fluid-filled spaces that surround the unmyelinated nerve terminal. A myelin sheath surrounds the fiber as it exits the corpuscle. Pacinian corpuscles are quite large (up to 1 mm in diameter) and resemble a sliced onion in histologic sections (Figs 10–1 and 10–2). They are found in the dermis beneath both glabrous and hairy skin and are especially numerous in the dermis of the digits. Pacinian corpuscles are also found in the periosteum of bones and in mesenteries. This receptor has a rapid adaptation time and has been associated with the detection of vibrations. The pacinian corpuscle is not

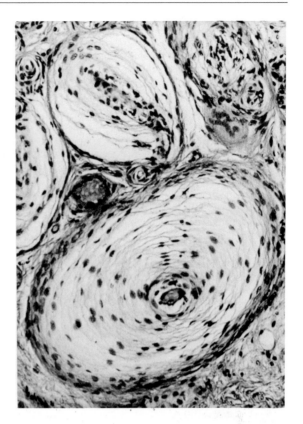

Figure 10–2. Photomicrograph of transverse sections of human pacinian corpuscles. Observe the concentric layers of connective tissue surrounding the centrally disposed unmyelinated nerve. H&E stain, $\times$ 320.

an important detector of pressure as is commonly stated, because it rapidly adapts (ceases discharging action potentials) to sustained stimuli.

Heat, Cold, & Pain

Cold receptors consist of slender myelinated fibers that penetrate the basement membrane of the epidermis, lose their Schwann cell investment, and then branch among the cells of the basal layer. They respond best to temperatures of 25–30 °C. Krause's endings are not the cold receptors, as previously thought. Warm receptors appear to be nonmyelinated fibers that respond maximally at 40–42 °C. Pain receptors (**nociceptors**) have been difficult to identify. It seems they are represented by thinly myelinated fibers that lose their myelin sheaths before penetrating the basement membrane of the skin. The endings branch, accompanied by thin sheets of Schwann cell cytoplasm, and penetrate between the cells of the lower layers of the epidermis (Fig 10–1). Round, clear vesicles and large, dense-core vesicles are present in these endings, but no synaptic specializations are seen, and it is believed that these vesicles do not contain neurotransmitters.

THE PROPRIOCEPTOR SYSTEM

All human striated muscles contain encapsulated proprioceptors known as **muscle spindles** (Fig 10–1). These structures are about 1.5 mm long and consist of a connective tissue capsule surrounding a fluid-filled space that contains from 2 to 20 specialized myofibers known as **intrafusal fibers.** These are easily distinguished from the majority of tension-producing **extrafusal fibers.** Within each spindle are one or 2 longer, thicker myofibers and several shorter, thinner fibers. Both types of fiber lose their cross-striations in their equatorial region, and many nuclei accumulate here. In the larger fibers, so many nuclei accumulate that a distinct swelling of the fiber is apparent. These fibers are called **nuclear bag fibers.** In the smaller fibers, the nuclei form a single row in the center of the cell, and these fibers are therefore known as **nuclear chain fibers.** A single, large-diameter myelinated afferent (sensory) nerve fiber penetrates the spindle. The myelin sheath is lost, and the nerve fiber branches extensively. Each branch encircles the equatorial region of intrafusal muscle fibers several times, forming the **primary sensory ending** or **annulospiral ending.** One or more smaller afferent nerves enter the spindle and innervate the ends of intrafusal fibers, mainly the nuclear chain fibers. These are the **secondary sensory endings,** also known as **flower-spray endings.** Each of the intrafusal fibers also receives a motor innervation via small (gamma) motor neurons.

Muscle spindles detect changes in length of extrafusal muscle fibers and relay this information to the spinal cord, where reflexes of varying complexity are activated to maintain posture and to regulate the activity of opposing muscle groups involved in motor activities such as walking. The simple, monosynaptic reflex known as the "knee-jerk" reflex illustrates an elementary function of the muscle spindle. When the patellar tendon is tapped, the quadriceps group of extensor muscles is stretched, including the contained muscle spindles. Stretching of the intrafusal fibers leads to generation of action potentials in sensory endings, principally the annulospiral endings. Sensory fibers synapse in the spinal cord with motor neurons that innervate the surrounding extrafusal muscle fibers. The motor neurons discharge action potentials that cause the extrafusal fibers to contract. Thus, there is a feedback mechanism to counteract stretch with contraction and maintain muscle fibers at a given length. The gamma motor efferents serve to maintain the sensitivity of the system at different lengths. (Details can be found in a textbook of physiology.)

In tendons, near the insertion sites of muscle fibers, a connective tissue sheath encapsulates a number of large bundles of collagen fibers that are continuous with collagen fibers comprising the myotendinous junction. Sensory nerves penetrate the connective tissue capsule, lose their Schwann cell covering, and arborize into an extensive network that envelops the collagen fibers of the tendon (Fig 10–1). These structures, known as **Golgi tendon organs,** are sensory receptors located in series with respect to the extrafusal muscle fibers. If a muscle (and its tendon) is stretched excessively, the muscle relaxes. This effect is mediated by Golgi tendon organs whose central endings synapse on inhibitory interneurons in the spinal cord.

Within the connective tissues of joints, sensory receptors include free nerve endings, Ruffini's corpuscles, and a few pacinian corpuscles. These receptors sense and relay spatial information to the central nervous system.

The structures mentioned above are sensitive to increases in tension and permit blind persons to know the exact position of their limbs and thereby regulate the amount of effort required to perform movements that call for variable amounts of muscular force.

THE CHEMORECEPTOR SYSTEM

Taste

Taste is a sensation perceived by **taste buds,** receptors principally located on the tongue but also present in smaller numbers on the soft palate and laryngeal surface of the epiglottis. Lingual taste buds are embedded within the stratified epithelium of the circumvallate, foliate, and fungiform papillae. Filiform papillae of the tongue do not possess taste buds. There are about 2000 taste buds on the human tongue. The position of taste buds on the 3 types of papillae is indicated in Fig 10–3, and the distribution of papillae on the tongue is shown in Fig 10–6.

Each ovoid taste bud is 50–80 μm high and 30–50 μm in diameter and consists of 30–80 spindle-shaped cells. Chemicals enter through the **taste pore,** a small aperture providing access to the receptor cells (Figs 10–4 and 10–5).

Taste buds are composed of at least 4 types of cells, which can be distinguished with the electron microscope. **Type I,** sustentacular, or "dark" cells are the most numerous. These are slender cells extending from the basal lamina to the taste pore, where

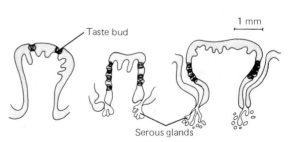

Fungiform papilla   Foliate papilla   Circumvallate papilla

Figure 10–3. Position of the taste buds on the 3 types of gustatory papillae. (Redrawn and reproduced, with permission, from Schmidt R [editor]: *Fundamentals of Sensory Physiology.* Springer-Verlag, 1978.)

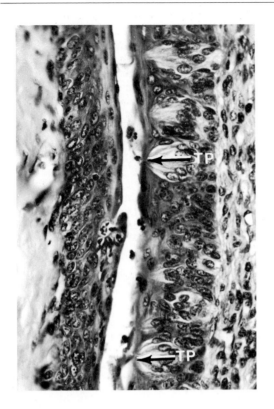

Figure 10–4. Photomicrograph of a section of a circumvallate papilla of the tongue, showing the taste buds embedded in the epithelial layer. TP, taste pore. H&E stain, × 400.

they display numerous microvilli. These cells contain numerous fine filaments that are thought to account for their dark appearance. Type I cells possess electron-opaque granules that probably store glycosaminoglycans which are later released into the taste pore. **Type II,** or "light," cells are the next most abundant. These cells are more rounded than type I cells; the cytoplasm contains fewer filaments; and numerous profiles of smooth endoplasmic reticulum are seen. Type II cells also have apical microvilli that project into the taste pore, but the function of these cells is not known. **Type III** cells resemble type II cells in many respects, but type III cells are characterized by the presence of numerous 40- to 60-nm vesicles resembling synaptic vesicles in their basal cytoplasm. Dendritic processes of sensory nerves are found in close proximity to these accumulations of synaptic vesicles (Fig 10–5). This is the basis for assigning taste reception to the type III cell. A relatively undifferentiated **basal cell** is found in taste buds. The basal cell is probably the precursor of the more specialized cells of the taste bud. Type I taste bud cells have a life span of about 10 days, whereas type II cells turn over more slowly. The life history of taste receptors (type III cells) remains to be elucidated.

Four fundamental taste sensations have been described in humans: acid, bitter, sweet, and salty. It is known that H^+ ions determine the sensation of sourness, but the chemical basis of the other sensations is unclear. For example, D-leucine tastes sweet, and L-leucine tastes bitter. Putting small drops of solutions

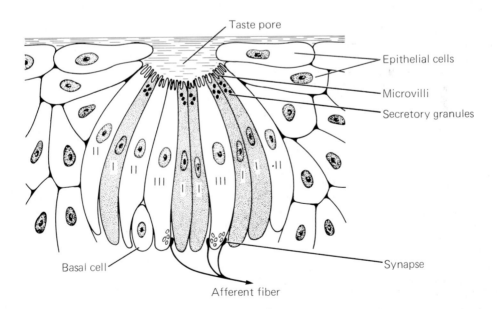

Figure 10–5. Structure and innervation of a taste bud. Four types of cells are shown. Type I cells are dark and possess apical secretory granules. The function of the light type II cells is not known. The sensory cell is the type III cell with its basally located synaptic vesicles and associated afferent nerve endings. Basal cells proliferate and give rise to the other cells. Only one afferent fiber is shown but, in reality, about 50 fibers innervate a single taste bud.

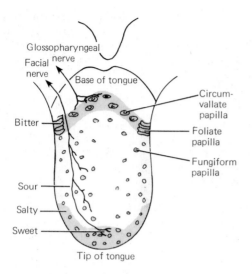

Figure 10–6. Diagram summarizing the distribution of gustatory papillae, their innervation, and the regions of maximum sensitivity to the different qualities on the human tongue. (Redrawn and reproduced, with permission, from Schmidt R [editor]: *Fundamentals of Sensory Physiology.* Springer-Verlag, 1978.)

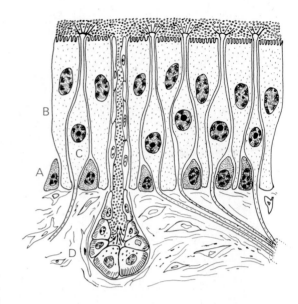

Figure 10–7. Olfactory mucosa showing the 3 cell types and the gland. *A:* basal cells; *B:* supporting cells; *C:* olfactory cells; *D:* Bowman's gland.

with different tastes on the fungiform papillae shows that some papillae are insensitive to some tastes whereas others are able to transmit more than one taste sensation. No structural differences have been described that might explain the differences in sensitivity of the taste buds to various substances. The secretions of serous glands (Ebner's glands) located at the bases of some lingual papillae (Fig 10–3) may serve to wash away gustatory stimuli, thus preserving sensitivity to new stimuli.

Receptors for the 4 basic taste modalities are not evenly distributed in the tongue, so some regions of this organ are more sensitive to certain tastes than to others. The distribution of taste bud–containing papillae on the lingual surface and their innervation are illustrated in Fig 10–6.

Olfaction

The olfactory chemoreceptors are located in a specialized area of the mucous membrane in the roof of the nasal cavity, the **olfactory epithelium.** In humans, it is about 10 cm^2 in area and up to 100 μm in thickness. This is a pseudostratified columnar epithelium composed of 3 types of cells:

The **supporting cells** have broad, cylindric apexes and narrower bases. On their free surface are microvilli which are submerged in the layer of a fluid consisting of both serous and mucous secretions that covers the entire epithelial surface. Well-developed junctional complexes bind the supporting cells to the adjacent olfactory cells. The cells contain a light yellow pigment that is responsible for the color of the olfactory mucosa (Fig 10–7).

The **basal cells** are small, are spherical or cone-shaped, and form a single layer at the base of the epithelium. They have branching processes that extend between the other cells in the epithelium.

Between the basal cells and the supporting cells are the **olfactory cells,** bipolar neurons distinguished from the supporting cells by the position of their nuclei, which lie below the nuclei of the supporting cells. Their apexes possess dilated areas from which arise 6–20 cilia (Fig 10–8). These cilia are long and nonmotile and are considered to be receptors, ie, the structures that respond to odoriferous substances by generating a receptor potential. Ciliary proximal segments show the usual 9 plus 2 microtubule axoneme. In the distal part of the cilium (70% of its length), all microtubules are single instead of the 9 double microtubules found in other cilia. These cilia are thought to be sensitive to chemical stimuli, and their presence in large numbers serves to considerably increase the receptor surface (Fig 10–9). The afferent axons of these neurons unite in small bundles that are directed toward the central nervous system. In the lamina propria of the olfactory mucosa, in addition to the abundant vessels and nerves, tubuloalveolar glands (Bowman's glands) containing both serous and mucous cells are observed (Fig 10–7). The excretory ducts of these glands open onto the epithelial surface, and the continuous flow of their secretion cleans the apical portion of the olfactory cells. In this manner, compounds that stimulate olfaction are constantly removed, thus keeping the receptors in a state of readiness to respond to new stimuli.

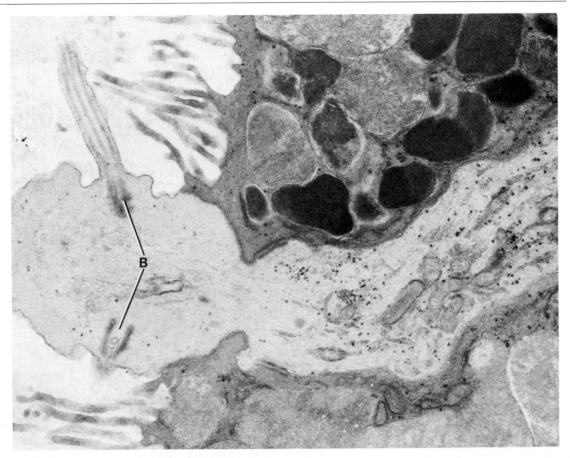

Figure 10–8. Electron micrograph of a section of olfactory mucosa from a frog. In the center is a pale olfactory cell and its terminal dilatation with 2 basal bodies (B) from which cilia emerge. × 28,000. (Courtesy of KR Porter.)

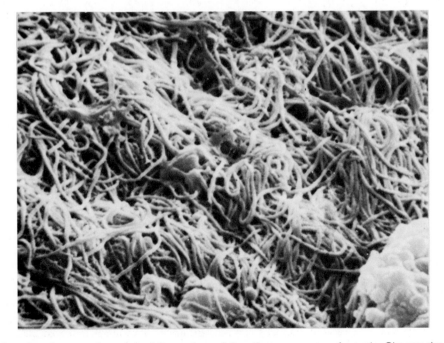

Figure 10–9. Scanning electron micrograph of the surface of the olfactory mucosa of a turtle. Observe the dense net of cilia covering its surface. × 6600. (Courtesy of PP Graziadei.)

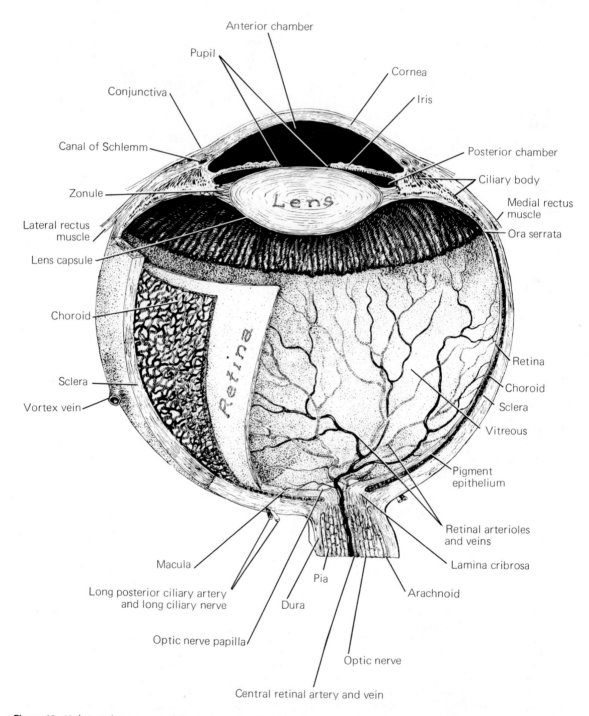

Figure 10–10. Internal structures of the human eye. (Redrawn from an original drawing by Paul Peck and reproduced, with permission, from *The Anatomy of the Eye.* Courtesy of Lederle Laboratories.)

THE EYE

The eye is a complex and highly developed photosensitive organ that permits an accurate analysis of the form, light intensity, and color reflected from objects. The eyes are located in protective bony structures of the skull—the **orbits.** Each eye includes a tough, fibrous globe to maintain the shape of the eye, a lens system to focus the image, a layer of photosensitive cells, and a system of cells and nerves whose function it is to collect, process, and transmit visual information to the central nervous system. Each eye is composed of 3 concentric layers: (1) an external layer that consists of the **sclera** and the **cornea;** (2) a middle layer—also called the **vascular layer** or **uveal tract**—consisting of the **choroid, ciliary body,** and **iris;** and (3) an inner layer of nerve tissue, the **retina,** which consists of an outer pigment epithelium (Fig 10–11) and an inner retina proper. The photosensitive retina proper communicates with the central nervous system through the **optic nerve** (Figs 10–10 and 10–11) and extends forward to the **ora serrata.**

The **lens** of the eye is a biconvex transparent structure held in place by a circular system of fibers, the **zonule of Zinn,** which extends from the lens into a thickening of the middle layer called the **ciliary body,** and by close apposition to the vitreous on its posterior side (Figs 10–10 and 10–11). Partially covering the anterior surface of the lens is an opaque pigmented expansion of the middle layer called the **iris.** The round hole in the middle of the iris is the **pupil** (Fig 10–10).

The eye contains 3 compartments: the **anterior chamber,** which occupies the space between the cornea and the iris and the lens; the **posterior chamber,** between the iris, ciliary process, zonular attachments, and the lens; and the **vitreous space** behind the lens and zonular attachments and surrounded by the retina (Figs 10–10 and 10–11). Both the anterior and the posterior chambers contain a protein-poor fluid called **aqueous humor.** The vitreous space is filled by a viscous, gelatinous substance called the **vitreous body.**

The blood supply of the eye arises from the ophthalmic artery and is divided into 2 almost completely independent systems. The first system supplies the optic nerve and the inner retina. These are the vessels that can be visualized with the ophthalmoscope. A second system supplies the vascular layer. The outer parts of the retina, including the photoreceptors, receive their blood supply from the choriocapillary layer of the choroid.

Note that the terms outer (external) and inner (internal) refer to the gross structure of the eye. Inner denotes a structure closer to the center of the globe, while outer means closer to the surface of the eyeball.

External Layer or Tunica Fibrosa

The opaque white posterior five-sixths of the external layer of the eye is the **sclera,** forming in the human a segment of a sphere roughly 22 mm in diameter (Figs 10–10 and 10–11). The sclera consists of tough, dense connective tissue made up mainly of flat collagen bundles intersecting in various directions—all bundles parallel to the surface of the organ—a moderate amount of ground substance, and a few fibroblasts. The external surface of the sclera—the **episclera**—is connected by a loose system of thin collagen fibers to a dense layer of connective tissue called **Tenon's capsule.** It comes into contact with the loose conjunctival stroma at the junction of the cornea with the sclera, also called the **limbus.** Between Tenon's capsule and the sclera is **Tenon's space.** It is because of this loose space that the eyeball can make rotating movements in all directions. Between the sclera and the choroid is a thin layer of loose connective tissue rich in melanocytes, fibroblasts, and elastic fibers called the **suprachoroidal lamina.** The sclera is relatively avascular.

In contrast to the posterior five-sixths of the eye, the anterior one-sixth—the **cornea**—is colorless and transparent (Figs 10–10 and 10–11). A transverse section of the cornea shows that it consists of 5 layers: epithelium, Bowman's membrane, stroma, Descemet's membrane, and endothelium (Fig 10–12). The corneal epithelium is stratified, squamous, and nonkeratinized and consists of 5 or 6 layers of cells. In the basal part of the epithelium there are numerous mitotic figures responsible for the remarkable regenerating capacity of the cornea. The turnover time for these cells is approximately 7 days. The surface corneal cells show microvilli protruding into the space filled by the precorneal tear film, a protective layer of lipid and glycoprotein, about 7 μm in thickness. The cornea has one of the richest sensory nerve supplies of any eye tissue.

Beneath the corneal epithelium lies a thick homogeneous layer 7–12 μm in thickness. It consists of collagen fibers crossing at random and a condensation of the intercellular substance, but no cells are found (Fig 10–13). This is **Bowman's membrane,** which contributes greatly to the stability and strength of the cornea.

The **stroma** is formed by many layers of parallel collagenous bundles that cross at approximately right angles to each other. The collagen fibrils within each lamella are parallel to each other and run the full width of the cornea. Between the several layers, the cytoplasmic extensions of fibroblasts are flattened like the wings of a butterfly. Both cells and fibers of the stroma are immersed in an amorphous metachromatic glycoprotein substance rich in chondroitin sulfate. Although the stroma is avascular, migrating lymphoid cells are normally present in the cornea.

Descemet's membrane is a thick (5–10 μm in thickness) homogeneous structure composed of fine collagenous filaments organized in a 3-dimensional network (Fig 10–12B).

The **endothelium** of the cornea is a simple squamous epithelium. These cells possess organelles characteristic of cells engaged in active transport and protein synthesis for secretion, which may relate to the synthesis and maintenance of Descemet's membrane.

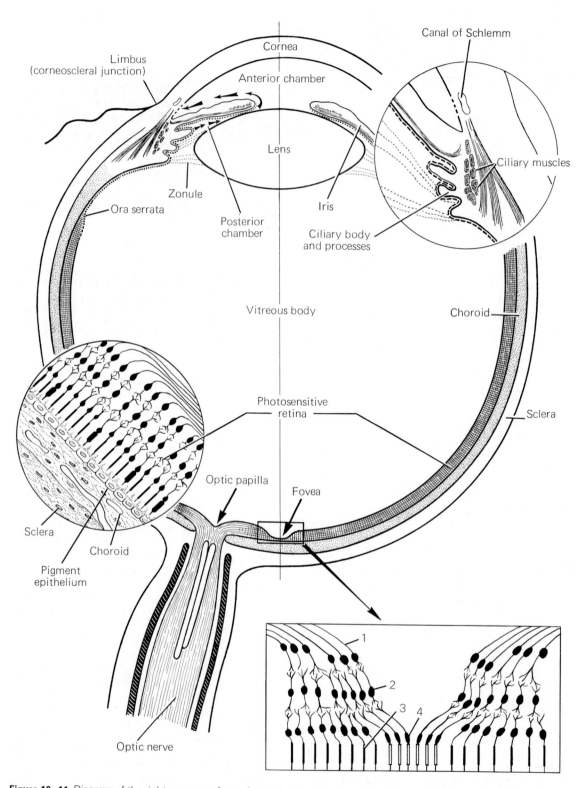

Figure 10–11. Diagram of the right eye, seen from above, showing the structure of the eye, retina, fovea, and ciliary body. Arrows in the anterior chamber show the direction of flow of aqueous humor. An enlarged diagram of the fovea is shown at lower right. 1, axons of ganglion cells; 2, bipolar cells; 3, rods; 4, cones. (Modified and reproduced, with permission, from Ham AW: *Histology,* 6th ed. Lippincott, 1969.)

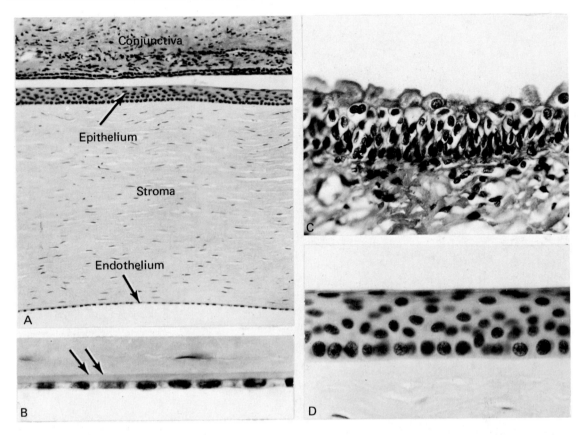

Figure 10–12. Photomicrographs of a transverse section of cornea. *A:* The cornea and conjunctiva seen at low magnification. × 80. *B:* The posterior corneal epithelium—also called endothelium (arrows indicate Descemet's membrane). × 400. *C:* Conjunctival epithelium. × 300. *D:* Anterior corneal epithelium. Note the smooth contour of the surface of this epithelium. × 400.

The corneal endothelium and epithelium are responsible for maintaining the transparency of the cornea. Both layers are capable of transporting sodium ions toward their apical surfaces. Chloride ions and water follow passively, and therefore the corneal stroma is maintained in a relatively dehydrated state. This, along with the regular orientation of the very thin collagen fibrils of the stroma, accounts for the transparency of the cornea.

The **corneoscleral junction** or **limbus** is an area of transition from the transparent collagenous bundles of the cornea to the white opaque fibers of the sclera. It is highly vascularized, and its blood vessels assume an important role in corneal inflammatory processes. The cornea—an avascular structure—receives its metabolites by diffusion from adjacent vessels and from the fluid of the anterior chamber of the eye. In the region of the limbus in the stromal layer, irregular endothelium-lined channels, the trabecular meshwork, merge to form the **canal of Schlemm** (Figs 10–10 and 10–11), which drains fluid from the anterior chamber of the eye. The canal of Schlemm communicates externally with the venous system.

Middle or Vascular Layer

The middle (vascular) layer of the eye consists of 3 parts: choroid, ciliary body, and iris (Fig 10–10). These 3 parts are known collectively as the uveal tract.

A. Choroid: The choroid is a highly vascularized coat. Between its blood vessels is found loose connective tissue rich in fibroblasts, macrophages, lymphocytes, mast cells, plasma cells, collagen fibers, and elastic fibers. Melanocytes are abundant in this layer and give it its characteristic black color. The inner layer of the choroid is richer in small vessels than the outer layer and is called the **choriocapillary layer.** It has an important function in nutrition of the retina, and damage to this tissue causes serious damage to the retina. A thin (3–4 μm), amorphous hyaline membrane separates the choriocapillary layer from the retina. This is known as **Bruch's membrane** and extends from the **optic disk** to the ora serrata. The optic disk, also called **optic papilla,** is the region where the optic nerve enters the eyeball (Fig 10–11).

Bruch's membrane is formed of 5 different layers. The central layer is composed of a network of elastic fibers. This network is lined on its 2 surfaces by layers

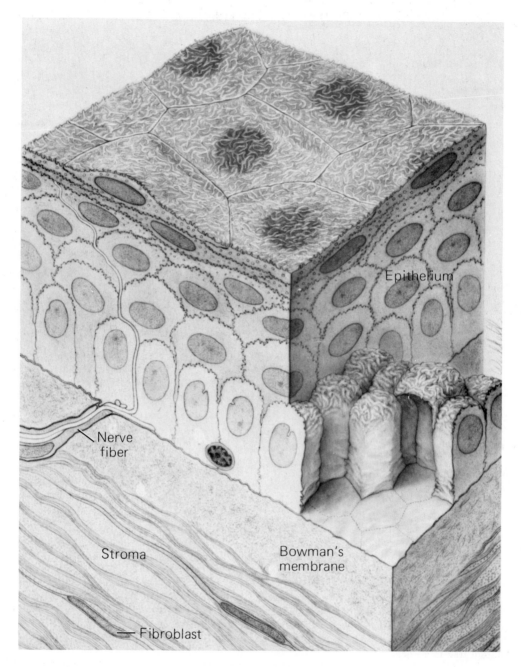

Figure 10–13. Tridimensional drawing of the cornea. (Reproduced, with permission, from Hogan MJ, Alvarado JA, Weddell JE: *Histology of the Human Eye.* Saunders, 1971.)

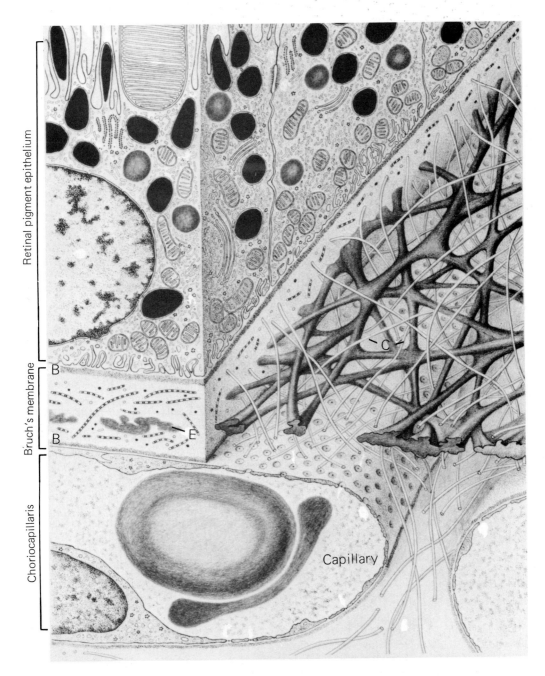

Figure 10–14. Tridimensional drawing showing the constitution of Bruch's membrane and its relation to the pigment cell layer and choriocapillary layer. B, basal lamina; E, elastic fibers; C, collagen fibers. (Slightly modified and reproduced, with permission, from Hogan MJ, Alvarado JA, Weddell JE: *Histology of the Human Eye.* Saunders, 1971.)

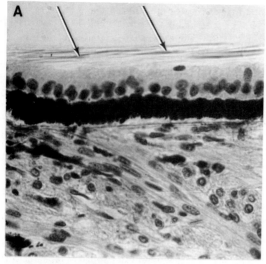

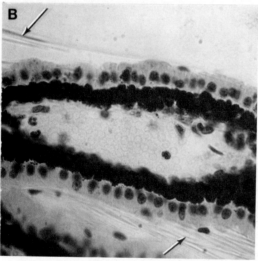

Figure 10–15. Photomicrographs of a ciliary body. *A:* Note the double layer, of which one consists of pigmented cells. *B:* The ciliary process is covered by epithelium on both sides. Arrows indicate zonular fibers. H&E stain, × 400.

of collagen fibers that are covered by the basal lamina of the capillaries of the choriocapillary layer on one side and basal lamina of the pigment epithelium on the other side (Fig 10–14). (See below, under Retina, for a description of the pigment epithelium.) The choroid is bound to the sclera by means of a loose layer of connective tissue rich in melanocytes called the **suprachoroidal lamina.**

B. Ciliary Body: The ciliary body is an anterior expansion of the choroid at the level of the lens (Figs 10–10 and 10–11). It constitutes a continuous thickened ring which lies at the inner surface of the anterior portion of the sclera. In transverse section, it forms a triangle. One of its faces is in contact with the vitreous, one with the sclera, and the third with the

lens and the posterior chamber of the eye. The histologic structure of the ciliary body is basically loose connective tissue (rich in elastic fibers, vessels, and melanocytes) surrounding the **ciliary muscle** (Fig 10–11). This structure is composed of 3 bundles of smooth muscle fibers that insert on the sclera anteriorly and on different regions of the ciliary body posteriorly. One of these bundles has the function of stretching the choroid; another bundle, when contracted, relaxes the tension on the lens. These muscular movements are important in visual accommodation, as will be seen later in the discussion on the lens. The surfaces of the ciliary body that face the vitreous, posterior chamber, and lens are covered by the anterior extension of the retina (Fig 10–11). In this region, the retina consists of only 2 cell layers. The layer directly adherent to the ciliary body consists of simple columnar cells rich in melanin. It corresponds to the forward projection of the pigment layer of the retina. The second layer, which covers the first, is derived from the sensory layer of the retina and consists of simple nonpigmented columnar epithelium (Fig 10–15A).

C. Ciliary Processes: The ciliary processes are ridgelike extensions of the ciliary body that have a loose connective tissue core, possess numerous fenestrated capillaries (see Chapter 12), and are covered by the 2 simple epithelial layers described above (Fig 10–15B). From the ciliary processes emerge fibers (zonule fibers) that insert into the capsule of the lens and anchor it in place. The apical ends of the epithelial cells are found at the junction between pigmented and nonpigmented cells. Thus, the cells meet each other head-to-head, and the basement membrane of the outer, pigmented cells is adjacent to the main mass of the ciliary body, while the basement membrane of the inner, nonpigmented cells is adjacent to the posterior chamber. It is in this basement membrane that the zonular fibers have their origin. The apical ends of the epithelial cells are joined by desmosomes, and elaborate tight junctions are found around the apical surfaces of epithelial cells of both layers. The unpigmented inner layer of cells has extensive basal infoldings and interdigitations characteristic of ion-transporting cells (see Chapter 4). These cells actively transport certain constituents of plasma into the posterior chamber, thus forming the **aqueous humor.** This fluid has an inorganic ion composition similar to plasma but has less than 0.1% protein (plasma has about 7% protein). Aqueous humor flows toward the lens and passes between it and the iris, reaching the anterior chamber of the eye (see arrows in Fig 10–11). Once in the anterior chamber, it proceeds to the angle formed by the cornea with the basal part of the iris. It penetrates the tissue of the limbus in a series of labyrinthine spaces (the trabecular meshwork) and finally reaches the irregular canal of Schlemm, lined by endothelial cells (Figs 10–10 and 10–11). This structure communicates with small veins of the sclera through which the aqueous humor escapes. Any impediment to the drainage of aqueous humor caused by an obstruction in the outflow channels results in an increase in intraocular pressure, causing **glaucoma.**

D. Iris: The iris is an extension of the choroid that partially covers the lens, leaving a round opening in the center called the **pupil** (Fig 10–10). The anterior surface of the iris is irregular and rough, with grooves and ridges; the posterior surface is smooth. The anterior surface is formed by a discontinuous layer of pigment cells and fibroblasts. Beneath this layer is a poorly vascularized connective tissue with few fibers and many fibroblasts and melanocytes. The next layer is rich in blood vessels embedded in loose connective tissue. The posterior surface of the iris is covered by 2 layers of epithelium that also cover the ciliary body and its processes. The inner epithelium, in contact with the posterior chamber, is heavily pigmented with melanin granules. The outer epithelial cells have tonguelike extensions of their basal region directed radially and filled with myofilaments that overlap,

creating the **dilator pupillae muscle** of the iris. The heavy pigmentation prevents the passage of light into the interior of the eye except through the pupil.

The function of the abundant melanocytes or melanin-containing pigment cells in several regions of the eye is to keep stray light rays from interfering with image formation. The melanocytes of the stroma of the iris are responsible for the color of the eyes, ie, the color of the iris. Thus, if the layer of pigment in the interior region of the iris consists of only a few cells, the light reflected from the black pigment epithelium present in the posterior surface of the iris will be blue. As the amount of pigment increases, the iris assumes various shades of greenish-blue, gray, and finally brown. Albinos have almost no pigment, and the pink color of their irises is due to the reflection of incident light from the blood vessels of the iris.

The iris contains smooth muscle bundles disposed in circles concentric with the pupillary margin, form-

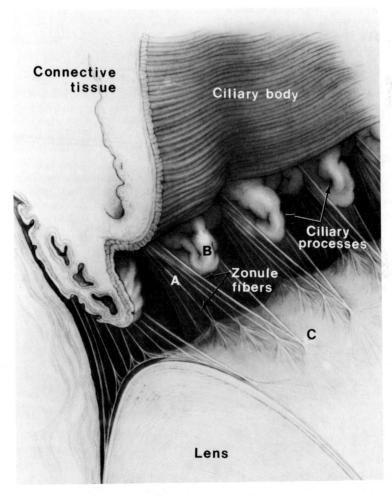

Figure 10–16. Anterior view of the ciliary processes showing the zonules attaching to the lens. Zonules form columns (A) on either side of the ciliary processes (B), which meet on a single site (C) as they attach to the lens. (Reproduced, with permission, from Hogan MJ, Alvarado JA, Weddell JE: *Histology of the Human Eye.* Saunders, 1971.)

ing the **sphincter pupillae muscle** of the iris. The dilator and sphincter muscles have sympathetic and parasympathetic innervation, respectively.

Lens

This biconvex structure is characterized by great elasticity, a feature that it loses with age as the lens hardens. The lens has 3 principal components:

A. Lens Capsule: The lens is enveloped by a thick (10–20 μm), homogeneous, refractile, carbohydrate-rich capsule coating the outer surface of the epithelial cells. It is elastic and consists mainly of collagen type IV and amorphous glycoprotein.

B. Subcapsular Epithelium: This consists of a single layer of cuboidal epithelial cells present only on the anterior surface of the lens. The lens increases in size and grows throughout life as new lens fibers develop from cells located at the equator of the lens. The cells of this epithelium exhibit many interdigitations with the lens fibers. Their cytoplasm has few organelles and stains lightly. They are bound together by gap junctions.

C. Lens Fibers: These are elongated and appear as thin flattened structures. They are highly differentiated cells derived from cells of the subcapsular epithelium. They eventually lose their nuclei and other organelles and become greatly elongated, attaining dimensions of 7–10 mm in length, 8–10 μm in width, and 2 μm in thickness. These cells are filled with a group of proteins called **crystallins.** Lens fiber production continues throughout life but at an ever-decreasing rate.

The lens is held in place by a radially oriented group of fibers, the **zonule,** which inserts on one side on the lens capsule and on the other on the ciliary body (Fig 10–16). Zonular fibers are similar to the microfibrils of elastic fibers. This system is important in the process known as **accommodation,** which permits focusing on near and far objects by changing the curvature of the lens. Thus, when the eye is at rest or gazing at distant objects, the lens is kept stretched by the zonule in a plane perpendicular to the optical axis. To focus on a near object, the ciliary muscles contract, resulting in forward displacement of the choroid and ciliary body. Consequently, the tension exerted by the zonule is relieved and the lens becomes thicker, thus keeping the object in focus.

With advancing age, the elasticity of the lens is reduced, making accommodation for near objects difficult. This is a normal aging process (presbyopia), which can be corrected by wearing glasses with convex lenses. If the lens becomes opaque, the condition is termed **cataract.** In older individuals, a brownish pigment accumulates in lens fibers, making them less transparent. Cataract may also be caused by excessive exposure to ultraviolet radiation. In diabetes mellitus, the high levels of glucose are thought to produce cataract.

Vitreous Body

The vitreous body occupies the region of the eye behind the lens. It is a transparent gel that consists of water (about 99%), collagen, and heavily hydrated glycosaminoglycans whose principal component is hyaluronic acid.

Retina

The retina, the inner layer of the globe, consists of 2 portions. The posterior portion is photosensitive; the anterior part is not photosensitive and constitutes the inner lining of the ciliary body and the posterior part of the iris (Figs 10–11 and 10–17). The retina derives from an evagination of the anterior cephalic vesicle or prosencephalon. This so-called **optic vesicle,** upon coming into contact with the surface ectoderm, gradually invaginates in its central region, forming a double-walled **optic cup.** In the adult, the outer wall gives rise to a thin membrane called the

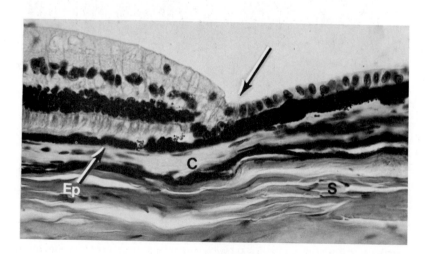

Figure 10–17. Photomicrograph of a section of retina in the transition (arrow) between the photosensitive *(left)* and blind *(right)* parts. This transition is called the ora serrata. Note the pigment epithelium (Ep), the choroid (C), and the sclera (S). H&E stain, × 200.

pigment epithelium; from the inner layer is derived the optical or functioning part of the retina—the **neural retina.**

The pigment epithelium consists of columnar cells with a basal nucleus. The basal regions of the cells adhere firmly to Bruch's membrane, and the cell membranes have numerous basal invaginations (Fig 10–23). Mitochondria are more abundant in the region of the cytoplasm near these invaginations. These 2 characteristics suggest an ion-transporting activity for this region.

The lateral cell membranes show cell junctions with conspicuous zonulae occludentes and zonulae adherentes at their apexes as well as desmosomes and gap junctions. These morphologic details indicate that the apical and basal regions of this epithelial sheet are sealed off and that intercellular communication exists. The existence of an electrical potential difference resulting from ion transport between the 2 surfaces of this epithelium can be accounted for by these junctional specializations.

The cell apex has abundant extensions of 2 types: slender microvilli and cylindric sheaths that invest the tips of the photoreceptors. Neither type of extension is anatomically joined to the photoreceptors, so that these regions can become separated, as occurs in a **detachment of the retina,** a common and serious disorder in humans (currently being treated effectively by laser surgery). The cytoplasm of pigmented epithelial cells has abundant smooth endoplasmic reticulum, believed to be a site of vitamin A esterification and transport to the photoreceptors. Melanin granules are numerous in the apical cytoplasm and microvilli. Melanin is synthesized in these cells by a mechanism similar to that described for the melanocytes in the skin (see Chapter 19). This dark pigment has the function of absorbing light after the photoreceptors have been stimulated.

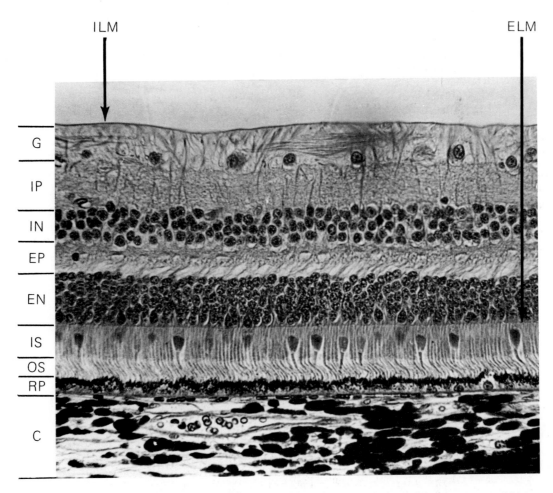

Figure 10–18. Section of the retina of a monkey. Light enters from the top and traverses the following layers: ILM, internal limiting membrane; G, ganglion cell layer; IP, internal plexiform layer; IN, internal nuclear layer (bipolar neurons); EP, external plexiform layer; EN, external nuclear layer (nuclei of rods and cones); ELM, external limiting membrane; IS, inner segments of rods (narrow lines) and cones (triangular dark structures); OS, outer segments of rods and cones; RP, retinal pigment epithelium; C, choroid. × 655.

The cell apex has numerous dense vesicles of variable shape that represent various stages in the phagocytosis and digestion of the tips of photoreceptor outer segments. The structure of these cells and the shedding of their tips are discussed below (Fig 10–23).

The optical part of the retina—the posterior or photosensitive part—is a more complex structure containing at least 15 types of neurons, and these cells form at least 38 distinct kinds of synapses with one another. The optical retina consists of the following layers: (1) an outer layer of photosensitive cells, the **rods** and **cones** (Figs 10–11, 10–18, and 10–19); (2) an intermediate layer of **bipolar neurons,** which connects the rods and cones to the ganglion cells; and (3) an internal layer of **ganglion cells,** which establishes contact with the bipolar cells through its dendrites and sends axons to the central nervous system. These axons converge at the optic papilla, forming the **optic nerve.**

Between the layer of rods and cones and the bipolar cells, a region called the **external plexiform** or **synaptic layer** exists where synapses between these 2 types of cells occur. The region where the synapses between the bipolar and ganglion cells are established is called the **internal plexiform layer** (Fig 10–19). The retina has an inverted structure, for the light will first cross the ganglion layer and then the bipolar layer to reach the rods and cones.

A needle inserted through the posterior part of the eyeball would pass through the sclera, the choroid, the pigment epithelium of the retina, the rods and cones, the bipolar layer, and the ganglion layer to enter the vitreous.

The structure of the retina will now be examined in greater detail. The rods and cones are polarized neurons; at one pole is a single photosensitive dendrite and at the other are synapses with cells of the bipolar layer (Figs 10–19 and 10–20). These photosensitive cells assume the form of a rod or cone, giving these cells their names. These cells can be divided into outer and inner segments, a nuclear region, and a synaptic region. The outer segments are modified cilia and contain stacks of flattened membrane-limited saccules with a flattened disklike shape. The photosensitive

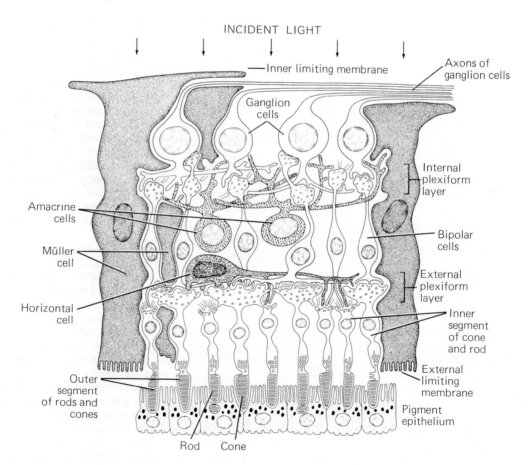

INCIDENT LIGHT

Inner limiting membrane

Axons of ganglion cells

Ganglion cells

Internal plexiform layer

Amacrine cells

Bipolar cells

Müller cell

External plexiform layer

Horizontal cell

Inner segment of cone and rod

External limiting membrane

Outer segment of rods and cones

Pigment epithelium

Rod   Cone

Figure 10–19. Schematic drawing of the 3 layers of retinal neurons. The arrows represent the direction of the light path. The stimulation generated by the incident light on rods and cones proceeds in the opposite direction. (Redrawn and reproduced, with permission, from Boycott and Dowling: *Proc R Soc Lond* [*Biol*] 1966;166:80.)

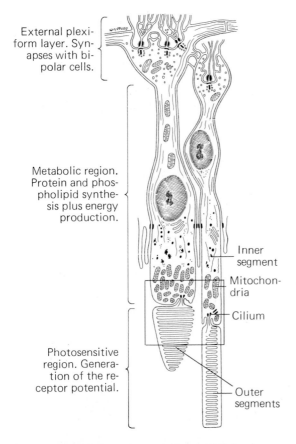

External plexi-
form layer. Syn-
apses with bi-
polar cells.

Metabolic region.
Protein and phos-
pholipid synthe-
sis plus energy
production.

Inner
segment

Mitochon-
dria

Cilium

Photosensitive
region. Genera-
tion of the re-
ceptor potential.

Outer
segments

Figure 10–20. The ultrastructure of the rods *(right)* and cones *(left)*. The enclosed region is illustrated in the electron micrograph in Fig 10–21. (Redrawn and reproduced, with permission, from Chevremont M: *Notions de Cytologie et Histologie.* S.A. Desoer Editions [Liège], 1966.)

pigment of the retina is in the membrane of these saccules. Both rod cells and cone cells pass through a thin layer called the **external limiting membrane,** which has been found to be a series of junctional complexes between photoreceptors and glial cells of the retina (Müller cells) (Fig 10–24). The nuclei of the cones are generally disposed near the limiting membrane, while rod nuclei lie near the center of the inner segment.

The **rod cells** are thin, elongated cells (50 × 3 μm) composed of 2 portions as shown in Figs 10–19 and 10–20. The external photosensitive rod-shaped portion is composed mainly of numerous (600–1000) flattened membranous disks piled up like a stack of coins. The disks in rods are not continuous with the plasma membrane. The **outer segment** is separated from the **inner segment** by a constriction. Just below this constriction there is a basal segment from which a cilium arises and passes to the outer segment. The inner segment is rich in glycogen and has a remarkable accumulation of mitochondria, most lying near the

constriction (Figs 10–20 and 10–21). This local accumulation of mitochondria is related to the production of energy necessary for the visual process and protein synthesis. Polyribosomes are present in large numbers below the mitochondrial region of the inner segment and are involved in protein synthesis. Some of these proteins migrate to the outer segment of the rod cells, where they are incorporated into membranous disks.

The flattened disks of the rod cells contain the pigment called **visual purple** or **rhodopsin,** which is bleached by light and initiates the visual stimulus. This substance is globular in form and is located in the outer surface of the lipid bilayer of the flattened membranous disks. It has been estimated that the human retina has approximately 120 million rods. They are extremely sensitive to light and are considered to be the receptors used when low levels of light are present, such as during the period of dusk or at night. The outer segment is the site of photosensitivity, whereas the inner segment contains the metabolic machinery necessary for the biosynthetic and energy-producing processes of these cells.

Radioautographic studies show that proteins of the vesicles of the rods are synthesized in the polyribosome-rich inner segment of these cells. From there, they migrate to the outer segment and aggregate at its basal region, where they are incorporated into membranes formed by a double layer of phospholipids producing flattened disks (Figs 10–20 and 10–21). These structures gradually migrate to the cell apex, where they are shed, phagocytized, and digested by the cells of the pigment epithelium (Figs 10–22 and 10–23). It has been calculated that in the monkey approximately 90 vesicles per cell are produced daily. The whole process of migration, from assembly at the basal cell region to apical shedding, takes 9–13 days. In **hereditary retinal dystrophy** in the rat, the vesicles shed from the rods are not phagocytized, probably as a result of a dysfunction of the pigment epithelium, and are instead deposited at the surface of the pigment layer.

The **cone cells** are also elongated (60 × 1.5 μm) neurons. Each human retina has about 6 million cone cells. They have a structure similar to that of the rods, with outer and inner segments, basal body with cilium, and an accumulation of mitochondria and polyribosomes (Fig 10–20). The cones differ from the rods in their conical form and the structure of their outer segments. This region is also composed of stacked membranous disks; however, they are not independent of the outer plasma membrane but arise as invaginations of this structure (Fig 10–20). In cones, newly synthesized protein is not concentrated in recently assembled disks (as it is in rods) but is distributed uniformly throughout the outer segment. There are at least 3 functional types of cones, which cannot be distinguished by their morphology. Each type contains a variety of the cone photopigment called **iodopsin.** The maximum sensitivity of each cone type is in the red, green, or blue region of the visible spectrum,

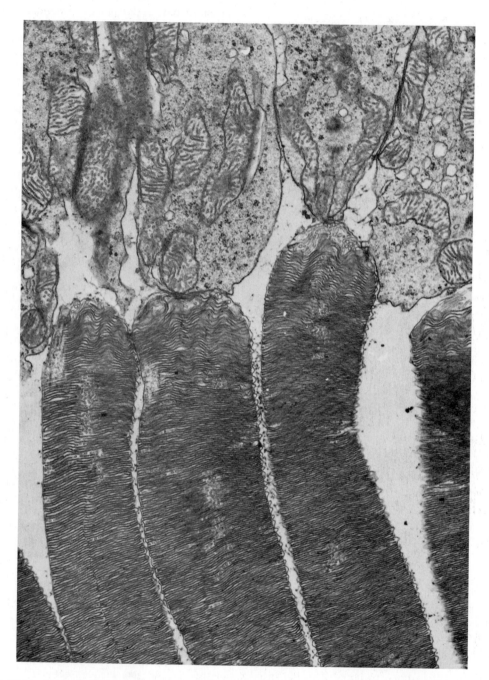

Figure 10–21. Electron micrograph of a section of the retina of a mouse. In the lower part of the picture are the outer segments. This photosensitive region consists of parallel membranous flat disks. Mitochondrial accumulation occurs in the inner segment. × 10,000. (Courtesy of KR Porter.)

respectively. The cones, sensitive only to light of a higher intensity than that required to stimulate the rods, are believed to permit better visual acuity than the rods.

The layer of bipolar cells consists of 2 types of cells (Fig 10–19): (1) **diffuse bipolar cells,** which have synapses with 2 or more photoreceptors; and (2) **monosynaptic bipolar cells,** which establish contact with the axon of only one cone photoreceptor and only one ganglion cell. There are, therefore, a certain number of cones which transmit their impulses directly to the central nervous system.

The cells of the ganglion layer, besides establishing contact with the bipolar cells, project their axons to a specific region of the retina where they come together to form the **optic nerve** (Fig 10–19). This region is devoid of receptors and is therefore called the **blind spot** of the retina, the **papilla of the optic nerve,** or the **optic nerve head** (Fig 10–11). The **ganglion cells** are typical nerve cells with a large euchromatic nucleus, basophilic Nissl substance, etc. These cells, like the bipolar cells, are also classified as diffuse or monosynaptic types in their connections with other cells.

Besides these 3 main types of cells (photoreceptors, bipolar cells, and ganglion cells), other types of cells are distributed more diffusely in the layers of the retina:

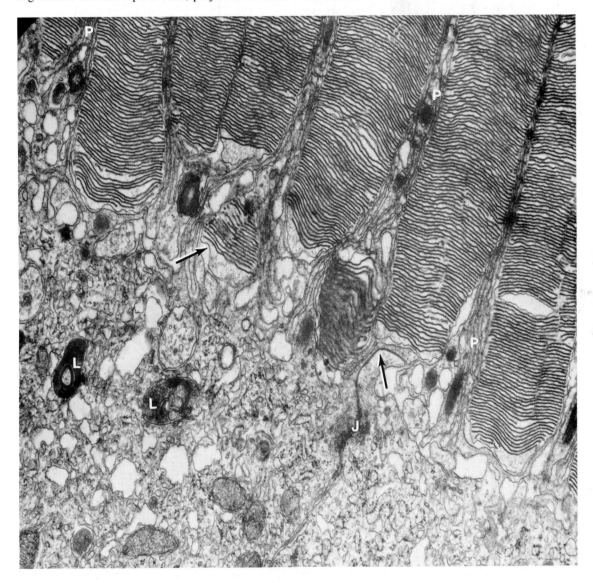

Figure 10–22. Electron micrograph of the interface between the photosensitive and pigmented layer in a rat retina. Below are portions of 2 pigment epithelial cells revealing junctional specializations between their lateral plasmalemmas (J). Above the pigment cells are the tips of several outer segments of rod cells that interdigitate with apical processes of the pigment epithelium (P). The large vacuoles containing flattened membranes (arrows) have been shed from the tips of the rods. Lysosomal vesicles are indicated by an L.

(1) Horizontal cells (Fig 10–19) establish contact between different photoreceptors. Their exact function is not known, but it is possible that they act to integrate stimuli.

(2) Amacrine cells are various types of neurons that establish contact between the ganglion cells. Their function is also obscure.

(3) Supporting cells are neuroglia that possess, in addition to the astrocyte and microglial cell types, some large, extensively ramified cells called **Müller cells.** The processes of these cells bind together the neural cells of the retina and extend from the inner to the outer limiting membranes of the retina (Fig 10–19). They contain abundant microfilaments and glycogen in their cytoplasm and are known to have a high metabolic rate. The outer limiting membrane is a zone of adhesion (tight junctions) between photo-

receptors and Müller cells. Müller cells are functionally analogous to neuroglia in that they serve to support, nourish, and insulate the retinal neurons and fibers (Fig 10–24).

Retinal Histophysiology

Light passes through the layers of the retina to the rods and cones, where it is absorbed, thus initiating a series of reactions that result in what we call vision. This is an extraordinarily sensitive process. There is experimental evidence to suggest that a single photon is enough to trigger the production of a receptor potential in a rod. Light acts to bleach the visual pigments, and this photochemical process is amplified by mechanisms that cause the local production of responses which are subsequently transmitted to the central nervous system.

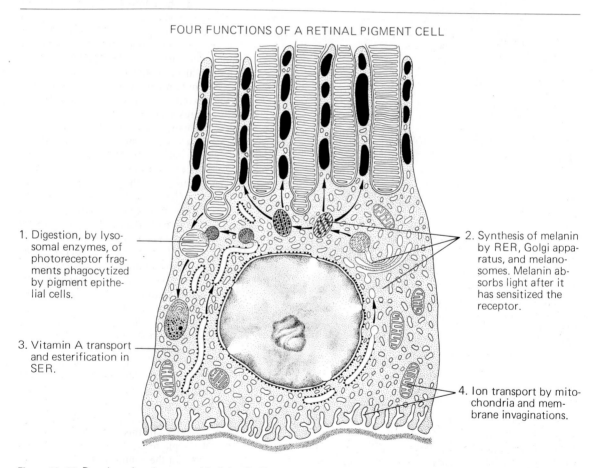

FOUR FUNCTIONS OF A RETINAL PIGMENT CELL

1. Digestion, by lysosomal enzymes, of photoreceptor fragments phagocytized by pigment epithelial cells.

2. Synthesis of melanin by RER, Golgi apparatus, and melanosomes. Melanin absorbs light after it has sensitized the receptor.

3. Vitamin A transport and esterification in SER.

4. Ion transport by mitochondria and membrane invaginations.

Figure 10–23. Drawing of a pigment epithelial cell. Observe that the apical portion has abundant cell processes that fill the spaces between the outer segments of the photosensitive cells. The membrane of the basal region has invaginations into the cytoplasm. This is a cell type with several functions. One of them is the synthesis of melanin granules (by a process described in Chapter 19) that absorb stray light in the eye chamber. This is depicted on the right side of the figure, which shows the organelles that participate in melanin synthesis. On the left side of the figure, lysosomes containing enzymes synthesized in the rough endoplasmic reticulum coalesce with the phagocytized apical parts of the photoreceptors, digesting them. Besides these activities, these cells are probably active in ion transport, since they maintain a potential between the 2 surfaces of the epithelial membrane. The relatively well developed smooth endoplasmic reticulum probably participates in the processes of vitamin A esterification. SER, smooth endoplasmic reticulum; RER, rough endoplasmic reticulum.

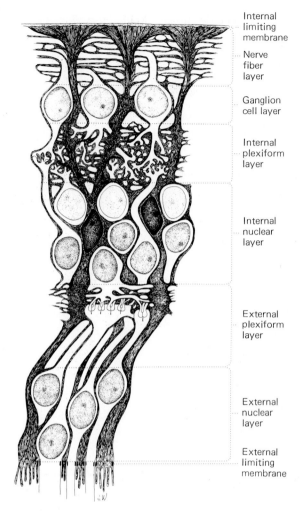

Internal limiting membrane

Nerve fiber layer

Ganglion cell layer

Internal plexiform layer

Internal nuclear layer

External plexiform layer

External nuclear layer

External limiting membrane

Figure 10–24. An illustration revealing the close association of Müller cells with neural elements in the sensory retina. Müller cells (dark fibrous cells) appear to be structurally and functionally equivalent to astrocytes of the central nervous system in that they envelop and support the neurons and nerve processes of the retina. (Reproduced, with permission, from Hogan MJ, Alvarado JA, Weddell JE: *Histology of the Human Eye.* Saunders, 1971.)

The visual pigment of rods, called **rhodopsin,** is composed of an aldehyde of vitamin A (called retinal) bound to specific proteins called opsins. Cones contain 3 (not yet completely identified) different pigments (iodopsins) in humans, thus providing a possible chemical basis for the classic tricolor theory of color vision. The rods are known to be very sensitive to light and are the receptors used for low levels of illumination. They have a low resolution and consequently form images without clear details. They are not sensitive to colors. On the other hand, cones have a higher threshold but are responsible for sharp images and color vision.

When light strikes rhodopsin molecules, retinal undergoes isomerization from the 11-*cis* form to the all-*trans* form. This change results in the dissociation of retinal from opsin, a reaction termed "bleaching." Bleaching of the visual pigment incorporated in the membrane disks increases the calcium conductance of the disk membranes and promotes a diffusion of calcium to the intracellular space of the outer segment of the photoreceptor. This calcium acts on the cell membrane, reducing its permeability to sodium ions and promoting cell hyperpolarization. The electrical signal produced by closing these sodium channels spreads to the inner segment and through gap junctions to neighboring cells.

In a second step, the visual pigment is reassembled and the calcium ions are transported back into the disks by an energy-consuming process. The energy requirement would seem to account for the abundance of mitochondria near the photosensitive site of rods and cones. Contrary to what happens in other receptors where action potentials are generated through cell depolarization, the rods and cones are hyperpolarized by light. This signal is transmitted to the bipolar amacrine and horizontal cells and then to the ganglion cells. Only the ganglion cells generate action potentials along their axons, which relay the information to the central nervous system.

The retina is a poorly vascularized structure containing few capillaries, which are found mainly in the ganglion and bipolar cell layers. In the photosensitive cell layer, capillaries are almost nonexistent. This poor vascularization accounts for the high glycolytic activity of this tissue. The clinical observation that the retina is damaged when it becomes detached suggests that the photosensitive cells derive their metabolites from the choriocapillary layer. The superficial localization of the vessels of the retina provides for their easy observation with an ophthalmoscope. This examination is of great value in the diagnosis and evaluation of disorders that affect blood vessels such as diabetes mellitus and hypertension.

At the posterior pole of the optical axis lies the **fovea,** a shallow depression in whose center the retina is very thin. This is because the bipolar and ganglion cells accumulate in the periphery of this depression, so that its center consists only of cone cells (Fig 10–11). Cone cells in the fovea are long and narrow and thus resemble rod cells in shape. This is an adaptation to permit closer packing of cones, thereby increasing visual acuity. In this area, blood vessels do not cross over the photosensitive cells. Light falls directly on the cones in the central part of the fovea, which helps account for the extremely precise visual acuity of this region.

Light not absorbed by the photoreceptors is absorbed by the pigment cells of the retinal pigment epithelium and the choroid.

The structure of the retina varies according to the region studied. The fovea has only cones, and the blind spot or papilla has no receptors (Fig 10–11). Other structural variations of physiologic significance are also observed in the retina. The number of ganglion cells per unit area is such an example. In the periphery of the retina, these cells are relatively few in number—hundreds of cells per square millimeter—which is in sharp contrast to the fovea, where the cells are counted in hundreds of thousands per square millimeter. Thus, vision at the peripheral part of the retina is much less sharp than at or near the fovea.

Although the retina has approximately 126 million receptors, not all the information gathered by receptors is relayed to the central nervous system. This is because the optic nerve does not have more than 1 million axons. Much of the information collected by the photoreceptors is selected and processed during its flow through the bipolar and ganglion cells. These cells integrate and code the information obtained, sending to the central nervous system a summary of the data.

ACCESSORY STRUCTURES OF THE EYE

Conjunctiva

The conjunctiva is a thin, transparent mucous membrane that covers the anterior portion of the eye up to the cornea and the internal surface of the eyelids. It has a stratified columnar epithelium with numerous goblet cells, and its lamina propria is composed of loose connective tissue (Fig 10–12).

Eyelids

Eyelids (Fig 10–25) are movable folds of tissue that serve to protect the eye. The skin of the lids is loose and elastic, permitting extreme swelling and subsequent return to normal shape and size. The **tarsal plates,** which lie within the eyelids and function as flexible supports, consist of dense fibrous and elastic tissue. They are covered posteriorly by conjunctiva and fuse medially and laterally to form the **medial and lateral palpebral tendons (ligaments),** which attach to the orbital bones. The **orbital septum** is the fascia lying posterior to the orbicularis oculi muscle and is the barrier between the lid and the orbit.

The **orbicularis oculi** muscle, supplied by the seventh cranial nerve, is roughly circular. Its function is to close the lids. The **levator palpebrae** muscle, supplied by the third cranial nerve, inserts into the tarsal plate and the skin and serves to elevate the lid. The superior tarsal muscle (of Müller), supplied by sympathetic nerves, originates in the levator muscle and inserts at the superior edge of the tarsus, coursing deep to the levator aponeurosis.

Three types of glands in the lid are the meibomian glands and the glands of Moll and Zeis. The meibomian glands are long sebaceous glands in the tarsal plate. They do not communicate with the hair follicles. There are about 25 in the upper lid and 20 in the lower lid, appearing as yellow vertical streaks deep to the conjunctiva. The meibomian glands produce a sebaceous substance that creates an oily layer on the surface of the tear film. This helps to prevent rapid evap-

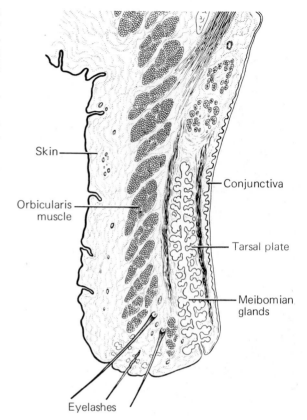

Figure 10–25. Diagram illustrating the structure of the eyelid.

oration of the normal tear layer. The glands of Zeis are smaller, modified sebaceous glands connected with the follicles of the eyelashes. The sweat glands of Moll are unbranched sinuous tubules that begin in a simple spiral and not in a glomerulus as do ordinary sweat glands. They empty their secretion into the follicles of the eyelashes.

The blood supply to the lids is derived mainly from ophthalmic and lacrimal arteries. The lymphatics drain into the preauricular, parotid, and submaxillary lymph glands.

Lacrimal Apparatus

The lacrimal apparatus (Figs 10–26 and 10–27) consists of the lacrimal gland, canaliculi, lacrimal sac, and nasolacrimal duct. The **lacrimal gland** is a tear-secreting gland located in the anterior superior temporal portion of the orbit. It consists of several separate glandular lobes with 6–12 excretory ducts that connect the gland to the superior conjunctival fornix. (Fornices are the conjunctiva-lined recesses between the lids and the eyeball.) It is a tubulo-alveolar gland that usually has distended lumens. It is composed of columnar-shaped cells of the serous type resembling the parotid acinar cells. They show lightly stained

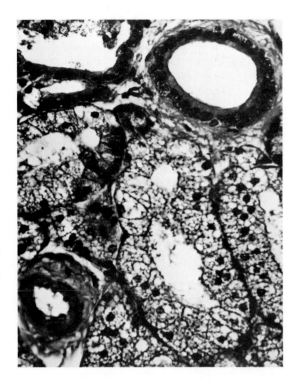

Figure 10–26. Photomicrograph of a section of a human lacrimal gland. A duct is shown in the upper right region. In the center is the secretory portion. H&E stain, × 350.

secretory granules, and a basal lamina separates them from the surrounding connective tissue. Well-developed myoepithelial cells surround the secretory portions of this gland. The secretion of the gland passes down over the cornea and the bulbar and palpebral conjunctiva, moistening the surfaces of these structures. They drain into the **lacrimal canaliculi** through the **lacrimal puncta,** round apertures about 0.5 mm in diameter on the medial aspect of both the upper and lower lid margins (Fig 10–27). The canaliculi are about 1 mm in diameter and 8 mm long. They join to form a common canaliculus just before opening into the lacrimal sac. The canaliculi are lined by a thick stratified squamous epithelium. Diverticuli of the common canaliculus may be part of the normal structure and are frequently susceptible to fungal infections. The **lacrimal sac** is the dilated portion of the lacrimal drainage system that lies in the bony lacrimal fossa. The **nasolacrimal duct** is the downward continuation of the lacrimal sac. It opens into the inferior meatus lateral to the inferior turbinate. Both the lacrimal sac and the nasolacrimal duct are lined with pseudostratified ciliated epithelium.

The tears pass into the puncta by capillary attraction. The combined forces of the capillary attraction in the canaliculi, gravity, and the pumping action of the orbicularis oculi muscle on the lacrimal sac cause the flow of tears down the nasolacrimal duct into the nose and nasopharynx. The lacrimal glands produce a fluid secretion rich in the enzyme lysozyme. The main functions of this fluid are to moisten the surface of the eye and to hydrolyze the cell walls of certain species of bacteria.

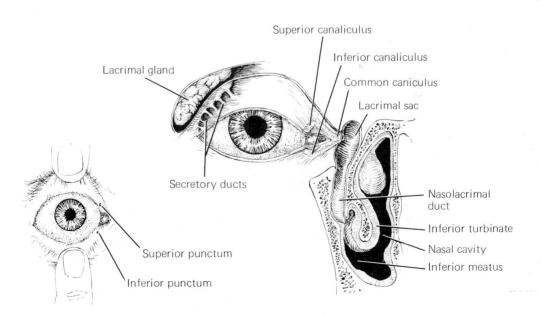

Figure 10–27. The lacrimal drainage system. (Redrawn with modifications and reproduced, with permission, from Thompson: Radiography of the nasolacrimal passageways. *Med Radiogr Photogr* 1949;25:66.)

THE EAR, OR VESTIBULOCOCHLEAR APPARATUS

The functions of the vestibulocochlear apparatus (Fig 10–28) are related to equilibrium and hearing. It consists of 3 parts: (1) the **external ear,** which receives the sound waves; (2) the **middle ear,** where these waves are transmitted from air to bone and by bone to the internal ear; and (3) the **internal ear,** where these vibrations are transduced to specific nerve impulses that pass via the acoustic nerve to the central nervous system. The internal ear also contains the vestibular organ, which functions to maintain equilibrium.

External Ear

The **auricle** (or **pinna**) consists of an irregularly shaped plate of elastic cartilage covered by tightly adherent skin on all sides.

The **external auditory meatus** is a somewhat flattened canal extending from the surface into the temporal bone. Its internal limit is the tympanic mem-

brane. A stratified squamous epithelium continuous with the skin lines the canal. Hair follicles, sebaceous glands, and a type of modified sweat gland—the **ceruminous glands**—are found in the submucosa. Ceruminous glands are coiled tubular glands that produce a brownish, semisolid mixture of fats and waxes—the cerumen (earwax). Hairs and cerumen probably have a protective function. The wall of the external auditory meatus is supported by elastic cartilage in its outer third, while the temporal bone provides support for the inner part of the canal.

Across the deep end of the external auditory meatus lies an oval membrane, the **tympanic membrane** (eardrum). Its external surface is covered by a thin layer of epidermis and, on its inner surface, by simple cuboidal epithelium continuous with the lining of the tympanic cavity (see below). Between the 2 epithelial coverings is a tough connective tissue layer composed of collagen and elastic fibers and fibroblasts. The anterior upper quadrant of the tympanic membrane is flaccid and more transparent, since the connective tissue layer is much thinner here. This region is known

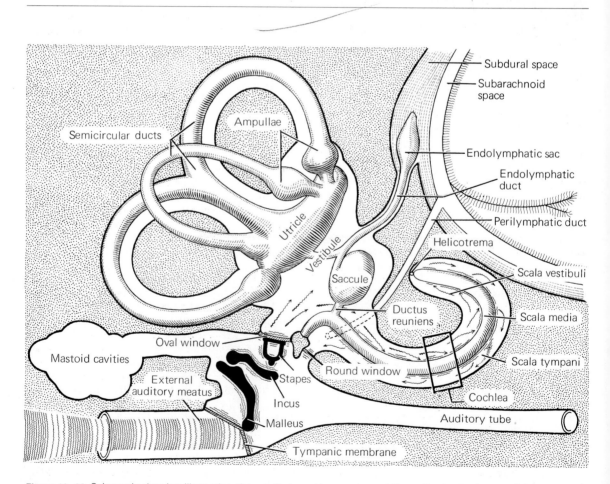

Figure 10–28. Schematic drawing illustrating the vestibulocochlear organ and the path of sound waves in the external, middle, and internal ear. (Redrawn and reproduced, with permission, from Best CH, Taylor NB: *The Physiological Basis of Medical Practice,* 8th ed. Williams & Wilkins, 1966.)

as **Schrapnell's membrane.** The tympanic membrane is the structure that transmits sound vibrations to the ossicles of the middle ear (Fig 10–28).

Middle Ear

The middle ear, or tympanic cavity, in the interior of the temporal bone, is an irregular space that lies between the tympanic membrane and the bony surface of the internal ear. It communicates anteriorly with the pharynx by the **auditory tube (eustachian tube)** and posteriorly with the air-filled cavities of the mastoid process of the temporal bone. The middle ear is lined by simple squamous epithelium resting on the thin lamina propria strongly adherent to the subjacent periosteum. Near the auditory tube and in its interior, the simple epithelium that lines the middle ear is gradually transformed into pseudostratified columnar ciliated epithelium. The walls of the tube are usually collapsed, but the tube opens during the process of swallowing, thus balancing the pressure of the air in the middle ear with atmospheric pressure. In the medial bony wall of the middle ear are 2 oblong regions devoid of bone and covered by membranes; these are the **oval** and **round windows** (Fig 10–28), which will be described later.

The tympanic membrane is connected to the oval window by a series of 3 small bones—the **auditory ossicles: malleus, incus,** and **stapes** (Fig 10–28)— that transmit the mechanical vibrations generated in the tympanic membrane to the inner ear. The malleus inserts itself in the tympanic membrane and the stapes in the membrane of the oval window. These bones are articulated by synovial joints, and like all structures of this cavity they are covered by simple squamous epithelium. In the middle ear, 2 small muscles are present that insert themselves in the malleus and stapes. They have a function in sound conduction, as will be seen later.

Internal Ear

The internal ear is composed of 2 **labyrinths** (see Table 10–1 for a summary of the terminology). The **bony labyrinth** consists of a series of spaces within the petrous portion of the temporal bone that house the **membranous labyrinth** (Fig 10–28). The membranous labyrinth is a continuous, epithelium-lined series of cavities of ectodermal origin. It derives from the auditory vesicle developed from the ectoderm of the lateral part of the embryo's head. During embryonic development, this vesicle invaginates into the subjacent connective tissue, loses contact with the cephalic ectoderm, and moves deeply into the rudiments of the future temporal bone. During this process, it undergoes a complex series of changes in form, giving rise to 2 specialized regions of the membranous labyrinth: the **utricle** and the **saccule.** From the utricle, **semicircular ducts** take their origin, while from the saccule, the elaborate **cochlear duct** is formed. In each of these areas, the epithelial lining becomes specialized to form sensory structures such as the **maculae** of the utricle and saccule, the **cristae** of the

Table 10–1. Terminology applied to the 2 labyrinths of the internal ear.

Bony Labyrinth	Membranous Labyrinth
Vestibule	Saccule
	Utricle
Semicircular canals	Semicircular ducts
Cochlea	Cochlear duct (scala media)

semicircular ducts, and the **organ of Corti** of the cochlear duct.

The **bony labyrinth** consists of spaces in the temporal bone. There is a central irregular cavity, the **vestibule,** housing the saccule and the utricle. Posteriorly, 3 **semicircular canals** enclose the semicircular ducts, while the anterolaterally directed **cochlea** contains the cochlear duct (Fig 10–28).

The cochlea is about 35 mm in total length and consists of 2.5 turns around a bony core known as the **modiolus.** The modiolus has spaces within it containing blood vessels and the cell bodies and processes of the acoustic branch of the eighth cranial nerve (spiral ganglion) (Fig 10–33). Extending laterally from the modiolus is a thin bony ridge, the **osseous spiral lamina.** This structure extends farther across the cochlea in the basal turns than it does at the apex (Fig 10–32).

The bony walls of the vestibule and semicircular canals are lined by several layers of flattened connective tissue cells that form a mesothelium. From this layer, thin trabeculae, consisting of fine fibrils and fibroblasts, extend to the outer walls of the utricle, saccule, and semicircular ducts and serve to support these parts of the membranous labyrinth. Blood vessels are also found in this connective tissue.

The bony labyrinth is filled with **perilymph,** which is similar in ionic composition to extracellular fluids elsewhere but has a very low protein content. The membranous labyrinth contains **endolymph,** which is characterized by its low-sodium and high-potassium content. The protein concentration in endolymph is low.

Histology of the Membranous Labyrinth

A. Saccule and Utricle: These structures are composed of a thin sheath of connective tissue lined by simple squamous epithelium. The membranous labyrinth is bound to the periosteum of the osseous labyrinth by thin strands of connective tissue that also contain blood vessels supplying the epithelia of the membranous labyrinth. In the wall of the saccule and utricle, one can observe small regions, called **maculae,** of differentiated neuroepithelial cells innervated by branches of the vestibular nerve (Fig 10–29). The macula of the saccule lies in its floor, whereas that of the utricle occupies the lateral wall. The maculae are thus oriented perpendicularly to one another. Maculae in both locations have basically the same histologic structure. They consist of a thickening of the wall and possess 2 types of receptor cells, some sup-

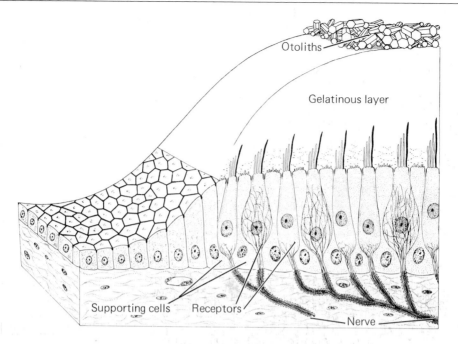

Figure 10–29. The structure of maculae.

porting cells, and the afferent and efferent nerve endings.

Receptor cells (**hair cells**) are characterized by the presence of 40–80 long, rigid stereocilia, which are actually highly specialized microvilli (Fig 10–29). They are arranged in rows of increasing length, with the longest being about 100 μm in length and located adjacent to a cilium. The cilium has a basal body and the usual 9 + 2 arrangement of microtubules in its proximal portion, but the central 2 microtubules soon disappear. This cilium is usually called a kinocilium, but it probably is immotile. Hair cells have a dense terminal web, numerous mitochondria, a well-developed Golgi complex, and an abundance of smooth endoplasmic reticulum. The 2 types of hair cells are distinguished by the form of their afferent innervation. Type I cells have a large, cup-shaped ending surrounding most of the base of the cell, while type II receptors have many small afferent endings. Both types have efferent nerve endings, which are probably inhibitory.

The supporting cells disposed between the receptors are columnar in shape with their nucleus at the base of the cell and microvilli on their apical surface (Fig 10–29). Covering this neuroepithelium is a thick, gelatinous glycoprotein layer, probably secreted by the supporting cells, with surface deposits of crystals composed mainly of calcium carbonate and called **otoliths (otoconia)** (Figs 10–29 and 10–30).

B. Semicircular Ducts: These structures have the same general form as the corresponding parts of the bony labyrinth. The receptor areas, present in their **ampullae** (Fig 10–28), have an elongated ridgelike

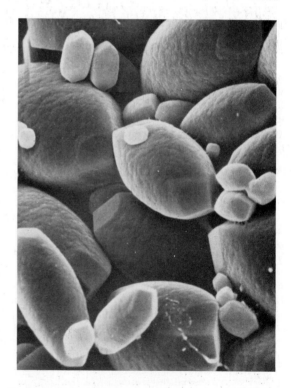

Figure 10–30. Scanning electron micrograph of the surface of a pigeon's macula showing the otoliths. (Courtesy of DJ Lim.)

form and are called **cristae ampullares.** The ridge is oriented perpendicularly to the long axis of the duct. Cristae are structurally similar to maculae, but their glycoprotein layer is thicker, has a conical form called a **cupula,** and is not covered by otoliths. The cupula extends across the ampullae, establishing contact with its opposite wall (Fig 10–31).

C. Endolymphatic Duct and Sac: The endolymphatic duct initially has a simple squamous epithelial lining. As it nears the endolymphatic sac, it gradually changes to tall columnar epithelium composed of 2 cell types, one of which has microvilli on its apical surface and abundant pinocytotic vesicles and vacuoles. It has been suggested that these cells are responsible for the resorption of endolymph and the endocytosis of foreign material and cellular remnants which may be present in endolymph.

D. Cochlear Duct: This structure, a diverticulum of the saccule, is highly specialized as a sound receptor. It is about 35 mm long and is surrounded by specialized perilymphatic spaces. When observed in histologic sections, the cochlea (bony labyrinth) appears to be divided into 3 spaces: the **scala vestibuli** above the cochlear duct (**scala media**) and the **scala tympani** below (Fig 10–32). The cochlear duct ends blindly at the apex of the cochlea and contains endolymph. The other 2 scalae contain perilymph and are in reality one long tube beginning at the **oval window** and terminating at the **round window** (Fig 10–28). They are in communication at the apex of the cochlea via an opening known as the **helicotrema.**

The cochlear duct has the following histologic structure (Fig 10–32). The **vestibular (Reissner's) membrane** consists of 2 layers of squamous epithelium, one derived from the cochlear duct and the other from the lining of the scala vestibuli. Cells of both layers are joined by extensive tight junctions that help preserve the very high ionic gradients across this membrane. The **stria vascularis** is an unusual vascularized epithelium located in the lateral wall of the cochlear duct. It consists of 3 types of cells: marginal, intermediate, and basal. Marginal cells have many deep infoldings of their basal plasma membranes, and numerous mitochondria are found here. These characteristics indicate that marginal cells are ion- and water-transporting cells, and it is generally believed that these cells are responsible for the characteristic ionic composition of endolymph.

The **organ of Corti** contains hair cells that can respond to different sound frequencies. It rests on a thick layer of amorphous ground substance containing fibrils related to keratin—the **basilar membrane**—formed by cells of the organ of Corti as well as mesothelial cells lining the scala tympani. It should be noted that the basilar membrane is about 100 μm wide in the basal turn of the cochlea and 500 μm wide in the apical turn. Supporting and hair (receptor) cells of the organ of Corti rest on the basilar membrane. Many different types of supporting cells and 2 types of hair cells can be distinguished. Three to 5 rows of **outer hair cells** can be seen, depending on the distance from

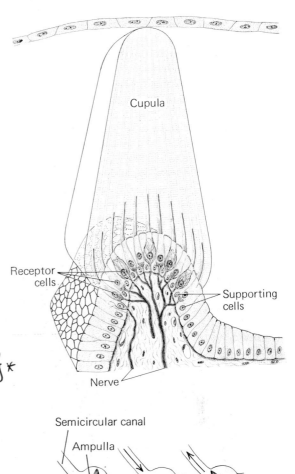

Cupula

Receptor
cells

Supporting
cells

Nerve

Semicircular canal

Ampulla

Rest   Acceleration

Figure 10–31. *Top:* Schematic drawing of the structure of the crista ampullaris. *Bottom:* Movements of the cupula in an ampullary crista during rotational acceleration. Arrows indicate direction of fluid movement. (Redrawn and reproduced, with permission, from Wersäll J: Studies on the structure and innervation of the sensory epithelium of the cristae ampullares in the guinea pig. *Acta Otolaryngol [Stockh] Suppl* 1956;**126:**1.)

the base of the organ, and a single row of **inner hair cells** is present. Both types of hair cells are columnar with basally located nuclei, numerous mitochondria, and distinctive cisternae of smooth endoplasmic reticulum aligned beneath the lateral plasma membranes. The most characteristic feature of these cells is the W-shaped (outer hair cells) or linear (inner hair cells) array of stereocilia (Fig 10–33). The stereocilia increase in height from one side of the array to the other. A basal body is found in the cytoplasm adjacent to the tallest stereocilia. In contrast to vestibular receptors, no kinocilium is present. This imparts a symmetry to the hair cell that is important in sensory transduction. In addition, the apical cytoplasm contains numerous fine filaments that impart stiffness to this part of the cell, a region termed the **reticular lamina.**

The tips of the tallest stereocilia of the inner hair cells are embedded in the **tectorial membrane,** a glycoprotein-rich secretion of certain cells of the spiral limbus (Fig 10–32).

Of the supporting cells, the **pillar cells** should be singled out for special mention. Pillar cells contain a large number of microtubules that seem to impart stiffness to these cells. They outline a triangular space between outer and inner hair cells—the **inner tunnel**

(Fig 10–32). This structure is of importance in sound transduction, as discussed below.

Both outer and inner hair cells have afferent and efferent nerve endings, although the inner hair cells have by far the greater afferent innervation. The functional significance of this difference is not understood. The cell bodies of the bipolar afferent neurons of the organ of Corti are located in the modiolus and constitute the spiral ganglion (Fig 10–32).

Histophysiology of the Inner Ear

A. Vestibular Functions: Increase or decrease in the velocity of circular movement—angular acceleration or deceleration—causes a flow of fluid in the semicircular ducts as a consequence of the inertia of the endolymph. This induces a corresponding move-

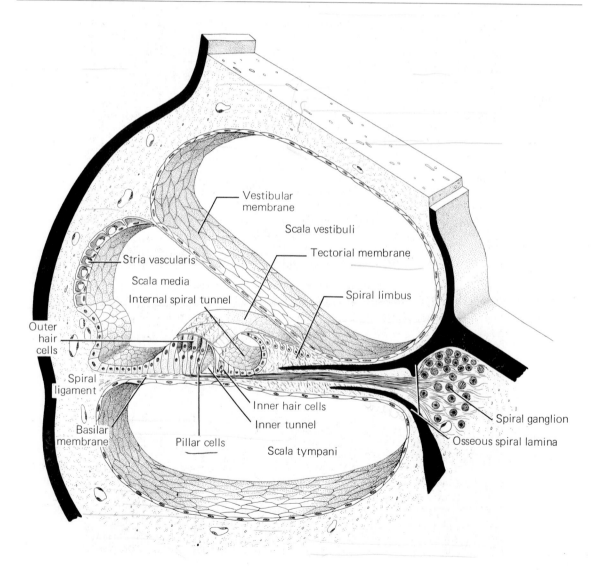

Figure 10–32. The structure of the cochlea. (Redrawn and reproduced, with permission, from Bloom W, Fawcett DW: *A Textbook of Histology,* 9th ed. Saunders, 1968.)

ment of the cupula that covers the crista ampullaris and results in bending of the stereocilia on the sensory cells. Measurement of electrical impulses along vestibular nerve fibers indicates that movement of the cupula in the direction of the kinocilium results in excitation of the receptors, accompanied by action potentials in the vestibular nerve fibers. Movement in the opposite direction inhibits neuronal activity.

When uniform movement returns, acceleration ceases, the cupula returns to its normal position, and excitation or inhibition of the receptors no longer occurs (Fig 10–31). The mechanism of transformation of mechanical into electrical energy is still unknown.

The semicircular ducts respond to fluid displacement and therefore body position following angular accelerations. The maculae of the saccules and the

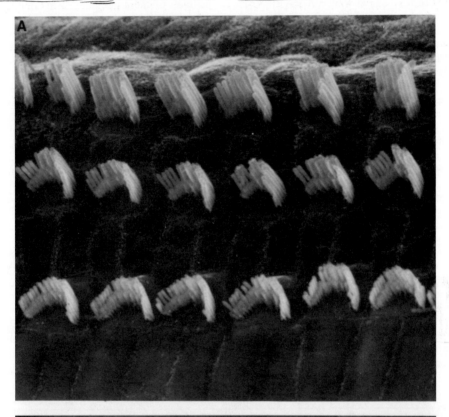

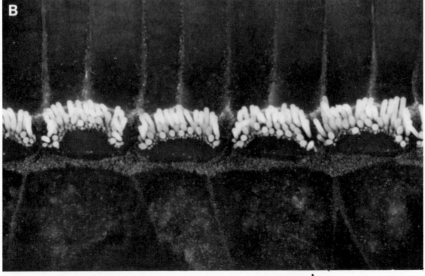

Figure 10–33. Scanning electron micrograph of the 3 rows of outer hair cells *(A)* and the single row of inner hair cells *(B)* in the middle turn of the cat cochlear duct. × 2700. (Courtesy of P Leake.)

utricles respond to *linear* accelerations. By virtue of their greater density, the otoliths are displaced when there is a change in the position of the head. This displacement is transferred to the underlying hair cells via the gelatinous otolithic membrane. Deformation of stereocilia of the hair cells results in action potentials that are carried to the central nervous system by the vestibular branch of the eighth cranial nerve. Maculae are thus sensitive to the force of gravity on the otoliths. The vestibular apparatus is important for the perception of movement and orientation in space and for the maintenance of equilibrium or balance.

B. Auditory Functions: Sound waves impinging on the tympanic membrane set the auditory ossicles into motion. The large difference in area of the tympanic membrane as compared to the footplate of the stapes ensures efficient transmission of mechanical motion from air to the fluids of the inner ear. Two striated skeletal muscles are found in the middle ear—the **tensor tympani** muscle (attached to the malleus) and the **stapedius** muscle (attached to the stapes). Loud sounds result in reflex contractions of these muscles, which limit excursions of the tympanic membrane and the stapes; this helps prevent damage to the inner ear. These reflexes are too slow to guard against sudden loud sounds, such as gunshots.

The following is a step-by-step explanation of how sound waves are converted to electrical impulses in the inner ear (Fig 10–28). Sound waves are longitudinal waves having compression and rarefaction phases. The compression phase causes the stapes to move inward. Since the fluids of the inner ear are almost incompressible, a pressure change is transmitted across the vestibular membrane and the basilar membrane, causing them to be deflected downward toward the scala tympani. This pressure change also causes the covering of the round window to bulge outward, thereby relieving the pressure change. Because the tips of the pillar cells form a pivot, downward deflection of the basilar membrane is converted into lateral shearing of stereocilia of hair cells against the tectorial membrane. The tips of stereocilia are deflected toward the modiolus and away from the position of the basal body. This deflection may hyperpolarize the cells, or it may have no effect. During the rarefaction phase of the sound wave, everything is reversed—the stapes moves outward, the basilar membrane moves upward toward the scala vestibuli, and stereocilia of hair cells are bent toward the stria vascularis and toward the position of the basal body. Deflection in this direction sets up depolarizing generator potentials in the hair cells that result in release of a neurotransmitter (chemical nature unknown) which causes the production of action potentials in bipolar neurons of the spiral ganglion (excitation). The key to frequency discrimination is the fact that the basilar membrane responds with maximal displacement at different places along its length, depending on the frequency of the sound. High frequencies are detected at the basal end of the membrane, while low frequencies result in maximal movement of the basilar membrane in the apex of the organ of Corti. This **tonotopic** localization can be correlated with the width and stiffness of the basilar membrane—the narrow basilar membrane, with greater stiffness at the base, responds best to high-frequency sounds. Maximal displacement of the basilar membrane at the threshold of hearing is very small; 0.1 nm is a commonly quoted figure for a 3000-Hz tone.

REFERENCES

Cutaneous & Other Sensory Mechanisms

Barker D: The morphology of muscle receptors. In: *Handbook of Sensory Physiology*. Vol III/2. Hunt C (editor). Springer-Verlag, 1974.

Beidler LM (editor): Olfaction. In: *Handbook of Sensory Physiology*. Vol 4. Springer, 1971.

Beidler LM (editor): Taste. In: *Handbook of Sensory Physiology*. Vol 4. Springer, 1971.

Chouchkov CV: Cutaneous receptors. In: *Advances in Anatomy, Embryology and Cell Biology*. Vol 54. Springer-Verlag, 1978.

Graziadei PPC: The olfactory mucosa of vertebrates. In: *Handbook of Sensory Physiology*. Vol IV/1. Beidler LM (editor). Springer-Verlag, 1971.

Iggo A, Andres KH: Morphology of cutaneous receptors. *Annu Rev Neurosci* 1982;**5**:1.

Keverne EB: Chemical senses: Smell. In: *The Senses*. Barlow HB, Mollon JD (editors). Cambridge Univ Press, 1982.

Loo SK: Fine structure of the olfactory epithelium in some primates. *J Anat* 1977;**123**:135.

Lowenstein WR (editor): Principles of receptor physiology. In: *Handbook of Sensory Physiology*. Vol 1. Springer, 1971.

Moulton DG: Dynamics of cell populations in the olfactory epithelium. *Trans NY Acad Sci* 1974;**237**:52.

Moulton DG: The olfactory pigment. In: *Handbook of Sensory Physiology*. Vol IV/1. Beidler LM (editor). Springer-Verlag, 1971.

Murray RG: The ultrastructure of taste buds. In: *The Ultrastructure of Sense Organs*. Friedman J (editor). North Holland Publishing Co, 1973.

Schmidt RF (editor): *Fundamentals of Sensory Physiology*. Springer-Verlag, 1978.

Zotterman Y (editor): *Sensory Function of the Skin in Primates*. Pergamon Press, 1976.

The Eye

Bok D, Hall MO: The role of the retinal pigment epithelium in the etiology of inherited retinal dystrophy in the rat. *J Cell Biol* 1971;**49**:664.

Botelho SY: Tears and the lacrimal gland. *Sci Am* (Oct) 1964;**211**:78.

Dowling JE: Organization of vertebrate retinas. *Invest Ophthalmol* 1970;**9**:665.

Duke-Elder S, Wybar KC: *System of Ophthalmology: The Anatomy of the Visual System*. Mosby, 1961.

Farnsworth PN et al: Ultrastructure of rat eye lens fibers. *Invest Ophthalmol* 1974;**13**:274.

Hogan MJ et al: *Histology of the Human Eye*. Saunders, 1971.

McDevitt D (editor): *Cell Biology of the Eye*. Academic Press, 1982.

Miller WH (editor): *Molecular Mechanisms of Photoreceptor Transduction*. Academic Press, 1981.

Orzalesi N, Riva A, Testa F: Fine structure of the human lacrimal gland. *J Submicrosc Cytol* 1971;**3**:283.

Schwartz EA: First events in vision: The generation of responses in vertebrate rods. *J Cell Biol* 1982;**90**:271.

Stell WK: The morphological organization of the vertebrate retina. In: *Physiology of Photoreceptor Organs*. Vol 7. Fuortes MGF (editor). Springer, 1972.

Streeten BW et al: Immunohistochemical comparison of ocular zonules and the microfibrils of elastic tissue. *Invest Ophthalmol Vis Sci* 1981;**21**:130.

Young RW: Visual cells and the concept of renewal. *Invest Ophthalmol* 1976;**15**:700.

The Ear

Anson BJ, Donaldson JA: *Surgical Anatomy of the Temporal Bone and Ear*. Saunders, 1973.

Hinojosa R, Rodriguez-Echandia EL: The fine structure of the stria vascularis of the cat inner ear. *Am J Anat* 1966;**118**:631.

Hudspeth AJ: The hair cells of the inner ear. *Sci Am* (Jan) 1983;**248**:54.

Kimura RS: The ultrastructure of the organ of Corti. *Int Rev Cytol* 1975;**42**:173.

Lim DJ: Cochlear anatomy related to cochlear micromechanics: A review. *J Acoust Soc Am* 1980;**67**:1686.

Rosenhall U, Engström B: Surface structures of the human vestibular sensory regions. *Acta Otolaryngol (Stockh)* 1974;**319**:3.

Soudijn ER: Scanning electron microscopy of the organ of Corti. *Ann Otol Rhinol Laryngol* 1976;**86**:16.

Steel KP: The tectorial membrane of mammals. *Hear Res* 1983;**9**:327.

Wersäll J, Flock A, Lundquist P-G: Structural basis for directional sensitivity in cochlear and vestibular sensory receptors. In: *Sensory Receptors. Cold Spring Harbor Symp Quant Biol* 1965;**30**.

Muscle tissue is responsible for most types of body movement. It consists of groups of elongated muscle cells, each of which contains great numbers of contractile cytoplasmic filaments. Most muscle cells are of mesodermal origin, and their differentiation occurs mainly by a gradual process of lengthening, with simultaneous synthesis of myofibrillar proteins.

Three types of muscle tissue may be distinguished in mammals on the basis of morphologic and functional characteristics (Fig 11–1). **Smooth muscle** consists of collections of fusiform cells which, in the light microscope, do not show striations. Their contraction process is slow and not subject to voluntary control. **Skeletal muscle** is composed of bundles of very long cylindric multinucleated cells that show cross-striations. Their contraction is quick, forceful, and usually under voluntary control. **Cardiac muscle** also has cross-striations and is composed of elongated or branched individual cells that lie parallel to each other. At sites of end-to-end contact are the **intercalated disks,** structures found only in cardiac mus-

cle. Cardiac muscle contraction is involuntary, vigorous, and rhythmic.

We shall see in this chapter that each type of muscle tissue has a structure adapted to its physiologic role.

Some muscle cell organelles have names different from their counterparts in other cells. Thus, the cytoplasm of muscle cells (excluding the myofibrils) is called **sarcoplasm,** and the smooth endoplasmic reticulum is called **sarcoplasmic reticulum**. The **sarcolemma** is the cell membrane or plasmalemma. Muscle cells are surrounded by a distinct collagenous basal lamina and a fine net of reticular fibers. In current usage, the sarcolemma is often called simply the **cell membrane,** or **plasmalemma.**

SKELETAL MUSCLE

Skeletal muscle consists of bundles of very long (up to 30 cm) cylindric multinucleated cells with a

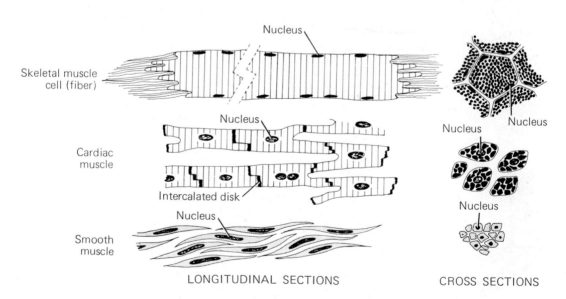

Figure 11–1. Diagram of the structure of the 3 muscle types. *Above:* Skeletal muscle. *Center:* Cardiac muscle. *Below:* Smooth muscle. The drawings at right show these muscles in cross section. Skeletal muscle is composed of large, elongated, multinucleated units (fibers). Cardiac muscle is composed of irregular branched cells bound together longitudinally by intercalated disks. Smooth muscle is an agglomerate of fusiform cells. The packing between cells may be more or less dense depending on the amount of extracellular connective tissue.

diameter of 10–100 μm called **muscle fibers.** Multinucleation results from the fusion of embryonic mononucleated myoblasts (muscle stem cells). The oval nuclei are usually found at the periphery of the cell under the cell membrane. This characteristic nuclear location is helpful in distinguishing skeletal muscle from cardiac and smooth muscle, which have centrally located nuclei.

Organization of Skeletal Muscle as an Organ

The masses of fibers that make up the different types of muscle are not grouped in random fashion but are arranged in regular bundles surrounded by an external sheath of dense connective tissue surrounding the entire muscle called the **epimysium** (Fig 11–2). From the epimysium, thin septa of connective tissue extend inward, surrounding bundles of fibers within a muscle. The connective tissue around each bundle of muscle fibers is called **perimysium.** Each bundle of perimysium-bound fibers is known as a **fascicle.** Each muscle fiber is surrounded by a delicate layer of connective tissue composed mainly of a basal lamina and reticular fibers, the **endomysium** (Figs 11–2 and 11–13). The epimysium, perimysium, and endomysium are all true connective tissue structures, complete with collagen, elastic fibers, fibroblasts, and blood vessels.

The connective tissue not only binds the muscle fibers together and permits some freedom of movement among them but also binds muscle tissue to the structures (tendon, periosteum, skin, aponeurosis, etc) with which it comes in contact.

One of the most important roles of connective

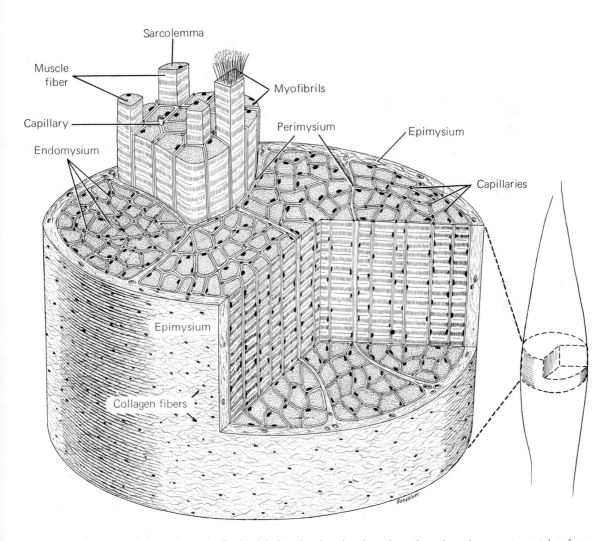

Figure 11–2. Structure of skeletal muscle. To the right is a drawing showing where the enlarged segment was taken from a muscle.

tissue is that of mechanical transmission of the forces generated by contracting muscle cells. In most instances, individual muscle cells do not extend from one end of a muscle to the other. The force of contraction generated by these cells is therefore transmitted by the ensheathing connective tissue.

Blood vessels penetrate the muscle within the connective tissue septa and form a rich capillary network that runs between and parallel to the muscle fibers. The capillaries are of the continuous type. Lymphatics are found in the connective tissue.

Some muscles taper off at their extremities, where a myotendinous junction is formed. Analysis of this transitional region with the aid of the electron microscope reveals that collagen fibers of the tendon insert themselves into complex infoldings of the plasmalemma of the muscle fibers present at this zone. Normally, each individual muscle fiber has on its surface a motor nerve ending, the so-called **motor end-plate,** whose structure is shown in Fig 11–12 and will be described in detail later in this chapter.

Organization of Skeletal Muscle Fibers

As observed with the light microscope, longitudinally sectioned muscle cells or muscle fibers, when stained with hematoxylin and eosin, show cross-striations composed of alternating light and dark bands (Fig 11–3). The darker bands are called **A bands** (**anisotropic**, ie, birefringent in polarized light) (Fig 11–4); the lighter bands are called **I bands** (**isotropic**, ie, does not alter polarized light). Each I band is bisected by a dark tranverse line, the **Z line.** The smallest repetitive subunit of the contractile apparatus, the **sarcomere**, extends from Z line to Z line (Figs 11–4 and 11–5) and is about 2.5 μm long in resting muscle.

The sarcoplasm of each muscle fiber is filled with long cylindric filamentous bundles called **myofibrils.** The myofibrils, which have a diameter of 1–2 μm and run parallel to the long axis of the muscle fiber, are composed of an end-to-end chainlike arrangement of sarcomeres (Figs 11–5 and 11–6). As a consequence of the lateral registration of sarcomeres in

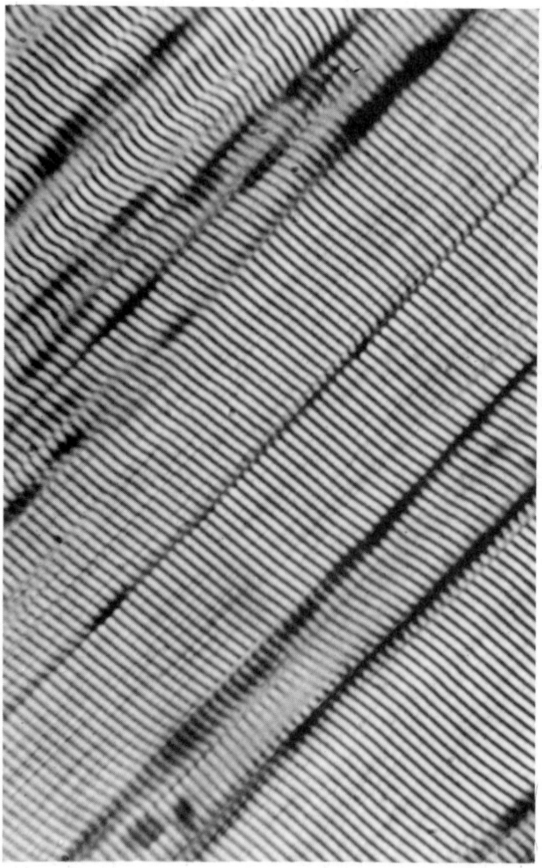

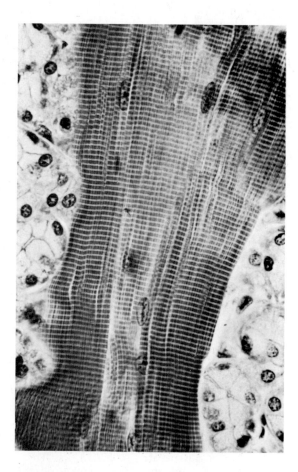

Figure 11–3. Photomicrograph of a section of the tongue of a rat, showing the transverse (cross) striations of the skeletal muscle fibers cut longitudinally. × 700.

Figure 11–4. Photomicrograph of a section of skeletal muscle observed with the polarizing microscope. The A bands appear as bright birefringent stripes. This is due to the highly ordered myosin molecules of thick filaments. The I bands are dark. × 700.

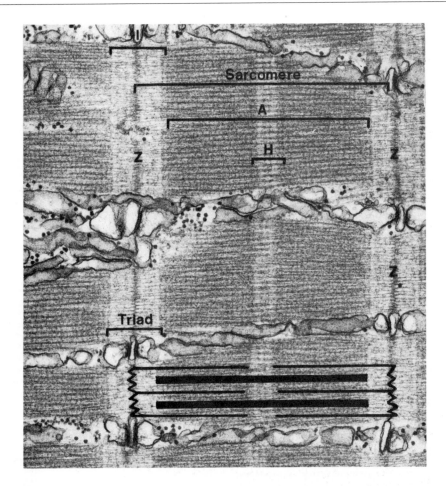

Figure 11–5. Electron micrograph of skeletal muscle of a tadpole. Observe the sarcomere, with its A, I, and H bands and Z line. The position of the thick and thin filaments in the sarcomere is shown schematically in the lower part. As illustrated above, triads in amphibian muscle are aligned with the Z line in each sarcomere. However, in mammalian muscle, each sarcomere exhibits 2 triads, one at each A–I band interface (see Fig 11–11). × 35,700. (Courtesy of KR Porter.)

adjacent myofibrils, the entire muscle fiber exhibits a characteristic pattern of transverse striations.

Electron microscopic studies reveal that the sarcomere pattern described above is due mainly to the presence of 2 types of filaments—thick and thin filaments—disposed parallel to the long axis of the myofibrils in a symmetric pattern.

The thick filaments are 1.6 μm long and 15 nm thick; they occupy the A band, the central portion of the sarcomere. The thin filaments run between and parallel to the thick filaments and have one end attached to the Z line (Figs 11–5 and 11–6). Thin filaments are 1.0 μm long and 8 nm wide. As a result of this arrangement, the I bands consist of the portions of the thin filaments that are not overlapping the thick filaments. The A bands are mainly composed of thick filaments in addition to portions of overlapping thin filaments. Closer observation of the A band shows the presence of a lighter zone in its center, the **H band** (Figs 11–5 and 11–6). The H band is that portion of

the A band that consists of only thick filaments. Bisecting the H band is the **M line,** a region where lateral connections are made between adjacent thick filaments (Fig 11–6[8]). The major protein of the M line is creatine kinase. Phosphocreatine is a storage form of high-energy phosphate groups. Creatine kinase catalyzes the transfer of a phosphate group from phosphocreatine to ADP, thus maintaining the supply of ATP necessary for muscle contraction.

Thin and thick filaments overlap for some distance within the A band. As a consequence, a cross section in the region of filament overlap shows each thick filament surrounded by 6 thin filaments in the form of a hexagon (Figs 11–6[9] and 11–7).

Striated muscle filaments contain at least 4 main proteins: actin, tropomyosin, troponin, and myosin. Thin filaments are composed of the first 3 proteins, while thick filaments consist primarily of myosin. Myosin and actin together represent 55% of the total protein of striated muscle.

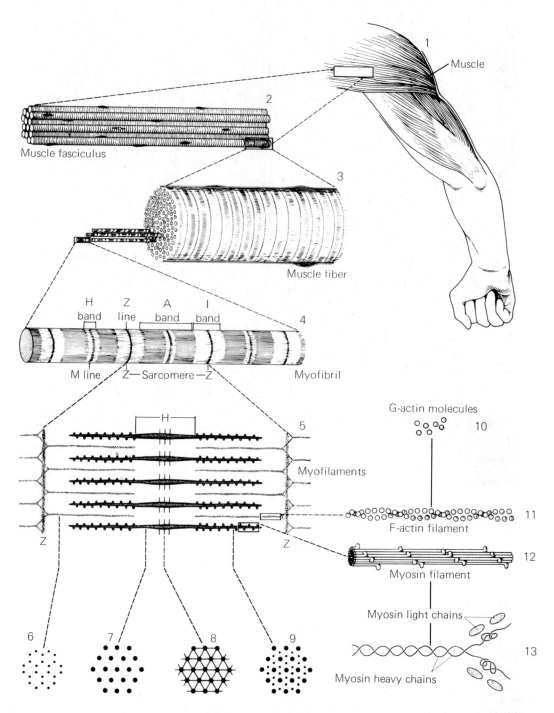

Figure 11–6. Diagram illustrating the structure and position of the thick and thin filaments in the sarcomere. The molecular structure of these components is shown at right. (Drawing by Sylvia Colard Keene. Reproduced, with permission, from Bloom W, Fawcett DW: *A Textbook of Histology,* 9th ed. Saunders, 1968.)

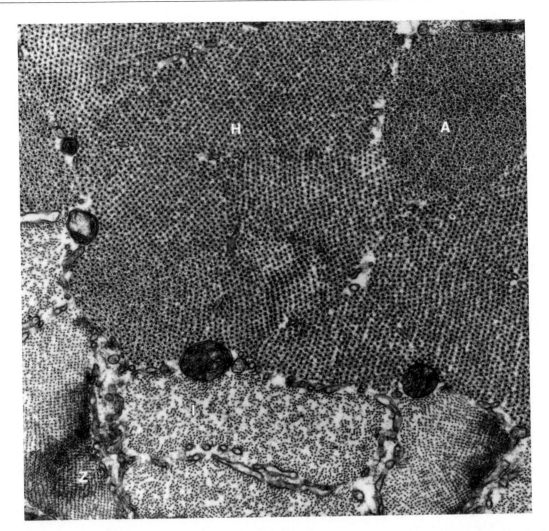

Figure 11–7. Oblique section of skeletal muscle myofibrils illustrating some of the features diagrammed in Fig 11–6. Z, Z line; I, I band (compare with Fig 11–6[6]); A, A band (compare with Fig 11–6[9]); H, H band (compare with Fig 11–6[7]). × 36,000.

Actin is present as long filamentous (F-actin) polymers consisting of 2 strands of globular (G-actin) monomers (MW 42,000), 5.6 nm in diameter, twisted around each other in a double helical formation (Fig 11–6[10, 11]). A notable characteristic of all G-actin molecules is their structural asymmetry. When G-actin molecules polymerize to form F-actin, they bind back to front, producing a filament with distinguishable polarity (Fig 11–8). Each G-actin monomer contains a binding site for myosin (Fig 11–9). Actin filaments, which anchor perpendicularly on the Z line, exhibit opposite polarity on each side of the Z line (Fig 11–6). The protein α actinin, a major component of the Z line, is thought to anchor the actin filaments to this region. α Actinin and desmin (an intermediate filament protein) are believed to tie adjacent sarcomeres together, thus keeping myofibrils in register.

Tropomyosin is a long, thin molecule about 40 nm in length containing 2 polypeptide chains (MW 35,000 each) in the form of an alpha helix. These polypeptide chains are coiled one around the other. Tropomyosin molecules are bound head to tail, forming filaments that run over the actin subunits alongside the outer edges of the groove between the 2 twisted actin strands (Fig 11–8).

Troponin is a complex of 3 subunits: **TnT,** which strongly attaches to tropomyosin; **TnC,** which binds calcium ions; and **TnI,** which inhibits the actin-myosin interaction. A troponin complex is attached at one specific site on each tropomyosin molecule (Fig 11–8).

In thin filaments, each tropomyosin molecule spans 7 G-actin molecules and has one troponin complex bound to its surface (Fig 11–8).

Myosin is a much larger complex (MW ~

THE DISASSEMBLED COMPONENTS OF THE THIN FILAMENT

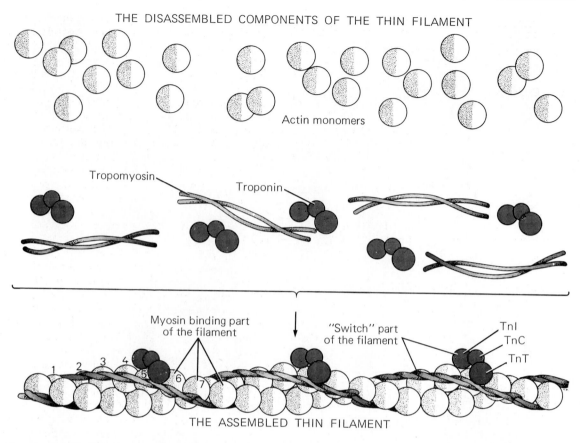

Actin monomers

Tropomyosin

Troponin

Myosin binding part of the filament

"Switch" part of the filament

TnI
TnC
TnT

THE ASSEMBLED THIN FILAMENT

Figure 11–8. Schematic representation of the thin filament, showing the spatial configuration of the 3 major protein components—actin, tropomyosin, and troponin. The individual components in the top half of the drawing are shown in polymerized form in the bottom half. The globular actin molecules are polarized (dark and light areas) and polymerize in one direction. Observe that each tropomyosin molecule extends over 7 actin molecules. TnI, TnC, TnT, see text.

500,000). Myosin can be dissociated into 2 identical heavy chains (MW 200,000 each) and 2 pairs of light chains (MW 20,000 and 16,000), each of which is present as 2 copies in the myosin complex. Myosin heavy chains are thin, rodlike molecules (150 nm long and 2–3 nm thick) made up of 2 heavy chains twisted together. Small, globular projections at one end of each heavy chain form the heads, which have ATP binding sites as well as the enzymatic capacity to hydrolyze ATP (ATPase activity) and the ability to bind to actin. The 4 light chains are associated with the head (Fig 11–6). When subjected to brief proteolysis, myosin heavy chains can be cleaved into 2 fragments, **light** and **heavy meromyosin.** The light fragment represents the greater part of the rodlike portion of the molecule; heavy meromyosin represents its globular projection plus a small part of the rod. Several hundred myosin molecules are arranged within each thick filament with their rodlike portions overlapping and their globular heads directed toward either end. A bare zone in the middle, which corresponds to the H band, represents a region of myosin overlap

consisting of only the rodlike part of the molecule (Fig 11–6[5]).

Analysis of thin sections of striated muscle shows the presence of cross-bridges between thin and thick filaments. These bridges are known to be formed by the head of the myosin molecule plus a short part of its rodlike portion. These bridges are considered to be directly involved in the transduction of chemical into mechanical energy (Fig 11–9).

Contraction Mechanism

Resting sarcomeres consist of partially overlapping thick and thin filaments. During contraction, both the thick and thin filaments retain their original length. Since contraction is not due to a shortening of individual filaments, it must be due to an increase in the amount of overlap between the filaments. This **sliding filament** hypothesis of muscle contraction proposed by Huxley has received the most widespread acceptance.

The following is a brief scheme of how actin and myosin interact during a contraction cycle: At rest,

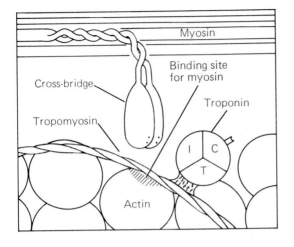

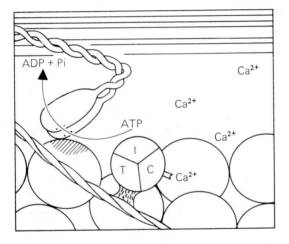

Figure 11–9. Initiation of muscle contraction occurs by the binding of Ca²⁺ to the TnC unit of troponin, which exposes the myosin binding site on actin (cross-hatched area). In a second step, the myosin head binds to actin and the ATP breaks down into ADP, yielding energy, which produces a movement of the myosin head. As a consequence of this change in myosin, the bound thin filaments slide over the thick filaments. This process, which repeats itself many times during a single contraction, leads to a complete overlap of the actin and myosin and, concomitantly, a shortening of the whole myofiber. (Reproduced, with permission, from Ganong WF: *Review of Medical Physiology*, 12th ed. Lange, 1985.)

ATP binds to the ATPase site on the myosin heads, but the rate of hydrolysis is very slow. Myosin requires actin as a cofactor in order to rapidly break down ATP and release energy. In a resting muscle, myosin cannot associate with actin, because the binding sites for myosin heads on actin molecules are blocked by the troponin-tropomyosin complex on the F-actin filament (Fig 11–9, top). However, when sufficiently high concentrations of calcium ions are available ($> 1 \times 10^{-6}$ mol/L), they bind to the TnC subunit of

troponin. The spatial configuration of the 3 troponin subunits changes and drives the tropomyosin molecule deeper into the groove of the actin helix (Fig 11–9). This exposes the myosin binding site on the globular actin components, so that actin is free to interact with the head of the myosin molecule. The binding of calcium ions to the TnC unit corresponds to the stage at which myosin-ATP is converted into the active complex. As a result of bridging between the myosin head and the G-actin subunit of the thin filament, the ATP is split into ADP and Pi, and energy is released. This activity leads to a deformation or bending of the head and a part of the rodlike portion (hinge region) of the myosin (Fig 11–9). Since the actin is bound to the myosin, movement of the myosin head pulls the actin past the myosin filament. The result is that the thin filament is drawn farther into the A band. Although a large number of myosin heads extend from the thick filament, at any one time during the contraction only a small number of heads align with available actin binding sites. However, as the bound myosin heads move the actin, they provide for alignment of new actin-myosin bridges. The old actin-myosin bridges only detach after the myosin binds a new ATP molecule; this action also resets the myosin head and prepares it for another contraction cycle. If no ATP is available, the actin-myosin complex becomes stable; this accounts for the extreme muscular rigidity (**rigor mortis**) that occurs after death. A single muscle contraction is the result of hundreds of bridge-forming and bridge-breaking cycles. The contraction activity that leads to a complete overlap between thin and thick filaments continues until Ca²⁺ ions are removed and the troponin-tropomyosin complex again covers the myosin binding site.

During contraction, the I band decreases in size as thin filaments penetrate the A band. Concomitantly, the H band—the part of the A band with only thick filaments—diminishes in width as the thin filaments completely overlap the thick filaments. A net result is that each sarcomere, and consequently the whole cell (fiber), is greatly shortened.

Sarcoplasmic Reticulum

As described above, muscle contraction depends on the availability of Ca²⁺ ions, while muscle relaxation is related to an absence of Ca²⁺. The sarcoplasmic reticulum (SR) specifically regulates calcium ion flow, which is necessary for rapid contraction and relaxation cycles. Cytologically, the sarcoplasmic reticulum system consists of a branching network of smooth endoplasmic reticulum cisternae that surrounds each myofibril (Fig 11–13). Following a neurally mediated depolarization of the sarcoplasmic reticulum membrane, Ca²⁺ ions concentrated within the sarcoplasmic reticulum cisternae are passively released into the vicinity of the overlapping thick and thin filaments, whereupon they bind to troponin and allow bridging between actin and myosin. When the membrane depolarization ends, the sarcoplasmic reticulum acts as a calcium sink and actively transports the Ca^{2+} back into the cisternae, which results in cessation of contractile activity.

Using cell homogenization and differential centrifugation, it has been possible to isolate the sarcoplasmic reticulum. In vitro, isolated sarcoplasmic reticulum acts as a **relaxation factor** that inhibits muscle contraction. This inhibition, related to the removal of available Ca^{2+} by the vesicular portions of the sarcoplasmic reticulum, demonstrates the existence of an active calcium transport mechanism in the sarcoplasmic reticulum membrane.

Transverse Tubule System

The depolarization of the sarcoplasmic reticulum membrane, which results in the release of Ca^{2+} ions, is initiated at a specialized myoneural junction on the surface of the muscle cell (structure described below). Surface-initiated depolarization signals would have to diffuse throughout the cell to effect Ca^{2+} release from internal sarcoplasmic reticulum cisternae. In larger muscle cells, the diffusion of the depolarization signal would lead to a wave of contraction, wherein peripheral myofibrils would contract prior to more centrally positioned myofibrils. To provide for a uniform contraction, skeletal muscle possesses a system of **transverse (T) tubules.** These fingerlike invaginations of the sarcolemma form a complex anastomosing network of tubules that encircle both A-I junctions of each sarcomere in every myofibril (Figs 11–10, 11–11, and 11–13).

Adjacent to opposite sides of each T tubule are expanded **terminal cisternae** of the sarcoplasmic reticulum. This specialized complex, consisting of SR–T tubule–SR components, is known as the **triad** (Figs 11–5, 11–11, and 11–13). At the triad, depolarization of the sarcolemma-derived T tubules is transmitted to the sarcoplasmic reticulum.

Innervation

In order to contract, each skeletal muscle fiber normally requires innervation by a motor nerve branch. Myelinated motor nerves branch out within the perimysial connective tissue, where each nerve gives rise to several terminal twigs. At the site of innervation, the nerve loses its myelin sheath and forms a dilated termination (terminal bouton) that sits within a trough

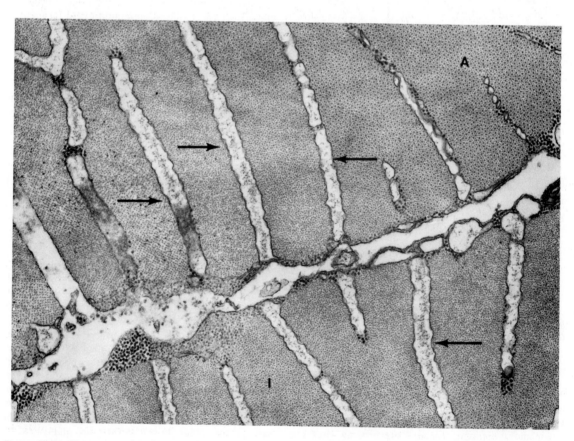

Figure 11–10. Electron micrograph of a transverse section of fish muscle, showing the surface of 2 cells limiting an intercellular space. Observe the invaginations of the sarcolemma, forming the tubules of the T system (arrows). The dark, coarse granules in the cytoplasm *(lower left)* are glycogen particles. At upper right (A), the section passes through the A band showing thick and thin filaments. At lower left (I), the I band is sectioned showing only thin filaments. × 60,000. (Courtesy of KR Porter.)

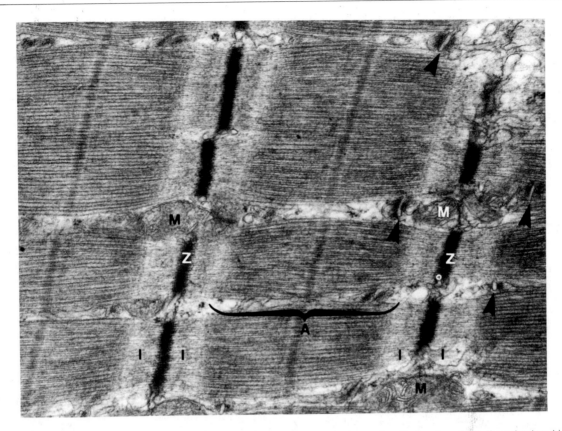

Figure 11–11. Electron micrograph of a longitudinal section of the skeletal muscle of a monkey. Note the mitochondria (M) between adjacent myofibrils. The arrowheads indicate triads—2 for each sarcomere in this muscle—located at the A-I band junction. A, A band; I, I band; Z, Z line. × 40,000. (Reproduced, with permission, from Junqueira LCU, Salles LMM: *Ultra-Estrutura e Função Celular.* Edgard Blücher, 1975.)

on the muscle cell surface (Fig 11–12). This structure is called the **motor end-plate** or **myoneural junction.** At this site the axon is covered by a thin cytoplasmic layer of Schwann cells. Within the axon terminal are numerous mitochondria and synaptic vesicles, the latter containing the neurotransmitter **acetylcholine** (described in Chapter 9). Between the axon and the muscle is a space, the **synaptic cleft,** in which lies an amorphous basal lamina matrix. At the junction, the sarcolemma is thrown into numerous deep **junctional folds.** In the sarcoplasm below the folds lie several myonuclei, numerous mitochondria, ribosomes, and glycogen granules.

When an action potential invades the motor end-plate, acetylcholine is liberated from the axon terminal, diffuses through the cleft, and binds to acetylcholine receptors in the sarcolemma of the junctional folds. Binding of the transmitter makes the sarcolemma more permeable to sodium, which results in **membrane depolarization.** Excess acetylcholine is hydrolyzed by the enzyme cholinesterase bound to the collagenous matrix of the synaptic cleft basal lamina. Acetylcholine breakdown is necessary to avoid prolonged contact of the transmitter with receptors present in the sarcolemma.

The depolarization initiated at the motor end-plate is propagated along the surface of the muscle cell and deep into the fibers via the transverse tubule system. At each triad, the depolarization signal is passed to the sarcoplasmic reticulum and results in the release of Ca^{2+}, which initiates the contraction cycle. When depolarization ceases, the Ca^{2+} is actively transported back into the sarcoplasmic reticulum cisternae and the muscle relaxes.

Evidence has firmly established that the myoneural disorder **myasthenia gravis,** characterized by a progressive muscular weakness, is an autoimmune disease. In myasthenics, circulating antibodies bind to acetylcholine receptors in the junctional folds and inhibit normal nerve-muscle communication.

A single nerve may innervate one muscle fiber or may branch and be responsible for innervating up to 160 or more muscle fibers. In the case of multiple innervation, a single nerve fiber and all the muscles it innervates are called a **motor unit.** Striated muscles do not show degrees of contraction—they either con-

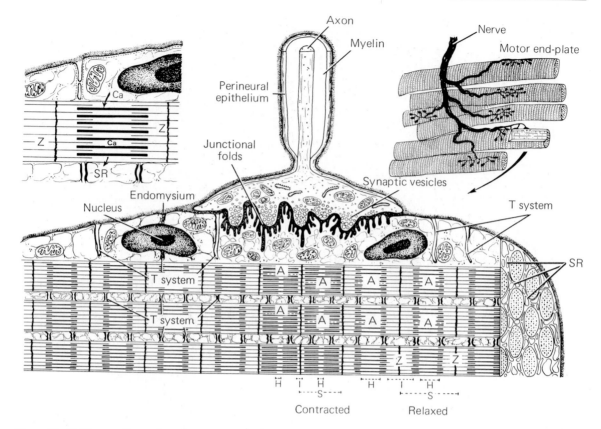

Figure 11–12. Diagram illustrating the ultrastructure of the motor end-plate and the mechanism of muscle contraction. The upper right drawing shows branching of a small nerve with a motor end-plate for each muscle fiber. The structure of one of the bulbs of an end-plate is highly enlarged in the central drawing. Observe that the axon terminal bud contains synaptic vesicles. The region of the muscle cell membrane covered by the terminal bud exhibits clefts and ridges called **junctional folds.** The axon loses its myelin sheath and dilates, establishing close, irregular contact with the muscle fiber. Muscle contraction begins with the release of acetylcholine from the synaptic vesicles of the end-plate. This neurotransmitter causes a local increase in the permeability of the sarcolemma. This process is propagated to the rest of the sarcolemma, including its invaginations, all of which constitute the T system, and is transferred to the sarcoplasmic reticulum (SR). The increase of permeability in this organelle liberates calcium ions that trigger the sliding filament mechanism of muscle contraction. Thin filaments slide between the thick filaments and reduce the distance between the Z lines. This produces a reduction in the size of all bands except the A band.

tract all the way or not at all. In order to vary the force of contraction, not all the fibers within a muscle bundle should contract at the same time. Since muscles are broken up into motor units, the firing of a single nerve will elicit a contraction that is proportionate to the number of fibers innervated by that "motor unit." Thus, the number of motor units and the variable size of each unit can control the intensity of a muscle contraction. The size of motor units within a given muscle is dependent upon the delicacy of movement required by that muscle. For example, because of the fine control required by eye muscles, each of their fibers is innervated by a different nerve fiber. However, in larger muscles exhibiting coarser movements, such as those of the limb, a single nerve fiber innervates a motor unit that consists of over 100 individual muscle fibers.

System of Energy Production

Skeletal muscle cells are highly adapted for discontinuous production of mechanical work through release of chemical energy and must have depots of energy to cope with bursts of activity. The most readily available energy is stored in the form of ATP and phosphocreatine, both of which are energy-rich phosphate compounds. Chemical energy is also available in glycogen depots, which constitute about 0.5–1% of muscle weight. Muscle tissue produces energy to be stored in phosphocreatine and ATP from the breakdown of fatty acids and glucose. In the resting muscle or during its recovery after contraction, the major substrate is fatty acids. Fatty acids are broken down to acetate by the process called β-oxidation. This set of enzymes is located in the mitochondrial matrix. Acetate is then further oxidized by the citric acid cycle,

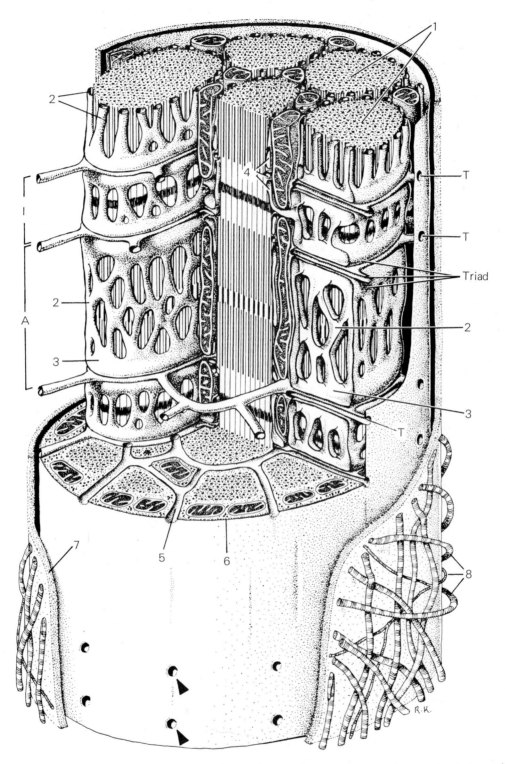

Figure 11–13. Diagram of a segment of mammalian skeletal muscle. The sarcolemma and muscle fibrils are partially cut, showing the following components: The invaginations of the T system (T and 5) occur at the level of transition between the A and I bands twice in every sarcomere. They associate with terminal cisternae of the sarcoplasmic reticulum (3), forming **triads.** Abundant mitochondria (4) lie between the myofibrils. The cut surface of the myofibrils (1) shows the thin and thick filaments. Surrounding the sarcolemma are a basal lamina (7) and reticular fibers (8). (Reproduced, with permission, from Krstić RV: *Ultrastructure of the Mammalian Cell.* Springer-Verlag, 1979.)

with the resulting energy being conserved in the form of ATP. Fatty acids are the main energy source in skeletal muscles of "endurance" athletes such as long-distance runners. When skeletal muscles are subjected to short-term ("sprint") exercise, they rapidly metabolize glucose (coming mainly from muscle glycogen stores) to lactate, thus causing an oxygen debt that is repaid during the recovery period. It is the lactate formed during this form of exercise that causes cramping and pain in skeletal muscles.

From the morphologic, histochemical, and functional point of view, we may classify skeletal muscle fibers into 3 types: red, white, and intermediate. **Red fibers** have a high content of myoglobin and cytochrome, which are responsible for the dark red color. They contract at a slower rate than white fibers but are capable of continuous and vigorous activity. Their energy derives mainly from oxidative phosphorylation, and these fibers thus contain great numbers of mitochondria. These are the fibers in the breast muscles of migrating birds and mammalian limbs. The long muscles of the human back, adapted for long, slow, posture-maintaining contractions, are also an example of red muscle. **White fibers** have a low content of myoglobin and cytochrome and fewer mitochondria. They are larger in diameter than red fibers. The breast muscles of chickens and turkeys as well as the extraocular muscles of the human eye consist of these fibers. They contract rapidly but cannot support continuous heavy work. The energy for their activity is derived mainly from anaerobic glycolysis. **Intermediate fibers** have characteristics between the 2 extremes described above. In humans, skeletal muscles are frequently composed of mixtures of these 3 types of fibers, as shown in Fig 11–14.

The differentiation of muscle into red, white, and intermediate fiber types is controlled by its innervation. In experiments where the nerves to red and white fibers are cut, crossed, and allowed to regenerate, the myofibers change their morphology and physiology in order to conform to the innervating nerve. Simple denervation of muscle will lead to fiber atrophy and paralysis.

Other Components of the Sarcoplasm

Glycogen is found in abundance in the sarcoplasm in the form of coarse granules (Fig 11–10). It serves as a depot of energy that is mobilized during muscle contraction.

Another component of the sarcoplasm is **myoglobin**, an oxygen-binding protein similar to hemoglobin that is principally responsible for the dark red color of some muscles. Myoglobin acts as an oxygen storage pigment and is present in great amounts in the muscle of deep-diving ocean mammals (eg, seals and whales). Muscles that must maintain activity for prolonged periods usually are red and have a high content of myoglobin.

Mature muscle cells have negligible amounts of rough endoplasmic reticulum and ribosomes, an observation that is consistent with the low level of protein synthesis occurring in this tissue.

Muscle spindles are described in Chapter 10.

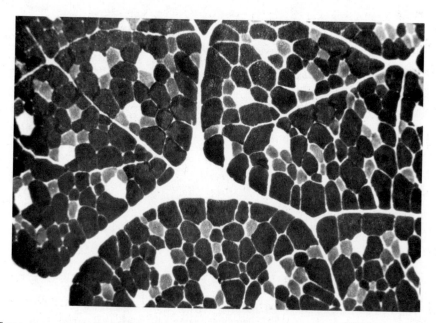

Figure 11–14. Transverse section of a striated muscle of the eye (rectus lateralis), stained by the histochemical technique for demonstrating myosin ATPase, showing 3 types of fibers in the muscle. This method shows that white fibers are large and dark-staining (high ATPase activity), red fibers are small and appear gray, and intermediate fibers are seen as pale areas in the section. (Reproduced, with permission, from Khan MA et al: A calcium-citrophosphate technique for the histochemical localization of myosin ATPase. *Stain Technol* 1972;47:277.)

CARDIAC MUSCLE

During development, the splanchnic mesoderm cells of the primitive heart tube align into chainlike arrays. Rather than fusing into syncytial cells like skeletal muscle, the cardiac cells form complex junctions between their extended processes. Cells within a chain often bifurcate or branch and bind to cells in adjacent chains. Consequently, the heart consists of tightly knit bundles of cells, interwoven in such fashion as to provide for a characteristic wave of contraction that leads to a "wringing out" of the heart ventricles.

Mature cardiac muscle cells are approximately 15 μm in diameter and from 85 to 100 μm in length. They exhibit a cross-striated banding pattern identical to that of skeletal muscle. However, unlike multinucleated skeletal muscle, each cardiac muscle cell possesses only one or 2 centrally located euchromatic nuclei. Surrounding the muscle cells is a delicate sheath of endomysial connective tissue in which lies a rich capillary network.

A unique and distinguishing characteristic of cardiac muscle is the presence of darkly staining transverse lines that cross the chains of cardiac cells at irregular intervals (Fig 11–15). These **intercalated disks** represent junctional complexes found at the interface between adjacent cardiac myocytes (Figs 11–16, 11–17, and 11–18). These junctions may appear as straight lines or may exhibit a steplike morphology. Two regions can be distinguished in the steplike junctions—a **transverse portion,** which runs across the fibers at right angles, and a **lateral portion** running parallel to the myofilaments. There are 3 main junctional specializations within the disk. **Fascia adherens,** the most prominent membrane specialization in transverse portions of the disk, serves as anchoring sites for actin filaments of the terminal sarcomeres. Essentially they represent **hemi (half) Z bands. Maculae adherentes** (desmosomes) bind the cardiac cells together to prevent their pulling apart under constant contractile activity. On the lateral portions of the disk, **gap junctions** provide ionic continuity between adjacent cells (Fig 11–18). The significance of ionic coupling is that chains of individual cells behave as a syncytium, allowing the signal to contract to pass in a wave from cell to cell.

The structure and function of the contractile proteins in cardiac cells is virtually the same as in skeletal muscle (Fig 11–19). The T tubule system and sarcoplasmic reticulum, however, are not as regularly arranged in the cardiac myocytes. The T tubules are

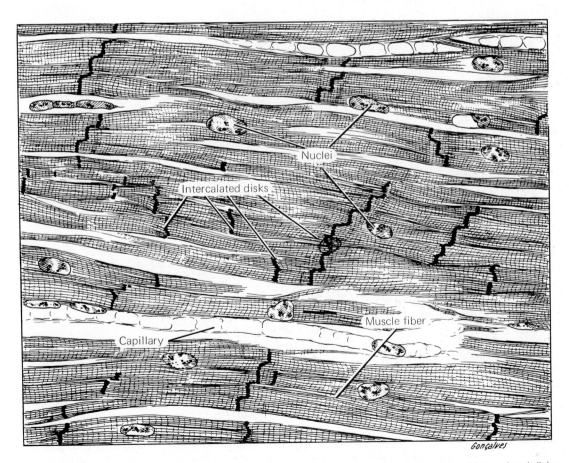

Figure 11–15. Diagram of a section of heart muscle. Observe the presence of central nuclei and intercalated disks.

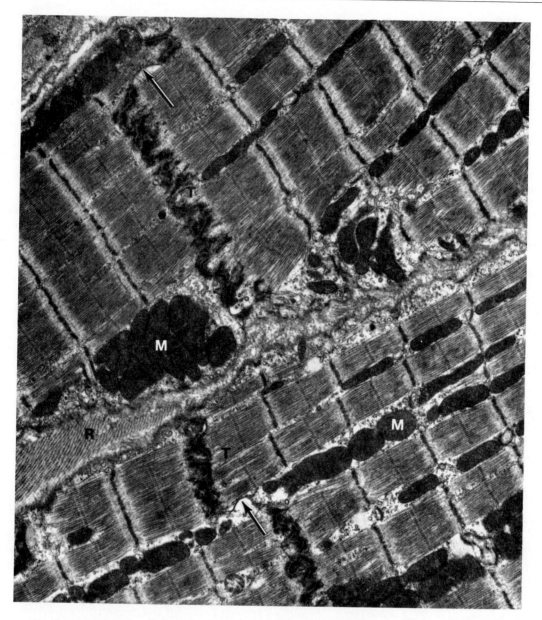

Figure 11–16. Longitudinal section of portions of 2 cardiac muscle cells. The transversely oriented parts of the intercalated disk consist of a fascia adherens and numerous desmosomes (T). The longitudinal parts (arrows) contain gap junctions. Mitochondria (M) are numerous. Reticular fibers (R) are seen between the 2 cells. × 18,000. (Reproduced, with permission, from Junqueira LCU, Salles LMM: *Ultra-Estrutura e Função Celular*. Edgard Blücher, 1975.)

more numerous and larger in ventricular muscle than in skeletal muscle. Cardiac T tubules are found at the level of the Z band rather than at the A-I junction, as in skeletal muscle. The sarcoplasmic reticulum is not as well developed and wanders irregularly through the myofilaments. As a consequence, discrete myofibrillar bundles are not present.

Triads are not common in cardiac cells, since the T tubules are generally associated with only one lateral expansion of sarcoplasmic reticulum cisternae. Thus,

heart muscle characteristically possesses **diads** composed of one T tubule and one sarcoplasmic reticulum cisterna.

Cardiac muscle cells contain numerous mitochondria, which occupy 40% or more of the cytoplasmic volume (Fig 11–19). This is a reflection of the need for continuous aerobic metabolism in heart muscle. By comparison, only about 2% of a skeletal muscle fiber is occupied by mitochondria. Fatty acids, transported to cardiac muscle cells by lipoproteins, are the

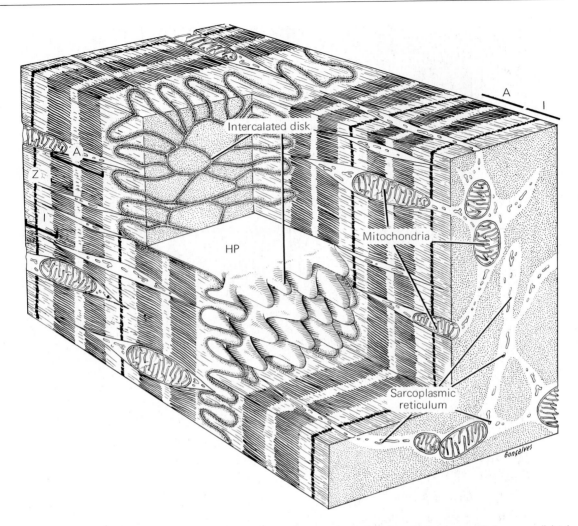

Intercalated disk

Mitochondria

HP

Sarcoplasmic
reticulum

Gonsalves

Figure 11–17. Ultrastructure of heart muscle in the region of an intercalated disk. Contact between cells is accomplished by interdigitation in the vertical region and is smooth in the horizontal plane (HP). (Redrawn and reproduced, with permission, from Marshall JM: The heart. In: *Medical Physiology,* 13th ed. Vol 2. Mountcastle VB [editor]. Mosby, 1974. Based on the results of Fawcett DW, McNutt NS: *J Cell Biol* 1969;**42**:1; modified from Poche R, Lindner E: *Z Zellforsch Mikrosk Anat* 1955;**43**:104.)

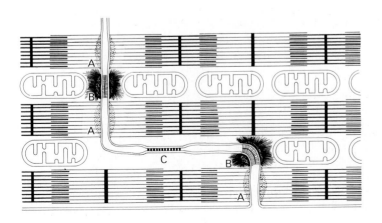

Figure 11–18. Diagrammatic representation of junctional specializations making up the intercalated disk. **Fascia (or zonula) adherens** (A) in the transverse portions of the disk serve to anchor actin filaments of the terminal sarcomeres to the plasmalemma. **Macula adherens,** or **desmosomes** (B), found primarily in the transverse portions of the disk, bind cells together, preventing their separation during contraction cycles. **Gap junctions** (C), restricted to lateral portions of the disk—that area subjected to the least stress—ionically couple cells and provide for the spread of contractile depolarization.

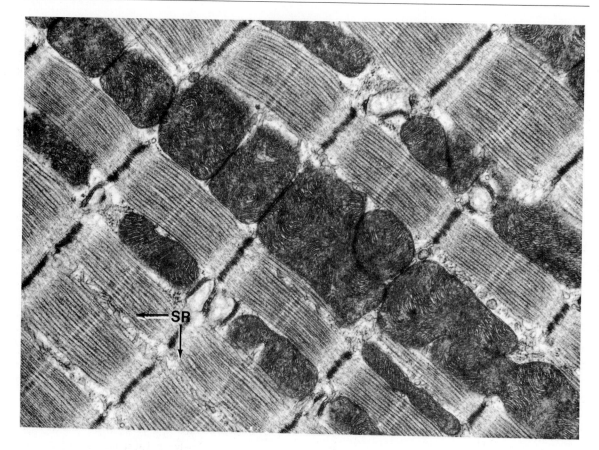

Figure 11–19. Electron micrograph from a longitudinal section of heart muscle. Observe the striation pattern and the alternation of myofibrils and mitochondria rich in cristae. Note the sarcoplasmic reticulum (SR), the specialized calcium-storing smooth endoplasmic reticulum. × 30,000.

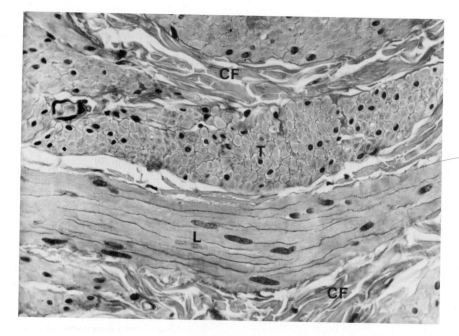

Figure 11–20. Photomicrograph of a section of urinary bladder. Smooth muscle cells are sectioned transversely (T) and longitudinally (L). Note the collagen fibers (CF) around the bundles of smooth muscle cells. H&E stain, × 400.

major fuel of the heart. Fatty acids are stored as triglycerides in the numerous lipid droplets seen in cardiac muscle cells. A small amount of glycogen is present, which can be broken down to glucose and utilized for energy production during periods of stress. Lipofuscin pigment granules (aging pigment), often seen in long-lived cells, are found near the nuclear poles of cardiac muscle cells.

A few differences in structure exist between atrial and ventricular muscle. The arrangement of myofilaments is the same in the 2 types of cardiac muscle, but atrial muscle has markedly fewer T tubules, and the cells are somewhat smaller. At both poles of cardiac muscle nuclei, and in association with Golgi complexes in this region, membrane-limited granules, each about $0.2 - 0.3$ μm in diameter, are found. These granules are most abundant in muscle cells of the right atrium (approximately 600/cell), but they are also found in the left atrium, the ventricles, and several other places in the body. These atrial granules contain the high-molecular-weight precursor of a hormone known as **atrial natriuretic factor,** auriculin, or atriopeptin. When the intravascular volume is expanded, the prohormone is secreted, a carboxy-terminal fragment is cleaved off, and this fragment (approximately 30 amino acids) forms the active hormone. Atrial natriuretic factor acts on the kidneys to cause sodium and water loss (natriuresis and diuresis). This hormone thus opposes the actions of aldosterone and antidiuretic hormone, whose effects on kidneys result in sodium and water conservation.

The rich autonomic nerve supply to the heart and the rhythmic impulse-generating and conducting structures are dealt with in Chapter 12.

SMOOTH MUSCLE

Smooth muscle is composed of elongated, nonstriated cells (Fig 11–20), each of which is enclosed

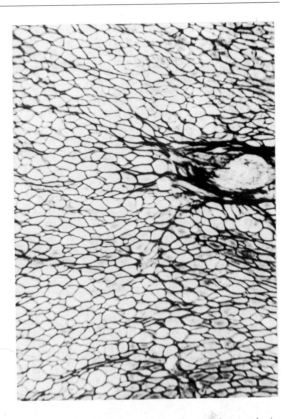

Figure 11–22. Transverse section of smooth muscle impregnated with silver to stain the reticular fibers. These structures form a network that surrounds the muscle cells not stained by this method. At right, an arteriole surrounded by thicker collagen fibers. × 300.

by a basal lamina and a network of reticular fibers (collagen type III) (Figs 11–21 and 11–22). The latter 2 components constitute the endomysium, which serves to combine the force generated by each smooth muscle fiber into a concerted action, eg, peristalsis in the intestine. Other components of smooth muscle, considered as an organ, are blood vessels and nerves.

Smooth muscle cells are fusiform; ie, they are largest at their midpoints and taper toward their ends. They may be from 30 μm up to 200 μm in length (pregnant uterus). Each cell has a single nucleus located in the center of the broadest part of the cell. To achieve closest packing, the narrow part of one cell lies adjacent to the broad part of neighboring cells (Fig 11–21). When such an arrangement is viewed in cross section, one sees a range of diameters with only the largest profiles containing a nucleus (Fig 11–20). When smooth muscle contracts, the borders of the cell become scalloped and the nucleus becomes folded or has the appearance of a corkscrew.

Concentrated at the poles of the nucleus are mitochondria, free ribosomes, cisternae of rough endoplasmic reticulum, and the Golgi complex.

The characteristic contractile activity of smooth

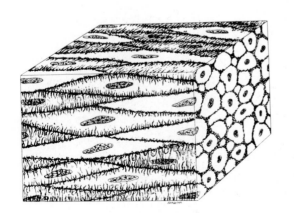

Figure 11–21. Diagram of a segment of smooth muscle. All cells are surrounded by a net of reticular fibers. In cross section, these cells exhibit variable diameters.

muscle is related to the structure and organization of its actin and myosin filaments, which do not exhibit the paracrystalline organization present in striated muscles (Fig 11–23). In smooth muscle cells, bundles of myofilaments crisscross obliquely through the cell, forming a latticelike network. These bundles consist of 5- to 7-nm thin filaments containing actin and tropomyosin, and 12- to 16-nm thick filaments consisting of myosin. Unlike the myosin filaments in skeletal muscle, which have a bare central region with myosin heads on each end, smooth muscle myosin has heads all along its length with bare regions at the ends of the filaments. This morphologic feature reflects polarity differences in the organization of myosin molecules. Much greater actin ''overlap'' and a concomitantly greater degree of contraction are possible in smooth muscle as a result of the molecular organization of the myosin filaments. Both structural and biochemical studies reveal that smooth muscle actin and myosin contract by a sliding filament mechanism similar to that which occurs in striated muscles.

Calcium ions control the contraction of smooth muscles, but the site of control is not troponin. Rather, myosin light chain phosphorylation is believed to be the controlling factor. A rudimentary sarcoplasmic reticulum is present in most smooth muscle cells and consists of a closed system of membranes, similar to the sarcoplasmic reticulum of striated muscles. T tubules are not present in smooth muscle cells.

Smooth muscle cells have an elaborate array of 10-nm intermediate filaments coursing through their cytoplasm. **Desmin** (skeletin) has been identified as the major protein of intermediate filaments in all smooth muscles, and **vimentin** occurs as an additional component in vascular smooth muscle. Two types of **dense bodies**—membrane-associated and cytoplasmic—are seen in smooth muscle. Both contain α actinin and are thus similar to the Z lines of striated muscles. Both thin filaments and intermediate filaments insert into dense bodies that may serve to transmit contractile force to adjacent smooth muscle cells and their surrounding endomysium.

The degree of innervation in a particular bundle of smooth muscle is dependent upon both the function and size of that muscle. Smooth muscle is innervated by both sympathetic and parasympathetic nerves of the autonomic system. Elaborate neuromuscular junctions similar to those in skeletal muscle are not present

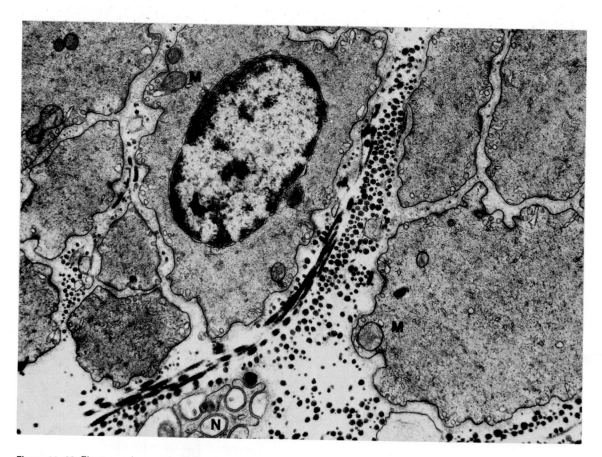

Figure 11–23. Electron micrograph of a transverse section of smooth muscle. The cells have variable diameters and many pinocytotic vesicles on their surface. Thick and thin filaments are not organized into myofibrils. There are few mitochondria (M). Between the cells are collagen fibrils and a small unmyelinated nerve (N). × 6650.

in smooth muscle. Frequently, autonomic nerve axons terminate in a series of dilatations in the endomysial connective tissue. Within these dilatations are vesicles containing either acetylcholine (cholinergic nerves) or norepinephrine (noradrenergic nerves). The dilatations may be as close as 10–20 nm from the surface of the muscle, or they may lie at greater distances (100 nm or more). In the latter case, excitation of the muscle depends upon long-range diffusion of the neurotransmitters through the intervening connective tissue.

In general, smooth muscle occurs in large sheets such as in the walls of hollow viscera, as in the intestines, uterus, and ureters. Their cells possess abundant gap junctions and a relatively poor nerve supply. These muscles function in syncytial fashion and are called **visceral** or **unitary smooth muscles.** In contrast, the **multiunit smooth muscles** have a rich innervation and can produce very precise and graded contractions as occur in the iris of the eye.

Smooth muscle usually has spontaneous activity in the absence of nervous stimuli. Its nerve supply therefore has the function of modifying activity and not initiating it, as in skeletal muscle. Smooth muscle receives both adrenergic and cholinergic nerve endings that act antagonistically, stimulating or depressing its activity. In some organs, the cholinergic endings activate and the adrenergic nerves depress, while in others the reverse occurs.

In addition to contractile activity, smooth muscle cells have also been shown to synthesize collagen, elastin, and proteoglycans, extracellular products normally associated with the function of fibroblasts (see Chapter 5). The elaborate rough endoplasmic reticulum and well-developed Golgi complex are organellar correlates reflecting this synthetic behavior. The collagen produced by smooth muscle cells is collagen type III (reticular fibers), and this explains why in the Ehlers-Danlos syndrome type IV (in which deficiency of the synthesis of collagen type III occurs), ruptures of the intestinal and aortic walls occur. (See Table 5–3.)

REGENERATION OF MUSCLE TISSUE

The 3 types of adult muscle exhibit varying potentials for regeneration after injury.

Cardiac muscle has practically no regenerative capacity beyond early childhood. Defects or damage (eg, infarcts) in heart muscle are generally replaced by proliferation of connective tissue, forming myocardial scars.

In skeletal muscle, although the nuclei in the syncytium are incapable of undergoing mitosis, the tissue undergoes extensive regeneration. The source of regenerating cells is believed to be the **satellite cells.** Satellite cells are a sparse population of mononucleated spindle-shaped cells which lie within the basal lamina that surrounds each mature myofiber and, because of their intimate apposition with the myofiber surface, can be identified only with the electron microscope. They are considered to be inactive myoblasts that persist after muscle differentiation. Following injury or certain other stimuli, the normally quiescent satellite cells become activated, proliferate, and fuse to form new skeletal muscle fibers. A similar activity of satellite cells has been implicated in muscle hypertrophy, where they fuse with their ''parent fibers'' to increase muscle mass following extensive exercise.

Smooth muscle is also capable of a modest regenerative response. Following injury, viable mononucleated smooth muscle cells undergo mitosis and provide for the replacement of the damaged tissue.

REFERENCES

Ashton FT, Somlyo AV, Somlyo AP: The contractile apparatus of vascular smooth muscle: Intermediate high voltage stereo electron microscopy. *J Mol Biol* 1975;**98**:17.

Bagby RM: Organization of contractile/cytoskeletal elements. In: *Biochemistry of Smooth Muscle*. Vol 1. Stephens NL (editor). CRC Press, 1983.

Bourne GH (editor): *The Structure and Function of Muscle*. Academic Press, 1972.

Bülbring E, Bolton TB (editors): Smooth muscle. *Br Med Bull* 1979;**35**:127.

Campion DR: The muscle satellite cell: A review. *Int Rev Cytol* 1984;**87**:225.

Cantin M, Genest J: The heart as an endocrine gland. *Sci Am* (Feb) 1986;**254**:76.

Challice CE, Viragh S (editors): *Ultrastructure of the Mammalian Heart*. Academic Press, 1973.

Cohen C: The protein switch of muscle contraction. *Sci Am* (Nov) 1975;**233**:36.

DeBold AJ: Atrial natriuretic factor: A hormone produced by the heart. *Science* 1985;**230**:767.

Devine CE, Somlyo AV, Somlyo AP: Sarcoplasmic reticulum and excitation-contraction coupling in mammalian smooth muscles. *J Cell Biol* 1972;**52**:690.

Fawcett DW: The sarcoplasmic reticulum of skeletal and cardiac muscle. *Circulation* 1961;**24**:336.

Franzini-Armstrong C, Peachey LD: Striated muscle: Contractile and control mechanisms. *J Cell Biol* 1981;**88**:166.

Gabella G, Blundell D: Nexuses between smooth muscle cells of the guinea-pig ileum. *J Cell Biol* 1979;**82**:239.

Gauthier GF, Padykula HA: Cytological studies of fiber types in skeletal muscle: A comparative study of the mammalian diaphragm. *J Cell Biol* 1966;**28**:333.

Heuser JE, Reese TS: Evidence for recycling of synaptic vesicle membrane during transmitter release at the frog neuromuscular junction. *J Cell Biol* 1973;**57**:315.

Huxley HE: The mechanism of muscular contraction. *Science* 1969;**164**:1356.

Huxley HE: Molecular basis of contraction in cross-striated muscles and relevance to motile mechanisms in other cells. In: *Muscle and Nonmuscle Motility*. Vol 1. Stracher A (editor). Academic Press, 1983.

Ishikawa H: Fine structure of skeletal muscle. In: *Cell and Muscle Motility*. Vol 4. Dowben RM, Shay JW (editors). Plenum Press, 1983.

Jones PA, Scott-Burden T, Gevers W: Glycoprotein, elastin and collagen secretion by rat smooth muscle cells. *Proc Natl Acad Sci USA* 1979;**76**:353.

MacLennan DH, Campbell KP: Structure, function and biosynthesis of sarcoplasmic reticulum proteins. *Trans Int Biol Soc* 1979;**4**:148.

Mannherz HG, Goody RS: Proteins of contractile systems. *Annu Rev Biochem* 1976;**45**:427.

Martonosi AN: The regulation of cytoplasmic calcium concentration in muscle and nonmuscle cells. In: *Muscle and Nonmuscle Motility*. Vol 1. Stracher A (editor). Academic Press, 1983.

McNutt NS, Fawcett DW: Myocardial ultrastructure. In: *The Mammalian Myocardium*. Langer GA, Brady AJ (editors). Wiley, 1974.

Rash JE, Hudson CS, Ellisman MH: Ultrastructure of acetylcholine receptors at the mammalian neuromuscular junction. In: *Cell Membrane Receptors for Drugs and Hormones: A Multidisciplinary Approach*. Straub RW, Bolis L (editors). Raven Press, 1978.

Small JV, Sobieszek A: Contractile and structural proteins of smooth muscle. In: *Biochemistry of Smooth Muscle*. Vol 1. Stephens NL (editor). CRC Press, 1983.

Somlyo AP, Somlyo AV: Ultrastructure of smooth muscle. In: *Methods in Pharmacology*. Daniel EE, Paton DM (editors). Plenum Press, 1975.

Somlyo AV: Bridging structures spanning the junctional gap at the triad of skeletal muscle. *J Cell Biol* 1979;**80**:743.

Sommer JR, Johnson EA: A comparative study of Purkinje fibers and ventricular fibers. *J Cell Biol* 1968;**36**:497.

Stracher A (editor): *Muscle and Nonmuscle Motility*. Vol 1. Academic Press, 1983.

Circulatory System

12

The circulatory system consists of the blood and lymphatic vascular systems. The blood vascular system is composed of the following structures: (1) the **heart,** whose function is to pump the blood; (2) a series of efferent vessels, the **arteries,** which become smaller as they branch and whose function it is to carry the blood and, with it, nutrients and oxygen to the tissues; (3) a diffuse network of thin tubules—the **capillaries**—which anastomose profusely and through whose walls the interchange between blood and tissues takes place; and (4) the **veins,** which represent the convergence of the capillaries into a system of larger channels that convey products of metabolism, CO_2, etc, toward the heart.

The lymphatic vascular system begins in blind-ended tubules, the lymphatic capillaries, which anastomose to form vessels of steadily increasing size and terminate in the blood vascular system, emptying into the large veins near the heart. The function of the lymphatic system is to return to the blood the fluid of the tissue spaces, which, on entering the lymphatic capillaries, contributes to formation of the liquid part of the lymph and, by passing through the lymphoid organs, contributes to the circulation of lymphocytes and other immunologic factors.

By distributing hormones and nutrients to the cells and tissues of the body, the circulatory system, along with the nervous system, contributes to the integrated functioning of the entire organism.

GENERAL STRUCTURE OF BLOOD VESSELS

All blood vessels have a number of structural features in common, although in the smallest vessels (capillaries and venules) the 3 tunics (described below) are greatly simplified. Blood vessels are structurally adapted according to physiologic requirements. Thus, pulmonary arteries (low-pressure system) have thinner walls than systemic arteries (high-pressure system) such as the carotid or renal arteries.

It should also be noted that there are no absolute criteria for distinguishing between large arteries, medium-sized arteries, and arterioles. Blood vessels constitute a continuous system, and intermediates in the classification are to be expected.

Tunics

Blood vessels are usually composed of the following layers (Fig 12–1):

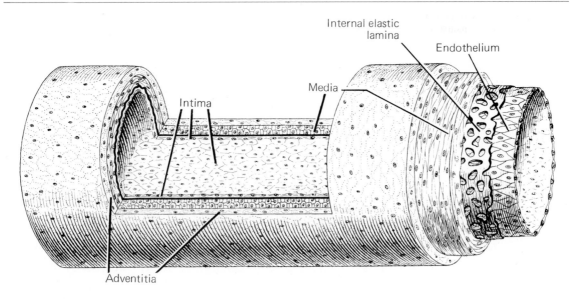

Figure 12–1. Drawing of a medium-sized artery (muscular artery) showing its layers. In the usual histologic preparations, the layers appear thicker than shown here. Experimental work suggests, however, that the drawing is more closely similar to the in vivo architecture of the vessel. After death, the vessel contracts, the layers become thicker, and the lumen becomes smaller and corrugated.

(1) Tunica intima: The intima consists of a layer of **endothelial cells** lining the vessel's interior surface. These cells rest on a basal lamina. (See under Capillaries, below, for a description of endothelial cells.) Beneath the endothelium is the **subendothelial layer,** consisting of loose connective tissue that may contain occasional smooth muscle cells. Both the connective tissue fibers and smooth muscle cells, when present, tend to be arranged longitudinally.

(2) Tunica media: The media consists chiefly of concentric layers of helically arranged smooth muscle cells (Fig 12–2). Interposed among the smooth muscle cells are variable amounts of elastic fibers and lamellae, collagen fibers, and proteoglycans. Smooth muscle cells are the cellular source of this extracellular matrix. In arteries, the media is separated from the intima by an **internal elastic lamina.** This lamina, composed of elastin, has gaps **(fenestrae)** that allow substances to diffuse to and nourish cells deep in the vessel wall. In larger arteries, a thinner **external elastic lamina** is often found separating the media from the outer tunica adventitia. In capillaries and postcapillary venules, the media is represented by cells called **pericytes** (see under Capillaries, below).

(3) Tunica adventitia: The adventitia consists principally of longitudinally oriented collagenous and elastic fibers (Fig 12–2). Collagen in the adventitia is only of type I, while in the media, collagen is mainly of type III. The adventitial layer gradually becomes continuous with the enveloping connective tissue of the organ through which the vessel is running.

Vasa Vasorum

In large vessels, vasa vasorum ("vessels of the vessel") branch profusely in the adventitia and the outer part of the media. The vasa vasorum provide metabolites to the adventitia and the media in larger vessels, since the layers are too thick to be nourished by diffusion from the lumen. These vessels are less frequent in arteries than in veins. The greater abundance of vasa vasorum in veins can be attributed to the paucity of oxygen and nutritional substances in venous blood. Vasa vasorum can arise from branches of the artery which they supply, or they can arise from neighboring arteries.

Lymphatics are present in arteries only in the adventitia, but they can penetrate the media of veins. This difference in distribution is probably related to differences in transmural pressures. The higher pressure across an arterial wall would tend to collapse a lymphatic capillary located near the arterial lumen, rendering it useless.

Innervation

Most blood vessels that contain smooth muscle in their walls are supplied with a profuse network of unmyelinated sympathetic nerve fibers (vasomotor nerves) whose neurotransmitter is norepinephrine. Discharge of norepinephrine from these nerves results in vasoconstriction. These efferent nerves generally do not enter the media of arteries, and thus the neurotransmitter must diffuse for several micrometers to affect smooth muscle cells of the media. Gap junctions

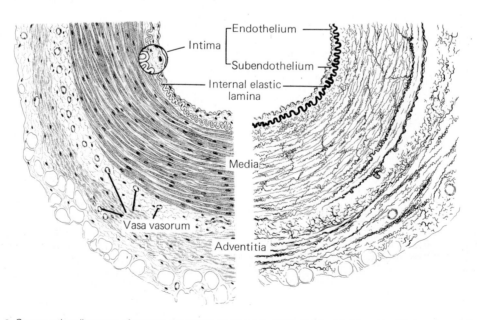

Figure 12–2. Comparative diagrams of a muscular artery prepared by H&E staining *(left)* and by Weigert's staining method for elastic structures *(right)*. The media is composed of a mixture of smooth muscle cells, collagen, and elastic fibers. The adventitia and the outer part of the media have small blood vessels (vasa vasorum) and elastic and collagenous fibers.

between smooth muscle cells of the media propagate the response to the neurotransmitter to the inner layers of muscle cells. In veins, nerve endings are found in both the adventitia and the media, but the overall density of innervation is less than that encountered in arteries. Arteries in skeletal muscle also receive a cholinergic vasodilator nerve supply.

Afferent (sensory) nerve endings in arteries include the baroreceptors (stretch receptors) in the carotid sinus and the arch of the aorta as well as chemoreceptors of the carotid and aortic bodies.

SPECIFIC STRUCTURE OF BLOOD VESSELS

It is customary to divide the circulatory system into the **macrovasculature** (vessels > 0.1 mm in diameter) and the **microvasculature** (vessels visible only with the light microscope). The microvasculature is particularly important because of its participation in the interchange between the circulatory system and surrounding tissues in inflammatory processes.

A description of the structure of the circulatory system, beginning with the simplest structures and proceeding to the more complex, follows.

Capillaries

Capillaries are composed of a single layer of **endothelial cells** of mesenchymal origin rolled up in the form of a tube, bounding a cylindric space. The average diameter of capillaries is small, varying from 7 to 9 μm. Their length usually varies from 0.25 mm to 1 mm, the higher value being characteristic of muscle tissue. In a few instances (adrenal cortex, renal medulla), capillaries may be up to 50 mm long. The total length of capillaries in the human body has been estimated at 96,000 km (60,000 miles). When cut transversely, their walls are observed to consist of portions of one or more cells (Fig 12–3). The external

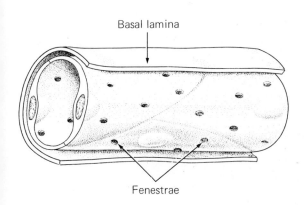

Basal lamina

Fenestrae

Figure 12–3. Diagram of the structure of a capillary with fenestrae in its wall. The sectioned portion at left is composed of 2 endothelial cells. Not all capillaries have perforated walls. The basal lamina surrounds the capillary.

surfaces of these cells usually rest on a basal lamina, a product of endothelial origin.

In general, endothelial cells are polygonal and about 10 × 30 μm when viewed face on. They are elongated in the direction of blood flow. The nucleus causes the cell to bulge into the capillary lumen. A small Golgi complex is present at the nuclear poles; a few mitochondria are evident; and free ribosomes as well as a few cisternae of rough endoplasmic reticulum are seen. Intermediate filaments (9–11 nm in diameter) are found in the perinuclear region. The presence of abundant microfilaments in endothelial cell cytoplasm is believed to be related to the proposed contractility of endothelial cells (Fig 12–4). The cell tapers toward the margins, where it may be 0.2 μm or less in thickness. Junctions of the zonula occludens type are present between most endothelial cells and are of physiologic importance. Such junctions offer variable permeability to macromolecules that play a significant role in normal physiologic or pathologic conditions. Junctions between endothelial cells of venules are the loosest. It is at this location that the characteristic loss of fluid from the circulatory system occurs during the inflammatory response, leading to edema formation.

At various locations along capillaries and small venules, there are mesenchymal cells with long cytoplasmic processes that partially surround the endothelial cells. These **pericytes** are enclosed in their own basal lamina, which may fuse with that of the endothelial cells. These perivascular cells have great potential for transformation into other cells. Pericytes contain myosin, actin, and tropomyosin, which strongly suggests that these cells also have a contractile function. Pericytes constitute the tunica media of these small vessels.

A thin layer of collagen fibers encompasses capillaries and postcapillary venules. This is the equivalent of the adventitia of larger blood vessels. Thus, even the smallest vessels of the cardiovascular system conform to the general architecture outlined above.

Capillaries can be grouped into 4 types depending on the structure of the endothelial cells and the presence or absence of a basal lamina.

(1) The **continuous,** or **somatic, capillary** (Fig 12–5) is characterized by the lack of fenestrae (openings) in its wall. This type of capillary is found in all kinds of muscle tissue, connective tissue, exocrine glands, and nervous tissue. Numerous pinocytotic vesicles, approximately 70 nm in greatest diameter, are present on both surfaces of muscle capillaries as well as appearing as isolated vesicles in the cytoplasm of these cells; these vesicles are responsible for the transport of macromolecules, in both directions, across the endothelial cell. Few or no pinocytotic vesicles are encountered in the continuous capillaries supplying most parts of the nervous system. This feature, in part, accounts for the existence of the **blood-brain barrier** (see Chapter 9).

(2) Fenestrated, or **visceral, capillaries** are characterized by the presence of large fenestrae in the

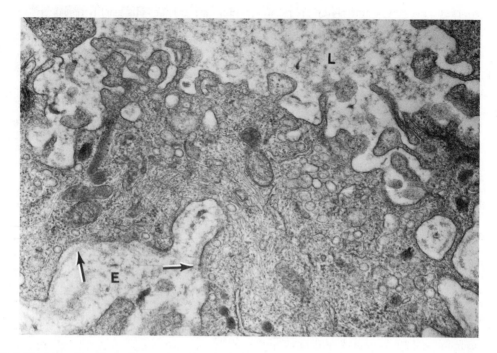

Figure 12–4. Electron micrograph of a section of a continuous capillary. Observe the ruffled appearance of its interior surface, the large and small pinocytotic vesicles, and numerous microfilaments in the cytoplasm. L, lumen of the capillary; E, its outer surface. The arrows show the basal lamina. Reduced slightly from × 30,000.

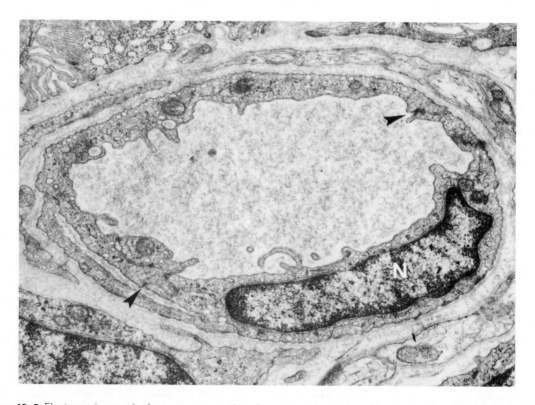

Figure 12–5. Electron micrograph of a transverse section of a continuous capillary. Note the nucleus (N) and the junctions between neighboring cells (arrowheads). Numerous pinocytotic vesicles are evident. × 10,000.

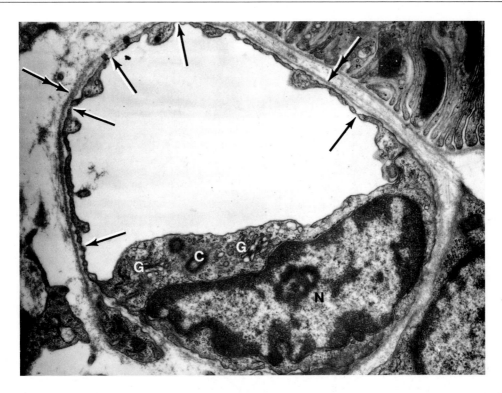

Figure 12–6. A fenestrated capillary in the kidney. Arrows indicate fenestrae closed by diaphragms. In this cell the Golgi complex (G), nucleus (N), and 2 centrioles (C) can be seen. Note the continuous basal lamina on the outer surface of the endothelial cell (double arrows). × 20,000. (Courtesy of J Rhodin.)

walls of endothelial cells. These fenestrae are 60–80 nm in diameter and are closed by a diaphragm that is thinner than a cell membrane and does not have the trilaminar structure of a "unit" membrane (Figs 12–3 and 12–6). A continuous basal lamina is present. Fenestrated capillaries are encountered in tissues where rapid interchange of substances occurs between the tissues and the blood, as is the case with the kidney, intestine, and endocrine glands. It has been shown that macromolecules injected into the bloodstream can cross the capillary wall through these fenestrae to enter the tissue spaces. This seems to be as important a mechanism of transcapillary transport as the transport due to pinocytosis (see Chapter 4).

(3) The third type of capillary is again a fenestrated capillary, but in this case no diaphragms are present to close the openings (Fig 4–3A). A very thick basal lamina separates this endothelium from the overlying epithelial cells (podocytes). This type of capillary is characteristic of the renal glomerulus (see Chapter 20).

(4) The fourth type of capillary, the **sinusoidal capillary** (Fig 15–17), has the following characteristics: (a) a tortuous path and a greatly enlarged diameter (30–40 μm), which slows the circulation of blood; (b) the presence of multiple fenestrations (no diaphragms) in the endothelial cell wall (Figs 15–17 and 17–17A); (c) the presence around the wall of cells with phagocytic activity; and (d) the absence of a continuous basal lamina. Sinusoidal capillaries are found mainly in the liver and in hematopoietic organs such as the bone marrow and spleen. These details suggest that interchange between blood and tissues is greatly facilitated by the structure of the capillary wall.

As illustrated in Fig 12–7, capillaries anastomose freely, forming a rich network interconnecting the small arteries and veins. The arterioles branch into small vessels surrounded by a discontinuous layer of smooth muscle, the **metarterioles.** These branch into capillaries that form a network with a high surface area to facilitate exchange of materials between the tissues and blood. Constriction of metarterioles helps to regulate but does not completely stop the circulation in capillaries, and it maintains pressure differences in the 2 systems. A simple ring of smooth muscle cells, or sphincter, exists at the point of origin of capillaries from the metarteriole. This **precapillary sphincter** can completely stop the blood flow within the capillary. The entire network does not always function simultaneously, and the number of functional and open capillaries depends not only on the state of contraction of the metarterioles but also on arteriovenous anastomoses that enable the arterioles to empty directly into venules, as illustrated in Fig 12–7. These interconnections are abundant in skeletal muscle and the skin of the hands and feet. When vessels of the arteriovenous anastomosis contract, all the blood must

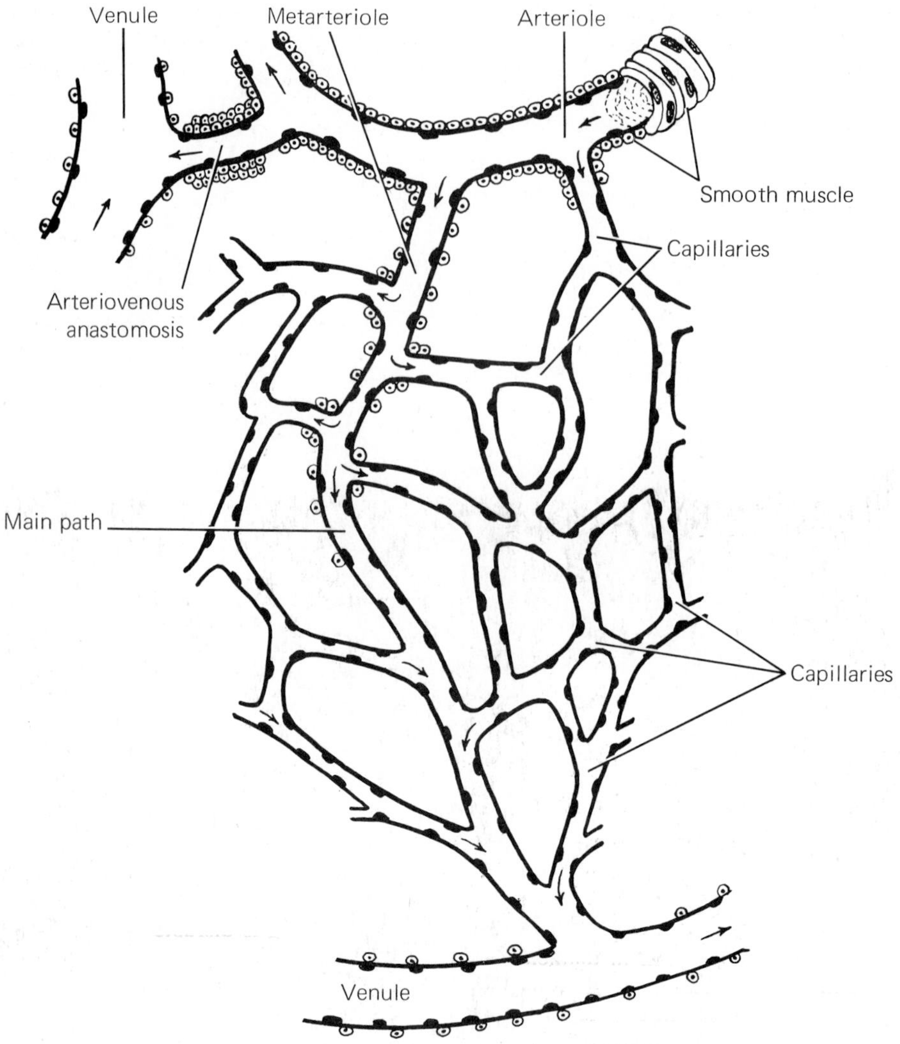

Figure 12–7. Branching of an arteriole to form a capillary network terminating in a venule. The continuous layer of smooth muscle of the arteriole becomes discontinuous in the metarterioles. In an arteriovenous anastomosis, blood passes directly from the arterial to the venous system. When blood pressure is lowered—as a result of the opening of the arteriovenous anastomosis or of contraction of the metarterioles—blood flow may be restricted to the main paths as indicated by arrows in the drawing. It is thus possible to regulate the extent of the capillary network utilized in a given territory. (Reproduced, with permission, from Copenhaver WM, Bunge RP, Bunge MB: *Bailey's Textbook of Histology*, 16th ed. Williams & Wilkins, 1972.)

pass through the capillary network. When it relaxes, some blood flows directly to a vein instead of circulating in the capillaries. Capillary circulation is controlled by neural and hormonal stimulation.

The richness of the capillary network is related to the metabolic activity of the tissues and represents a transition zone between the high-pressure system (arterial) and low-pressure system (venous). Tissues with high metabolic rates such as the kidney, liver, and cardiac and skeletal muscle have an abundant capillary network; the opposite is true of tissues with low metabolic rates such as smooth muscle and dense connective tissue.

An idea of the importance of the capillaries can be gained by noting that in the human body the surface area of the capillary network approaches 6000 m². Its total diameter is approximately 800 times larger than the aorta. A unit volume of fluid within a capillary is exposed to a larger surface area than the same volume in the other parts of the system. The flow of blood in the aorta averages 320 mm/s; in the capillaries, about 0.3 mm/s. The capillary system can thus be compared with a lake where a full-flowing river enters and leaves; because of their thin walls and slow blood flow, the capillaries are a favorable place for the exchange of water, solutes, and macromolecules between blood and tissues.

Functions of capillaries: Capillaries perform at least 3 important functions. They serve as (1) a selective permeability barrier, (2) a synthetic and metabolic system, and (3) a nonthrombogenic container for blood.

A. Permeability: Capillaries (and postcapillary venules) are often referred to as **exchange vessels,** since it is at these sites that oxygen, carbon dioxide, substrates, and metabolites are transferred from blood to the tissues and vice versa. Permeability of capillary walls varies with the size and charge of the permeating molecules and with the structure of the endothelial cell. The mechanism by which interchange of materials between blood and tissues occurs is controversial. Interpreting results of physiologic experiments, researchers have postulated the existence of 2 sizes of pores in capillary walls. The smaller pores are thought to have a diameter of 9–11 nm and the larger pores a diameter of 50–70 nm. Three possible morphologic equivalents of these "physiologic pores" are (1) intercellular junctions and clefts between neighboring endothelial cells, (2) fenestral diaphragms in fenestrated capillaries, and (3) large numbers of pinocytotic vesicles thought to cross the endothelial cells of most capillaries.

It is generally agreed that small hydrophobic and hydrophilic molecules (eg, oxygen, carbon dioxide, glucose) can diffuse or be actively transported across the plasmalemma of capillary endothelial cells. These substances are then transported by diffusion to the opposite cell surface where they are discharged into the extracellular space. Water and some other hydrophilic molecules, less than 1.5 nm in diameter and below 10,000 in molecular weight, can cross the capillary wall by diffusing through the intercellular junctions (paracellular pathway). The **intercellular junction** is now believed to be the morphologic counterpart of the **small pore** postulated by physiologic studies. The **large pore** of the physiologist is almost certainly represented morphologically by the **fenestrae** or **pinocytotic vesicles** of endothelial cells.

In abnormal states such as inflammation or injection of snake or bee venom, capillary and postcapillary venular permeability is greatly increased. These conditions apparently alter the permeability of the junctions between endothelial cells. Under such circumstances, electron-dense colloidal substances can be observed to pass from capillary and small venule lumens into surrounding tissues by traversing the endothelial cell junctions. Leukocytes may leave the bloodstream by passing between endothelial cells and entering the tissue spaces by a process called **diapedesis.** Opening of these junctions seems to be mediated by locally liberated pharmacologically active substances, such as histamine and bradykinin, that increase vascular permeability and can also play a conspicuous role in inflammation.

The observation that some drugs, given intravenously, do not reach the brain, whereas such penetration occurs in almost all other tissues of the body gave rise to the concept of the **blood-brain barrier.** This phenomenon was initially studied by intravenous administration of dyes that readily escape from capillaries to surrounding tissues. Careful study of brain capillaries showed that not only do they lack fenestrae and have few pinocytotic vesicles, but that occluding junctions between their endothelial cells do not permit the passage of macromolecules used as tracers. These properties would appear to explain the barrier. Other blood-tissue barriers of physiologic importance are the blood-ocular barrier, blood-thymus barrier, blood-nerve barrier, and blood–testicular seminiferous tubule barrier.

B. Metabolic Functions: Capillary endothelial cells can metabolize a wide variety of substrates. Although lung capillaries have been the most intensively studied, the results presented here are not restricted to pulmonary capillaries.

1. Activation – Conversion of angiotensin I to angiotensin II (see Chapter 20).

2. Inactivation – Conversion of bradykinin, serotonin, prostaglandins, norepinephrine, thrombin, etc, to biologically inert compounds.

3. Lipolysis – Breakdown of lipoproteins to yield triglycerides (energy) and cholesterol (substrates for steroid hormone synthesis and membrane structure).

C. Nonthrombogenic Function: Platelets do not normally adhere to an intact endothelium. This is due, in part, to the ability of endothelial cells to release prostacyclin (prostaglandin I_2). This arachidonic acid derivative is a powerful inhibitor of platelet aggregation and thus thrombus (clot) formation. If the endothelial lining is disrupted, the underlying collagen of the basal lamina is an important stimulus for clot formation.

Arteries

Arteries are classified according to their size into (1) arterioles; (2) muscular arteries of medium or large diameter; and (3) large elastic arteries. In general, the walls of arteries are thicker than the walls of veins when vessels of the same overall diameter are compared.

Arterioles are generally less than 0.5 mm in diameter and have relatively narrow lumens. The lumen is lined by endothelial cells similar to those described above for continuous capillaries. An important difference is the presence of rod-shaped granules, about 3 μm long but only 0.1 μm wide. These are the **Weibel-Palade granules** found only in endothelial cells of vessels larger than capillaries. These granules store components of the blood coagulation mechanism known as von Willebrand's factor (factor VIII). Deficiency of this group of proteins results in impaired platelet adhesion to injured endothelium and in prolonged bleeding. The subendothelial layer is very thin, and an internal elastic lamina is lacking except in the largest arterioles. The media is muscular and generally composed of 1–5 circularly arranged layers of smooth muscle cells. The adventitia is thin and shows no external elastic lamina (Fig 12–8).

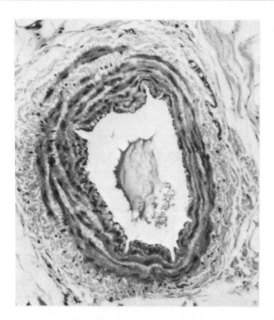 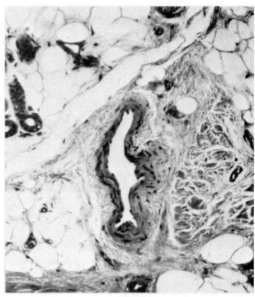

Figure 12–8. Photomicrographs of sections of a small artery *(left)* and a venule *(right)*. Without special staining (eg, Weigert's), elastin is not as apparent in this artery as it is in the artery in Fig 12–10. H&E stain, × 100.

Most of the named arteries in the human body are **muscular arteries** (Figs 12–2 and 12–8 to 12–10). The intima is similar to that described for arterioles except that the subendothelial layer is somewhat thicker and a few smooth muscle cells may be present. An internal elastic lamina is prominent (Figs 12–9 and 12–10). The media may contain up to 40 layers of smooth muscle cells, although the number of layers diminishes as the artery becomes smaller. These cells are intermingled with variable numbers of elastic lamellae (depending on the size of the vessel) as well as collagen fibers and proteoglycans. An external elastic lamina is present in larger muscular arteries. The

adventitia consists of collagenous and elastic fibers, a few fibroblasts, and adipose cells. Lymphatics, vasa vasorum, and nerves are also found in the adventitia, and these structures may penetrate to the outer part of the media.

Large elastic arteries include the aorta and its large branches. They have a yellowish color owing to the accumulation of elastin in the media. This type of artery has the following characteristics: (1) The intima, thicker than the corresponding tunic of a muscular artery, is lined by endothelial cells. In the electron microscope, the endothelial cells show microvilli, pinocytotic vesicles, rough endoplasmic reticulum,

Internal elastic lamina

Media

Adventitia

Figure 12–9. Photomicrograph of a section of a muscular artery stained by Weigert's method for elastic structures. × 110.

microfilaments, intercellular junctions, and lysosomes. Endothelial cells undergo continuous turnover, and replacements arise from preexisting cells by mitosis. In medium- and large-sized arteries, a folded endothelium whose cells bulge into the lumen of this vessel is often observed. This sometimes occurs as a result of postmortem contraction of the muscle of the arteries. The subendothelial layer is thick. The connective tissue fibers of the subendothelial layer display a longitudinal orientation and play an important role in the distortion of the endothelial layer of cells during rhythmic contractions and dilations of the vessel. An internal elastic lamina may not be evident, since it is similar to the elastic laminae of the next layer. (2) The media consists of a series of concentrically arranged perforated elastic laminae whose number increases with age (40 in the newborn; 70 in the adult). Elastic structures, once formed, usually become metabolically inert as shown by radioautographic studies, especially in older animals. These laminae exhibit a progressive increase in thickness by deposition of elastin. Between the elastic laminae are smooth muscle cells, collagen fibers, and ground substance consisting mainly of chondroitin sulfate. (3) The tunica adventitia does not show an external limiting lamina, is relatively underdeveloped, and contains elastic and collagen fibers.

Histophysiology of arteries. The large arteries are also called **conducting arteries,** since their major function is transporting blood away from the heart. These arteries also serve to smooth out the large fluctuations in pressure created by the heartbeat. During ventricular contraction **(systole),** the elastic laminae of conducting arteries are stretched and reduce the pressure change. During ventricular relaxation **(diastole),** ventricular pressure drops to a low level, but the elastic rebound of conducting arteries helps maintain arterial pressure. As a consequence, arterial pressure and blood flow decrease and become less variable as the distance from the heart increases (Fig 12–11).

The function of medium-sized arteries, also known as **distributing arteries,** is to furnish blood to the various organs. The muscular layer in distributing arteries, by contracting or not contracting owing to local chemical or more generalized neural input, can control the flow of blood to various organs.

Blood vessels undergo progressive and gradual changes from birth to death, and it is difficult to say where the normal growth processes end and the processes of involution begin. Each artery exhibits its own aging pattern. The artery that changes most precociously, beginning at 20 years of age, is the coronary. Other arteries begin to be modified only after age 40. When the media of an artery is weakened by an embryonic defect, disease, or lesion, the wall of the artery gives way, dilating extensively. As this process progresses, it becomes an **aneurysm** and might result in rupture of the wall. The importance of collagen type III in arterial structure is illustrated by the observation that in type IV Ehlers-Danlos syndrome (a genetic deficiency of the synthesis of collagen type

III), the main cause of death is spontaneous aortic rupture.

Atherosclerotic lesions are characterized by focal thickening of the intima, proliferation of smooth muscle cells and extracellular connective tissue elements, and deposition of cholesterol in smooth muscle cells and macrophages. When heavily loaded with lipid, these cells are referred to as ''foam cells'' and form the macroscopically visible fatty streaks and plaques that characterize **atherosclerosis.** These changes may extend to the inner part of the tunica media. The thickening may become so great as to occlude the vessel. Coronary arteries are among those most prone to atherosclerosis. It should be noted that uniform thickening of the intima is believed to be a normal phenomenon of aging.

Certain arteries irrigate only definite areas of specific organs, and obstruction results in necrosis (death of the tissues owing to lack of metabolites). These are **infarcts** that occur commonly in the heart, kidneys, cerebrum, and certain other organs. In other regions, such as the skin, arteries anastomose frequently, and the obstruction of one artery does not lead to tissue necrosis, because blood flow is maintained.

The polypeptide **angiotensin** contributes to the regulation of blood pressure by binding initially to vascular endothelial cells. It is believed that this endothelial stimulus is later transmitted to arterial smooth muscle cells, stimulating their contraction and consequent increase in blood pressure. Support for this hypothesis comes from morphologic studies which reveal that endothelial cells exhibit processes that extend across the internal elastic lamina and contact the smooth muscle cells.

Carotid Bodies

Small structures encountered near the bifurcation of the common carotid artery act as chemoreceptors sensitive to low oxygen tension, high carbon dioxide concentration, and low pH of arterial blood. Carotid bodies consist of glomus cells (type I cells) and sheath cells (type II cells) surrounded by a rich vascular supply whose capillaries are of the fenestrated type. Most of the nerves of the carotid body (95% in the rat) are afferent fibers. The glomus cells contain numerous dense-core vesicles that store the catecholamine dopamine. It remains controversial whether the glomus cell or the afferent nerve endings are the principal chemoreceptor element. Aortic bodies and jugular glomeruli are similar in structure to the carotid body and are thought to have a similar function.

Arteriovenous Anastomosis

Direct communications between arterial and venous circulation are often observed. These arteriovenous anastomoses are distributed throughout the body and generally occur in small vessels. The luminal diameters of anastomotic vessels vary depending on the physiologic condition of the organ. Changes in diameter serve to regulate the circulation in particular

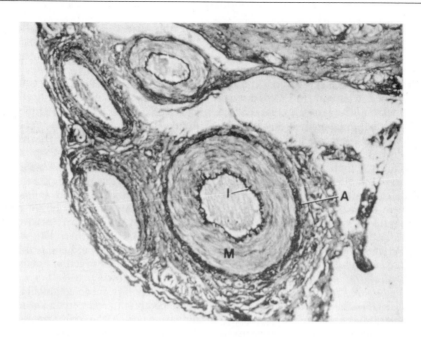

Figure 12–10. Photomicrograph of 2 small arteries *(right)* and veins *(left).* The arteries have thicker walls than the veins. In the arteries, elastin is present as an internal elastic lamina (I) and as dispersed elastic fibers in the adventitia (A). Between the elastin-containing structures is the thick muscular media (M), which is not evident in the veins. Weigert's stain, × 150.

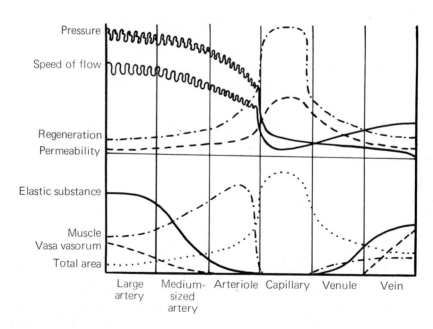

Figure 12–11. Relationship between the characteristics of blood circulation and the structure of the blood vessels. The arterial blood pressure and rapidity of flow decrease and become more constant as distance from the heart gradually increases. This coincides with a reduction in number of elastic fibers and an increase in the number of smooth muscle cells in the arteries. The graphs illustrate the gradual changes in vessel structure and their biophysical properties. Regenerative capacity and permeability are highly developed in the capillaries. (Reproduced, with permission, from Cowdry EV: *Textbook of Histology.* Lea & Febiger, 1944.)

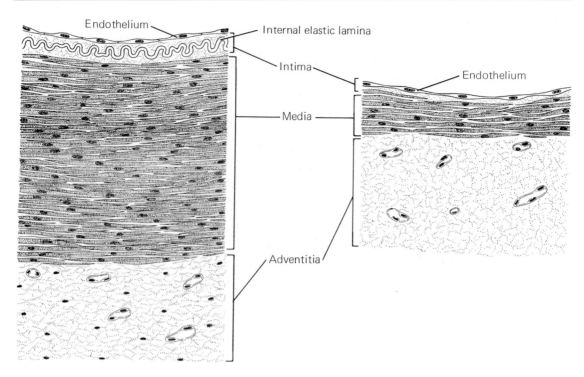

Figure 12–12. Diagram comparing the structure of a muscular artery *(left)* and accompanying vein. Note that the tunica intima and tunica media are highly developed in the artery but not in the vein.

areas (Fig 12–7). Using the technique of injecting microspheres of a certain size that obliterate the capillaries, it is possible to calculate that about one-third of the blood flow in the ear of a rabbit can pass through arteriovenous anastomoses. Besides these direct communications, more complex structures, **glomera,** occur—mainly in fingerpads, fingernail beds, and ears. In these structures, the arterioles that establish continuity with venules lose their internal elastic membranes and acquire a thick layer of concentrically arranged smooth muscle cells. This muscle layer forms a sheath that partially or completely surrounds the lumen of a vessel. Contraction of this layer can promote the complete or partial transitory closure of blood vessels. These structures have an important role in control of the circulation in various organs and participate in several physiologic phenomena such as menstruation, erection, thermoregulation, and regulation of blood pressure. The arteriovenous anastomoses are richly innervated by the sympathetic and parasympathetic nervous systems. Control of this activity appears to be mainly neural.

Veins

When considered as a functional unit, all of the veins can be classified as capacitance vessels because more than 70% of the total blood volume is in this portion of the cardiovascular system at any one time. As with arteries, it is customary to arbitrarily classify the veins into venules and veins of small, medium, and large size.

Venules are small, with a diameter of 0.2–1 mm. They are characterized by an intima composed of endothelium; a thin media that may consist of from none to a few cell layers of smooth muscle; and an adventitial layer, which is the thickest layer and is composed of connective tissue rich in collagenous fibers. Venules have thin walls (Fig 12–10) when compared with an artery of comparable overall diameter. Venules with luminal diameters up to 50 μm have the structure and other biologic features of capillaries such as participation in inflammatory processes and interchange of metabolites between blood and tissues.

With the exception of the main trunks, most veins are **small** or **medium-sized veins** and have a diameter of 1–9 mm. The intima usually has a thin subendothelial layer, but this may at times be absent. The media consists of small bundles of smooth muscle cells intermixed with collagenous and reticular fibers and a delicate network of elastic fibers. The collagenous adventitial layer, rich in collagen fibers, is well developed (Fig 12–12).

Large veins have a well-developed tunica intima. The media is much thinner, with few layers of smooth muscle cells and abundant connective tissue. The adventitial layer is the thickest and best developed tunic in veins. Cardiac muscle is present in the adventitia

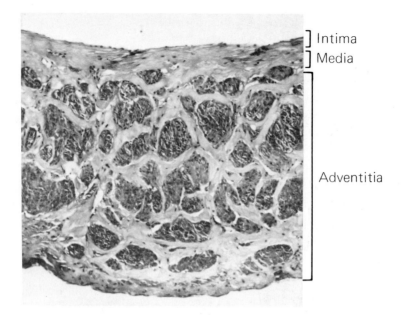

Figure 12–13. Photomicrograph of a section of a large vein. Observe the well-developed adventitia with characteristic longitudinal smooth muscle bundles. H&E stain, × 100.

of the venae cavae and pulmonary veins for a short distance before they empty into the heart. In large, unsupported abdominal veins (eg, mesenteric vein) or in other large veins that lie below the level of the heart, the adventitia frequently contains longitudinal bundles of smooth muscle (Fig 12–13). This adventitial muscle serves to strengthen the wall and prevent distention of the vessel. The circular and longitudinal arrangement of smooth muscle in these vessels may oppose the action of gravity by providing a peristaltic pumping of the blood up to the heart. In contrast to arteries, small or medium-sized veins have valves in their interior. These structures consist of 2 semilunar folds of the tunica intima that project into the lumen. They are composed of elastic connective tissue and lined on both sides by endothelium. The valves are especially numerous in veins of the limbs (arms and legs). They direct the venous blood toward the heart. The propulsive force of the heart is reinforced by contraction of skeletal muscles that surround these veins.

Heart

The heart is a muscular organ that contracts rhythmically, pumping the blood through the circulatory system. Its walls consist of 3 tunics: the internal, or **endocardium;** the middle, or **myocardium;** and the external, or **pericardium.** The heart has a fibrous central region, the **fibrous skeleton,** which serves as the base of the valves as well as the site of origin and insertion of the cardiac myocytes.

The **endocardium** is homologous with the intima of blood vessels. It consists of a single layer of squamous endothelial cells resting on a thin subendothelial layer of loose connective tissue containing elastic and collagenous fibers as well as some smooth muscle cells. Between the endocardium and the myocardium is a layer of connective tissue often termed the **subendocardial layer,** which consists of veins, nerves, and branches of the impulse-conducting system of the heart (Purkinje cells).

The **myocardium** is the thickest of the tunics of the heart and consists of cardiac muscle cells (see Chapter 11) arranged in layers that surround the heart chambers in a complex spiral manner. A large number of these layers insert themselves on the fibrous cardiac skeleton. The arrangement of these muscle cells is extremely varied, so that in histologic preparations of a small area, cells are seen oriented in many directions. The muscle cells of the heart are grouped into 2 populations: contractile cells and impulse-generating and -conducting cells that generate and conduct the electrical signal initiating the heartbeat.

Epicardium is the serous covering of the heart, forming the visceral layer of the pericardium. Externally, it is covered by simple squamous epithelium (mesothelium) supported by a thin layer of connective tissue. A subepicardial layer consisting of loose connective tissue contains veins, nerves, and nerve ganglia. The adipose tissue that generally surrounds the heart accumulates in this layer.

The **fibrous skeleton of the heart** is composed of dense connective tissue. Its principal components are the **septum membranaceum,** the **trigona fibrosa,** and the **annuli fibrosi.** These structures consist of a dense connective tissue, with thick collagen fibers oriented in various directions. Certain regions contain nodules of fibrous cartilage.

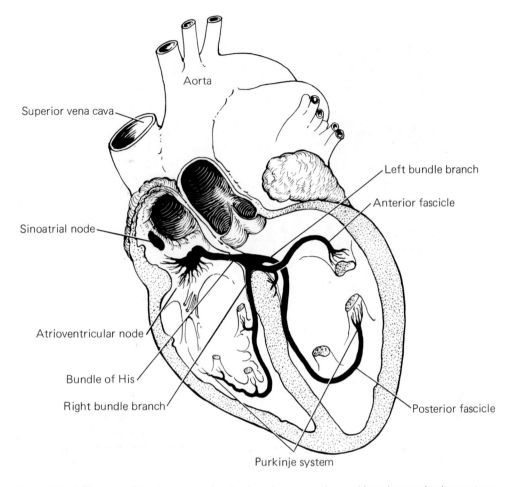

Figure 12–14. Diagram of the heart showing the impulse-generating and impulse-conducting system.

The **cardiac valves** consist of a central core of dense fibrous connective tissue lined on both sides by an endothelial layer. Their bases are attached to the annuli fibrosi of the fibrous skeleton.

Impulse-Generating & -Conducting System of the Heart; Innervation

The impulse-generating and conducting system of the heart consists of several structures that make it possible for the atria and ventricles to beat in succession and permit the heart to function as an efficient pump. The **sinoatrial node** (of Keith and Flack) is the "pacemaker" of the heart, since it has the most rapid rhythmic activity (Fig 12–14). It is located close to the entrance of the superior vena cava into the right atrium. The nodal cells are modified cardiac muscle cells, smaller than atrial muscle cells and with fewer myofibrils. Nodal cells are concentrically arranged around a large nodal artery. Some authors describe internodal tracts of specialized cells that conduct the electrical depolarization of the sinoatrial node to the **atrioventricular node** (of Tawara). This mass of spe-

cialized cardiac muscle cells lies beneath the endocardium of the septal wall of the right atrium. The nodal cells are similar to those of the sinoatrial node. In addition, there are large arterioles present as well as considerable amounts of adipose tissue. The **atrioventricular bundle of His** is formed by **Purkinje cells** (Fig 12–15) that penetrate the fibrous skeleton and then divide to form the **right** and **left bundle branches.** The left bundle again divides to form 2 fascicles. These bundles of Purkinje cells travel in the subendocardial layer to the apex of the heart, where they reverse their direction and begin giving off side branches that make contact with ordinary ("working") cardiac muscle cells via gap junctions. Owing to this arrangement, the stimulus for ventricular contraction is rapidly conducted to the apex of the heart, which must contract first to eject blood from the ventricles. Then, the wave of contraction sweeps toward the base of the heart (pulmonary valve and aortic valve).

Purkinje cells have a diameter considerably greater than ordinary cardiac muscle cells (30 μm versus 15

Connective tissue

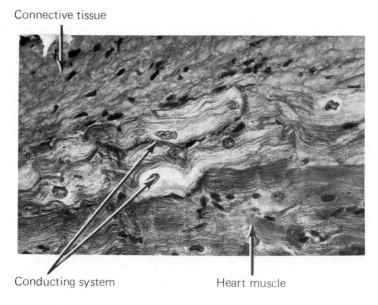

Conducting system   Heart muscle

Figure 12–15. The Purkinje cells of the conducting system of the heart are characterized by a reduced number of myofibrils present mainly in the periphery of the muscle cell. The light area around the nuclei of the conducting cells is due to local accumulation of glycogen. H&E stain, × 400.

μm) but are somewhat shorter (20–50 μm versus 80 μm). It is the greater diameter of Purkinje cells that is responsible for the rapid conduction of electrical activity. Purkinje cells have one or 2 centrally placed nuclei, an abundance of glycogen, and few peripherally disposed myofibrils. These cells are united longitudinally by intercalated disks.

Both the parasympathetic and the sympathetic divisions of the autonomic system contribute to innervation of the heart and form widespread plexuses at the base of the heart. In the regions close to the sinoatrial and atrioventricular nodes, ganglionic nerve cells and nerve fibers are present. It is known that these nerves do not affect generation of the heartbeat, a process attributed to the sinoatrial (pacemaker) node. These nerves do affect heart rhythm, whereby stimulation of the parasympathetic division (vagus nerve) promotes a slowing of the heartbeat, whereas stimulation of the sympathetic nerve accelerates the rhythm of the pacemaker.

Lymphatic Vascular System

Besides blood vessels, the human body has a system of thin-walled channels lined with endothelium that collects fluid from the tissue spaces and returns

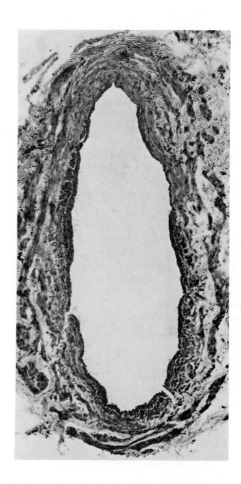

Figure 12–16 (at right). Section of the thoracic duct. H&E stain. × 200. (Reproduced, with permission, from Junqueira LC, Carneiro J: *Histologie.* Schiebler TH, Peiper U [translators]. Springer-Verlag, 1984.)

it to the blood. This fluid is called lymph; in contrast to the blood, it circulates in only one direction, ie, toward the heart.

The **lymphatic capillaries** originate in the various tissues as thin, blind-ended vessels. They consist of a single layer of endothelium. Lymphatic capillaries do not have fenestrations in their endothelial cells or a zonula occludens between neighboring cells, and they have practically no basal lamina. These thin vessels ultimately converge and end up as 2 large trunks, the **thoracic duct** and the **right lymphatic duct,** which empty into the junction of the left internal jugular vein with the left subclavian vein and into the confluence of the right subclavian vein and the right internal jugular vein. Interposed in the path of the lymphatic vessels are lymph nodes, whose morphology and functions are discussed in Chapter 15. With rare exceptions such as the nervous system and the bone marrow, a lymphatic system is found in almost all organs.

The larger lymphatic vessels have a structure similar to that of veins except they have thinner walls and lack a clear-cut separation between the 3 layers (intima, media, and adventitia). Like veins, they have numerous internal valves. These valves are, however, more numerous in lymphatic vessels. Between the valves the lymphatic vessels are dilated and assume a nodular, or beaded, appearance.

As in veins, lymphatic circulation is aided by the action of external forces (eg, contraction of surrounding skeletal muscle) on their walls. These forces act discontinuously, and unidirectional lymph flow occurs mainly as a result of the presence of many valves in these vessels. Contraction of smooth muscle in the walls of larger lymphatic vessels also helps propel lymph toward the heart.

The **lymphatic ducts** of large size (thoracic duct and right lymphatic duct) have a structure similar to that of a vein with a reinforcement of smooth muscle in the middle layer. In this layer, the muscle bundles are longitudinally and circularly arranged, with longitudinal fibers predominating (Fig 12–16). The adventitia is relatively underdeveloped. As with arteries and veins, large lymphatic ducts contain vasa vasorum and a rich neural network.

REFERENCES

Bruns RR, Palade GE: Studies on blood capillaries. 1. General organization of blood capillaries in muscle. 2. Transport of ferritin molecules across the wall of muscle capillaries. *J Cell Biol* 1968;**37**:244, 277.

Challice CE, Virágh S (editors): *Ultrastructure of the Mammalian Heart.* Academic Press, 1973.

Clementi F, Palade GE: Intestinal capillaries. 1. Permeability to peroxidase and ferritin. *J Cell Biol* 1969;**41**:33.

Cliff WJ: *Blood Vessels.* Cambridge Univ Press, 1976.

Cryer A (editor): *Biochemical Interactions at the Endothelium.* Elsevier Science, 1983.

Fishman AP (editor): Endothelium. *Ann NY Acad Sci* 1982; **481**:1. [Entire volume.]

Hüttner I, Boutet M, More RH: Gap junctions in arterial endothelium. *J Cell Biol* 1973;**57**:247.

Johnson PC: *Peripheral Circulation.* Wiley, 1978.

Joyce NE et al: Contractile proteins in pericytes. *J Cell Biol* 1985;**100**:1387.

Karnovsky MJ: The ultrastructural basis of capillary permeability studied with peroxidase as a tracer. *J Cell Biol* 1967;**35**:213.

Lauweryns JM, Boussauw L: The ultrastructure of lymphatic valves in the adult rabbit lung. *Z Zellforsch* 1973;**143**:149.

Leak LV: Normal anatomy of the lymphatic vascular system. In: *Handbuch der Allgemeine Pathologie.* Meessen H (editor). Springer-Verlag, 1972.

McDonald DM, Mitchell RA: The innervation of glomus cells, ganglion cells and blood vessels in the rat carotid body; A quantitative ultrastructural analysis. *J Neurocytol* 1975;**4**:177.

McNutt NS, Fawcett DW: Myocardial ultrastructure. In: *The Mammalian Myocardium.* Langer GA, Brady TW (editors). Wiley, 1974.

Papp M et al: An electron microscopic study of the central lacteal in the intestinal villus of the cat. *Z Zellforsch Mikrosk Anat* 1962;**57**:475.

Rhodin JAG: Architecture of the vessel wall. In: *Handbook of Physiology.* Section 2: Cardiovascular System. Vol 2. American Physiological Society, 1980.

Richardson JB, Beaulines A: The cellular site of action of angiotensin. *J Cell Biol* 1971;**51**:419.

Simionescu N: Cellular aspects of transcapillary exchange. *Physiol Rev* 1983;**63**:1536.

Somlyo AP, Somlyo AV: Excitation and contraction in vascular smooth muscle. In: *Structure and Function of the Circulation.* Vol 3. Schwartz CJ, Werthessen NT, Wolf S (editors). Plenum Press, 1981.

Thaemert JC: Fine structure of the atrioventricular node as viewed in serial sections. *Am J Anat* 1973;**136**:43.

Thorgeirsson G, Robertson AL Jr: The vascular endothelium: Pathobiologic significance. *Am J Pathol* 1978;**93**:802.

Truex RC: Structural basis of atrial and ventricular conduction. *Cardiovasc Clin* 1974;**6**:1.

Wagner D, Marder J: Biosynthesis of von Willebrand protein by human endothelial cells: Processing steps and their intracellular localization. *J Cell Biol* 1984;**99**:2123.

Williams MC, Wissig SL: The permeability of muscle capillaries to horseradish peroxidase. *J Cell Biol* 1975;**66**:531.

Wissig SL: Identification of the small pore in muscle capillaries. *Acta Physiol Scand [Suppl]* 1979;**463**:33.

Wissig SL, Williams MC: The permeability of muscle capillaries to microperoxidase. *J Cell Biol* 1978;**76**:341.

Woolf N: *Pathology of Atherosclerosis.* Butterworth, 1982.

Zetter BR: The endothelial cells of large and small blood vessels. *Diabetes* 1981;**30(Suppl 2)**:24.

13

Blood Cells

Blood consists of the cells and fluid contained in the closed circulatory system that flow in a regular unidirectional movement, propelled mainly by the rhythmic contractions of the heart. An adult human male has about 5.5 L of blood. Blood is made up of 2 parts: **formed elements,** or blood cells, and **plasma,** the liquid phase in which the former are suspended. The formed elements are **erythrocytes,** or red blood cells; **platelets;** and **leukocytes,** or white blood cells. Blood is a specialized connective tissue consisting of cells and an abundant fluid extracellular interstitium.

If blood is removed from the circulatory system, it will clot. This clot contains formed elements and a clear yellow liquid called **serum,** which separates from the coagulum during the phenomenon of coagulation. Blood serum is equivalent in composition to plasma except that it lacks **fibrinogen** and some other protein factors necessary for clot formation and contains **serotonin** in increased amounts.

Blood collected and kept from coagulating by the addition of anticoagulants (heparin, citrate, etc) separates, when centrifuged, into layers that reflect its heterogeneity (Fig 13–1). The **hematocrit** is an estimation of the volume of packed erythrocytes per unit volume of blood. The normal value is 40–50% in the adult male, 35–45% in the adult female, approximately 35% in a child up to age 10 years, and 45–60% in the newborn. In pregnancy, this value is diminished by physiologic hemodilution. The hematocrit is normally higher in venous blood than in arterial blood because of the hydration of red cells and their increase in size.

The translucent, yellowish, and somewhat viscous supernatant obtained when the hematocrit is measured is the plasma of the blood. The formed elements of the blood separate into 2 easily distinguishable layers. The lower layer represents 42–47% of the entire volume of blood present in the hematocrit tube. It is red and is made up of erythrocytes. The layer immediately above (1% of the blood volume), which is white or grayish in color, is called the **buffy coat** and consists of leukocytes. This separation occurs because the leukocytes are less dense than the erythrocytes. Covering the leukocytes is a fine layer of platelets not distinguishable by the naked eye.

Leukocytes, some of which are phagocytic, constitute one of the chief defenses against infection and

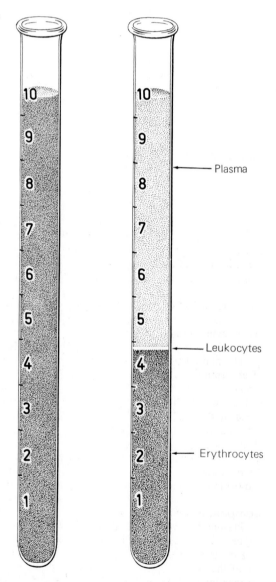

Figure 13–1. Hematocrit tubes with blood. *Left:* Before centrifugation. *Right:* After centrifugation. In the centrifuged tube, the red blood cells represent 43% of the blood volume. Between the sedimented red blood cells and the supernatant light-colored plasma is a thin layer of leukocytes called the buffy coat.

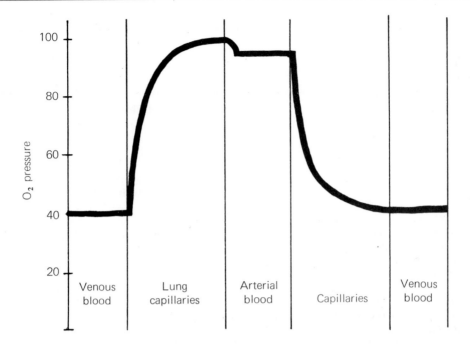

Figure 13–2. Blood oxygen content in each type of blood vessel. The amount of oxygen (O_2 pressure) is highest in lung capillaries and in arteries and decreases in tissue capillaries, where exchange takes place between blood and tissues.

circulate through the body via the blood vascular system. By crossing the capillary wall, these cells become concentrated rapidly in the tissues and participate in the inflammatory response. The blood vascular system is also the vehicle for the transport of oxygen (O_2) (Fig 13–2) and carbon dioxide (CO_2); O_2 is bound mainly to the hemoglobin of the erythrocytes, whereas CO_2, in addition to being bound to the proteins of the erythrocytes (mainly hemoglobin), is also carried in solution in the plasma as CO_2 or in the form of HCO_3^-.

The plasma transports metabolites from their site of absorption or synthesis, distributing them to different areas of the organism. It also transports the residues of metabolism, which are removed from the blood by the excretory organs. Blood, being the distributing vehicle for the hormones, permits the exchange of chemical messages between distant organs for normal cellular function. It further participates in the regulation of body temperature and in acid-base and osmotic balance.

Composition of Plasma

Plasma is an aqueous solution containing substances of small or large molecular weight comprising 10% of its volume. The plasma proteins account for 7% of the volume and the inorganic salts for 0.9%; the remainder of the 10% consists of several organic compounds of different origin—amino acids, vitamins, hormones, lipoproteins, etc.

Through the capillary walls, the low-molecular-weight components of plasma are in equilibrium with the interstitial fluid of the tissues. The composition of plasma is usually an indicator of the mean composition of the extracellular fluids in general.

Plasma proteins can be separated in the ultracentrifuge or by electrophoresis into **albumin; alpha, beta,** and **gamma globulins;** and **fibrinogen.** Albumin is the main component and has a fundamental role in maintaining the osmotic pressure of the blood. The gamma globulins are antibodies and are called **immunoglobulins.** Fibrinogen is necessary for the formation of fibrin in the final step of coagulation.

Several substances insoluble or only slightly soluble in water can be transported by the plasma because they combine with albumin or with the alpha and beta globulins. For example, lipids are insoluble in the plasma but combine with the hydrophobic portions of protein molecules. Since the protein molecules also have hydrophilic parts, the lipid-protein complex is soluble in water.

Staining of Blood Cells

Blood cells are generally studied in smears or films prepared by spreading a drop of blood thinly over a microscope slide (Fig 13–3). The blood should be evenly distributed over the slide and allowed to dry rapidly in air. In such films the cells are clearly visible and distinct from one another. Their cytoplasm is spread out, thus facilitating observation of their nuclei and cytoplasmic organization.

Blood smears are routinely stained with special dye mixtures first discovered by Dimitri Romanovsky and modified by other investigators. In 1891, Romanovsky observed that a mixture of solutions of

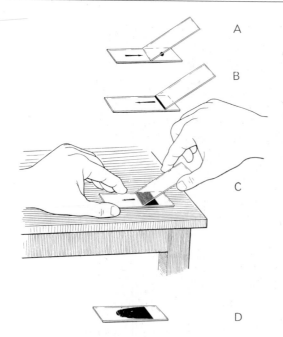

Figure 13-3. Preparation of a blood smear. *A:* A drop of blood is placed on a microscope slide. A second slide is moved over the first at an angle of 45 degrees. *B:* When the slide edge touches the blood drop, the blood spreads along the edge. *C:* With a uniform movement of the oblique slide, a thin film of blood is spread on the horizontal fixed slide. *D:* After air drying, slides are fixed and stained.

philia (yellowish-pink); and (4) affinity for a complex dye present in the mixture—incorrectly thought to be neutral—is known as **neutrophilia** (salmon-pink to lilac).

FORMED ELEMENTS OF BLOOD

Erythrocytes

Most mammalian erythrocytes (red blood cells) are described as biconcave disks without nuclei (Fig 13–4). When suspended in an isotonic medium, human erythrocytes are 7.8 μm in diameter, 2.6 μm thick at the rim, and 0.8 μm thick in the center. However, when dried and stained to make a routine blood film, they shrink to 7.2–7.4 μm in diameter and 1.9 μm in thickness at the rim (Fig 13–5). The biconcave shape provides erythrocytes with a large surface-to-volume ratio, thus facilitating gas exchange.

The normal concentration of erythrocytes in blood is approximately 3.9–5.5 million/μL in women and 4.1–6 million/μL in men (Table 13–1).

Erythrocytes with diameters greater than 9 μm are called **macrocytes,** and those with diameters less than 6 μm are called **microcytes.** The presence of a high percentage of erythrocytes varying greatly in size is called **anisocytosis.**

methylene blue and eosin in certain proportions stained the nuclei of leukocytes and malarial parasites purple. Other components of the cell may stain pink owing to eosin binding, or shades of red-blue resulting from the binding of **azures.** Azures are oxidation products of methylene blue and are positively charged (as is methylene blue). Positively charged dyes are known as basic dyes. Eosin is a negatively charged dye and is therefore called an acidic dye. Thus, some information about the net charge of cellular constituents is obtained by observing their affinity for acidic or basic dyes.

Stains currently used to study blood cells differ slightly in the proportion of their components and in the way methylene blue is oxidized. They are named for the investigator who first introduced the modification. Leishman's, Wright's, and Giemsa's stains are examples of modified stains collectively known as Romanovsky-type mixtures.

After application of a Romanovsky-type mixture, blood cell types can be distinguished based on 4 staining characteristics representing the affinity of cellular structures for the respective dyes of the mixture: (1) affinity for methylene blue (a basic dye) is known as **basophilia** (purple); (2) affinity for the azures is known as **azurophilia** (red-blue); (3) affinity for the eosin (an acidic stain) is known as **acidophilia** or **eosino-**

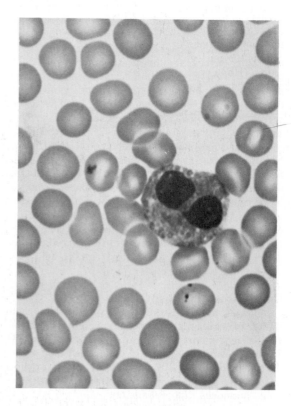

Figure 13-4. Photomicrograph of a Leishman-stained human blood smear. There are numerous erythrocytes and one granulocyte (eosinophil) present. × 1300.

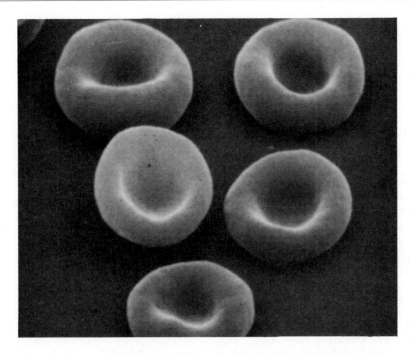

Figure 13–5. Scanning electron micrograph of normal human erythrocytes. Note their biconcave shape. × 6500.

The erythrocyte is quite flexible, and this property permits it to adapt to the irregular shape and small diameter of capillaries. Observations in vivo show that, when traversing the angles of capillary bifurcations, erythrocytes containing normal adult hemoglobin (HbA) are easily deformed and frequently assume a cuplike shape. As a consequence of a single amino acid substitution in the beta chain of hemoglobin A (Glu → Val), the altered hemoglobin (HbS) becomes insoluble at low oxygen tensions and crystallizes into long rods. This results in the clinical syndrome called **sickle cell anemia.** Erythrocytes containing these long rods are distorted (Fig 13–6) and very inflexible, and when forced through narrow

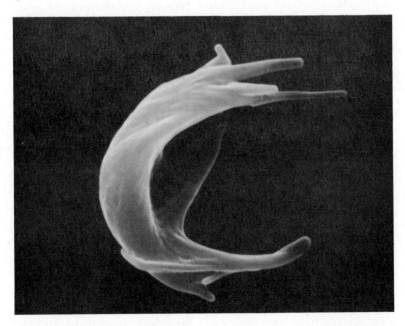

Figure 13–6. Scanning electron micrograph of a distorted red blood cell from a person who is homozygous for the HbS gene (sickle cell anemia). × 6500.

Table 13–1. Size and number of human blood cells.

Cell	Size	Number*
Erythrocytes	6.5–8 μm (mean = 7.5 μm)	4.1–6 × 10⁶/μL (males) 3.9–5.5 × 10⁶/μL (females)
Leukocytes		6000–10,000/μL
Neutrophil	12–15 μm	60–70%
Eosinophil	12–15 μm	2–4%
Basophil	12–15 μm	0–1%
Lymphocyte	6–18 μm	20–30%
Monocyte	12–20 μm	3–8%
Platelets	2–4 μm	200,000–400,000/μL

*Some references give these values per cubic millimeter (mm^3). Microliters and cubic millimeters are identical units.

apertures such as those encountered in the spleen (see Chapter 15), they rupture, and anemia is a consequence.

Erythrocytes are surrounded by a plasmalemma, which, because of its ready availability, is the best-known membrane of any cell. It consists of about 40% lipid (phospholipids, cholesterol, glycolipids, etc), 50% protein, and 10% carbohydrate. About half of the proteins span the lipid bilayer and are known as **integral membrane proteins** (see Chapter 3). A well-studied erythrocyte integral membrane protein is glycophorin, which has 16 complex oligosaccharide chains exposed at the external surface of the cell. The composition and sequence of 5 N-terminal amino acids of glycophorin, exposed at the extracellular surfaces of erythrocytes, determine the MN blood group to which an individual belongs. Glycophorin has no other known function. The ABO blood group determinants are terminal sugars of oligosaccharides on membrane glycoproteins and glycolipids. Several **peripheral** proteins are associated with the inner surface of the erythrocyte membrane, including spectrin and actin, which seem to serve as a membrane skeleton determining the unusual shape of the red blood cell (Fig 3–4A). Spectrin and actin are bound to certain erythrocyte integral membrane proteins via other peripheral membrane proteins known as ankyrin and protein 4.1. These membrane-associated proteins also permit the flexibility of the membrane necessary for the large changes in shape that occur when the erythrocyte passes through capillaries. Because red blood cells are not rigid, the viscosity of blood remains low.

The red cell membrane also acts as a semipermeable barrier, maintaining differences in the concentrations of sodium and potassium between the plasma and the interior of the cell. This is due to ATP-dependent active transport molecules in the membrane that are specific for sodium and potassium. Anion channels identified with the protein 3 tetramer are also present. If placed in a hypotonic medium, erythrocytes swell, become spherical, and lose hemoglobin to the surrounding fluid. This phenomenon is called **hemolysis.** The resulting (virtually pure) membranes are called **ghosts** and are the starting material for studies of membrane structure. On the other hand, if erythrocytes are submitted to hypertonic conditions, the cells shrink irregularly, leaving protuberances on their surfaces, resulting in **crenated** red blood cells.

In their interiors, erythrocytes contain a 33% solution of **hemoglobin,** the oxygen-carrying protein that accounts for their acidophilia. In addition, there are enzymes of the glycolytic and hexose monophosphate shunt pathways of glucose metabolism.

The hemoglobin molecule (a conjugated protein) consists of 4 subunits, each containing a heme group covalently linked to a polypeptide. The heme group is a porphyrin derivative containing ferrous iron (Fe^{2+}).

Owing to variations in each polypeptide chain attached to the heme, various types of hemoglobin can be distinguished, several of which are considered normal: hemoglobins A_1 (HbA₁), A_2, (HbA₂), and F (HbF) are found normally in postnatal life.

HbA₁ represents 97% of the normal hemoglobin in adults; HbA₂ represents 2%. HbF (fetal hemoglobin; 1%) is the predominant hemoglobin of the fetus—around 80% of the hemoglobin in newborns—and decreases progressively to lower levels until the eighth postnatal month, when it represents a small percentage similar to that found in adults.

Combined with oxygen or carbon dioxide, hemoglobin forms **oxyhemoglobin** or **carbaminohemoglobin,** respectively. These combinations are reversible, which is the basis for the gas-transporting capability of hemoglobin. However, the combination of hemoglobin with carbon monoxide (**carboxyhemoglobin**) is irreversible, resulting in reduced capacity to transport oxygen.

Erythrocytes recently released by the bone marrow into the bloodstream often contain ribosomal RNA (rRNA), which, in the presence of supravital dyes (eg, brilliant cresyl blue), can be precipitated and stained. Under these conditions, the younger erythrocytes, which are called **reticulocytes,** may have a few granules or a netlike structure in their cytoplasm (Figs 14–2 and 14–5). Reticulocytes normally constitute about 1% of the total number of circulating red blood cells, since that is the rate at which erythrocytes are replaced daily by the bone marrow. Increased numbers of reticulocytes indicate increased demand for oxygen-carrying capacity, which may be due to hemorrhage or recent ascent to high altitude. The process by which reticulocytes are released from the bone marrow into the circulation is not completely understood.

Red blood cells lose their mitochondria, ribosomes, and many cytoplasmic enzymes during maturation from reticulocytes to adult erythrocytes, a process that takes 24–48 hours. This breakdown of organelles and enzymes is not mediated by lysosomal enzymes. Instead, a group of ATP-dependent enzymes, present in the cytoplasm, are responsible for the disappearance of proteins and organelles during erythrocyte development. The source of energy for erythrocytes is glucose, 90% of which is anaerobically degraded to lactate. The remaining 10% is aerobically utilized through the hexose monophosphate pathway. Erythrocytes do not synthesize hemoglobin, since they do not have a nucleus or other organelles necessary for protein synthesis.

Erythrocytes of humans survive in the circulation for about 120 days. This is measured by labeling young erythrocytes with ^{14}C-glycine or ^{15}N-glycine and determining their survival. Worn-out erythrocytes are removed from the circulation by macrophages of the spleen and bone marrow. The signal for removal seems to be the appearance of defective complex oligosaccharides attached to integral membrane proteins of the plasmalemma. Sialic acid is removed from the ends of these molecules, but how this is timed so exactly is not yet understood.

Sometimes—mainly in disease states—nuclear fragments (containing DNA) remain in the erythrocyte after extrusion of its nucleus, which occurs late in its development (see Chapter 14). These nuclear remnants are Feulgen-positive and stain with basic dyes. Often they take the form of one or 2 small granules (1 μm in size) and are called **Howell-Jolly bodies.** When they appear as circular filaments, they are called **Cabot rings.**

Leukocytes

On the basis of the type of granule in their cytoplasm and the shape of the nucleus, white blood cells are classified into 2 groups: (1) **Granulocytes** (polymorphonuclear leukocytes) possess **specific granules,** ie, granules that specifically bind either the neutral, acidic, or basic component of the Romanovsky-type dye mixture. In addition, the nucleus has 2 to several lobes. Granulocytes include the **neutrophils, eosinophils,** and **basophils.** (2) **Agranulocytes** (mononuclear leukocytes) do not have specific granules, but they do have several to many granules that are azurophilic; ie, they bind the azure dyes of the stain. The nucleus is round or indented. This group includes the **lymphocytes** and **monocytes.**

The size and frequency (differential count) of blood leukocytes are presented in Table 13–1.

Leukocytes are involved in the cellular and humoral defense of the organism against foreign material. They are spherical, nonmotile cells when in suspension in the circulating blood but are capable of becoming flattened and motile on encountering a solid substrate. Leukocytes may leave the capillaries by passing between endothelial cells and penetrating the connective tissue **(diapedesis).** The population of leukocytes in connective tissue is so great that they are considered normal cellular components of that tissue.

The number of leukocytes per microliter of blood in the normal adult is 6000–10,000; at birth, it varies between 15,000 and 25,000, and by the fourth day it falls to 12,000. At 4 years, the average is around 8000 with a maximum normal limit of 12,000. The white count reaches normal adult values at about 12 years of age. There is a qualitative variation within the white cell population depending on age; thus, at birth there is a preponderance of neutrophils, but by the second week lymphocytes constitute around 60% of the leukocytes and predominate during infancy until age 4, when the granulocytes and lymphocytes are equal in number. There follows a progressive increase in the percentage of granulocytes, and at age 14–15 years the percentages typical of the adult (60–70%) are reached. Not only the percentage but also the absolute number of each cell type per unit of blood volume must be taken into consideration when studying physiologic and pathologic variations in the number of blood cells.

Neutrophils (Polymorphonuclear Leukocytes)

These cells, which constitute 60–70% of circulating leukocytes, develop in the bone marrow and are released into the circulation. They are 12–15 μm in diameter, with a nucleus consisting of 2–5 lobes (usually 3 lobes) linked to each other by fine threads of chromatin (Fig 13–7). The immature neutrophil (band form) has a nonsegmented nucleus in the shape of a horseshoe.

The nuclei of all granulocytes have a similar chromatin pattern, in which dense masses of heterochromatin are distributed on the inner surface of the nuclear envelope (Fig 13–8). Zones of loosely arranged euchromatin are located mainly in the center of the nucleus. Nucleoli are not present.

Neutrophils with more than 5 lobes are called **hypersegmented** and represent old cells. Although under normal conditions the maturation of the neutrophil parallels the increase in the number of nuclear lobes, this relationship is not absolute. In some pathologic conditions, young cells appear with 5 or more lobes.

In the living neutrophil, the shape of the nucleus is variable. The chromatin bridges that unite the nuclear lobes frequently change position and vary in number. Therefore, for the same cell, the number of lobes is variable from time to time depending on the moment when it is observed.

In females, the inactivated X chromosome appears as an appendage ("drumstick") on one of the lobes of the nucleus (Fig 13–7). However, in only a few neutrophils will this be obvious.

The abundant cytoplasm of the neutrophil contains 2 types of granules of different sizes and staining properties. The more abundant granules are the **specific granules,** which are stained a salmon-pink color by Romanovsky-type dyes (Fig 13–7). Since the size of these granules lies close to the limit of resolution of the optical microscope, individual specific granules are not easily seen in routine blood smears. However, their presence is indicated by the salmon-pink color of the cytoplasm. Most neutrophil specific granules are spherical (0.1 μm in diameter), but a few rod-shaped forms (0.1 $\times$ 1 μm) can be seen in the electron microscope. Specific granules are surrounded by a typical unit membrane and have been shown to contain alkaline phosphatase, collagenase,

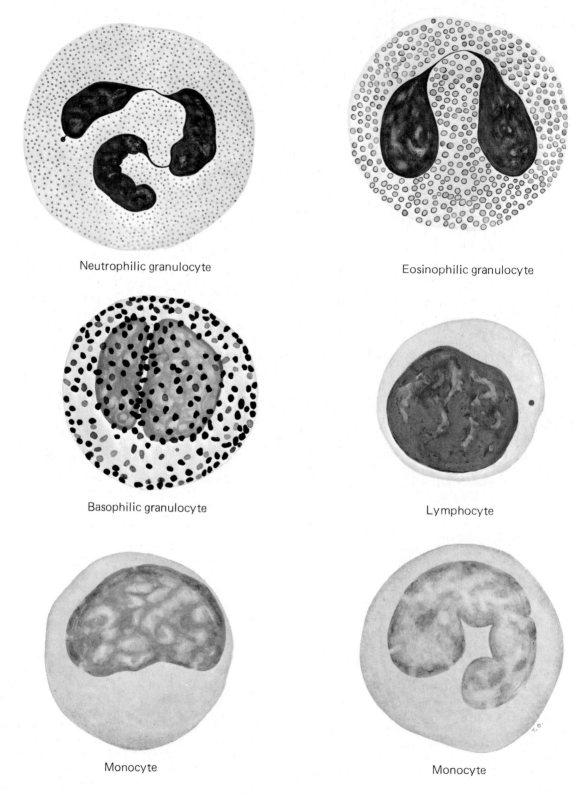

Neutrophilic granulocyte

Eosinophilic granulocyte

Basophilic granulocyte

Lymphocyte

Monocyte

Monocyte

Figure 13–7. The 5 types of human leukocytes. The drawings were made from blood smears stained by the Romanovsky technique. (This illustration is reproduced in color on p x.)

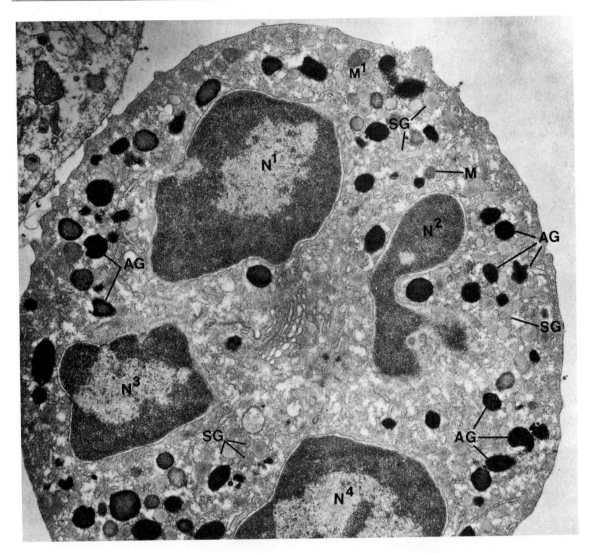

Figure 13–8. Electron micrograph of a human neutrophil stained for peroxidase. The cytoplasm contains 2 types of granules: the small, pale, peroxidase-negative specific granules (SG) and the larger, dense, peroxidase-positive azurophilic granules (AG). The nucleus is lobulated (N^1–N^4), and the Golgi complex (G) is small. Rough endoplasmic reticulum and mitochondria (M) are not abundant, since this cell is in the terminal stage of its differentiation. × 27,000. (Reproduced, with permission, from Bainton DF: Selective abnormalities of azurophil and specific granules of human neutrophilic leukocytes. *Fed Proc* 1981;**40:**1443.)

lactoferrin, some poorly characterized basic proteins called phagocytins, and two-thirds of the total neutrophil lysozyme.

The second granule population in neutrophils consists of **azurophilic granules** about 0.5 μm in diameter that stain a deep reddish-purple owing to a metachromatic shift when the azure dyes are bound. These granules are primary lysosomes and contain the enzymatic activities listed in Table 13–2.

In fully differentiated neutrophils, approximately one-third of the granules are azurophilic, while the remainder are specific granules.

The cytoplasm also contains a few mitochondria,

a small Golgi complex, a rudimentary rough endoplasmic reticulum, a few free ribosomes, and considerable amounts of glycogen. Glycogen is broken down to yield energy via the glycolytic and hexose monophosphate shunt pathways of glucose oxidation. The citric acid (Krebs) cycle is less important, as might be expected in view of the paucity of mitochondria in these cells. The ability of neutrophils to survive in an anaerobic environment is highly advantageous, since they can kill bacteria and help clean up debris in poorly oxygenated regions such as necrotic tissue.

Neutrophils are short-lived cells with a half-life in blood of 6–7 hours and a life span of 1–4 days in

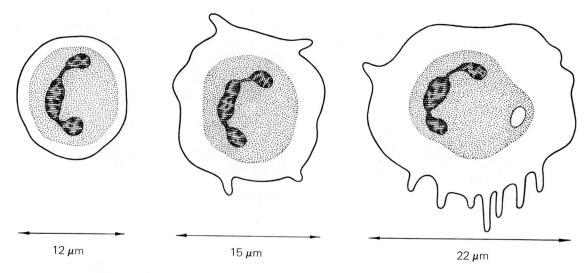

Figure 13–9. Neutrophils undergo a process called "expansion" when in contact with a solid surface. Filopodial processes spread out from the hyaloplasm; at the same time, the cell increases its diameter with no increase in volume as a result of flattening on the substrate.

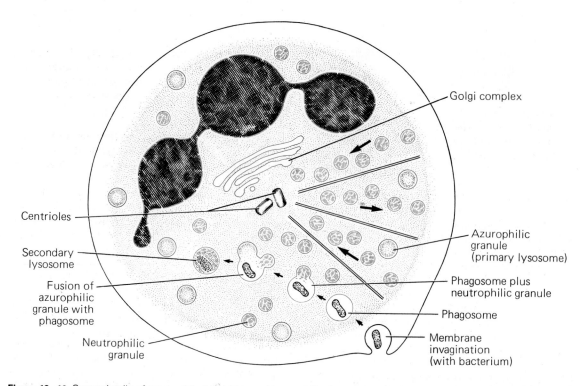

Figure 13–10. Some details of neutrophil ultrastructure. Neutrophilic granules move constantly; microtubules radiate from the centrioles. The direction of this movement is indicated by larger arrows. The lower part of the figure shows the process of intracellular digestion of a phagocytized bacterium (smaller arrows). Neutrophil specific granules fuse with the phagosome, providing molecules that kill the bacterium. Later, azurophilic granules fuse with this vacuole and introduce the acid hydrolases that digest the bacterium.

Table 13–2. Granule composition in human granulocytes.

Cell	Specific Granules	Azurophilic Granules
Neutrophils	Alkaline phosphatase Collagenase Lactoferrin Lysozyme (2/3)	Acid phosphatase α-Mannosidase Arylsulfatase β-Galactosidase β-Glucuronidase Cathepsin 5′ Nucleotidase Elastase Collagenase Myeloperoxidase Lysozyme (1/3) Acidic mucosubstances Cationic antibacterial proteins
Eosinophils	Acid phosphatase Arylsulfatase β-Glucuronidase Cathepsin Phospholipase RNAase Myeloperoxidase Basic protein	
Basophils	Eosinophil chemo- tactic factor Heparin Histamine Peroxidase	

connective tissues. They die thereafter, whether or not they have engaged in phagocytosis. Because of this short life span, there is no need to produce additional granules; therefore, the protein synthetic apparatus is poorly developed.

Neutrophils constitute the first line of defense against invasion by microorganisms, especially bacteria. They are active phagocytes of small particles and have sometimes been called microphages to distinguish them from macrophages, which take up larger particles. These cells are inactive and spherical while circulating but change shape upon adhering to a solid substrate, over which they migrate via pseudopodia. The cells move at a speed of 19–36 μm/min. Following adhesion to a supporting surface, these granulocytes undergo a process called "expansion" or spreading, characterized by the emission of cytoplasmic processes in various directions that are transformed into fringes of hyaloplasm (cytoplasm without granules), attaining a diameter of 20 μm. It is interesting to note that the granules keep a distance of 3–5 μm from the cell boundary where ruffling of the membrane is occurring (Fig 13–9). In this process, the base of the cell does not adhere to the substrate but maintains itself above the surface and touches the substrate only with filamentous projections of the hyaloplasm.

The particle to be phagocytized by the neutrophil is surrounded by pseudopodia that fuse around it (Fig 13–10); thus, the particle eventually occupies a vacuole (phagosome) delimited by a membrane derived from the cell surface. Immediately thereafter, specific granules fuse with and discharge their contents into the phagosome. By means of proton pumps in the phagosome membrane, the pH of the vacuole is lowered to about 4.0. Then the azurophilic granules (primary lysosomes) discharge their enzymes into the acid environment, where killing and digestion of the bacterium is accomplished.

During phagocytosis, a burst of oxygen consumption occurs and leads to hydrogen peroxide formation. Together with myeloperoxidase and halide ions, a powerful cytotoxic system is formed. This system may act by adding bulky halide groups (Cl^-, I^-) to essential proteins, thereby interfering with their function. Strong oxidizing agents are also formed (eg, hypochlorite) that can inactivate proteins. These agents are effective against bacteria, fungi, viruses, and mammalian cells. Lysozyme has the function of specifically cleaving a bond in the peptidoglycan that forms the cell wall of some gram-positive bacteria, thus causing their death. Lactoferrin avidly binds iron, and since this is a crucial element in bacterial nutrition, lack of available iron leads to bacterial death. The acid environment of phagocytic vacuoles can itself cause the death of certain microorganisms. Thus, a combination of these mechanisms will kill most microorganisms.

Lysosomal enzymes of the azurophilic granules hydrolyze the dead bacterium to its constituent small molecules. These diffuse out of the cell and provide a small amount of nutrients to surrounding tissues.

Eosinophils

Eosinophils are much less numerous than neutrophils, constituting only 2–4% of leukocytes in normal blood. The cell has a diameter of 12–15 μm and contains a characteristic bilobed nucleus (Fig 13–7). The endoplasmic reticulum, Golgi complex, and mitochondria are poorly developed (Fig 13–11). Glycogen particles are relatively abundant. The main identifying characteristic is the presence of many large, refractile specific granules that are stained by eosin. These granules are 0.5–1.5 μm in length and 0.3–1 μm in width. There are about 200 specific granules per cell.

Eosinophil specific granules are surrounded by a unit membrane. A crystalline core (**internum**) lies parallel to the long axis of the granule (Fig 13–11). It is composed of a protein (MW 9200) containing a large number of arginine residues and called the major basic protein. This protein constitutes 50% of the total granule protein and accounts for the eosinophilia of these granules. The major basic protein also seems to function in the killing of parasitic worms such as schistosomes. The less dense material surrounding the internum is known as the **externum** or **matrix** and consists of the enzymes listed in Table 13–2. Eosinophil myeloperoxidase is different from that found in neutrophils in that it has little antibacterial activity.

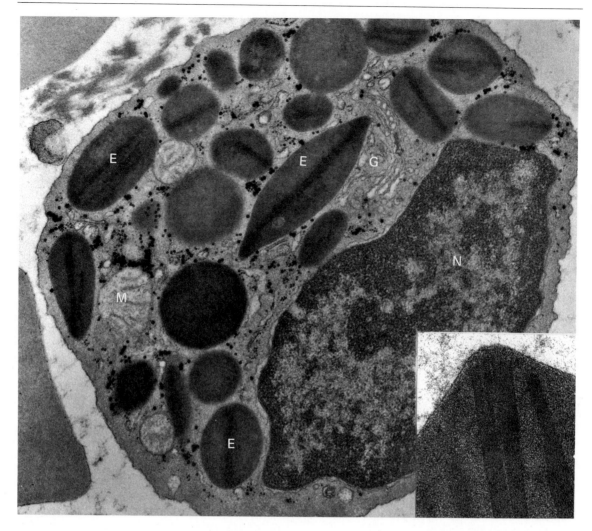

Figure 13–11. Electron micrographs of rabbit eosinophil. Observe a nuclear lobe (N), the Golgi complex (G), a mitochondrion (M), and the eosinophil specific granules (E). × 21,500. The inset shows a higher magnification of a specific granule revealing its crystalloid organization. × 132,000. (Courtesy of DF Bainton and MG Farquhar.)

Thus, in the eosinophil, the specific granules are primary lysosomes, whereas in neutrophils, azurophilic granules fulfill the function of primary lysosomes.

An increase in the absolute number of eosinophils in blood (**eosinophilia**) is associated with allergic reactions and infections by helminthic parasites. In tissues, eosinophils are found in the connective tissues underlying epithelia of the skin, bronchi, gastrointestinal tract, uterus, and vagina and surrounding the parasitic worms. A major function of eosinophils is phagocytosis and disposal of antigen-antibody complexes formed as part of the allergic response in asthma and hay fever. These cells can inactivate mediators of inflammation such as the leukotrienes (SRS-A) and histamine. Eosinophils also assist in killing helminths. Specific granules fuse with phagocytic vacuoles, and the soluble hydrolases in the matrix digest the phagocytized material. The internum remains intact in the vacuole for a long time.

Corticosteroids (hormones from the adrenal cortex) produce a rapid fall in the number of blood eosinophils; however, these hormones have no effect on bone marrow eosinophils. Corticosteroids probably interfere with the release of granulocytes from the bone marrow into the bloodstream.

Basophils

Basophils make up less than 1% of blood leukocytes and therefore are difficult to locate in smears of normal blood. They are about 12–15 μm in diameter and have a less heterochromatic nucleus than other granulocytes. The nucleus is divided into irregular lobes, but this is usually obscured by the overlying specific granules.

The specific granules (0.5 μm in diameter) stain metachromatically with the basic dye of the Romanovsky-type mixture (Fig 13–7). This staining is due to the presence of heparin. There are fewer specific

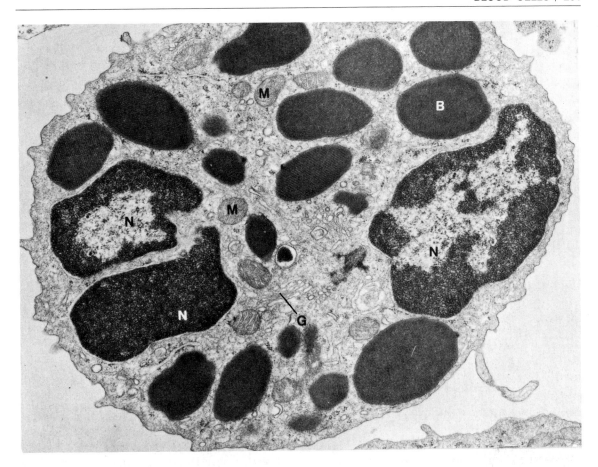

Figure 13–12. Electron micrograph of a rabbit basophil. The lobulated nucleus (N) appears as 3 separated portions. Note the basophilic granules (B), the mitochondria (M), and the Golgi complex (G). × 16,000. (Reproduced, with permission, from Terry RW, Bainton DF, Farquhar MG: *Lab Invest* 1969;**21**:65.)

granules in basophils when compared with the granule content of the other granulocytes. They are also more irregular in size and shape. When viewed with the electron microscope, each granule is surrounded by a unit membrane, and a lamellar or spherical substructure is present (Fig 13–12). Basophil specific granules contain heparin and histamine and are capable of generating leukotrienes (SRS-A), which cause slow contraction of smooth muscles. Basophils may supplement the functions of mast cells in immediate hypersensitivity reactions by migrating into connective tissues under special circumstances.

There is some similarity between granules of basophils and those of mast cells (see Chapter 5). Both are metachromatic and contain heparin and histamine. In response to certain antigens, basophils can liberate their granule content, as happens with the mast cell (see Chapter 5). Despite the similarities they present, mast cells and basophils are not the same, for in the same species they have different ultrastructural appearances and they originate from different stem cells in the bone marrow. Under certain conditions, basophils constitute the major cell type in an inflam-

matory site. This condition has been called **cutaneous basophil hypersensitivity.** Like the other granulocytes, basophils are capable of ameboid movement and phagocytosis, although they are not very active in this respect.

Lymphocytes

These are spherical cells with diameters of 6–8 μm. Lymphocytes with these dimensions are known as **small lymphocytes** (Fig 13–7). In the circulating blood there occurs a small number of **medium-sized lymphocytes** and **large lymphocytes** with diameters up to 18 μm. This distinction has functional significance in that the larger lymphocytes are thought to be cells activated by specific antigens. These cells will differentiate into effector T or B lymphocytes (see below).

The small lymphocyte, predominant in the blood, has a spherical nucleus, sometimes with an indentation. Its chromatin is condensed and appears as coarse clumps, so that the nucleus is intensely stained in the usual preparations, a characteristic that facilitates the identification of the lymphocyte (Figs 13–7 and

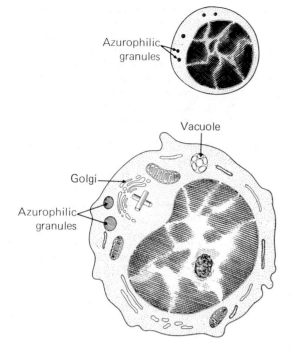

Azurophilic granules

Vacuole

Golgi

Azurophilic granules

Figure 13–13. A medium lymphocyte as seen with the light microscope *(above)* and the electron microscope *(below)*. Cytoplasmic organelles are scanty. Small lymphocytes have even less cytoplasm.

13–13). In blood smears, the nucleolus of the lymphocyte is not visible, but it can be demonstrated by special staining techniques and with the electron microscope.

The cytoplasm of the small lymphocyte is scanty, and in blood smears it appears as a thin rim around the nucleus. It is slightly basophilic, assuming a light blue color in stained smears (Fig 13–7). It may contain azurophilic granules that stain purple by Romanovsky-type mixtures. The cytoplasm of the small lymphocyte has a few mitochondria and a small Golgi complex associated with a pair of centrioles but contains many free ribosomes and polyribosomes (Fig 13–14).

In addition to their difference in size, the criteria that serve to distinguish large and small lymphocytes are that large ones have (1) an abundance of cytoplasm, greater numbers of polyribosomes, and a few cisternae of rough endoplasmic reticulum; (2) fewer coarse heterochromatin clumps in their nuclei; (3) visible nucleoli within more euchromatic nuclei; and (4) more mitochondria and larger Golgi complexes.

Although morphologically similar, lymphocytes of blood constitute a heterogeneous cell population. Experimental evidence, based on studies of electrophoretic mobility, surface topography, histologic localization, buoyant density, and responsiveness to mitogens, suggests the existence of several subgroups of lymphocytes with different and characteristic im-

munologic functions. They vary in life span; some lymphocytes live only a few days while others survive in the circulating blood for many years.

A fundamental division of lymphocytes into 2 classes can be made on the basis of their site of differentiation and their possession of distinctive integral membrane proteins. Precursor cells originate in the bone marrow in late fetal life, and slow proliferation of these precursor cells continues during postnatal life. Differentiation into immunocompetent cells occurs in the bone marrow and in the thymus (see Chapter 15).

In the early 1960s, experiments using chicken embryos revealed one of the anatomic sites of lymphocyte differentiation. The **bursa of Fabricius** is a mass of lymphoid tissue associated with the cloaca of birds. When this tissue is destroyed in the embryo (either surgically or by the administration of high levels of testosterone), chickens lack the ability to produce immunoglobulins (IgM, IgG, etc) against specific antigens. In other words, **humoral immunity** is impaired. The number of lymphocytes found in specific areas in lymph nodes and spleen is profoundly reduced, leading to the designation of these regions as bursa-dependent areas. The lymphocytes affected are called **B lymphocytes** or B cells. In mammals (including humans), it is generally believed that B lymphocytes acquire their differentiated characters in special microenvironments in the bone marrow.

Experiments on newborn mice demonstrated that removal of the **thymus** (see Chapter 15) resulted in profound deficiencies in **cellular immune responses**—responses that require the presence of living cells in contrast to humoral responses that depend on circulating immunoglobulins (Fig 15–6). An important example of a cellular immune response in humans is rejection of transplanted organs, such as skin or kidney. In thymectomized mice, the lymph nodes and spleen showed depletion of lymphocytes in areas different from those affected by removal of the bursa of Fabricius. These are the thymus-dependent areas, and the cells involved are called **T lymphocytes** or T cells.

The thymus and the bursa-equivalent in mammals (bone marrow) are called **primary** or **central lymphoid organs,** and lymphocytes differentiated in these organs colonize **secondary** or **peripheral** areas of the body where lymphoid tissues are found in diffuse, encapsulated, or organ form (see Chapter 15).

In blood, most lymphocytes (~ 80%) are T cells with a very long life. These cells have several functions. They can regulate the activity of other T cells or B cells both positively (**helper T cells**) and negatively (**suppressor T cells**). T cells elaborate several factors (**lymphokines**) that affect the behavior of macrophages, such as their movement toward inflammatory sites. Some T lymphocytes (**cytotoxic cells**) secrete substances that kill other cells, including tumor cells and foreign grafts. A far smaller percentage of circulating lymphocytes (~ 15%) are B cells, which, upon appropriate stimulation, divide several times and differentiate into plasma cells in tissues and produce immunoglobulins. Specific immunoglobulins (**opso-**

nins) coat bacteria and other invaders, making them more susceptible to phagocytosis by macrophages. Finally, there are a few lymphocytes in blood ($\sim$ 5%) that have neither T nor B lymphocyte surface antigens and are called **null cells.** These cells may be circulating stem cells.

Lymphocytes also display the phenomenon of **immunologic memory.** Each lymphocyte is primed to respond to only one antigen. Upon first encountering its specific antigen, the lymphocyte undergoes several cell divisions. Some of the resulting cells differentiate into **effector cells;** eg, a B lymphocyte will differentiate into a plasma cell that will secrete antibodies. Other cells remain inactive (**memory cells**) but are primed to respond more rapidly and to a greater extent upon subsequent exposure to the specific antigen.

Monocytes

These bone marrow–derived agranulocytes have diameters varying from 12 to 20 μm (Fig 13–7). The nucleus is oval, horseshoe-shaped, or kidney-shaped and is generally eccentrically placed. The chromatin is less condensed and has a more fibrillar arrangement than in the lymphocytes, this being the most constant characteristic of the monocyte (Fig 13–15). Owing to the delicate distribution of their chromatin, the nuclei of monocytes are more lightly stained than those of large lymphocytes, which are the blood cells with which they are most often confused, although the monocytes are generally larger (Fig 13–7). The nucleus of the monocyte usually contains 2 or 3 nucleoli that can be seen in blood smears stained by Romanovsky-type dyes.

The cytoplasm of the monocyte is basophilic and frequently contains very fine azurophilic granules, some of which are at the limits of optical microscopic resolution. These granules are distributed throughout the cytoplasm, giving it a bluish-gray color in stained smears. The azurophilic granules of the monocytes are lysosomes. In the electron microscope, one or 2 nucleoli are seen in the nucleus, and a small quantity of rough endoplasmic reticulum, polyribosomes, and many small elongated mitochondria are observed (Fig 13–15). A well-developed Golgi complex involved in the formation of the lysosomal granules is present in the cytoplasm. Microfilaments and microtubules

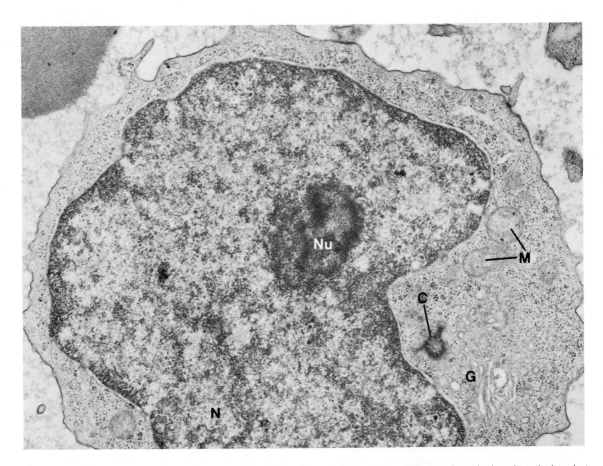

Figure 13–14. Electron micrograph of a human blood lymphocyte. This cell has little rough endoplasmic reticulum but contains a moderate quantity of free ribosomes. Observe the nucleus (N), the nucleolus (Nu), the centriole (C), the mitochondria (M), and the Golgi complex (G). Reduced from × 22,000. (Courtesy of DF Bainton and MG Farquhar.)

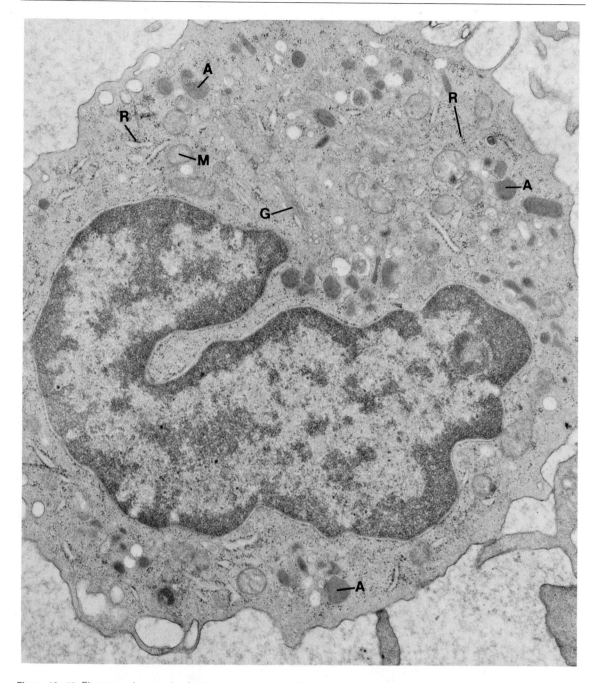

Figure 13–15. Electron micrograph of a human monocyte. Note the Golgi complex (G), the mitochondria (M), and the azurophilic granules (A). Rough endoplasmic reticulum is poorly developed. There are some free ribosomes (R). × 22,000. (Courtesy of DF Bainton and MG Farquhar.)

are usually observed in areas near the indentation of the nucleus. Many microvilli and pinocytotic vesicles are found at the cell surface.

Monocytes are found in the blood, where they represent the recently formed precursors of the mononuclear phagocyte system (see Chapter 5). After crossing capillary walls and entering connective tissues, monocytes differentiate into phagocytic cells. The half-life of the monocyte in the blood is 12–100 hours, and there is no strong evidence of recirculation after they enter connective tissues. In these tissues they interact with lymphocytes and play an essential role in the recognition and interaction of immunocompetent cells with antigen.

Platelets

Blood platelets (**thrombocytes**) are non-nucleated, disklike cell fragments $2-5$ μm in diameter. Platelets originate from the fragmentation of giant polyploid **megakaryocytes** residing in the bone marrow. Because of their tendency to agglutinate, platelet counts are difficult to derive; consequently, their reported normal concentration in human blood varies between wide extremes. Normal counts range from 200,000 to 400,000 per microliter of blood. Upon entering the bloodstream, platelets have a life span of about 10 days.

In stained blood smears, platelets often appear in clumps. Each platelet has a peripheral light blue–stained transparent zone, the **hyalomere,** and a central dense zone containing purple granules called the **granulomere.** Filopodial processes extending from the hyalomere produce an irregular conformation of the platelet surface.

Platelet ultrastructure is diagrammatically illustrated in Fig 13–16. These corpuscles contain a system of channels, called the **open canalicular system,** that connect to invaginations of the platelet plasma membrane (Fig 13–17). It is probable that this arrangement is of functional significance in facilitating liberation of active molecules stored in platelets. Around the periphery of the platelet lies a **marginal bundle** of microtubules that helps maintain the platelet's ovoid shape. In the hyalomere, there are also a number of electron-dense irregular tubes known as the **dense tubular system.** Actin-containing microfilaments in the hyalomere function in the elaboration of filopodia and surface projections during platelet movement and aggregation. A cell coat rich in glycosaminoglycans and glycoproteins, $15-20$ nm thick, lies outside the plasmalemma and is concerned with platelet adhesion.

The central granulomere possesses a variety of membrane-bound granules and a sparse population of mitochondria and glycogen particles (Figs 13–16 and 13–17). **Dense bodies (delta granules),** $250-300$ nm in diameter, contain calcium ions, pyrophosphate, ADP, and ATP. These granules also take up and store serotonin (5-hydroxytryptamine) from the plasma. **Alpha granules** are a little larger ($300-500$ nm in diameter) and contain fibrinogen, platelet-derived growth factor, and several other platelet-specific proteins. Recently, small vesicles, $175-250$ nm in diameter, have been shown to contain only lysosomal enzymes and have been termed **lambda granules.** Most of the azurophilic granules that are seen with the light microscope in the granulomere of platelets are alpha granules.

Platelet functions. The role of platelets in controlling hemorrhage can be summarized as follows.

A. Primary Aggregation: Discontinuities in the endothelium, produced by blood vessel lesions, are followed by adsorption of plasma proteins on the subjacent collagen. Immediately, platelets aggregate on this damaged tissue, forming a **platelet plug.**

B. Secondary Aggregation: Platelets of the plug release the content of their alpha and delta granules. ADP is a potent inducer of platelet aggregation.

C. Blood Coagulation: During platelet aggregation, factors from the blood plasma, damaged blood vessels, and platelets promote the sequential interaction (cascade) of approximately 13 plasma proteins, giving rise to a polymer, **fibrin,** that forms a tridimensional network of fibers trapping red cells, leukocytes, and platelets (**blood clot [thrombus]**). An inherited abnormality of one of the plasma proteins (factor VIII) results in the bleeding disorder known as **hemophilia.**

D. Clot Retraction: The clot that initially bulges into the blood vessel lumen contracts owing to the interaction of platelet actin, myosin, and ATP.

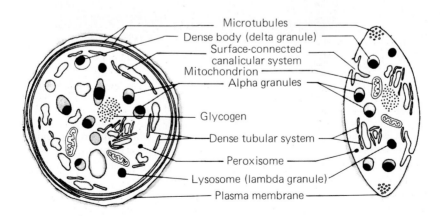

Microtubules
Dense body (delta granule)
Surface-connected canalicular system
Mitochondrion
Alpha granules
Glycogen
Dense tubular system
Peroxisome
Lysosome (lambda granule)
Plasma membrane

Figure 13–16. Diagrams of a human platelet in horizontal *(left)* and cross *(right)* section. (Reproduced, with permission, from Bentfeld-Barker ME, Bainton DF: Identification of primary lysosomes in human megakaryocytes and platelets. *Blood* 1982;59:472.)

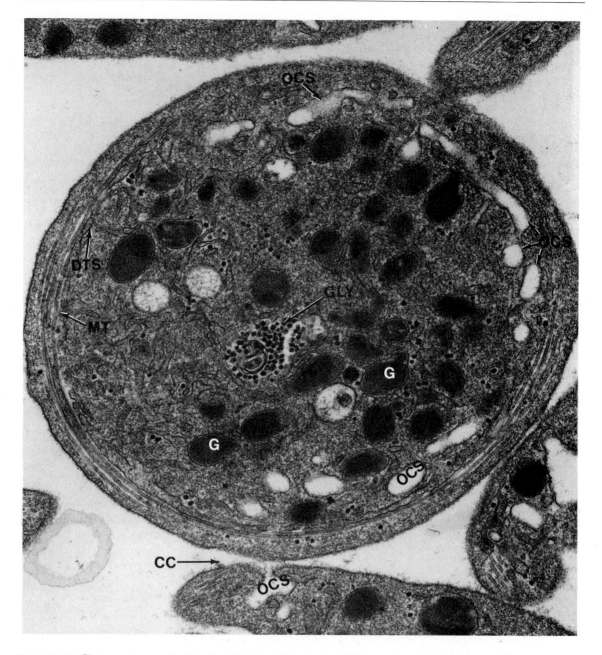

Figure 13–17. Electron micrograph of human platelets. CC, cell coat; OCS, open canalicular system; MT, microtubules; DTS, dense tubular system; G, granules; GLY, glycogen granules. × 40,740. (Courtesy of M Harrison.)

E. Clot Removal: Protected by the clot, the vessel wall is restored by new tissue formation. The clot is then removed, mainly by the proteolytic enzyme **plasmin** formed through the activation of the plasma proenzyme **plasminogen** by endothelium-produced **plasminogen activators.** Enzymes released from platelet lambda granules (lysosomes) also contribute to clot removal.

REFERENCES

Bainton DF: Sequential degranulation of the 2 types of polymorphonuclear leukocyte granules during phagocytosis of microorganisms. *J Cell Biol* 1973;**58**:249.

Bainton DF, Farquhar MG: Origin of granules in polymorphonuclear leukocytes: Two types derived from opposite faces of the Golgi complex in developing granulocytes. *J Cell Biol* 1966;**28**:277.

Bainton DF, Farquhar MG: Segregation and packaging of granule enzymes in eosinophilic leukocytes. *J Cell Biol* 1970;**45**:54.

Bainton DF, Ullyot JL, Farquhar MG: The development of neutrophilic polymorphonuclear leukocytes in human bone marrow. *J Exp Med* 1971;**134**:907.

Barr RD, Whang-Peng J, Perry S: Hemopoietic stem cells in human peripheral blood. *Science* 1975;**190**:284.

Bentfeld ME, Bainton DF: Cytochemical localization of lysosomal enzymes in rat megakaryocytes and platelets. *J Clin Invest* 1975;**56**:1635.

Bentfeld ME, Nichols BA, Bainton DF: Ultrastructural localization of peroxidases in leukocytes of rat bone marrow and blood. *Anat Rec* 1977;**187**:219.

Bessis M: *Living Blood Cells and Their Ultrastructure*. Springer, 1973.

Cline MJ: *The White Cell*. Harvard Univ Press, 1975.

Gowans JL: Differentiation of the cells which synthesize the immunoglobulins. *Ann Immunol* (Paris) 1974;**125**:201.

Kincade PW: Formulation of B lymphocytes in fetal and adult life. *Adv Immunol* 1981;**31**:177.

Marchesi VT: Stabilizing infrastructure of cell membranes. *Annu Rev Cell Biol* 1985;**1**:531.

Nichols BA, Bainton DF: Differentiation of human monocytes in bone marrow and blood: Sequential formation of 2 granule populations. *Lab Invest* 1973;**29**:27.

Smith JA: Molecular and cellular properties of eosinophils (a review). *Ric Clin Lab* 1981;**11**:181.

Stites DP et al (editors): *Basic & Clinical Immunology*, 5th ed. Lange, 1984.

Ullyot JL, Bainton DF: Azurophil and specific granules of blood neutrophils in chronic myelogenous leukemia: An ultrastructural and cytochemical analysis. *Blood* 1974;**44**:469.

Ullyot JL, Bainton DF, Farquhar MG: Cytochemical studies of human neutrophilic leukocyte granules. *J Histochem Cytochem* 1970;**18**:681.

Wintrobe MM et al: *Clinical Hematology*, 8th ed. Lea & Febiger, 1981.

Zucker-Franklin D et al: *Atlas of Blood Cells: Function and Pathology*. Vols 1 and 2. Lea & Febiger, 1981.

Mature blood cells have a relatively short life span, and consequently the population must be continuously replaced by the progeny of stem cells produced in the **hematopoietic organs.** In the earliest stages of embryogenesis, blood cells arise from the yolk sac mesoderm. Sometime later, the liver and spleen serve as temporary hematopoietic tissues, but by the second month, the clavicle has begun to ossify and begins to develop bone marrow in its core. As the prenatal ossification of the rest of the skeleton accelerates, the bone marrow becomes the predominant hematopoietic tissue.

After birth and on into childhood, erythrocytes and granular leukocytes, monocytes, and platelets are derived from stem cells localized in bone marrow. The origin and maturation of these cells are termed, respectively, "erythropoiesis," "granulopoiesis," "monocytopoiesis," and "megakaryocytopoiesis." Although their stem cells initially arise from the bone marrow, circulating lymphocytes are mainly derived from the mitotic activity of cells that reside in lymphatic organs.

Before attaining complete maturity and being released into the circulation, the blood cells go through specific stages of differentiation and maturation. Because these processes are continuous, cells with characteristics that are intermediate between 2 typical stages are frequently encountered in smears of blood or bone marrow.

It is probable that all of the formed elements of the blood originate from a single type of precursor cell (**unitarian** or **monophyletic theory**). In the past, some investigators favored the concept of more than one type of precursor cell (**polyphyletic theory**). The simplest polyphyletic theory postulates the existence of 2 stem cells: one for lymphocytes and the other for all other types of blood cells. The other extreme is the complete polyphyletic theory, which maintains that there is a primitive stem cell for each type of blood cell.

These theories represent an effort to resolve the difficulties of following the various stages of cell differentiation in bone marrow and lymphatic tissue. When cells at different stages of differentiation are arranged in a definite sequence—eg, in stratified squamous epithelium (skin, esophagus) or in the seminiferous tubules (testis)—it is easy to follow each cell through its various stages of differentiation. In the hematopoietic organs, cells develop in clusters (groups of cells of the same origin). Because cells within the clusters do not exhibit any regular organization, cells in specific stages of differentiation can be recognized only by morphologic characteristics. Since the immature cells of each blood cell type have more similarities among themselves than do the progeny that have reached a more highly differentiated stage, difficulties and controversies arise in identifying these less mature cells.

According to the widely accepted unitarian theory, all of the blood cells are derived from **pluripotential hematopoietic stem cells,** also known as **hemocytoblasts** or **transitional cells.** These cells have the capacity for self-renewal and differentiation into all types of mature blood cells. On average, half of the products of mitosis of stem cells remain as stem cells, while the other half of the progeny differentiate further to become **unipotential stem cells.** These cells are the precursors of only one type of mature blood cell, with the exception of the neutrophil-monocyte lineage, in which one unipotential stem cell can give rise to both types of cell.

Pluripotential stem cells divide infrequently—only often enough to maintain a steady-state supply of stem cells. It is the intermediate stages of cell differentiation that provide for expansion of the supply of precursors when called for in infections, hemorrhage, etc. Growth factors, such as **erythropoietin,** control the rate of proliferation of these intermediate stem cells.

At present, the morphology of this series of stem cells is uncertain. Several authors have proposed, as a candidate stem cell, a small ($7-15$ μm in diameter) cell with a large, euchromatic nucleus containing several nucleoli and with a small amount of basophilic cytoplasm. In other words, candidate stem cells have some features (size, basophilic cytoplasm, high nucleus:cytoplasm ratio) in common with lymphocytes. However, these 2 types of cells differ in the degree of condensation of their chromatin, stem cells having far less heterochromatin than lymphocytes.

Functionally, stem cells can be identified in experimental animals (mice) by their capacity to repopulate bone marrow after extensive cellular destruction and by their ability to grow and differentiate in semisolid culture media. When lethally irradiated mice receive bone marrow transplants from normal syngeneic donors, colonies derived from a single stem cell appear in their marrow and spleen and contain all types of mature blood cells. For these reasons, these pluripotential hematopoietic cells are also called **colony-forming unit (CFU) stem cells.**

BONE MARROW

Bone marrow is found in the medullary canals of long bones and in the cavities of spongy bones. Two types have been described according to their appearance on gross examination: **red, hematogenous, or active bone marrow,** whose color is due to the presence of numerous erythrocytes and their precursors in several phases of maturation; and **yellow bone marrow,** rich in adipose cells, which does not produce blood cells except upon conversion or transformation into red bone marrow induced by severe bleeding or hypoxia. In newborns, all of the bone marrow is red and is therefore active in the production of blood cells. As the child grows, most of the bone marrow changes into the yellow variety; in adults, red bone marrow is primarily found only in the flat bones (sternum, vertebrae, ribs, clavicles, bones of the pelvis, and diploë of the skull bones); in young adults, red marrow is found also in the proximal epiphyses of the femur and humerus.

Active (Red) Bone Marrow

As in hematopoietic tissues in general, red bone marrow is made up of a **stroma** and **hematopoietic cords,** profusely vascularized by sinusoidal capillaries. The stroma consists of at least 2 types of cells: **adventitial cells** and **macrophages.** Adventitial cells are not phagocytic, are highly branched, resemble fibroblasts in their cytologic features, and probably secrete the few reticular fibers seen in bone marrow. Processes of these cells are frequently seen just beneath the endothelium of marrow sinusoids as well as partially surrounding developing granulocytes. Macrophages are typically found at the center of **erythroblastic islands** where they are engaged in the transfer of iron to developing erythroblasts and the phagocytosis of extruded nuclei of mature erythrocytes.

Hematopoietic cords consist of related blood cells in the process of maturation. In mammals, hematopoietic cords are always separated from the lumens of sinusoids by the sinusoidal endothelium and by processes of adventitial cells. In other words, hematopoiesis in mammals is extravascular (Fig 14–1). Megakaryocytes are found closest to the sinusoids, while erythroblastic islands and granulopoiesis are seen farther away from these vessels.

When they reach maturity, blood cells enter the circulation by passing the sinusoids of the marrow cavity. Sinusoids consist of an endothelial lining with an incomplete basal lamina and adventitial cells that cover up to 60% of the outer surface. Developing blood cells penetrate the sinusoids by passing between adventitial cells, through the basal lamina (if present), and through discontinuities between endothelial lining cells.

The main functions of red bone marrow are production of blood cells, destruction of red blood cells, and storage of iron derived from the breakdown of hemoglobin.

Erythrocytes, granulocytes, monocytes, and platelets are released into the circulation as mature or nearly mature cells ready to perform their functions. Lymphocytes, on the other hand, are different. B lymphocytes acquire most of their specific characteristics in bone marrow but may require further differentiation

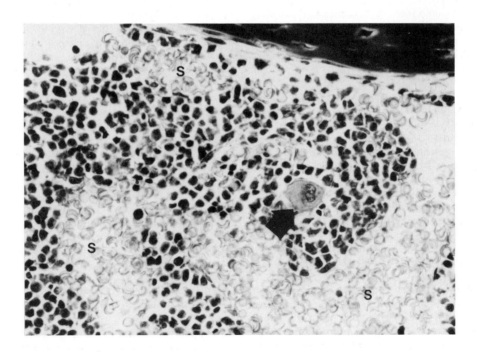

Figure 14–1. Section of active bone marrow showing the cell cords separated by sinusoidal capillaries (S). The arrow indicates a megakaryocyte. × 140.

in the periphery, probably in the spleen. T lymphocyte precursors arise in bone marrow but require the specific environment of the thymus to attain full maturity.

The destruction of old red blood cells is a function of macrophages in the spleen, liver, and bone marrow. Hemoglobin is broken down to yield (1) **globin,** which is quickly destroyed; (2) a porphyrin ring, which is converted to the bile pigment **bilirubin;** and (3) **iron,** which is transported by a plasma protein known as **transferrin.** Transferrin carries iron to red bone marrow, where the iron is reutilized by developing red blood cells.

Iron is stored in bone marrow as ferritin and hemosiderin in the cytoplasm of macrophages and early erythroblasts. Large amounts of ferritin and hemosiderin are also stored outside the bone marrow in hepatocytes, skeletal muscle fibers, and splenic macrophages.

Ferritin is an iron-containing protein consisting of 24 polypeptide subunits, each with a molecular weight of about 20,000 **(apoferritin).** Apoferritin forms a shell around a maximum of 4500 Fe^{3+} atoms. The whole particle has a diameter of 12 nm, and the iron core has a diameter of 5.5 nm. Under the electron microscope, each ferritin particle shows 4–6 electron-dense subunits, which permit its identification in electron micrographs.

Hemosiderin is a heterogenous complex consisting of iron (either bound to apoferritin or free), lysosomal enzymes, carbohydrates, and lipids. Hemosiderin is defined biochemically as water-insoluble iron, but cytologically it is the iron found in autophagic vacuoles called **siderosomes** (1–2 μm in diameter) seen in many types of cells including erythrocyte precursors and macrophages of erythroblastic islands.

Yellow Bone Marrow

In the yellow bone marrow there is a great predominance of adipose cells with an admixture of macrophages, undifferentiated mesenchymal cells, and reticular cells. Under stimulation (eg, hypoxia or hemorrhage), the undifferentiated cells may proliferate, giving rise to myeloid cells and transforming the yellow marrow into red marrow again.

Yellow bone marrow has 2 main functions: it is a storage organ, by virtue of its richness in fat; and it represents a reserve of hematopoietic tissue, becoming the site of production of cells in pathologic situations marked by frequent hemorrhages or excessive destruction of erythrocytes.

MATURATION OF ERYTHROCYTES

Stages in the differentiation and maturation of erythrocytic cells are the formation of **proerythroblasts, basophilic erythroblasts, polychromatophilic erythroblasts, orthochromatophilic erythroblasts** (normoblasts), **reticulocytes,** and finally **erythrocytes.** A **mature** cell is one that has differentiated to the state where it has acquired the capability to carry out all of its specific functions. The basic process in maturation is the synthesis of hemoglobin and the formation of a small corpuscle, the erythrocyte (red cell), which has the greatest possible area for the diffusion of oxygen (Fig 14–2).

During maturation of the cells of the erythrocytic series, the following major morphologic and histologic changes occur, corresponding to biochemical events of the developing erythroid cell: (1) cell volume decreases; (2) nucleoli diminish in size until they become invisible under the light microscope; (3) nuclear diameter decreases, and the chromatin becomes increasingly more dense until the nucleus presents a pyknotic appearance and is finally extruded from the cell; (4) there is a decrease in the number of polyribosomes (basophilia) and an increase in the amount of hemoglobin (acidophilia) within the cytoplasm; and (5) the quantity of mitochondria diminishes (Fig 14–2).

The number of cell divisions that intervene between the proerythroblast and the mature erythrocyte varies between 3 and 5. In the following description, the occurrence of 3 divisions is assumed (Fig 14–3).

Proerythroblast

Erythroid stem cells are induced to divide and differentiate into proerythroblasts under the influence of a hormone known as **erythropoietin** (see below). The first recognizable cell in the erythroid series is the proerythroblast. It is a large cell, 14–19 μm in diameter with a large, spherical nucleus occupying about 80% of the cell volume. Nuclear chromatin is lacy and not heavily stained. One or 2 nucleoli are easily visualized. The cytoplasm is basophilic because of the presence of numerous polyribosomes. With the light microscope, proerythroblasts are virtually identical to **myeloblasts,** the first cells in granulocyte differentiation. Using the electron microscope, **ferritin** can be demonstrated to be present in large quantities in the cytoplasm of proerythroblasts but not in myeloblasts.

Iron is supplied to proerythroblasts and their progeny by **transferrin,** a plasma protein that binds 2 atoms of Fe^{3+}. Erythroblasts possess plasma membrane receptors for transferrin; after binding, the receptor-transferrin complex is internalized by receptor-mediated endocytosis. The receptors are localized in coated pits commonly seen at the surfaces of proerythroblasts and later cells in this lineage (Fig 14–6). In CURL (see p 32), one of the iron atoms dissociates and is available for hemoglobin synthesis. The remaining transferrin-iron complex is recycled to the erythroblast cell surface, where it can take on another iron atom and reenter the erythroblast. Iron can also be transferred to erythroblasts by macrophages that form the centers of **erythroblastic islands**—groups of erythroblasts surrounding a phagocytic cell.

Basophilic Erythroblast

The proerythroblast continues to differentiate and then undergoes mitosis to form 2 basophilic erythroblasts. These cells are a bit smaller (12–17 μm in

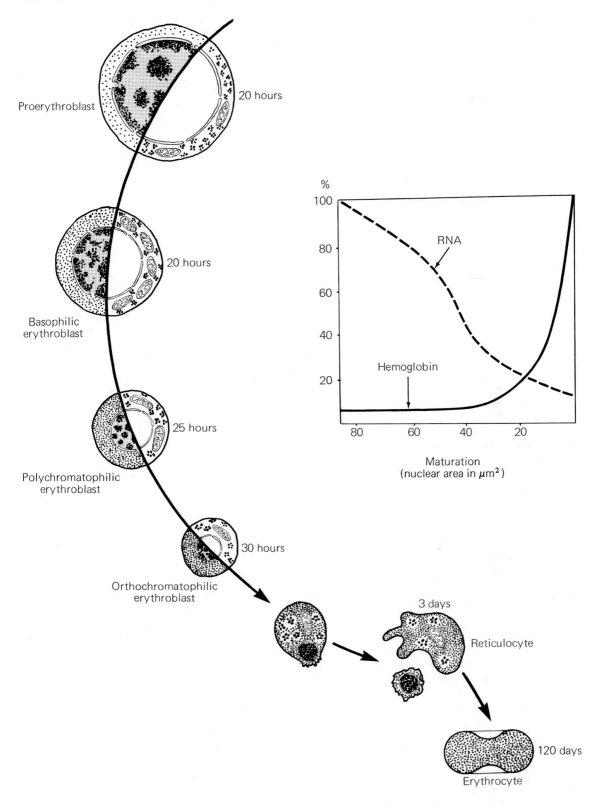

Figure 14–2. Summary of erythrocyte maturation. The stippled part of the cytoplasm shows that hemoglobin concentration increases continuously from the proerythroblast to the erythrocyte stage. There is also a decrease in nuclear volume and an increase in chromatin condensation, followed by extrusion of a pyknotic nucleus. In the graph, the highest recorded concentrations of hemoglobin and RNA were considered to be 100%. The times are average life spans.

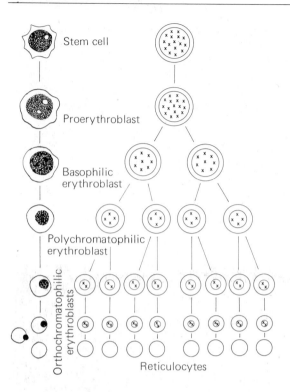

Figure 14–3. Radioautographic data on erythrocyte maturation obtained after a single labeling injection of ³H-thymidine. Silver granules in the radioautographs are represented by crosses. In each mitotic division, the number of silver granules per nucleus is reduced by half. In adult bone marrow, stem cells are few in number, and they rarely divide. The erythrocytes are normally produced by multiplication of proerythroblasts, basophilic erythroblasts, and polychromatophilic erythroblasts.

diameter) than the proerythroblast, and their cytoplasm is more basophilic owing to intense RNA synthesis in preparation for hemoglobin production (Figs 14–4, 14–5, and 14–6). Nucleoli can no longer be detected against the background of increasingly condensed nuclear chromatin. Chromatin commonly forms numerous small blocks that give the nucleus its characteristic "checkerboard" appearance. The cell also contains a small Golgi complex, a few cisternae of rough endoplasmic reticulum, numerous mitochondria, and a few microtubules and microfilaments. Hemoglobin synthesis is under way, but no trace of its presence is seen with the light microscope. Basophilic erythroblasts may divide one or 2 times; therefore, this stage of erythropoiesis is the most variable with respect to cell size and cell number.

Polychromatophilic Erythroblast

When the first patches of eosinophilia are visible, the cell is considered to be a polychromatophilic erythroblast (Figs 14–4 and 14–5). These small areas of eosinophilia are due to local accumulations of hemo-

globin. The diameter of the cell ranges from 12 to 15 μm. The nucleus is relatively smaller and more heterochromatic, but these cells are still capable of mitosis. The number of cytoplasmic organelles begins to decline.

Orthochromatophilic Erythroblast

When the degree of cytoplasmic acidophilia is approximately the same as that of mature erythrocytes, the cell is termed an orthochromatophilic erythroblast (Fig 14–5). This cell is the smallest of the nucleated erythrocyte precursors, usually measuring 8–12 μm in diameter. The nucleus is shrunken and extremely heterochromatic (**pyknotic**); eventually, it will be extruded. Orthochromatophilic erythroblasts are incapable of mitosis.

Reticulocytes

Microcinematography has demonstrated that at any given moment the orthochromatophilic erythroblast puts forth a series of cytoplasmic protrusions. During this activity, the nucleus is expelled encased in a thin layer of cytoplasm containing hemoglobin. The extruded nuclei, separated from the orthochromatophilic erythroblasts, are engulfed by bone marrow macrophages. Expulsion of nuclei may occur at an earlier maturation stage than the orthochromatophilic erythroblast, in which case the erythrocyte will be larger than normal and is called a **macrocyte.** Following loss of its nucleus, the remaining cell is called a **reticulocyte.** Under the electron microscope, it still contains 2 centrioles, some mitochondria, remnants of the Golgi complex, and polyribosomes. These last organelles synthesize the small quantity of hemoglobin (about 20%) necessary to complete the total hemoglobin content of the mature erythrocyte. Polyribosomes cannot be renewed because of the absence of a nucleus, so protein synthesis ceases within a short time.

The reticulocyte is capable of contracting, forming folds at certain points and projections at others. The reticulocyte enters the circulation by sending forth a pseudopodium that penetrates the wall of the sinusoidal capillary and ultimately passes into the lumen. The maturation period of reticulocytes in the circulation is 24–28 hours, with a total life span of approximately 72 hours. During this period, the remaining organelles are broken down by a soluble ATP-dependent enzyme known as **ubiquitin.** Lysosomal enzymes are not involved.

The reticulocyte differs from the erythrocyte in that it retains some RNA, thus showing a slight diffuse basophilia superimposed on the intense acidophilia of the hemoglobin. In blood smears stained by the usual methods, the reticulocyte appears larger than the erythrocyte, measuring approximately 9 μm in diameter.

When treated with supravital dyes such as cresyl blue, the ribonucleoprotein of the reticulocytes precipitates, forming a reticulum of variable appearance and size that stains dark blue (Fig 14–4). During this

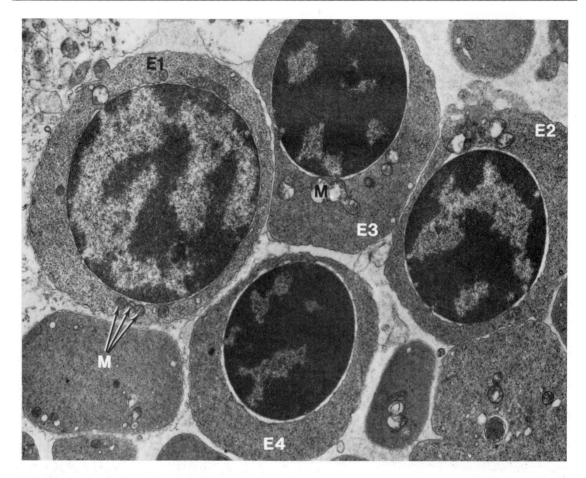

Figure 14–4. Electron micrograph of the bone marrow of a rat. Four erythroblasts in successive stages of maturation are seen (E1, E2, E3, and E4). As the cell matures, its chromatin becomes condensed and the accumulation of hemoglobin increases the electron density of the cytoplasm. Note the mitochondria (M). × 11,000.

period of maturation, all of the polyribosomes disperse into free single ribosomes.

Reticulocytes are young erythrocytes. They account for approximately 1% of the erythrocytes in normal circulating blood. When there is a physiologic demand for more oxygen, as after hemorrhage, the reticulocyte count will be higher.

Erythron

The erythron (Fig 14–7) is the total cell population of erythrocytes and their precursor cells and is a widely dispersed but functionally single organ. Its principal function is to supply the organism with the oxygen necessary for tissue metabolism. Moreover, it carries CO_2, a gas which is also transported dissolved in the plasma for elimination from the lungs.

The erythron can be divided into 2 functional compartments: (1) the **circulating** or **blood compartment,** represented by the erythrocytes in the blood; and (2) the **medullary compartment** or **erythropoietic pool,** the bone marrow sites where formation of new erythrocytes takes place. As can be seen by

reference to Fig 14–2, the development of an erythrocyte, from the first recognizable erythroid cell (proerythroblast) to the release of a reticulocyte into the circulating compartment, takes approximately 7 days.

The total number of erythrocytes in the circulation at any time is about 2.5×10^{13} cells. Since erythrocytes have an average life span of 120 days, this means that 200 billion cells are produced and destroyed per day—more than 2 million per second. Pluripotential stem cells provide a pool of unipotential stem cells committed to erythropoiesis, which multiply more or less rapidly under the influence of the hormone **erythropoietin.** Erythropoietin is a glycoprotein (MW 39,000); about 10% of its mass is carbohydrate. This hormone is synthesized in the kidney cortex, but the cell responsible for its synthesis is uncertain (Fig 14–7). It may be the epithelial cell (podocyte) of the renal glomerulus. Synthesis of erythropoietin is stimulated by any condition that causes a low partial pressure of oxygen in blood **(hypoxia).** Such conditions include hemorrhage, ascent to high altitude, and compromise of pulmonary function (eg,

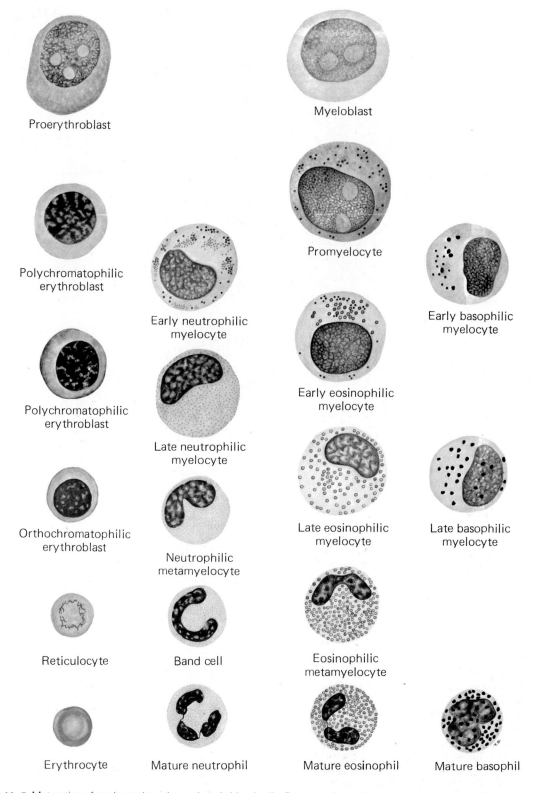

Figure 14–5. Maturation of erythrocytic and granulocytic blood cells. Romanovsky staining was used except for the reticulocyte, which was treated additionally with cresyl blue in order to precipitate and stain the RNA found in this cell. (This illustration is reproduced in color on p xi.)

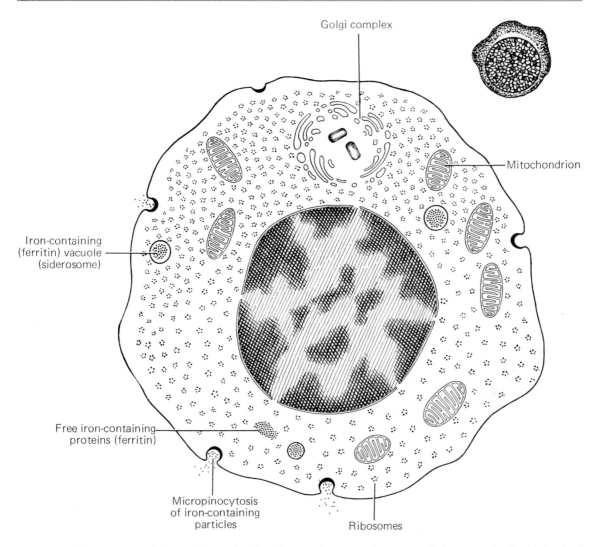

Figure 14 –6. Ultrastructure of a basophilic erythroblast. Its cytoplasm contains many polyribosomes for the synthesis of hemoglobin. The upper right drawing shows the structure of the same cell as seen in bone marrow smears. The light area near the nucleus contains the Golgi complex and the centrioles.

emphysema). The effects of erythropoietin include an increase in the rate of mitosis of erythroid progenitor cells, skipped mitoses in erythroid differentiation, increases in mRNA and tRNA synthesis, and shortening of the transit time from the medullary compartment to the circulating blood compartment. For example, under normal circumstances, reticulocytes reside in the bone marrow for about 3 days before they enter the circulation. Increased levels of erythropoietin reduce this time, resulting in increased reticulocyte counts in circulating blood.

Erythropoietin is also synthesized in extrarenal sites, notably the liver. Here, the cells responsible for erythropoietin production are probably Kupffer cells.

Numerous substances are essential for the proper functioning of the erythron and for the production of erythrocytes. Among these are iron, vitamin B_{12}, and folic acid.

Several hormones (eg, thyroxine, testosterone, cortisol) stimulate erythropoiesis, but the mechanisms of action are unknown and probably indirect. Injection of estrogens lowers the red cell count, and growth hormone acts directly upon the erythron, increasing the number of erythrocytes in the blood.

MATURATION OF GRANULOCYTES

The **myeloblast** is the most immature recognizable cell in the myeloid series and gives rise to the 3 types of granulocytes. The presence of azurophilic granules in the cytoplasm identifies a cell as a **promyelocyte.**

BONE MARROW

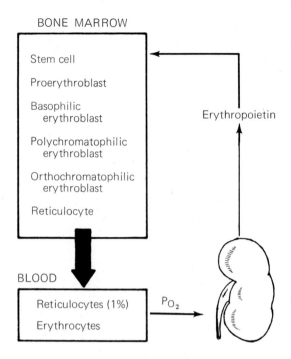

Figure 14–7. The erythron is composed of both the medullary and circulating blood compartments. Reticulocytes pass from the bone marrow to the blood, where they complete maturation into erythrocytes. A fall in blood oxygen tension (P$_{O_2}$) stimulates the kidney to produce a hormone, erythropoietin, which accelerates the mitotic rate and the maturation of red cells in the medullary compartment. Thus, the number of liberated reticulocytes and erythrocytes in the blood increases.

When the various specific cytoplasmic granules are fully developed, the cell is called a **neutrophilic, eosinophilic,** or **basophilic myelocyte** according to the staining characteristics of the granules. The subsequent stages of maturation are from the **myelocyte** to the **metamyelocyte,** then to the **band cell,** and finally to the **mature granulocyte** (neutrophilic, eosinophilic, or basophilic). Only the last 2 forms are normally seen in the circulation.

Myeloblast

The myeloblast is 10– 12 μm in diameter, with a large spherical nucleus that has a delicate chromatin network and 1– 3 nucleoli. Its cytoplasm is scanty and basophilic (Fig 14– 5). Examination with the electron microscope shows many mitochondria, ribosomes, and dispersed rough endoplasmic reticulum. No granules are present.

Promyelocyte

The promyelocyte is the same size as or larger than the myeloblast (up to 15 μm or more). The nucleus is generally spherical; its chromatin is coarser than in the myeloblast; and nucleoli are prominent (Fig 14– 5).

The cytoplasm of the promyelocyte is more basophilic than that of the myeloblast and contains azurophilic granules. These granules are different from the specific granules that appear in myelocytes, which develop in the next stage of maturation. They are derived from the **trans face** of the Golgi cisternae (Fig 14– 9). Azurophilic granules are around 500 nm in diameter and have a homogeneous density, are surrounded by a membrane, and contain lysosomal enzymes as well as myeloperoxidase. Rough endoplasmic reticulum and the Golgi complex are well developed.

Myelocyte

The myelocyte is 10– 12 μm in diameter. The nucleus is ovoid and usually eccentric, with coarse chromatin. Different stages in the development of the myelocyte can be identified depending on the nature of the specific granules, the appearance of the nucleus (from spherical to ovoid), and the relative size of its cytoplasm. A slight cytoplasmic basophilia and azurophilic granules are still encountered (Figs 14– 4, 14– 8, and 14– 9). The origin of specific granules differs from that of azurophilic granules in that the former arise from the **cis face** of the Golgi complex (Fig 14– 9).

What characterizes an immature cell of the granulocytic series as a myelocyte is the beginning of the appearance of the specific granules—**neutrophil, eosinophil,** and **basophil.** The 3 different lines of granulocytes in peripheral blood can be traced from this stage. The process of further maturation in each cell is characterized principally by changes in the size, shape, and appearance of the nucleus and by relative increases in the amount of cytoplasm. The specific granules appear first in the perinuclear region and later fill the cytoplasm. Neutrophil specific granules are about 200 nm in diameter and thus below the resolution limit of the light microscope. Their presence is indicated by a salmon-pink tint of the cytoplasm. Eosinophil and basophil specific granules are larger and individually visible as orange or dark purple granules, respectively. Myelocytes retain the ability to divide by mitosis.

Metamyelocyte

The metamyelocyte is characterized by a nucleus with a deep indentation, indicating the beginning of lobe formation. The chromatin pattern becomes denser, and azurophilic granules are still seen in the cytoplasm along with the population of specific granules. Azurophilic granules are synthesized only in the promyelocyte stage of granulopoiesis. Since several mitoses occur in the promyelocyte and myelocyte stages, the number of azurophilic granules becomes progressively reduced. During this stage of development, nuclear activity diminishes as the chromatin condenses into heterochromatin. Concomitantly, protein synthesis and related organelles (Golgi complex, ribosomes, and rough endoplasmic reticulum) are reduced. Glycogen accumulations are evident in the cytoplasm.

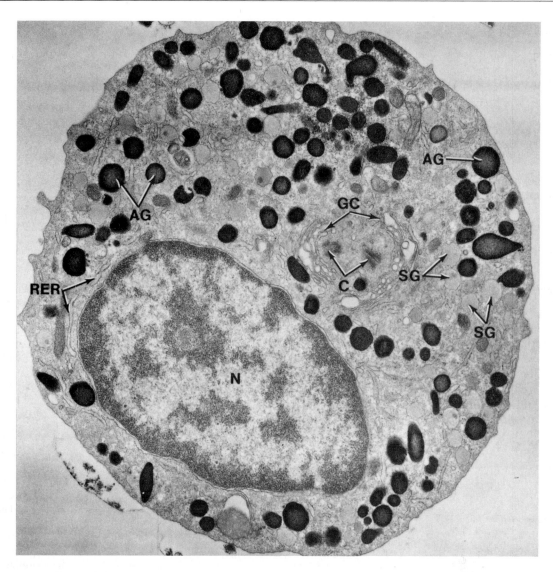

Figure 14–8. Neutrophilic myelocyte from normal human bone marrow treated with peroxidase. At this stage, the cell is smaller than the promyelocyte and the cytoplasm contains 2 different types of granules: (1) large, peroxidase-positive azurophilic granules (AG); and (2) the smaller specific granules (SG), which do not stain for peroxidase. Note that the peroxidase reaction product is present only in azurophilic granules and is not seen in the rough endoplasmic reticulum (RER) or Golgi cisternae (GC), which are located around the centriole (C). N, nucleus. × 15,000. (Courtesy of DF Bainton.)

The modifications that characterize the metamyelocytes are not easily identifiable in the basophil cell series, so that the basophilic metamyelocyte is not easily distinguished from mature basophils (Fig 14–5). Metamyelocytes do not divide.

Band Cell

Before assuming the lobate form typical of a mature cell, the granulocyte goes through an intermediate stage in which the nucleus appears as a curved rod (Fig 14–5). This cell may be found in the peripheral blood, and stimulation of granulocytopoiesis is associated with the appearance of larger than normal numbers of these cells in the peripheral blood. The normal percentage in blood is 3–5%. The appearance of large numbers of immature cells in the blood is called a "shift to the left" and is of clinical significance, usually indicating bacterial infection.

KINETICS OF NEUTROPHIL PRODUCTION

The time taken for a myeloblast to differentiate into a circulating neutrophil is determined by studying the pattern of ^{3}H-thymidine uptake and its subsequent

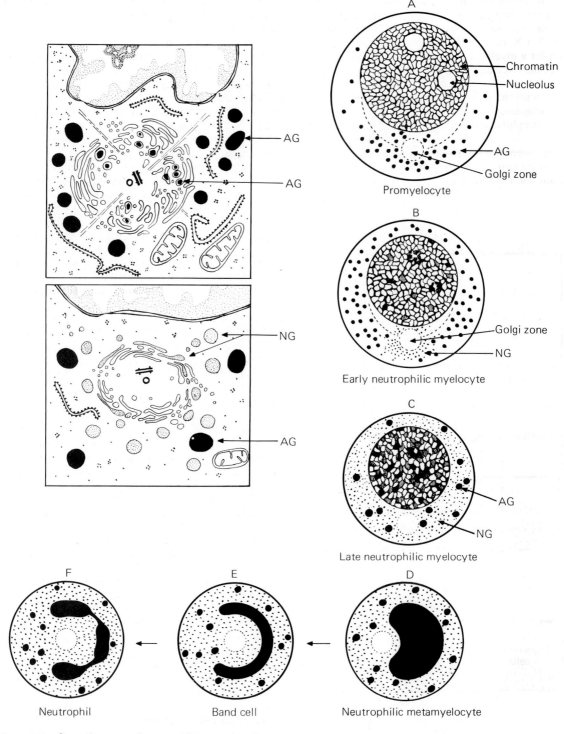

Figure 14–9. Several stages of neutrophil maturation. Note the changes in nuclear shape and structure. The light area close to the nucleus contains the Golgi complex and the 2 centrioles. This is the region where the neutrophilic granules (NG) and the azurophilic granules (AG) first appear. At upper left is shown the ultrastructure of the light juxtanuclear area. Both neutrophilic and azurophilic granules are formed in the cisternae of the Golgi complex. Observe that azurophilic granules are formed deep in the Golgi complex (the *cis* face) close to the centrioles, whereas the neutrophilic granules are formed later in the maturation process in the outer cisternae of the Golgi complex (the *trans* face). Note that during maturation the number of specific granules increases while the azurophilic granule population is reduced by cell division.

dilution in the several intermediate cells of this lineage. In humans, approximately 4.5×10^7 neutrophils per kilogram per hour are produced. A 70-kg man produces 7.5×10^{10} neutrophils per day. The total time taken for a myeloblast to emerge as a mature neutrophil in the circulation is about 11 days. Under normal circumstances, 5 mitotic divisions occur in the myeloblast, promyelocyte, and neutrophilic myelocyte stages of development.

Neutrophils pass through several functionally and anatomically defined compartments (Fig 14–10). (1) The **medullary formation compartment** can be subdivided into a mitotic compartment ($\sim$ 3 days) and a maturation compartment ($\sim$ 4 days). (2) A **med-**

ullary storage compartment acts as a buffer system, capable of releasing large numbers of mature neutrophils upon demand. Neutrophils remain in this compartment for about 4 days. (3) The **circulating compartment** consists of neutrophils suspended in plasma and circulating in blood vessels. (4) The **marginating compartment** is composed of neutrophils that are present in blood but do not circulate. These neutrophils are in capillaries, temporarily excluded from the circulation by vasoconstriction, or—especially in the lungs—at the periphery of vessels, adhering to the endothelium and not in the main bloodstream.

The latter 2 compartments are of about equal size, and there is a constant interchange of cells between the marginating and circulating compartments. The half-life of a neutrophil in these 2 compartments is 6–7 hours. The medullary formation and storage compartments are about 10 times as large as the circulating and marginating compartments.

Neutrophils (and other granulocytes) enter the connective tissues by passing through intercellular junctions found between endothelial cells of capillaries and postcapillary venules **(diapedesis).** The connective tissues form a fifth compartment for neutrophils, but its size is not known. Neutrophils reside here for 1–4 days and then die, whether or not they have performed their major function of phagocytosis.

Changes in neutrophil number in the peripheral circulation must be evaluated by taking all of these compartments into consideration. Thus, **neutrophilia,** an increase in the number of neutrophils in the circulation, does not necessarily imply an increase in neutrophil production. Intense muscular activity or administration of epinephrine causes neutrophils in the marginating compartment to move into the circulating compartment, with an apparent neutrophilia even though neutrophil production has not increased.

Neutrophilia may also result from liberation of greater numbers of neutrophils of the medullary storage compartment. This type of neutrophilia is transitory and is followed by a "recovery" period during which no neutrophils are released.

The neutrophilia that occurs during the course of bacterial infections is due to an increase in neutrophil production and a shorter stay of these cells in the medullary storage compartment. In such cases, immature forms such as band cells, neutrophilic metamyelocytes, and even myelocytes may appear in the bloodstream. The neutrophilia that occurs during infection is of longer duration than that which occurs as a result of intense muscular activity.

Control of Neutrophilopoiesis

The mechanism that stimulates the production of neutrophils by the bone marrow appears to be set in motion by a decrease in the number of these cells in the circulating compartment. This conclusion arises from the observation that destruction of neutrophils (eg, by the injection of an antineutrophil antibody) immediately stimulates the production of these cells. Leukapheresis, which consists of withdrawing blood

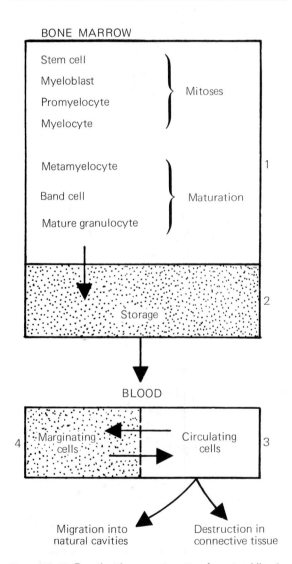

Figure 14–10. Functional compartments of neutrophils. *1:* Medullary formation compartment. *2:* Medullary reserve compartment. *3:* Circulating compartment. *4:* Marginating compartment. The size of each compartment is roughly proportionate to the number of cells.

and reinfusing it after removal of most of the leu-kocytes, also causes neutrophilia, which rules out the possibility that a substance liberated by dead neutrophils (present in experiments with antineutrophil antibody) stimulates the production of these cells by the bone marrow. The production of neutrophils is controlled by a humoral mechanism not yet identified.

MATURATION OF LYMPHOCYTES & MONOCYTES

Study of the precursor cells of lymphocytes and monocytes is difficult because these cells do not contain specific cytoplasmic granules or the nuclear lobulation that is present in granulocytes, both of which facilitate the distinction between young and mature forms. Lymphocytes and monocytes are distinguished mainly on the basis of size, chromatin structure, and the presence of nucleoli in smear preparations. As lymphocytic cells mature, their chromatin becomes more compact, nucleoli become less visible, and the cells decrease in size. In addition, subsets of the lymphocytic series acquire distinctive cell-surface antigens that can be detected by immunofluorescence techniques.

Lymphocyte

Circulating lymphocytes originate mainly in the thymus and the peripheral lymphoid organs (spleen, lymph nodes, tonsils, etc). However, it is now thought that *all* lymphocyte progenitor cells originate in the bone marrow. Some of these relatively undifferentiated lymphocytes migrate to the thymus, where they acquire the attributes of T lymphocytes. Subsequently, T lymphocytes populate specific regions of peripheral lymphoid organs. Other bone marrow lymphocytes remain in the marrow, differentiate into B lymphocytes, and then migrate to peripheral lymphoid organs where they inhabit their own special compartments. A large number of progenitor cells in bone marrow never differentiate further, and they die there. This is thought to be related to the elimination of ''forbidden'' or ''self'' clones of cells that are programmed to react against host antigens.

The first identifiable progenitor of lymphoid cells is the **lymphoblast,** a large cell capable of incorporating ^{3}H-thymidine and dividing 2–3 times to form **prolymphocytes.** These latter cells are smaller and have relatively more condensed chromatin but do not have any of the cell-surface antigens that mark prolymphocytes as T or B lymphocytes. In the thymus or bone marrow, these cells synthesize cell-surface antigens characteristic of their lineage, but they are not recognizable as distinct cell types by routine histologic procedures.

Monocyte

The **monoblast** is a committed progenitor cell that is virtually identical to the **myeloblast** in its morphology. Further differentiation leads to the **pro-monocyte,** a large cell (up to 18 μm in diameter) with a basophilic cytoplasm and a large, slightly indented nucleus. The chromatin is lacy, and nucleoli are evident. Promonocytes divide 2 times in the course of their development into **monocytes.** A large amount of rough endoplasmic reticulum is present, as is an extensive Golgi complex in which granule condensation can be seen to be taking place. These granules are **primary lysosomes,** which are observed as fine **azurophilic granules** in blood monocytes. Mature monocytes enter the bloodstream, circulate for about 8 hours, and then enter the connective tissues, where they mature into **macrophages** and function for several months.

ORIGIN OF PLATELETS

In adults, the platelets originate in the red bone marrow by fragmentation of the cytoplasm of mature **megakaryocytes.** These in turn arise by differentiation of the **megakaryoblasts.**

Megakaryoblast

The megakaryoblast is 15–50 μm in diameter and has a large ovoid or kidney-shaped nucleus with numerous nucleoli. The nucleus becomes highly polyploid (contains up to 30 times as much DNA as a normal cell) before cytoplasmic differentiation begins. The cytoplasm of this cell is homogeneous and intensely basophilic (Fig 14–11).

Megakaryocyte

The megakaryocyte is a giant cell (35–150 μm in diameter) with an irregularly lobulated nucleus, coarse chromatin, and no visible nucleoli (Figs 14–11 and 14–12). The cytoplasm contains numerous mitochondria, a well-developed rough endoplasmic reticulum, and an extensive Golgi complex. Alpha granules and vesicles containing lysosomal enzymes (lambda granules) are seen developing from Golgi vesicles and cisternae. With maturation of the megakaryocyte, numerous invaginations of the plasma membrane ramify throughout the cytoplasm, forming the **demarcation membranes.** This system delimits areas of megakaryocyte cytoplasm that will be shed as platelets after a complex and little understood process of membrane fusion occurs.

In smear preparations of bone marrow, it is possible to observe platelets still bound to the cytoplasm of the megakaryocyte and in various phases of separation. Furthermore, in cultures of megakaryocytes, the liberation of platelets can be observed under the microscope, which substantiates their megakaryocytic origin. In certain forms of **thrombocytopenic purpura,** a disease in which the number of blood platelets is reduced, platelets appear bound to the cytoplasm of the megakaryocytes, indicating a defect in the liberation mechanism of these corpuscles.

In observations carried out using platelets marked in vitro with radioactive isotopes and afterward rein-

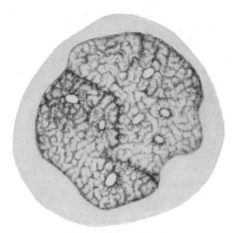

Megakaryoblast

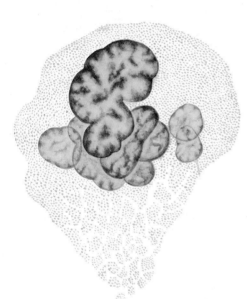

Megakaryocyte

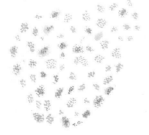

Platelets

Figure 14–11. Cells of the megakaryocytic series shown in a bone marrow smear with Romanovsky-type staining.

jected, the life span of these corpuscles was found to be approximately 10 days.

INTRAUTERINE HEMATOPOIESIS

There are 3 overlapping stages of intrauterine hematopoiesis: a **primordial** or **prehepatic phase,** a **hepatosplenothymic phase,** and a **medullolymphatic** or **definitive phase.**

When one of these stages is initiated, the predominant processes of the previous phase persist for some time, though gradually decreasing in importance (Fig 14–13).

All formed elements of the blood are of mesenchymal origin. In organs of dual embryonic origin such as the liver and thymus (endoderm and mesoderm), cells originating in the mesoderm are responsible for hematopoiesis.

Primordial or Prehepatic Phase

In humans, the first blood cells appear in the mesoderm of the yolk sac during the third week of intrauterine life. The **blood islands** consist of elongated clusters of mesenchymal cells. The endothelium of the first vessels originates in the most superficial cells of these islands; the innermost cells become spherical and differentiate into blood stem cells.

By the association of the endothelial cells of contiguous islands, the first blood vessels are formed. These vessels soon establish communication with those in the body of the embryo. This permits cells formed in the yolk sac to penetrate and circulate in the body of the embryo.

The blood stem cells of the yolk sac divide within the vessels to form **primitive erythroblasts,** which are larger than **definitive erythroblasts.** Cells that arise by primitive red cell erythropoiesis are larger than those that develop as a result of definitive erythropoiesis, and this process is known as **megaloblastic erythropoiesis.** The majority of erythroblasts formed in the yolk sac do not lose their nuclei, so that at this stage the red cells are predominantly nucleated. Only at the end of the primordial phase do enucleated erythrocytes appear as a result of extrusion of the erythroblast nucleus. In addition, the type of hemoglobin synthesized is unique (Gower I and II).

During the primordial phase, blood contains only the above-mentioned red cell series. No leukocytes or platelets are present.

Hepatosplenothymic Phase

This period begins in the second month, with hematopoiesis taking place in the liver and spleen. Subsequently, the thymus starts producing lymphocytes. In the mesenchyme that invades the endodermal primordium of the liver, precursor cells of granulocytes, megakaryocytes, and definitive erythroblasts appear. Of the latter, a large number reach the blood without losing their nuclei. Fetal hemoglobin (HbF) synthesis predominates during this period. The mechanisms un-

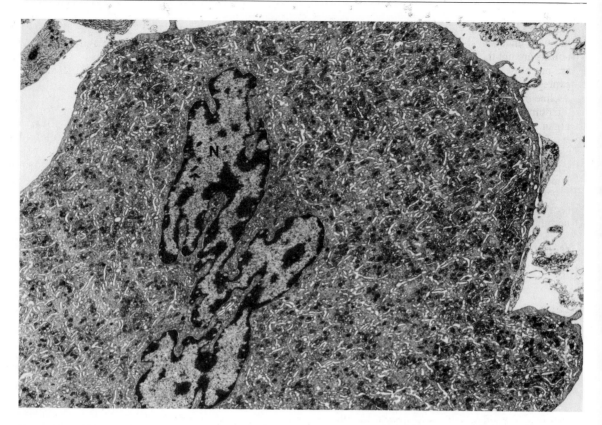

Figure 14–12. Electron micrograph of a megakaryocyte showing the lobulated nucleus (N) and numerous cytoplasmic granules. The demarcation membranes are visible as tubular profiles. × 4900. (Reproduced, with permission, from Junqueira LCU, Salles LMM: *Ultra-Estrutura e Função Celular.* Edgard Blücher, 1975.)

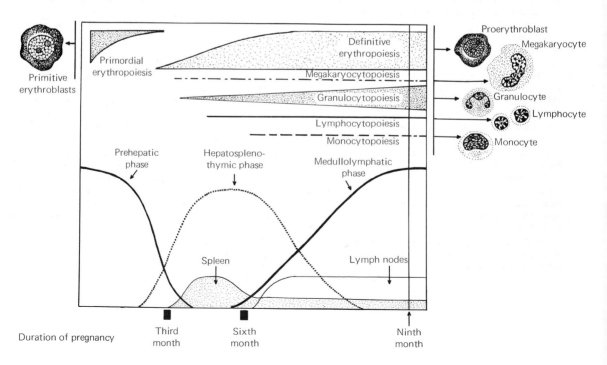

Figure 14–13. The main events in intrauterine hemocytopoiesis.

derlying switches in hemoglobin gene expression are not well understood. Changes in the site of erythropoiesis are not the main stimulus, since these changes are not closely synchronized with switching of gene expression. Although hepatic hematopoiesis begins to decline in the fifth month, it persists until some weeks after birth. In the adult, the liver is not a hematopoietic organ.

The spleen produces mainly cells of the red cell series and, in smaller quantity, granulocytes and platelets. Production of lymphocytes in the spleen becomes important as birth becomes imminent.

The thymus begins to form lymphocytes in the second month of intrauterine life and produces almost no other type of blood cell.

Medullolymphatic Phase

The clavicle is the first bone to show hematopoietic activity. Its bone marrow begins to function between the second and third month of intrauterine life. The marrow of other bones soon begins to function, and in the fourth month bone marrow hematopoiesis is significant.

The bone marrow shows great erythrocytic, granulocytic, and megakaryocytic activity. Lymphocytes and monocytes are also produced.

During this period—and close to birth—the lymph nodes (which since the beginning of their existence have been lymphocyte-producing organs) become very active. Before birth, the lymph nodes may show erythropoietic activity.

If the bone marrow should be injured or destroyed after birth, the liver and spleen can resume their hematopoietic functions (extramedullary hematopoiesis).

REFERENCES

Bainton DF, Farquhar MG: Segregation and packaging of granule enzymes in eosinophilic leukocytes. *J Cell Biol* 1970;**45**:54.

Bainton DF, Ullyot JL, Farquhar MG: The development of neutrophilic polymorphonuclear leukocytes in human bone marrow. *J Exp Med* 1971;**134**:907.

Barr RD, Whang-Peng J, Perry S: Hemopoietic stem cells in human peripheral blood. *Science* 1975;**190**:284.

Becker RP, DeBruyn PP: The transmural passage of blood cells into myeloid sinusoids and the entry of platelets into the sinusoidal circulation. *Am J Anat* 1976;**145**:183.

Behnke O: An electron microscope study of the rat megacaryocyte. 2. Some aspects of platelet release and microtubules. *J Ultrastruct Res* 1969;**26**:111.

Berman I: The ultrastructure of erythroblastic islands and reticular cells in mouse bone marrow. *J Ultrastruct Res* 1967;**17**:291.

Bessis MC, Breton-Gorius J: Iron metabolism in the bone marrow as seen by electron microscopy: A critical review. *Blood* 1962;**19**:635.

Caffrey RW, Everett NB, Rieke WO: Radioautographic studies of reticular and blast cells in the hematopoietic tissues of the rat. *Anat Rec* 1966;**155**:41.

Evatt BL, Levine RF, Williams NT: *Megakaryocyte Biology and Precursors: In Vitro Cloning and Cellular Properties.* Elsevier/North-Holland, 1981.

Gowans JL: Life-span, recirculation and transformation of lymphocytes. *Int Rev Exp Pathol* 1966;**5**:1.

Harrison PR: Analysis of erythropoiesis at the molecular level. *Nature* 1976;**262**:353.

Moore MAS, Metcalf D: Ontogeny of the haemopoietic system: Yolk sac origin of in vivo and in vitro colony-forming cells in the developing mouse embryo. *Br J Haematol* 1970;**18**:279.

Nichols BA, Bainton DF: Differentiation of human monocytes in bone marrow and blood: Sequential formation of two granule populations. *Lab Invest* 1973;**29**:27.

Nichols BA, Bainton DF, Farquhar MG: Differentiation of monocytes: Origin, nature and fate of their azurophil granules. *J Cell Biol* 1971;**50**:498.

Penington DG: The cellular biology of megakaryocytes. *Blood Cells* 1979;**5**:5.

Quesenberry P, Levitt L: Hematopoietic stem cells. *N Engl J Med* 1979;**301**:755.

Richter GW: The iron-loaded cell—the cytopathology of iron storage: A review. *Am J Pathol* 1978;**91**:361.

Tavassoli M, Yoffey JM: *Bone Marrow Structure and Function.* Liss, 1983.

Till JE, McCulloch EA: Hemopoietic stem cell differentiation. *Biochim Biophys Acta* 1980;**605**:431.

Ullyot JL, Bainton DF: Azurophil and specific granules of blood neutrophils in chronic myelogenous leukemia: An ultrastructural and cytochemical analysis. *Blood* 1974;**44**:469.

Weiss L: The hematopoietic microenvironment of the bone marrow: An ultrastructural study of the stroma in rats. *Anat Rec* 1976;**186**:161.

Weiss L, Chen L-T: The organization of hematopoietic cords and vascular sinuses in bone marrow. *Blood Cells* 1975;**1**:617.

Westen H, Bainton DF: Association of alkaline phosphatase−positive reticulum cells in bone marrow with granulocytic precursors. *J Exp Med* 1979;**150**:919.

Williams WJ et al (editors): *Hematology,* 3rd ed. McGraw-Hill, 1983.

Yoffey JM, Courtice FC: *Lymphatics, Lymph and Lymphoid Tissue,* 2nd ed. Harvard Univ Press, 1970.

15

Lymphoid System

The lymphoid system consists of cells, tissues, and organs that protect the internal environment against invasion and damage by foreign substances. Certain cells of this system are known as **immunocompetent cells,** since they have the capacity to distinguish between "self" (the organism's own molecules) and "nonself" (foreign substances) and to provide for the inactivation or destruction of foreign materials. **Immunity** is the term used to describe this protective response, and the lymphoid system is sometimes called the immune system.

In general, lymphoid tissues and organs consist of a framework of reticular fibers (type III collagen) secreted by "reticular cells," which are indistinguishable from fibroblasts. The "epithelial reticular cells" of the thymus are an exception to this generalization, as will be discussed below. Lymphocytes, macrophages, antigen-presenting cells, and plasma cells occupy spaces between the reticular cells and fibers. Each lymphoid organ or tissue has its own special organizational features; these will be described as each organ or tissue is discussed.

LYMPHOID TISSUE

Encapsulated & Unencapsulated Lymphoid Organs & Tissues

Lymphoid organs and tissues may be either encapsulated or unencapsulated, meaning that they have or do not have a connective tissue sheath surrounding the structure. Examples of the former include the spleen and lymph nodes. Unencapsulated lymphoid tissues include tonsils, Peyer's patches in the ileum, and lymphoid nodules found in the mucosa of the alimentary, respiratory, urinary, and reproductive tracts.

Cellular & Humoral Immunity

There are 2 different but related systems of immunity in mammals. The first is cellular immunity, in which living cells interact with and destroy foreign (nonself) cells. This category of immunity is mediated by thymus-derived lymphocytes (T cells), whose origin and functions are described in more detail below. The other broad class of immunity is called humoral immunity because specific circulating glycoproteins (immunoglobulins, antibodies) interact with foreign substances and promote their inactivation or destruction. Lymphocytes maturing in the bone marrow of mammals (B cells) differentiate into plasma cells after encountering a foreign substance. Plasma cells then synthesize and secrete large quantities of immunoglobulins. In most cases, B lymphocytes require the cooperation of T lymphocytes to produce antibodies. The cellular and humoral immune systems also require accessory cells, such as macrophages and antigen-presenting cells, for an optimal response to occur.

Central & Peripheral Lymphoid Organs

A central lymphoid organ is one in which lymphoid precursors undergo antigen-independent proliferation and acquire surface antigens that mark them as committed to either the cellular or humoral immune response. The thymus is the organ in which lymphocytes take on the capacity of participating in the cellular immune response. These cells are referred to as T lymphocytes. The progenitor cells for the humoral immune response are called B lymphocytes because they differentiate in a special microenvironment in the bone marrow of mammals.

Lymphocytes leave central lymphoid organs and populate specific regions of peripheral lymphoid organs. Peripheral organs include lymph nodes, spleen, Peyer's patches of the ileum, and diffuse, unencapsulated lymphoid tissue in the mucosa of the digestive, respiratory, urinary, and reproductive tracts.

Antigens & Antibodies

The foreign (nonself) substance encountered by the 2 immune systems acts as an antigen, ie, a substance that elicits a host response which may be cellular, humoral, or, most commonly, of both types. Antigens may be whole cells (bacteria, tumor cells) or macromolecules such as proteins, polysaccharides, or nucleoproteins. In any case, the specificity of the immune response is controlled by small molecular domains of the antigen called **antigenic determinants.** For proteins and polysaccharides, antigenic determinants consist of 4–6 amino acid or monosaccharide units. Therefore, a complex antigen such as a bacterial cell, having many antigenic determinants, will elicit a spectrum of humoral and cellular responses.

Antibodies are circulating plasma proteins (immunoglobulins, gamma globulins) which can interact specifically and noncovalently with the antigenic determinant that elicited their formation. Antibodies are secreted by plasma cells that arise by proliferation and differentiation of B lymphocytes. In humans, 5 classes of immunoglobulins are recognized.

IgG is the most abundant class and constitutes 75% of serum immunoglobulins. It also serves as a model for the other classes and, as such, will be described in more detail. IgG consists of 2 identical light chains, each with a molecular weight of 23,000, and 2 identical heavy chains with molecular weights of 50,000 each. Heavy chains have small amounts of covalently bound carbohydrate, but no carbohydrate is associated with the light chains. The chains are held together by noncovalent forces as well as by interchain disulfide bridges. The carboxy-terminal regions of the 2 heavy chains form the Fc region of the molecule. There are specific Fc receptors on some cells such as macrophages and mast cells. The amino-terminal regions of the light and heavy chains form the binding sites for antigens. These regions are variable in amino acid sequence and are thus responsible for the exquisite specificity of the immune response. IgG is the only immunoglobulin that crosses the placental barrier and is incorporated into the circulatory system of the fetus, thus protecting the newborn against infection.

IgA, with a molecular weight of 160,000 (monomeric form), is found in small amounts in serum. It is the main immunoglobulin found in tears, colostrum, and saliva, in nasal, bronchial, intestinal, and prostatic secretions, and in the vaginal fluid. Secretory IgA is composed of 2 molecules of monomeric IgA united by a polypeptide chain named **protein J** and combined with another protein known as the **secretory** or **transport component.** Secretory IgA has a molecular weight of 400,000 and, being resistant to several enzymes, can provide protection against proliferation of microorganisms in body secretions and aid in defense against penetration of the body by foreign molecules. IgA monomers and protein J are secreted by plasma cells of the mucous membranes lining the digestive, respiratory, and urinary passages, while the secretory component is synthesized by the mucosal epithelial cells.

IgM constitutes 10% of the serum immunoglobulins and usually exists as a pentamer with a molecular weight of 900,000. It is the dominant immunoglobulin in early immune responses and, together with IgD, is the major immunoglobulin found on the surfaces of B lymphocytes. These 2 classes of immunoglobulins exhibit both membrane-bound and circulating forms. Membrane-bound IgM and IgD serve as receptors for specific antigens. The result of this interaction is further differentiation of the B lymphocyte, resulting in the antibody-secreting plasma cell. IgM is also effective in activating the **complement system,** a group of plasma enzymes that have the capacity to lyse cells, including bacteria.

IgE usually exists as a monomer with a molecular weight of 190,000. This immunoglobulin has a great affinity for receptors located in the plasma membranes of mast cells and basophils. Immediately after its secretion by plasma cells, IgE attaches to these cells and practically disappears from the blood plasma. When the antigen that elicited the production of a certain IgE antibody is again encountered, the antigen-antibody complex formed on the surface of a mast cell or basophil triggers the production and liberation

of several biologically active substances, such as histamine, heparin, leukotrienes (slow-reacting substance of anaphylaxis, SRS-A), and ECF-A (eosinophil chemotactic factor of anaphylaxis). Thus, an **allergic reaction** is mediated by the activity of IgE and the antigens (**allergens**) that stimulate its production.

The properties and activities of **IgD** are not completely understood. It has a molecular weight of 180,000, and its concentration in blood plasma constitutes only 0.2% of the total of immunoglobulins. IgD is found on the plasma membranes of B lymphocytes (together with IgM) and is involved in the differentiation of these cells.

Differentiation of Lymphocytes

The plasma membranes of B lymphocytes have special forms of IgM and IgD embedded in the lipid bilayer as integral membrane proteins. These immunoglobulins serve as **receptors** for specific antigens. Cell membranes of T lymphocytes also contain antibodylike molecules that are the antigen receptors of this class of lymphocytes. Each lymphocyte carries only one kind of receptor, which can recognize only a few closely related antigenic determinants. Binding of an antigen to its receptor sets in motion the complex sequence of events that constitute the immune response. Acquisition of this specificity occurs in central lymphoid organs—thymus and bone marrow. At the same time, lymphocytes that could react against "self" antigens are destroyed.

In peripheral lymphoid organs, lymphocytes interact with the appropriate antigens, enlarge to form **lymphoblasts,** and then divide several times. Some of the division products differentiate into **effector cells.** B lymphocyte effector cells are **plasma cells** that secrete immunoglobulins into the surrounding connective tissues. Plasma cells rarely undergo cell division and live for only 2–3 days. However, in this time, they can produce several thousand immunoglobulin molecules per second. T lymphocyte effector cells are of several types. **Helper T cells** cooperate with B cells to stimulate the proliferation and differentiation of B cells into antibody-secreting plasma cells. The immune response to most antigens requires this cooperation, and these antigens are termed "thymus-dependent antigens." Immune responses can also be regulated by **suppressor T cells,** which act on helper T cells to moderate or inhibit their activities. **Cytotoxic T cells** are capable of lysing cells that bear antigens for which they are specific. Cells attacked include tumor cells and virus-infected cells. Proteins secreted by T lymphocytes and macrophages, called **lymphokines,** are responsible for regulating the proliferation of both B and T lymphocytes.

Some of the progeny of lymphocyte division do not become effector cells but are held in reserve as **memory cells.** These cells circulate in the blood and pass into lymphoid tissues via postcapillary venules (see below, under Histophysiology of Lymph Nodes), where they may reencounter the antigenic determinants that elicited their production. Since the number of memory cells is larger than the number of original effector cells, the secondary immune response is both more rapid and of greater magnitude. Memory cells recirculate for many years and provide an efficient surveillance system directed against foreign antigens.

Antigen-Presenting Cells

To be effective in an immune response, antigens must be processed and presented to effector cells. The molecular details of this activity are, as yet, uncertain. Several cells have been implicated in antigen presentation: follicular dendritic cells, some macrophages (including Kupffer cells of the liver), and Langerhans cells in the epidermis. Antigen-presenting cells are usually nonphagocytic, and they carry antigen-antibody complexes on their surfaces for long periods of time. Details about antigen-presenting cells will be provided as each organ or tissue is described.

THYMUS

The thymus is a central lymphoid organ situated in the mediastinum at about the level of the great vessels of the heart. It consists of incomplete lobules measuring about 0.5–2 mm in diameter and partially separated by septa derived from the connective tissue capsule that envelops the organ (Fig 15–1).

While other lymphoid organs originate exclusively from mesenchyme (mesoderm), the thymus has a dual embryologic origin. Its lymphocytes arise from mesenchymal cells which invade an epithelial primordium that takes its origin from the endoderm of the third and fourth pharyngeal pouches.

During intrauterine life, the thymus is colonized by lymphocyte-forming cells that come from blood islands of the yolk sac and probably also from hematopoietic cells in the liver. After birth, it is believed that colonizing cells originate only in the bone marrow.

The intense lymphocytic proliferation that takes place in the thymus during embryonic through prepubertal development pushes apart the epithelial cells. Since these cells are bound together by desmosomes, they remain attached to each other at the ends of their processes, creating an extensive network of stellate **epithelial reticular cells** (Figs 15–2 and 15–3).

Histology of the Thymus

Each lobule of the thymus consists of a peripheral zone of densely packed lymphocytes—the **cortex**—that surrounds a lightly staining central zone or **medulla** (Fig 15–1). Serial sections show that the cortical and medullary zones of a lobule are continuous with those of adjacent lobules. In the medulla are found **Hassall's corpuscles,** each consisting of several layers of flattened, concentrically arranged epithelial cells. These apparently degenerative bodies are characteristic of the thymic medulla (Fig 15–4). They increase in size and number throughout life.

Thymus Cells

Both the cortical and the medullary zones have the same cellular types, although in different proportions. The most abundant are T lymphocytes and their precursor cells in various stages of differentiation and maturation and the epithelial reticular cells (Fig 15–2). Besides these cells, the thymus has a few mesenchymal reticular cells and many macrophages. Myoid

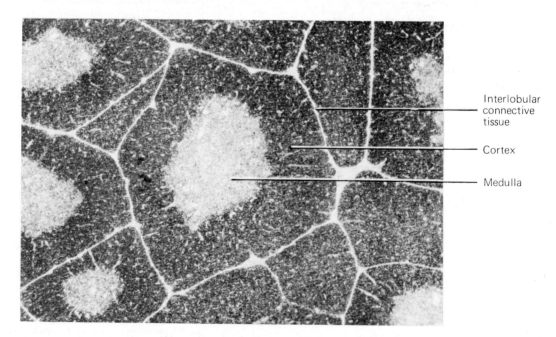

Interlobular connective tissue

Cortex

Medulla

Figure 15–1. Photomicrograph of the thymus. H&E stain, × 32.

cells, containing thick and thin filaments as well as Z-line materials, are seen in prenatal thymuses. Sarcomeres are not formed. Myoid cells are rarely seen in the postnatal thymus of humans.

Epithelial reticular cells have large oval nuclei containing lightly staining chromatin and one or 2 small nucleoli. Thin cytoplasmic processes of adjacent cells are joined by desmosomes (Fig 15–2). Bundles of tonofilaments in the cytoplasm are evidence of the epithelial origin of these cells (Fig 15–3). Dense granules are present that probably contain the secretory product of epithelial reticular cells. This secretory product may be one or more of a series of proteins and peptides which have been extracted from the thymus and which act to promote the differentiation of pre-T cells to mature T lymphocytes. Some of the better-characterized thymic hormones include serum thymic factor, thymic humoral factor, thymopoietin, and thymosin α_1.

Cortex

This zone is unique in that its blood supply consists only of capillaries and no other types of vessels. In the cortical zone, small lymphocytes predominate. These cells do not form nodules, as in other lymphoid organs, but are disposed in a continuous layer that passes from one lobule to the other. This area is a very active site of lymphocyte production. When lymphocyte precursors first enter the thymus from the bone marrow, they do not display any of the characteristic surface antigens of T lymphocytes. With time, some of these antigens are expressed, and maturing T lymphocytes move toward the medulla. Many cells die in the cortex and are phagocytized by macrophages before they can be released. The significance of this extensive cell death is not certain, but it has been suggested that it is concerned with the elimination of cells that could react to "self" antigens.

Epithelial reticular cells are less numerous in the cortical layer, and here their processes are generally very thin and long because of the distention that results from the intercalation of lymphocytes. In the cortical zone, the epithelial reticular cells envelop groups of lymphocytes multiplying in isolation from circulating antigens. Furthermore, they seem to form a complete covering at the periphery of the lobules and around

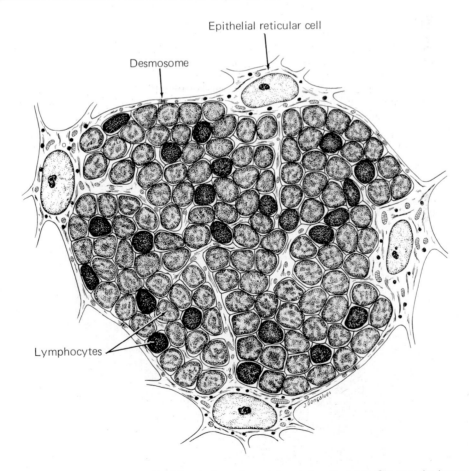

Figure 15–2. The relationship between epithelial reticular cells and thymic lymphocytes. Observe the long processes of epithelial reticular cells extending among the lymphocytes. Note the absence of reticular fibers.

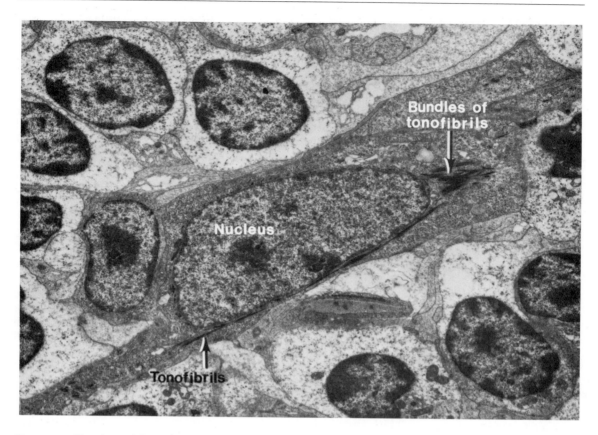

Figure 15–3. Thymic medulla seen under the electron microscope. An epithelial reticular cell runs diagonally across the figure. The nucleus has fine chromatin, and tonofibrils are present in the cytoplasm. × 7100.

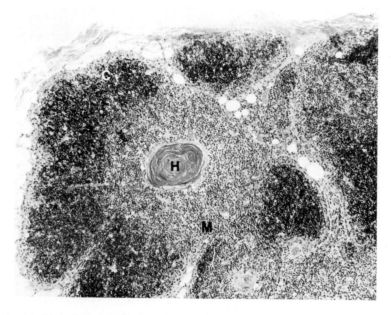

Figure 15–4. Photomicrograph of a human thymus, showing the dense cortical (C) and lighter medullary (M) zones. Near the center, one Hassall corpuscle (H) appears in the medulla. Connective tissue septa form incomplete lobules. H&E stain, × 118.

the blood and lymphatic vessels. These epithelial cells form a continuous layer that separates the thymic cortical parenchyma from the other histologic components of the organ, especially the vessels. Thus, between the epithelial cells and the capillaries, a space is encountered in which a basal lamina is seen and which also has macrophages. As a consequence of ensheathment of blood vessels by epithelial reticular cells, antigenic material has difficulty in passing through this **blood-thymus barrier** and in coming into contact with the developing and programmed T lymphocytes, although some antigens eventually do pass through. It has also been suggested that the dynamics of flow in this space direct these antigens toward the medulla of the organ and away from the cortex.

The blood-thymus barrier is present only in the cortical zone and is formed by the following layers: the blood capillary wall with its endothelial cells and basal lamina; a small amount of connective tissue containing some macrophages; the basal lamina of the epithelial reticular cells; and the cytoplasm of epithelial reticular cells. In the medullary zone, the epithelial reticular cell covering of vessels is incomplete, and there is no special barrier to the passage of molecules from the blood to the thymic parenchyma.

Medulla

The thymic medulla stains lightly because of the large number of epithelial reticular cells found there. Only about 5% of the total number of thymic lymphocytes are found in the medulla, but these cells are fully mature T lymphocytes and are generally smaller than the lymphocytes found in the cortex. They leave the thymus, via venules and efferent lymphatic vessels, to populate specific regions of peripheral lymphoid organs such as the spleen and lymph nodes.

The medulla also contains Hassall's corpuscles, which are a characteristic feature of the thymus (Fig 15–4). Hassall's corpuscles are 30–150 μm in diameter and consist of concentric layers of epithelial reticular cells. Some of these cells, mainly the innermost ones, degenerate and die. It is not rare to find Hassall's bodies with cores that consist of only cell remnants, sometimes calcified. The functional significance of Hassall's corpuscles is unknown.

Development & Involution of the Thymus

In relation to body weight, the thymus shows its maximum development immediately after birth and undergoes involution after puberty. In the newborn, it weighs 12–15 g; at puberty, 30–40 g; and in old age, 10–15 g.

The thymus is very sensitive to radiation, glucocorticoids produced by the adrenal cortex, infection, and disease. Thymuses observed at autopsies of children and adults who die after protracted illnesses are much smaller than normal.

Despite the processes of involution that accompany the passage of the years, the thymus remains capable of producing great numbers of lymphocytes

when stimulated. Involution begins in the cortical zone, which gradually becomes thinner. The medulla begins its process of involution only at puberty. Reticular cells of epithelial origin and Hassall's corpuscles are more resistant to involution than lymphocytes. The thymus never disappears completely; it is still present even in very old people and consists of reticular cells, Hassall's corpuscles, some lymphocytes, and a great amount of connective and adipose tissue.

Vascularization

Arteries enter the thymus through the capsule, branch, and penetrate the organ more deeply following the septa of connective tissue. Arterioles leave the septa to penetrate the parenchyma along the border between the cortical and medullary zones. These arterioles give off capillaries that penetrate the cortex describing an arched course, finally reaching the medulla where they drain into venules. The medulla is supplied with capillary branches of some arterioles located in the medullary-cortical border. The capillaries of the medulla drain into venules, which also receive the capillaries returning from the cortical zone.

Thymic capillaries have an endothelium without fenestrae and a very thick basal lamina (Fig 15–5). The endothelial cells have thin processes that perforate the basal lamina and may come in contact with epithelial reticular cells.

As mentioned earlier, cortical epithelial reticular cells surround all vessels of the thymic cortex and constitute a layer that separates the blood from the lymphocytes.

The medullary veins penetrate the connective tissue septa and leave the thymus through its capsule.

The thymus does not have afferent lymphatic vessels and does not constitute a filter for the lymph as do lymph nodes. The few lymphatic vessels encountered in the thymus are all efferent and localized in the walls of blood vessels and in the connective tissue of the septa and the capsule.

Histophysiology of the Thymus

It was observed as long ago as 1961 that thymectomy in newborn rats caused atrophy of other lymphoid organs and a decrease in the number of circulating lymphocytes. We now know that undifferentiated cells whose morphology is little understood migrate through the blood from the bone marrow to the **thymus,** where they proliferate, giving rise to **T lymphocytes.** As explained in Chapter 13, these lymphocytes are responsible for cell-mediated immune reactions such as delayed hypersensitivity and graft rejection, whereas **B lymphocytes,** arising in the bone marrow, differentiate into plasma cells that synthesize antibodies (immunoglobulins) and are thus responsible for the humoral immune response (Fig 15–6).

Leaving the thymus through the blood vessels in the medulla, T lymphocytes penetrate certain areas of other lymphoid organs called peripheral lymphoid organs. Those areas are called **thymus-dependent.** In mammals, the main thymus-dependent areas are the paracortical zone of lymph nodes and the periarterial sheaths in the white pulp of the spleen. On the other hand, B lymphocytes are found in lymphoid nodules of the spleen and lymph nodes as well as in Peyer's patches in the small intestine.

Both in the light microscope and in the electron microscope, B and T lymphocytes are morphologically indistinguishable. However, for each type of lymphocyte (B or T), there is a difference in the type of marker present on the surface membrane. These differences in markers are used to identify the 2 types of lymphocytes. They are shown in Table 15-1.

T lymphocytes are long-lived cells and constitute a population of cells comprising a portion of the lymphocytes of the thymus, most lymph and blood lymphocytes, and the lymphocytes found in all thymus-dependent zones.

Mitotic proliferation of lymphocytes is much higher in the cortical than in the medullary zone, being 5-10 times higher than in other lymphoid organs. The thymic mitotic rate is at its maximum at birth and decreases with age. However, only a small number of the lymphocytes produced daily in the thymus leave this organ. Most are destroyed and phagocytized within the thymus, a process whose significance is not yet fully understood.

Table 15-1. Surface markers of human T and B cells.

Marker	Method
T cells	
E rosettes	Binding of sheep red blood cells
Anti-T cell antibody	Direct or indirect immunofluorescence or cytotoxicity study
B cells	
Surface immunoglobulin	Direct immunofluorescence
EAC rosettes (complement receptor)	Binding of complement and IgM-coated sheep or ox red blood cells
Aggregated immunoglobulin	Direct or indirect immunofluorescence
Anti-B cell antibody	Direct or indirect immunofluorescence or cytotoxicity study

Thymectomy at Birth

When newborn animals are thymectomized—or in cases where the thymus does not develop during embryonic life—the following effects are observed: (1) There is no formation of T lymphocytes, with a consequent decrease in the number of lymphocytes in blood and lymph as well as a depletion of all thymus-dependent areas of lymphoid tissues and organs. (2) There is no delayed hypersensitivity reaction, and

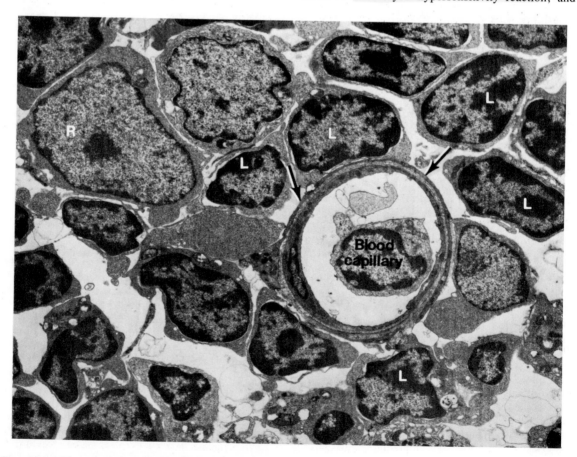

Figure 15-5. Electron micrograph of the thymic cortex. There is a blood capillary showing a thick basal lamina. Arrows point to epithelial reticular cells covering the blood vessel. Note the lymphocytes (L) and the reticular cell (R). × 28,500.

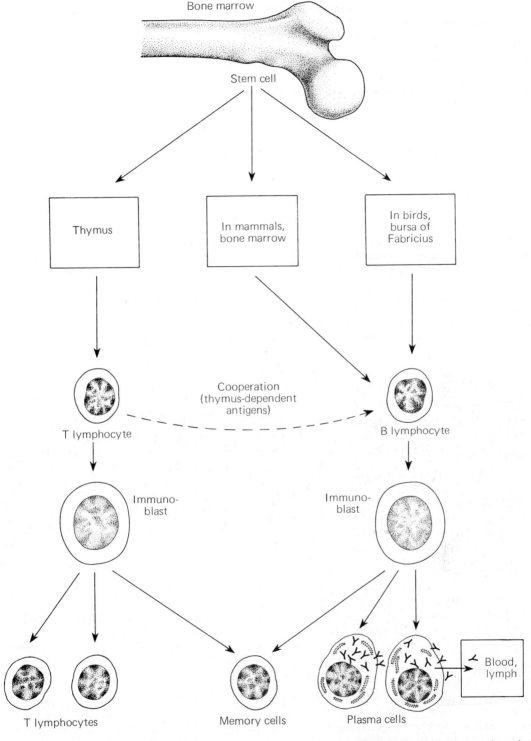

Figure 15–6. All lymphocytes originate from a stem cell, whose morphology is not clear. This cell migrates through the blood and invades the thymus, dividing many times to form T lymphocytes. In birds, the stem cells are "conditioned" to become B lymphocytes in the bursa of Fabricius, a lymphatic organ located in the cloaca. The mammalian equivalent of the bursa of Fabricius is probably the bone marrow itself. After encountering an antigen, the lymphocyte modulates into a larger cell—the immunoblast—which then proliferates and produces more T lymphocytes or plasma cells as the case may be. The so-called thymus-dependent antigens promote the transformation of B lymphocytes into plasma cells only when T lymphocytes are also present. This phenomenon is called cooperation between T cells and B cells in antibody production.

graft rejection does not occur. (3) After 3–4 months of age, the thymectomized animal becomes weak, loses weight, and dies. This has been called wasting or runt disease. Since this condition can be prevented by continuous injection of antibiotics or by keeping the thymectomized animals in a sterile environment, it is believed that death is due to widespread infections occurring simultaneously in several organs.

In humans, diseases with symptoms related to those seen in animal studies have been described, and in most cases, death occurs shortly after birth. One of the best-understood is **DiGeorge's syndrome,** which consists of congenital thymic aplasia, hypoparathyroidism, congenital heart disease, and defective cellular immunity. This disorder has been treated by transplanting fetal thymus into the patient as soon as possible after diagnosis.

On the other hand, the pool of B lymphocytes in thymectomized animals is nearly normal. They react to some antigens, producing plasma cells which synthesize antibodies. However, many antigens require both T and B lymphocytes for antibody formation. For these antigens, T lymphocytes are important for the differentiation of B lymphocytes into plasma cells. When injected into animals thymectomized immediately after birth, these antigens do not elicit the formation of antibodies and are thus called **thymus-dependent antigens** (Fig 15–6).

The generalized atrophy of lymphoid organs observed in animals thymectomized immediately after birth is believed to be due to lack of a humoral factor produced by the thymus, which stimulates the development of lymphoid tissue in general. This hypothesis is based on strong experimental evidence. For example, implantation of thymus fragments in a small box whose walls are permeable to fluids and small molecules but not to cells prevents the lymphoid atrophy of thymectomized newborn animals. It has been observed also that implantation of fragments of thymus whose lymphocytes have been destroyed by irradiation has the same protective effect. Epithelial reticular cells secrete a group of thymic hormones (thymopoietin, thymosin, and others) that have a trophic action on the lymphoid system and appear to promote the differentiation of T cells. The electron microscope shows, in the cytoplasm of these cells, small granules that are very similar to secretory granules of some endocrine glands.

Thymectomy in Adults

In adult animals, the effects of thymectomy are not as pronounced as in younger animals. There is usually a slight decrease in the number of blood lymphocytes as well as in the weight of the lymphoid organs. Since they are long-lived, the T lymphocytes that exist at the time of thymectomy maintain the pool of these circulating cells at a nearly normal level. On the other hand, since the trophic activity of the thymus is important only for the development of the lymphoid system, the lymphoid organs, once formed, are able to maintain themselves.

Thymus Grafting

In animals of any age, thymus grafting avoids the adverse effects of thymectomy. Studies of graft recipients whose cells have been labeled by chromosome markers show that there is an initial proliferation of lymphocytes from the graft. However, after the third week, lymphocytes divide for a few days but soon disappear entirely. The donor thymus then will be populated with host stem cells.

Hormones That Act on the Thymus

The thymus is subject to the effects of several hormones. Injections of some adrenocorticosteroids cause a reduction in lymphocyte number and mitotic rate. There is atrophy of the cortical layer of the thymus. Adrenocorticotropic hormone (ACTH) produced by the anterior pituitary achieves the same effect by stimulating the activity of the adrenal cortex.

Male and female sex hormones also accelerate thymic involution; castration has the reverse effect.

Pituitary growth hormone (somatotropin) stimulates thymic development in a nonspecific way, having a general effect on body growth.

ORGAN TRANSPLANTATION

Transplants are classified as **autografts** when the transplanted tissue or organ is taken from a different site on the same individual; **isografts** when the tissue or organ is taken from an identical twin; **homografts** or **allografts** when it is taken from an unrelated individual of the same species; and **heterografts** or **xenografts** when it is taken from an animal of a different species.

Autologous and isologous transplants take easily as long as an efficient blood supply is established. In such cases, there is no rejection, because the transplanted cells are genetically similar to those of the host and are composed of molecules that the organism recognizes as its own. For this reason, no antibodies are produced.

Homologous and heterologous transplants, on the other hand, contain cells whose membranes have constituents that are foreign to the host and are therefore recognized and treated as such. Transplant rejection is due mainly to the activity of **graft rejection cells** (Fig 15–7). These cells are T lymphocytes that penetrate the transplant and act locally, destroying the transplanted cells.

Homologous transplants are normally rejected. However, when this type of transplant is carried out between fraternal twins who shared the same placenta, the graft is not rejected. This was verified after observing that fraternal twin calves that had shared a single placenta, although having different blood groups, had erythrocytes from each other and did not develop an immunologic reaction. What occurs in these cases is that during embryonic life there is an exchange of blood between the animals. It is now known that an organism will never form antibodies

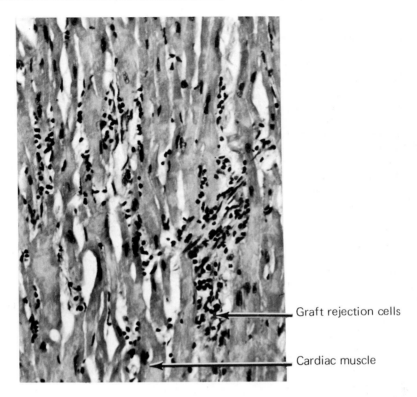

Graft rejection cells

Cardiac muscle

Figure 15–7. Photomicrograph of human myocardium from a transplanted heart. Among the cardiac muscle fibers that show degenerative changes there are many graft-rejecting cells. H&E stain, × 250.

against an antigen that was present in it before its immune system started functioning. Only the molecules that enter the body after the organism has become **immunocompetent** and has begun to synthesize antibodies are recognized as foreign and treated as antigens. In humans, the synthesis of antibodies begins a few days after birth. The infant is protected during the first few days of life mainly by antibodies received from the mother through the placenta. This is, therefore, a passive immunity that protects against infection until the child's own cells begin to produce antibodies.

LYMPH NODES

Lymph nodes are encapsulated spheroid or kidney-shaped organs composed of lymphoid tissue. They are distributed throughout the body, always along the course of the lymphatic vessels, which carry lymph into the thoracic and the right lymphatic ducts. They are found in the axillas and in the groin, along the great vessels of the neck, and in large numbers in the thorax, the abdomen, and especially in the mesentery. Lymph nodes constitute a series of in-line filters, whereby all tissue fluid–derived lymph is filtered by at least one node, prior to its return to the circulatory system. Kidney-shaped lymph nodes have a convex side and a depression, the hilum, through which the

arteries and nerves penetrate and the veins leave the organ. The shape and internal structure of lymph nodes vary greatly, but all have the basic pattern of organization described below and illustrated in Figs 15–8 and 15–9.

Lymph penetrates the lymph node through the **afferent lymphatic vessels,** which enter on the convex surface of the organ, and it exits through the **efferent lymphatic vessels** of the hilum (Fig 15–8). The flow of lymph through the node is unidirectional, being controlled by valves in the afferent and efferent vessels.

The capsule of dense connective tissue that covers lymph nodes sends trabeculae into their interior, dividing the parenchyma into incomplete compartments. A reticular tissue, consisting of a network of reticular fibers ensheathed by stellate reticular cells, unites with the connective tissue trabeculae and extends throughout the node, thus providing a scaffolding in which the immunocompetent cells are freely suspended.

Each lymph node consists of a **cortex,** situated beneath the capsule (except at the hilum), and a **medulla** that occupies the center of the organ and its hilum.

The cortex is composed of a **subcapsular sinus,** several **peritrabecular sinuses,** numerous **primary** or **secondary lymphoid nodules** (follicles), and the **paracortical** or **deep cortical areas.**

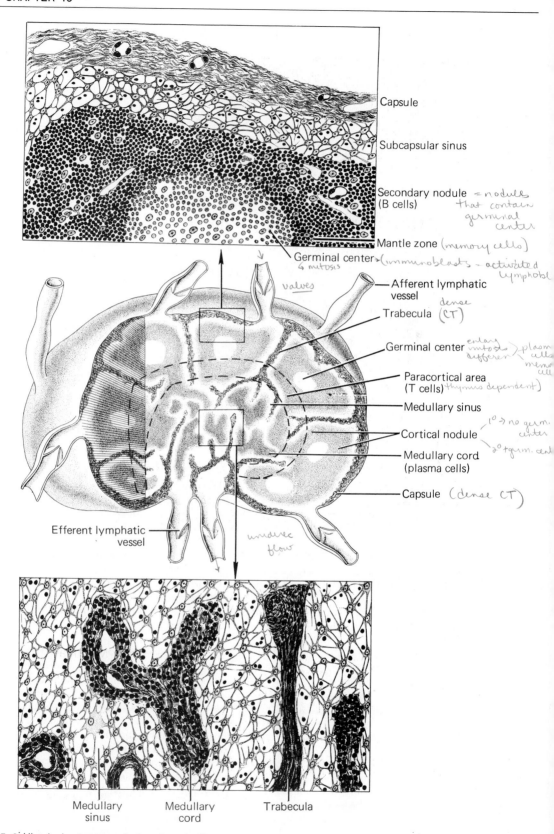

Capsule

Subcapsular sinus

Secondary nodule (B cells) *= nodules that contain germinal center*

Mantle zone *(memory cells)*

Germinal center→ *(immunoblasts - activated* *lymphobl* *↳ mitosis*

valves

Afferent lymphatic vessel

Trabecula *(CT)* *dense*

Germinal center *enlarg mitosis } plasm differen cells memor cell*

Paracortical area (T cells) *thymus dependent)*

Medullary sinus

Cortical nodule *1° → no germ. center* *2° ↑germ. cent*

Medullary cord (plasma cells)

Capsule *(dense CT)*

Efferent lymphatic vessel

undirec flow

Medullary sinus

Medullary cord

Trabecula

Figure 15–8. Histologic structure of a lymph node. The rectangular areas in the center drawing are magnified in the upper and lower drawings. The cortical layer is composed mainly of lymphatic nodules, whose germinal centers (lightly stained core of each nodule) are clearly seen in the center drawing.

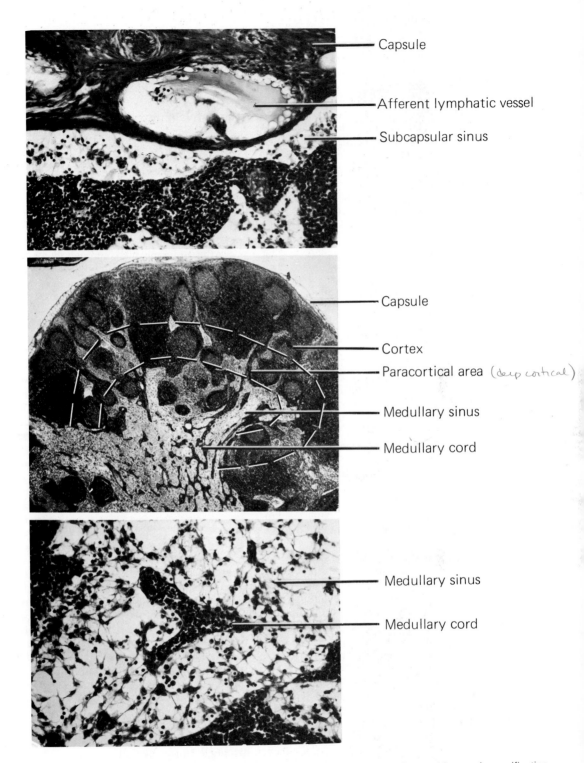

— Capsule

— Afferent lymphatic vessel

— Subcapsular sinus

— Capsule

— Cortex

— Paracortical area *(deep cortical)*

— Medullary sinus

— Medullary cord

— Medullary sinus

— Medullary cord

Figure 15–9. Photomicrographs of lymph nodes, reduced from × 30 *(middle)* and × 200 *(top* and *bottom)* magnification. H&E stain.

Sinuses of a lymph node are irregular spaces containing lymph that are incompletely lined by reticular cells and numerous macrophages (Figs 15–8 and 15–9). Reticular cells and their accompanying reticular fibers cross the sinuses, and macrophages also span these spaces. The complex architecture of sinuses serves to slow the flow of lymph through the node, thus facilitating uptake and digestion of foreign materials by macrophages.

Some of the lymphocytes in the cortex are organized into spherical or ellipsoid aggregations of cells, 0.2–1 mm in diameter, which are called primary nodules or follicles (Figs 15–8 and 15–9). The cells are mainly B lymphocytes, although some T lymphocytes are present, as are reticular cells and fibers, macrophages, and antigen-presenting cells (follicular dendritic cells). In histologic sections, nodules are strongly stained by hematoxylin as a consequence of the presence of a dense population of small lymphocytes that possess a basophilic nucleus with condensed chromatin and a narrow rim of cytoplasm. The interior of the nodule often shows a less densely stained region called the **germinal center** (Fig 15–8). This difference in staining of the central region is due to the presence of activated lymphocytes (**immunoblasts**) that have large, euchromatic nuclei as well as a larger amount of cytoplasm. Many cells in a germinal center are in mitosis. Germinal centers appear in a nodule when an antigen is present to which some of the lymphocytes can respond. The response consists of enlargement, mitosis, and differentiation into plasma cells. Some of the products of mitosis do not differentiate into plasma cells but remain as small lymphocytes known as **memory cells.** These cells are found mainly in the **mantle zone** of secondary nodules (Fig 15–8). The mantle zone is composed of those small lymphocytes which surround the germinal centers of secondary nodules. Nodules that contain germinal centers are termed secondary nodules, whereas those lacking germinal centers are called primary nodules.

Follicular dendritic cells are nonphagocytic cells with extensive, sheetlike cytoplasmic extensions. Their nuclei are irregular in shape, and few organelles indicative of secretion or phagocytosis (ie, rough endoplasmic reticulum or lysosomes) are present in their cytoplasm. These cells can trap antigens on their surfaces and ''present'' these antigens to B and T lymphocytes to produce an appropriate immunologic response.

Between adjacent nodules and between nodules and the medulla are more loosely arranged lymphocytes that constitute the paracortical or deep cortical area. Lymphocytes found in the paracortical region disappear when an animal has its thymus removed, especially if done at birth. This demonstrates that they are thymus-dependent, belonging to the population of T lymphocytes. Antigen-presenting cells, here called **dendritic cells** or **interdigitating cells,** are found in the paracortical areas of lymph nodes. Also found are the **high-endothelial venules,** which are described below.

The medulla consists of **medullary cords,** composed of closely packed lymphocytes and numerous plasma cells, and the intervening **medullary sinuses,** which receive and circulate the lymph from cortical sinuses (Fig 15–8). Medullary sinuses communicate with efferent lymphatic vessels through which lymph leaves the lymph node.

Histophysiology of Lymph Nodes

Lymph nodes can be compared to filters through which lymph flows and is cleared of foreign particles before its return to the blood circulatory system. Because lymph nodes are distributed throughout the body, lymph formed in tissues must cross at least one lymph node before entering the bloodstream. Each node receives lymph from a limited region of the body of which it is said to be a **satellite node.** Malignant tumors often metastasize via satellite nodes.

Afferent lymph enters through the convex surface of nodes and percolates through the subcapsular sinuses, passes to the peritrabecular and medullary sinuses, and leaves the lymph nodes by the efferent lymphatic vessels. As lymph flows through the sinuses, 99% or more of the antigens and other debris are removed by the phagocytic activity of macrophages that span the sinuses.

Almost all of the lymph traverses the nodule by flowing through the sinuses. However, a small amount, less than 1% of the volume, will penetrate the nodules. As lymph filters through the nodules, the bulk of the antigenic material is destroyed by macrophages. Some antigen, however, is trapped on the surface of specialized cells known as **follicular dendritic cells.** This bound antigen is not phagocytized but is exposed on the dendritic cell surface where it may be recognized and acted upon by immunologically competent lymphocytes. If a B cell recognizes the antigen, under appropriate conditions (which may necessitate the involvement of T cells), the B lymphocyte may be **activated.** Activated B lymphocytes migrate to the germinal center and undergo a series of cell divisions and transformations that lead to the production of immature **immunoblasts.** These in turn divide and give rise to **plasma cells** and **memory B lymphocytes.** Plasma cells leave the germinal center and migrate into the medullary cords. Here, these cells actively synthesize specific antibodies and release them into the lymph flowing through the medullary sinuses. Memory B cells, which can secrete some antibody and also bind some to their surface, leave the nodule and flow with the lymph to reenter the blood circulatory system. If in its travels the memory B cell encounters more of the stimulating antigen, it may leave the blood, enter the connective tissue, and differentiate into an immotile, secretory plasma cell. The presence of memory cells provides for a more rapid and more persistent immunologic response when an antigen is next encountered. This is called an anamnestic or secondary immune response.

As a consequence of infection and antigenic stimulation, affected lymph nodes enlarge, reflecting the formation of multiple germinal centers and active cell proliferation. In resting nodes, plasma cells constitute 1–3% of the cell population; however, their numbers are greatly increased in and they partially account for the enlargement of stimulated lymph nodes.

Cells in the lymph are returned to the bloodstream via the thoracic duct. Blood-borne lymphocytes, which are predominantly T cells, can repopulate the lymph nodes by leaving through specific venules in the paracortical zone of the lymph node. These vessels, **postcapillary,** or **high-endothelial, venules,** have an unusual endothelial lining consisting of tall cuboidal cells. Lymphocytes are capable of traveling between the endothelial cells of this vessel. Other lymphoid tissues, such as Peyer's patches of the ileum, also possess high-endothelial venules. It has been shown that certain lymphocytes preferentially recirculate through different lymphoid tissues. Thus, peripheral lymph nodes have more T lymphocytes than B lymphocytes, whereas the reverse is true of Peyer's patches. This "homing" behavior is due to complementary molecules on the lymphocytes and the endothelial cells of postcapillary venules. Each type of lymphocyte has a different integral membrane glycoprotein at its surface that binds to carbohydrates on endothelial cells. The carbohydrates present on endothelial cells vary according to anatomic site. This receptor-ligand interaction results in the differential localization of B and T lymphocytes mentioned above. Lymphocytes that pass between the endothelial cells of the venules penetrate the paracortical zone and medullary sinuses and leave the node via efferent lymphatics together with newly formed lymphocytes. In this way, most T lymphocytes recirculate many times. Recirculation of lymphocytes also occurs through venules found in the spleen, tonsils, and Peyer's patches of the ileum.

THE SPLEEN

The spleen is the largest accumulation of lymphatic tissue in the organism, and in humans it is the largest lymphatic organ in the circulatory system. Owing to its abundance of phagocytic cells and the close contact between the circulating blood and these cells, the spleen represents an important defense against microorganisms that penetrate the circulation and is also the site of destruction of many red cells. As is true of all other lymphatic organs, the spleen is a site of formation of activated lymphocytes, which pass into the blood. The spleen reacts promptly to antigens carried in the blood and is an important antibody-forming organ. While lymph nodes serve as immunologic filters of the lymph, the spleen is the immunologic filter of the blood.

General Structure

The spleen is surrounded by a capsule of dense connective tissue which sends out trabeculae that divide the parenchyma or **splenic pulp** into incomplete compartments (Fig 15–10). The medial surface of the spleen presents a hilum, where the capsule gives rise to a number of trabeculae which carry the nerves and arteries into the splenic pulp. Veins derived from the parenchyma and lymphatic vessels that originate in the trabeculae leave through the hilum. The splenic pulp has no lymphatic vessels.

The connective tissue of the capsule and of the trabeculae contains some smooth muscle cells. In hu-

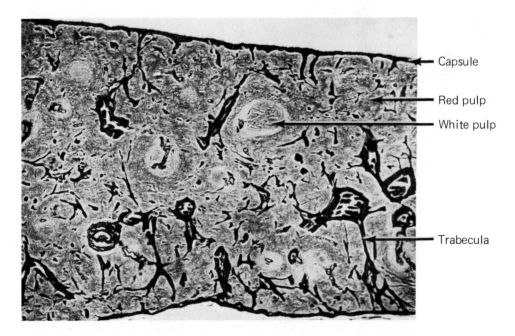

Figure 15–10. Photomicrograph of a silver-stained spleen section to show the general architecture of the organ. × 30.

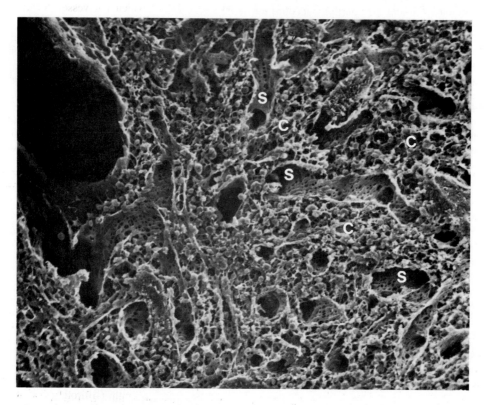

Figure 15–11. General view of splenic red pulp with a scanning electron microscope. Note the sinusoids (S) and the red pulp cords (C). × 360. (Reproduced, with permission, from Miyoshi M, Fujita T: Stereo-fine structure of the splenic red pulp: A combined scanning and transmission electron microscope study on dog and rat spleen. *Arch Histol Jpn* 1971;**33**:225.)

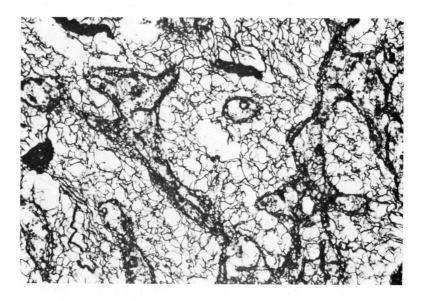

Figure 15–12. Photomicrograph of the network of splenic reticular fibers. Silver-stained section, × 200.

mans, these cells are not numerous. In certain other mammals (cat, dog, horse) they are quite abundant, and their contraction causes the expulsion of accumulated blood from the spleen, which has a spongy structure and serves to store blood cells.

Splenic Pulp

On the surface of a fresh or fixed slice cut through the spleen, one can observe white spots in the parenchyma with the naked eye. These are lymphatic nodules and are part of the **white pulp.** These nodules appear within the dark red tissue, rich in blood, called the **red pulp** (Figs 15–10, 15–11, 15–13, and 15–14). Examination under a low-power microscope reveals that the red pulp is composed of elongated structures, the **splenic cords** (Billroth's cords), which lie between the **sinusoids** (Fig 15–11).

All of the splenic pulp is supported by connective tissue containing reticular fibers. Fixed cellular elements of this tissue are the reticular cells and macrophages, and the function of the reticular fibers is that of support (Fig 15–12). Electron microscopy has demonstrated that the reticular fibers may be encased in extensions of reticular cells.

Blood Circulation

The splenic artery divides as it penetrates the hilum, branching out into vessels of various sizes that follow the course of the connective tissue trabeculae and are called **trabecular arteries.** When they leave the trabeculae to enter the parenchyma, the arteries are immediately enveloped by a sheath of lymphocytes. These vessels are known as the **central arteries** or **white pulp arteries.** Along its course, the lymphocytic sheath (white pulp) may thicken to form a number of lymphatic nodules in which the vessel occupies an eccentric position, although it is still called the central artery. During its course through the white pulp, the artery divides into numerous radial branches that supply the lymphatic tissue surrounding it.

After leaving the white pulp, the central artery, now called the pulp artery, subdivides to form straight **penicillar arterioles** with an outside diameter of approximately 25 μm. Near their termination, some of the penicillar arterioles are surrounded by a sheath of phagocytic cells whose function is to ingest blood-borne particles.

Beyond the sheath, the vessels continue as simple arterial capillaries that carry blood to the **sinusoids** (red pulp sinuses). These sinusoids occupy the area between the red pulp cords (Figs 15–11 and 15–13). The manner in which blood flows from the arterial capillaries of the red pulp to the interior of the sinusoids has not yet been completely explained. Some investigators consider that the capillaries open directly into the sinusoids; others maintain that the blood passes through the spaces between the red pulp cord cells and then moves on to be collected by the sinusoids (Figs 15–13 and 15–16). In the first instance, this would mean a **closed** circulation, as proposed by the supporters of the "closed theory," who maintain that the blood always remains inside the vessels. In the second case, the circulation would open into the parenchyma of the red pulp (Billroth's cords), and the

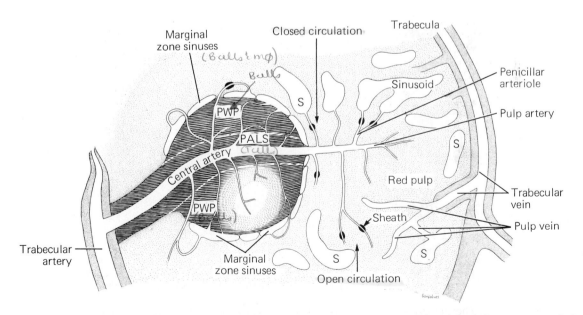

Figure 15–13. Schematic view of the blood circulation of the spleen. Theories of open and closed circulation are represented in this drawing. Splenic sinuses (S) are indicated. PALS, periarterial lymphatic sheath; PWP, peripheral white pulp. (Redrawn and reproduced, with permission, from Greep RO, Weiss L: *Histology,* 3rd ed. McGraw-Hill, 1973.)

blood would pass through the area between the cells in order to reach the sinusoids (**open** circulation). Others maintain that in a distended spleen, full of blood, the circulation would be open, whereas in a spleen with little blood the arterial capillaries would connect directly with the sinusoids, establishing a closed circulation. Current evidence suggests that the blood circulation in the human spleen is of the open type.

From the sinusoids, the blood proceeds to the red pulp veins that join together and enter the trabeculae, forming the **trabecular veins.** From these latter vessels originates the splenic vein, which emerges from the hilum of the spleen. The trabecular veins do not have individual muscle walls, ie, their walls are composed of trabecular tissue. They can be regarded as channels hollowed out in the trabecular connective tissue and lined by endothelium.

White Pulp

White pulp consists of lymphatic tissue arranged in sheaths around central arteries as well as lymphoid nodules appended to the sheaths. The lymphoid cells surrounding central arteries are mainly T lymphocytes and form the **periarterial lymphatic sheaths (PALS).** Lymphoid nodules consist of a preponderance of B lymphocytes (Figs 15–13, 15–14, and 15–15). As is the case with lymphatic tissue in general, reticular cells and reticular fibers are both present and form a 3-dimensional mesh. The spaces in this mesh are occupied mainly by lymphocytes and macrophages.

Between the white pulp and the red pulp lies a **marginal zone** consisting of many sinuses and of loose lymphoid tissue. In this zone there are few lymphocytes but many macrophages showing active phagocytosis. The marginal zone harbors an abundance of blood antigens and thus plays a major role in the immunologic activity of the spleen. Many of the pulp arterioles, derived from the central artery, extend out and away from the white pulp but then turn back and empty into the moatlike sinuses of the marginal zone that encircles the nodules. As a consequence of this drainage, which includes the added blood flow from vessels within the white pulp that also terminate in the marginal zone, this area plays a significant role in filtering the blood and launching an immune response. A large number of macrophages phagocytize and remove antigenic debris. **Dendritic cells** (interdigitating dendritic cells) in the marginal zone trap and present antigens to immunologically competent cells. The marginal zone is an ideal site for this activity, since not only are antigens removed from the blood here but also the T and B lymphocytes. As these lymphocytes leave the systemic circulation to penetrate the white pulp, they pass by the dendritic cells. If the appropriate B cells, T cells, and antigen are present, an immune response will be initiated. Activated B cells migrate to the center of the white pulp nodule and give rise to immunoblasts, plasma cells, and activated B cells. Plasma cells migrate to the cords of Billroth and release antibody into the blood of the sinuses.

The lymphocytes of the periarterial lymphatic sheath (PALS) are **thymus-dependent,** whereas the marginal zones and the nodules—the **peripheral white pulp**—are populated by B lymphocytes. Thus, the splenic white pulp has B and T lymphocytes segregated in 2 different sites.

Red Pulp

The red pulp is a reticular tissue with a special characteristic, ie, the presence of **splenic cords of**

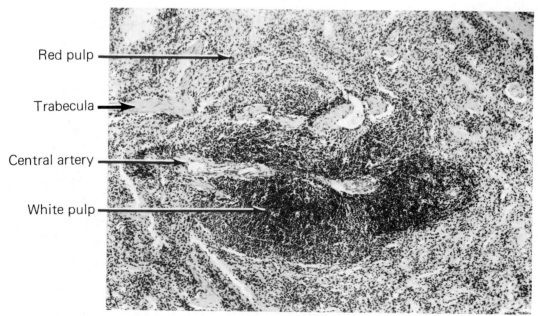

Figure 15–14. Photomicrograph of splenic white and red pulp. H&E stain, × 100.

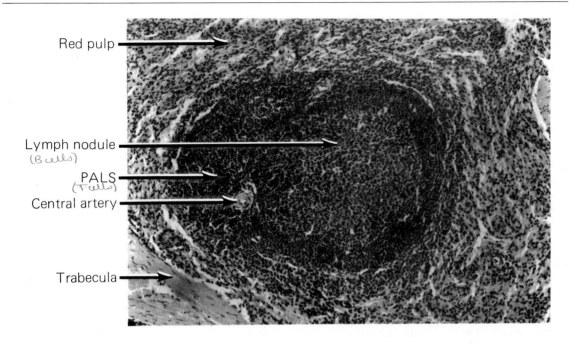

Red pulp

Lymph nodule
(B cells)

PALS
(T cells)
Central artery

Trabecula

Figure 15–15. Photomicrograph of the spleen, showing a lymphatic nodule (white pulp) surrounded by red pulp. × 150.

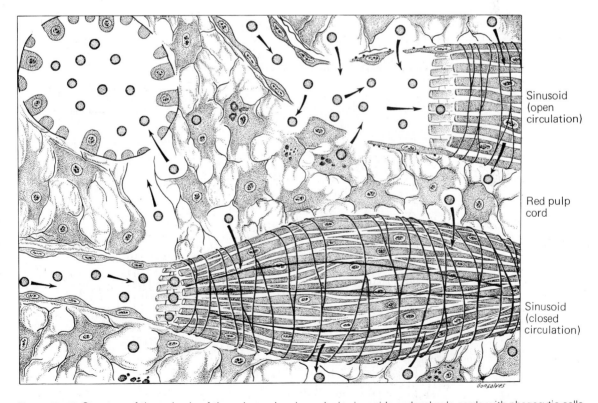

Sinusoid
(open
circulation)

Red pulp
cord

Sinusoid
(closed
circulation)

Figure 15–16. Structure of the red pulp of the spleen, showing splenic sinusoids and red pulp cords with phagocytic cells (some with phagocytized material). The relationship between reticular fibers and sinusoid lining cells is also shown. A sinusoid in cross section is shown at upper left. Both the open and closed theories of spleen blood circulation are illustrated.

Billroth. The cords consist of all the cells between the sinusoids.

The cords are continuous and of varying thickness according to the local distention of the sinusoids. Besides reticular cells, the splenic cords contain fixed and wandering macrophages, monocytes, lymphocytes, plasma cells, and many blood elements (erythrocytes, platelets, and granulocytes).

The **sinusoids** of the spleen differ from common capillaries in 3 ways: (1) they have a dilated, large, irregular lumen; (2) between their lining endothelial cells are spaces that permit exchange between the sinusoids and adjacent tissues; and (3) the basal lamina–like material is not continuous but forms barrel hoop–like rings around the endothelial walls.

The endothelial cells that line the splenic sinusoids are elongated, with their long axis parallel to the long axis of the sinusoids. These cells are enveloped in reticular fibers set mainly in a transverse direction, similar to the hoops of a barrel. The transverse fibers and those oriented longitudinally join to form a network enveloping the sinusoid cells (Fig 15–16). It was formerly thought that the endothelial cells of sinuses were phagocytic; however, it appears that the observed phagocytosis was due to processes of macrophages that had penetrated the spaces between adjacent endothelial cells.

The spaces between the cells of the splenic sinusoids are 2–3 μm in diameter or even smaller, so that only flexible cells are able to pass easily from the red pulp cords to the lumen of the sinusoids (Fig 15–17).

Sickle cell anemia is a molecular disease in which a glutamic acid residue in the β chain of normal hemoglobin is replaced by a valine residue. This results in profound changes in the conformation of hemoglobin molecules when they are exposed to hypoxic environments, as in the spleen. Under these conditions, hemoglobin "crystallizes" and forms long aggregates that deform the red blood cell into a characteristic "sickle" shape (Fig 13–6). These cells are not flexible and cannot pass between the endothelial cells lining the splenic sinusoids. Such cells are destroyed here, and an anemia results.

Histophysiology of the Spleen

The spleen is a lymphatic organ with special characteristics. Its best-known functions are (1) formation of lymphocytes, (2) destruction of erythrocytes, (3) defense of the organism against foreign particles that enter the bloodstream, and (4) storage of blood.

A. Production of Blood Cells: The white pulp of the spleen produces lymphocytes that migrate to the red pulp and reach the lumens of the sinusoids, where they are incorporated into the blood that is present

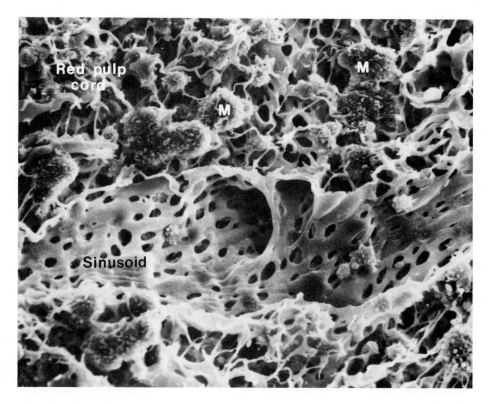

Figure 15–17. Scanning electron micrograph of the red pulp of the spleen, showing sinusoids, red pulp cords, and macrophages (M). × 1600. (Reproduced, with permission, from Miyoshi M, Fujita T: Stereo-fine structure of the splenic red pulp: A combined scanning and transmission electron microscope study on dog and rat spleen. *Arch Histol Jpn* 1971;**33**:225.)

there. In the fetus, the spleen also produces granulocytes (neutrophils, basophils, and eosinophils) and erythrocytes, but this activity ceases at the end of the fetal phase. In certain pathologic conditions (eg, leukemia), the spleen may recommence the production of granulocytes and erythrocytes, thus undergoing a process known as **myeloid metaplasia** (pathologic transformation of one kind of cell into another).

B. Destruction of Erythrocytes: Red blood cells have an average life span of 120 days, after which they are destroyed, mainly in the spleen. This phenomenon of the removal of degenerating erythrocytes also occurs in the bone marrow.

The macrophages of the red pulp cords engulf entire pieces of the erythrocytes that frequently fragment in the extracellular spaces. The engulfed erythrocytes are digested by lysosomes of the macrophages. The hemoglobin they contain is broken down into several parts. The protein part, globin, is hydrolyzed to amino acids that are reutilized for protein synthesis. Iron is released from heme and is transported in blood, in combination with transferrin, to the bone marrow, where it is reused in erythropoiesis. Iron-free heme is metabolized to bilirubin, which is excreted by liver cells in the bile.

C. Defense: Since it contains both B and T lymphocytes and macrophages, the spleen is important in body defense. In the same way that lymph nodes "filter" the lymph, the spleen is considered as a "filter" for the blood.

Under the stimulus of antigens, splenic B lymphocytes proliferate and give rise to antibody-producing plasma cells.

Of all the phagocytic cells of the organism, those of the spleen are most active in the phagocytosis of living particles (bacteria and viruses) and inert particles that find their way into the bloodstream. After the injection of trypan blue, the macrophages of the spleen are among the first to accumulate this dye.

When there is an excess of lipids in the blood plasma (hyperlipidemia), the macrophages of the spleen accumulate considerable quantities of these substances. In diabetes, hyperlipidemia is frequent, and for this reason large macrophages, their cytoplasm containing numerous lipid droplets, are common in the spleens of diabetics.

D. Blood Storage: Owing to the spongy structure of the red pulp, the spleen stores blood, which can be returned to the circulation to increase the volume of circulating blood. In animals with spleens composed of a capsule and trabeculae rich in smooth muscle, the organ is emptied by muscular contraction. Because the human spleen is poor in smooth muscle fibers, the storage and expulsion of blood depend on changes in the diameter of the blood vessels. It has been demonstrated that in humans the blood storage capacity of the spleen is very small.

UNENCAPSULATED LYMPHOID TISSUE

Lymphatic nodules—also called lymphatic follicles—can be found isolated in the loose connective tissue of several organs, mainly in the lamina propria of the digestive tract, upper respiratory tract, and urinary passages. Lymphatic nodules are especially common in the connective tissue underlying the line where 2 types of epithelia meet, eg, the gastroesophageal junction. Unencapsulated nodules have the same microscopic structure as nodules in the cortex of a lymph node. They are composed of densely packed lymphocytes, mainly B lymphocytes that differentiate into plasma cells upon appropriate antigenic stimulation. Plasma cells secrete IgA, which is transported through the overlying epithelium to provide protective antibodies at the luminal surface.

Peyer's patches are aggregates of unencapsulated nodules found in the lamina propria of the ileum. They are discussed more extensively in Chapter 16.

TONSILS

Tonsils are organs composed of aggregates of incompletely encapsulated lymphoid tissue that lie beneath but in contact with the epithelium of the digestive tract. According to their location, tonsils in the mouth and pharynx are called **palatine tonsils, pha-**

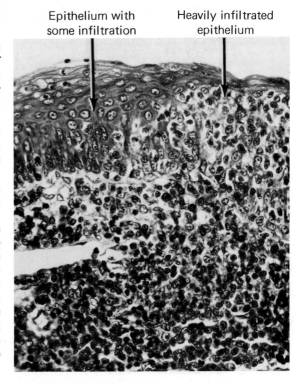

Epithelium with some infiltration   Heavily infiltrated epithelium

Figure 15–18. Photomicrograph of a palatine tonsil. The stratified squamous epithelium is infiltrated by lymphocytes. H&E stain, × 400.

ryngeal tonsil, and **lingual tonsils.** Tonsils produce lymphocytes, many of which cross the epithelium and are deposited in the mouth and pharynx.

Palatine Tonsils

The 2 palatine tonsils are located in the lateral walls of the oral part of the pharynx. The dense lymphoid tissue present in these tonsils forms, under the squamous stratified epithelium, a band that contains lymphatic nodules, generally with germinal centers. Each tonsil has 10–20 epithelial invaginations that penetrate the parenchyma deeply, forming the **crypts,** which contain in their lumens desquamated epithelial cells, live and dead lymphocytes, and bacteria. They may appear as purulent spots in tonsillitis (Figs 15–18 and 15–19).

Separating the lymphoid tissue from subjacent organs is a band of dense connective tissue called the **capsule** of the tonsil. This capsule usually acts as a barrier against spreading tonsillar infections.

Pharyngeal Tonsil

This is a single tonsil situated in the superoposterior portion of the pharynx. It is covered by ciliated pseudostratified columnar epithelium typical of the respiratory tract. Areas of stratified epithelium may also be observed.

The pharyngeal tonsil is composed of pleats of mucosa and shows diffuse lymphoid tissue and lymphatic nodules. It has no crypts.

The capsule of the pharyngeal tonsil is thinner than the capsules of the palatine tonsils.

Lingual Tonsils

The lingual tonsils are smaller and more numerous than the others. They are situated at the base of the tongue and are covered by squamous stratified epithelium. Each has a single crypt (Fig 16–1).

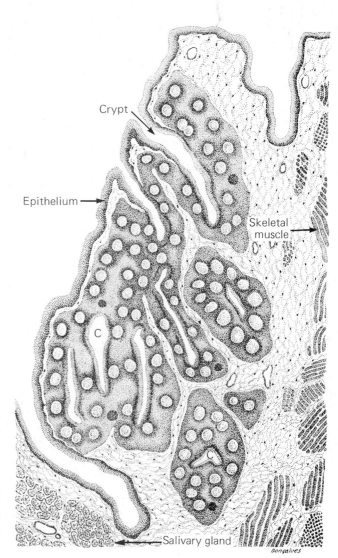

Figure 15–19. Palatine tonsil. There are numerous lymphatic nodules near the stratified squamous epithelium of the oropharynx. The light areas in the lymphoid tissue are germinal centers. Note the sections through the epithelial crypts (C).

REFERENCES

Anderson AO, Anderson NJ: Studies on the structure and permeability of the microvasculature in normal rat lymph nodes. *Am J Pathol* 1975;**80:**387.

Bach JF: Thymic hormones. *J Immunopharmacol* 1979;**1:**277.

Balfour BM et al: Antigen-presenting cells, including Langerhans cells, veiled cells, and interdigitating cells. *Ciba Found Symp* 1981;**84:**281.

Bearman RM, Levine GD, Bensch KG: The ultrastructure of the normal human thymus: A study of 36 cases. *Anat Rec* 1978;**190:**755.

Chen LL, Adams JC, Steinman RM: Anatomy of germinal centers in mouse spleen, with special reference to "follicular dendritic cells." *J Cell Biol* 1978;**77:**148.

Chen LT, Weiss L: Electron microscopy of the red pulp of human spleen. *Am J Anat* 1972;**134:**425.

Cordier AC, Haumont SM: Development of the thymus, parathyroids and ultimobranchial bodies in NMRI and nude mice. *Am J Anat* 1980;**157:**227.

Gowans JL, Knight EJ: The route of recirculation of lymphocytes in the rat. *Proc R Soc Lond [Biol]* 1964;**159:**257.

Haar JL: Light and electron microscopy of the human fetal thymus. *Anat Rec* 1974;**179:**463.

Hirasawa Y, Tokuhiro H: Electron microscopic studies on the normal human spleen, especially on the red pulp and the reticuloendothelial cells. *Blood* 1970;**35:**201.

Hoefsmit ECM: Macrophages, Langerhans cells, interdigitating and dendritic accessory cells: A summary. *Adv Exp Med Biol* 1982;**149:**463.

Ito T, Hoshino T: Fine structure of the epithelial reticular cells of the medulla of the thymus in the golden hamster. *Z Zellforsch Mikrosk Anat* 1966;**69:**311.

Klaus GGB et al: The follicular dendritic cell: Its role in antigen presentation in the generation of immunological memory. *Immunol Rev* 1980;**53:**3.

Lumb JR: Perspectives on the in vivo location of cellular interactions in the humoral immune response. *Annu Rev Microbiol* 1979;**33:**439.

Marrack P, Kappler J: The T cell and its receptor. *Sci Am* (Feb) 1986;**254:**36.

Paul WE: *Fundamental Immunology*. Raven Press, 1984.

Raviola E, Karnovsky MJ: Evidence for a blood-thymus barrier using electron opaque tracers. *J Exp Med* 1972;**136:**466.

Rouse RV, Weissman IL: Microanatomy of the thymus: Its relationship to T cell differentiation. *Ciba Found Symp* 1981;**84:**161.

Scollay RG, Butcher EC, Weissman IL: Thymus cell migration: Quantitative aspects of cellular traffic from the thymus to the periphery in mice. *Eur J Immunol* 1980;**10:**210.

Stevens SK, Weissman IL, Butcher EC: Differences in the migration of B and T lymphocytes: Organ-selective localization in vivo and the role of lymphocyte-endothelial cell recognition. *J Immunol* 1982;**128:**844.

Stites DP et al (editors): *Basic & Clinical Immunology*, 4th ed. Lange, 1984.

Weiss L: *The Cells and Tissues of the Immune System*. Prentice-Hall, 1972.

Weiss L: A scanning electron microscopic study of the spleen. *Blood* 1974;**43:**665.

16

Digestive Tract

The digestive system consists of the digestive tract (oral cavity, mouth, esophagus, stomach, small and large intestines, rectum, and anus) and its associated glands (salivary glands, liver, and pancreas). Its function is to obtain from ingested food the metabolites necessary for the growth and energy needs of the body. Before being stored or used as energy, food is digested and transformed into small molecules that can be easily absorbed through the lining of the digestive tract. However, a barrier between the environment and the internal milieu of the body must be maintained.

The first step in the complex process known as digestion occurs in the mouth, where food is ground by the teeth into smaller pieces and moistened by saliva, which also initiates the digestion of carbohydrates. Digestion continues in the stomach and small intestine. In the small intestine, the food—transformed into its basic components (amino acids, monosaccharides, free fatty acids, monoglycerides, etc)—is absorbed. Water absorption occurs in the large intestine, and as a consequence the undigested contents become semisolid.

GENERAL STRUCTURE OF THE DIGESTIVE TRACT

The entire gastrointestinal tract presents certain common structural characteristics. The digestive tract is a hollow tube composed of a lumen of variable diameter surrounded by a wall made up of 4 principal layers: the **mucosa,** the **submucosa,** the **muscularis externa,** and the **serosa.** The structure of these layers is summarized below and illustrated in Fig 16–1.

The **mucosa** is composed of (1) an **epithelial lining;** (2) a **lamina propria** of loose connective tissue rich in blood and lymph vessels and smooth muscle cells, sometimes containing also glands and lymphoid tissue; and (3) the **muscularis mucosae,** usually consisting of an inner circular and an outer longitudinal layer of smooth muscle cells separating the mucosa from the submucosa. The mucosa is frequently called a **mucous membrane.**

The **submucosa** is composed of loose connective tissue with many blood and lymph vessels and a **submucosal** (also called **Meissner's**) **nerve plexus.** It may also contain glands and lymphoid tissue.

The **muscularis externa** contains the following elements: (1) Smooth muscle cells, spirally oriented, divided into 2 sublayers according to the main direction the muscle cells follow. In the internal sublayer

(close to the lumen), the orientation is generally circular; in the external sublayer, it is mostly longitudinal. (2) The **myenteric** (or **Auerbach's**) **nerve plexus,** which lies between the 2 muscle sublayers. (3) Blood and lymph vessels in the connective tissue between the muscle sublayers.

The **serosa** is a thin layer composed of (1) loose connective tissue, rich in blood and lymph vessels and adipose tissue; and (2) simple squamous covering epithelium (mesothelium).

The main functions of the epithelial lining of the digestive tract are (1) to provide a selectively permeable barrier between the contents of the tract and the tissues of the body; (2) to facilitate the transport and digestion of food; (3) to promote the absorption of the products of this digestion; and (4) to produce hormones that affect the activity of the digestive system. Cells in this layer either produce mucus or are involved in digestion or absorption of food.

The abundant lymphoid nodules present in the lamina propria and in the submucosal layer protect the organism (in association with the epithelium) from bacterial invasion. The necessity for this immunologic support is obvious if one considers that—with the exception of the oral cavity, esophagus, and anal canal—the entire digestive tract is lined by a simple thin and vulnerable epithelium. Careful study of the lamina propria has demonstrated that there is a zone rich in macrophages and lymphoid cells just below the epithelium. Some of these lymphoid cells actively produce antibodies. These antibodies are mainly immunoglobulin A (IgA) and are bound to a secretory protein produced by the epithelial cells of the intestinal lining and secreted into the intestinal lumen (Fig 16–2). This complex is thought to have a protective activity against viral and bacterial invasion. It is significant that there are 20–30 IgA-secreting cells for every IgG-producing cell in this region and that IgM-secreting cells are 5 times more numerous than IgG cells.

The muscularis mucosae promotes the movement of the mucosa independently of other movements of the digestive tract and, as a consequence, increases its contact with the food. The contractions of the muscularis externa propel and mix the food in the digestive tract. Nerve plexuses coordinate this muscular contraction. They are composed mainly of nerve cell aggregates (multipolar visceral neurons) forming small parasympathetic ganglia. A rich network of pre- and postganglionic fibers of the autonomic nervous system and some visceral sensory fibers in these ganglia permit communication between them. The num-

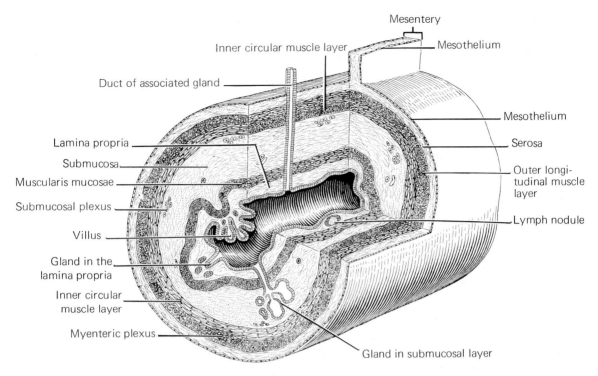

Figure 16–1. Schematic structure of a portion of the digestive tract with various possible components. (Redrawn and reproduced, with permission, from Bevelander G: *Outline of Histology,* 7th ed. Mosby, 1971.)

ber of these ganglia along the digestive tract is variable. They are more numerous in regions where motility is greatest.

In certain diseases such as Hirschsprung's disease or *Trypanosoma cruzi* infection (Chagas' disease), the digestive tract plexuses are severely injured and most of their neurons are destroyed. This results in disturbances of digestive tract motility with frequent dilatations in some areas. The fact that the digestive tract receives abundant innervation from the autonomic nervous system provides an anatomic explanation of the widely observed action of emotional disturbances

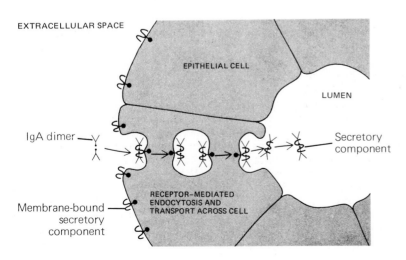

Figure 16–2. The mechanism by which the secretory component mediates the transport of a dimeric IgA molecule across an epithelial cell. The entire complex is transported from the extracellular fluid into the lumen of the epithelial tube. The secretory component is synthesized by the epithelial cell as a transmembrane glycoprotein and serves as a receptor on its basolateral surface for binding the IgA dimer. The secretory component–IgA complex enters the cell in an endocytotic vesicle, which crosses the cell and is exocytosed at the apical surface. The part of the secretory component that is bound to the IgA dimer is then cleaved from its transmembrane tail (black dot), thereby releasing the complex into the lumen. (Reproduced, with permission, from Alberts B et al: *Molecular Biology of the Cell.* Garland, 1983.)

on the digestive tract—a phenomenon of importance in psychosomatic medicine.

THE ORAL CAVITY

The oral cavity is lined with nonkeratinized stratified squamous epithelium. Its superficial cells are nucleated and have scanty granules of keratin in their interior. In the lips, a transition from nonkeratinized to keratinized epithelium can be observed. The lamina propria has papillae, similar to those in the dermis of the skin, and is continuous with a submucosa containing diffuse small salivary glands.

The roof of the mouth is composed of the hard and soft palates, both covered with the same type of stratified squamous epithelium. In the hard palate, the mucous membrane rests on bony tissue. The soft palate has a core of skeletal muscle and numerous mucous glands in its submucosa.

The palatine **uvula** is a small conical process that extends downward from the center of the lower border of the soft palate. It has a core of muscle and areolar connective tissue covered by typical oral mucosa.

1. THE TONGUE

The tongue is a mass of striated muscle covered by a mucous membrane whose structure varies according to the region studied. The muscle fibers cross one another in 3 planes. They are grouped in bundles, usually separated by connective tissue. The mucous membrane is strongly adherent to the muscle, because the connective tissue of the lamina propria penetrates the spaces between the muscular bundles. On the lower surface of the tongue, the mucous membrane is smooth. The dorsal surface is irregular, covered anteriorly by a great number of small eminences called **papillae.** The posterior one-third of the dorsal surface of the tongue is separated from the anterior two-thirds by a V-shaped boundary. Behind this boundary, the surface of the tongue shows small bulges composed mainly of small lymphatic aggregations of 2 types: (1) small collections of lymph nodules; and (2) the lingual tonsils, where lymph nodules aggregate around invaginations (crypts) of the mucous membrane (Fig 16–3).

Papillae

Papillae are elevations of the oral epithelium and

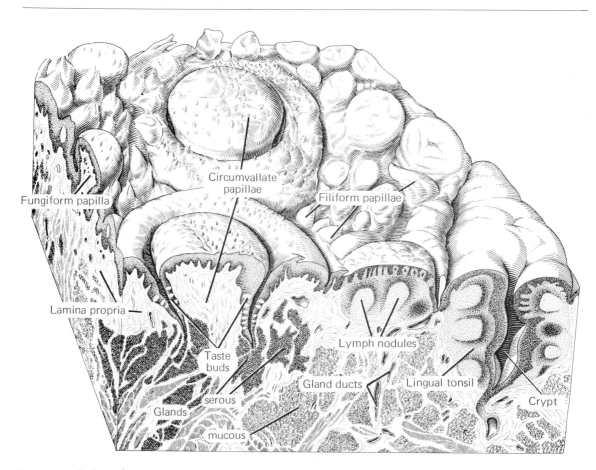

Figure 16–3. Surface of tongue on the region close to its V-shaped boundary between the anterior and posterior portions. Observe the lymph nodules, lingual tonsils, glands, and papillae. (After Braus.)

lamina propria that assume different forms and functions. There are 4 types:

A. Filiform Papillae: These papillae have an elongated conical shape, are quite numerous, and are present over the entire surface of the tongue. Their epithelium, which does not contain taste buds, is frequently partially keratinized (Fig 16– 3).

B. Fungiform Papillae: These resemble mushrooms in that they have a narrow stalk and a smooth-surfaced, dilated upper part (Fig 16– 3). These papillae, which contain scattered taste buds on their upper surfaces, are irregularly interspersed among the filiform papillae.

C. Foliate Papillae: These papillae are poorly developed in humans. They consist of 2 or more parallel ridges and furrows on the dorsolateral surface of the tongue. Ducts from serous glands drain into the bases of the furrows. Numerous taste buds are present in the walls of the furrows in animals such as the rabbit (Fig 10– 3).

D. Circumvallate Papillae: These are extremely large circular papillae whose flattened surfaces extend above the other papillae (Fig 16– 3). The 7– 12 circumvallate papillae are distributed in the "V" region in the posterior portion of the tongue. Numerous serous (von Ebner) glands drain their contents into the deep groove that encircles the periphery of each papilla. This "moatlike" arrangement provides a continuous flow of fluid over the great number of taste buds present along the sides of this papilla. This flow of secretions is important in removing food particles from the vicinity of the taste buds so that they can receive and process new gustatory stimuli. In addition to the serous glands associated with this type of papilla, other small mucous and serous glands dispersed throughout the lining of the oral cavity act in the same way to prepare the taste buds in other parts of the oral cavity—epiglottis, pharynx, palate, etc—to respond to taste stimuli. The appearance and location of taste buds within the epithelium of the papillae are illustrated in Figs 10– 3 and 10– 4. The distribution of the various types of papillae on the surface of the tongue is illustrated in Fig 10– 6.

2. THE PHARYNX

The pharynx represents a transition space between the oral cavity and the respiratory and digestive systems. It forms a communication between the nasal region and the larynx. The pharynx is lined by stratified squamous epithelium of the mucous type, except in those regions of the respiratory portions that are not subject to abrasion. In these latter areas, the epithelium is pseudostratified ciliated columnar with goblet cells.

The pharynx contains the tonsils (described in Chapter 15). The mucosa of the pharynx also has many small mucous glands in its dense connective tissue layer. Outside this layer are located the constrictor and longitudinal muscles of the pharynx.

3. TEETH & ASSOCIATED STRUCTURES

In adult humans, the 32 **permanent teeth** are disposed in 2 bilaterally symmetric arches in the maxillary and mandibular bones. There are 8 teeth in each quadrant: 2 incisors, 1 canine, 2 premolars, and 3 molars. The permanent teeth are preceded by 20 **deciduous** (baby) **teeth.** There are no deciduous precursors of the 12 permanent molar teeth.

Each tooth is composed of a portion that projects above the **gingiva** (or gum)—the **crown**—and one or more **roots** below the gingiva that hold the teeth in bony sockets called **alveoli,** one for each tooth (Fig 16– 4). The crown is covered by the extremely hard **enamel,** while roots are covered by **cementum.** These 2 coverings meet at the **neck** (or cervix) of the tooth. The interior of a tooth contains another calcified material called **dentin,** which surrounds a tissue-filled space known as the **pulp cavity** (Fig 16– 4). The pulp cavity extends to the apex of the root (the root canal), where an orifice (**apical foramen**) permits entrance and exit of blood vessels, lymphatics, and nerves of the pulp cavity. The **periodontal ligament** (or membrane) is a collagenous, fibrous structure inserted in the cementum that serves to fix the tooth firmly in its bony socket (alveolus).

Dentin

Dentin is a calcified tissue similar to bone but harder because of its higher content of calcium salts. It is composed mainly of collagen fibrils (type I), glycosaminoglycans, and calcium salts (70% of dry weight) in the form of crystals of **hydroxyapatite.** The organic matrix of dentin is secreted by **odontoblasts,** cells that line the internal surface of the tooth, separating it from the pulp cavity (Figs 16– 5 and 16– 7). The odontoblast is a polarized, slender cell, producing organic matrix only at the dentinal surface. The cytoplasm of each of these cells contains a nucleus at its base, a large Golgi complex, many ribosomes (both free and attached to rough endoplasmic reticulum), and secretion granules containing procollagen. Odontoblasts have slender, branched cytoplasmic extensions that penetrate perpendicularly through the width of the dentin—the **odontoblast processes** (Tomes fibers). These processes gradually become longer as the dentin becomes thicker, running in small canals called **dentinal tubules** that are extensively branched near the junction between dentin and enamel (Fig 16– 6). Odontoblast processes have a diameter of 3– 4 μm near the cell body but gradually become thinner at their distal ends. The space between the process of the cell and the tubule is full of tissue fluid.

The matrix produced by odontoblasts is initially unmineralized and is called **predentin** (Fig 16– 5). Mineralization of developing dentin begins when membrane-limited vesicles—**matrix vesicles**—appear. They contain fine crystals of hydroxyapatite that grow and serve as nucleation sites for further mineral deposition on the surrounding collagen fibrils.

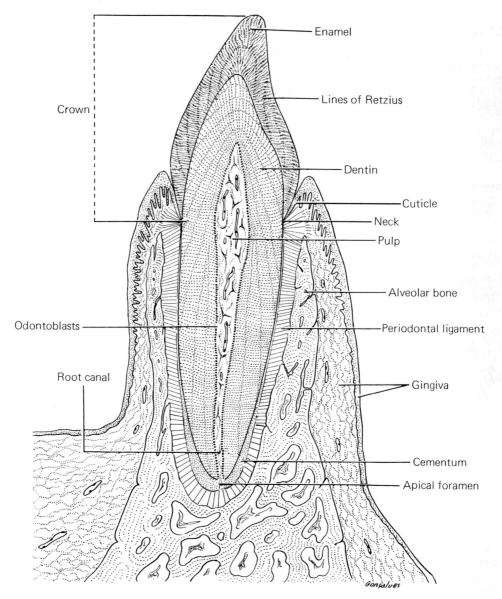

Figure 16–4. Diagram of a sagittal section from an incisor tooth in position in the mandibular bone. (Redrawn and reproduced, with permission, from Leeson TS, Leeson CR: *Histology,* 2nd ed. Saunders, 1970.)

In contrast to bone, dentin persists as a mineralized tissue for a long time after destruction of the odontoblasts. It is thus possible to maintain teeth whose pulp and odontoblasts have been destroyed by infection. In adult teeth, destruction of the covering enamel by erosion due to use or dental caries (tooth decay) usually triggers a reaction in the dentin that causes it to resume the synthesis of its components.

Enamel

Enamel is the hardest component of the human body and the richest in calcium. It consists of about 95% calcium salts (mainly hydroxyapatite), 0.5% or-

ganic material, and water as the remainder. Enamel is produced by cells of ectodermal origin, whereas most of the other structures of teeth derive from mesodermal or neural crest cells. The organic enamel matrix is not composed of collagen fibrils but consists of at least 2 heterogeneous classes of proteins called **amelogenins** and **enamelins.** The roles of these proteins in the organization of the mineral component of enamel are under intensive investigation.

Enamel consists of elongated rods or columns of hydroxyapatite crystals called **enamel rods** (prisms) that are bound together by **interrod enamel.** Interrod enamel differs from rod enamel only in the orientation

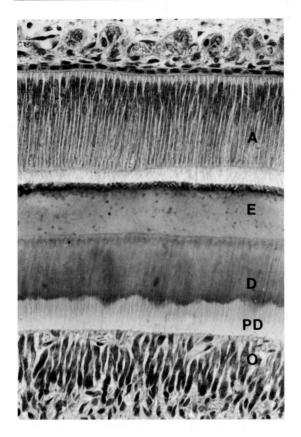

Figure 16–5. Photomicrograph of a section of an immature tooth, showing predentin (PD), dentin (D), and enamel (E). The ameloblasts (A) and the odontoblasts (O) are both disposed as palisades. Masson's stain, × 350.

of the hydroxyapatite crystals that form both structures. Each rod extends through the entire thickness of the enamel layer.

Enamel matrix is secreted by cells called **ameloblasts** (Fig 16–5). These tall, columnar cells possess numerous mitochondria in the region below the nucleus. Many profiles of rough endoplasmic reticulum as well as a well-developed Golgi complex are found above the nucleus. Each ameloblast has an apical extension, known as a **Tomes process,** containing numerous secretory granules. These granules contain the proteins that make up the enamel matrix.

Pulp

Tooth pulp consists of a loose connective tissue. Its main components are odontoblasts, fibroblasts, thin collagen fibrils, and a ground substance containing glycosaminoglycans (Fig 16–7).

Pulp is a highly innervated and vascularized tissue. Blood vessels and myelinated nerve fibers enter the apical foramen and divide into numerous branches. Some nerve fibers lose their myelin sheaths and extend for a short distance into the dentinal tubules. These sensory fibers are sensitive to pain, the only sensory modality recognized in teeth.

Associated Structures

The structures responsible for maintaining the teeth in the maxillary and mandibular bone consist of the **cementum, periodontal ligament, alveolar bone,** and **gingiva.**

A. Cementum: This tissue covers the dentin of the root and is similar in composition to bone, although haversian systems and blood vessels are absent. It is thicker in the apical region of the roots, and in this area there are cells with the appearance of osteocytes, the **cementocytes.** Like osteocytes, they are encased in lacunae that communicate through canaliculi. Like bony tissue, cementum is labile and reacts by resorption or production of new tissue according to the stresses to which it is subjected. When the periodontal ligament is destroyed, cementum undergoes necrosis and may be resorbed. Continuous production of cementum compensates for the normal growth that teeth undergo. This process maintains a close contact between the roots of the teeth and their sockets.

B. Periodontal Ligament: The periodontal ligament is composed of a special type of dense connective tissue whose fibers penetrate the cementum of the tooth and bind it to the bony walls of its socket—permitting, however, limited movements of the tooth. It serves as the periosteum of the alveolar bone. Its fibers are organized such that pressures exerted during mastication are supported by them. This avoids transmission of pressure directly to the bone—a process that would cause localized resorption of this structure.

Collagen of the periodontal ligament has characteristics that resemble those of immature tissue. It has a high protein turnover rate (as demonstrated by radioautography) and a large content of soluble collagen. The space between its fibers is filled with glycosaminoglycans. This high rate of collagen renewal in the periodontal ligament allows processes affecting protein or collagen synthesis—eg, protein or vitamin C deficiency—to cause atrophy of this ligament. As a consequence, teeth become loose in their sockets and in extreme cases may fall out. This relative plasticity of the periodontal ligament is important because it allows orthodontic intervention, which can produce extensive changes in the disposition of teeth in the mouth.

C. Alveolar Bone: This portion of bone is in immediate contact with the periodontal ligament. It is an immature type of bone (woven bone) in which the collagen fibers are not arranged in the typical lamellar pattern present in adult bone. Many of the collagen fibers of the periodontal ligament are arranged in bundles that penetrate this bone and the cementum, forming a connecting bridge between these structures. The bone closest to the roots of the teeth forms the socket. Vessels and nerves run through this alveolar bone to the apical foramen of the root to enter the pulp.

D. Gingiva: The gingiva is a mucous membrane firmly bound to the periosteum of the maxillary or mandibular bone. It is composed of stratified squamous epithelium and numerous connective tissue papillae. This epithelium is bound to the tooth enamel

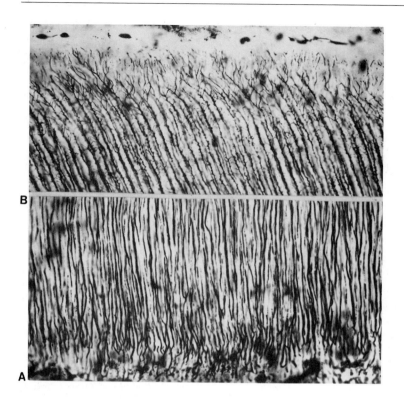

Figure 16–6 (at left). Photomicrograph of a section of a tooth, showing the odontoblast processes of the dentin. *A:* Initial portion. *B:* Terminal portion. These processes gradually get thinner and terminate by branching into delicate extensions. × 400.

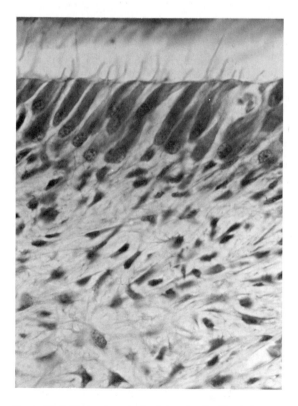

Figure 16–7. Photomicrograph of dental pulp. Fibroblasts are abundant. In the upper region are the odontoblasts, from which the odontoblast processes derive. H&E stain, × 400.

by means of a "cuticle" resembling a thick basal lamina and forms the **epithelial attachment of Gottlieb.** The epithelial cells are attached to the "cuticle" by hemidesmosomes. Between the enamel and the epithelium is a small deepening surrounding the crown called the gingival crevice.

Development of Teeth

At about 6 weeks of gestation, the basal layer of the oral epithelium (ectoderm) proliferates and bulges into the underlying ectomesenchyme derived from the neural crest (Fig 16–8A). A horseshoe-shaped band known as the **dental lamina** is formed in each jaw. A little later, 10 regions of intensified mitotic activity are noted in each dental lamina. These ectodermal outgrowths form caps over clumps of ectomesenchyme, and each collection of cells (tooth bud) will develop into a deciduous tooth. The intervening ectodermal cells later degenerate and disappear. The ectodermal component of a tooth bud forms the **enamel organ** responsible for the secretion of **enamel** (Fig 16–8B and C). The ectomesenchymal component forms the **dental papilla** from which will differentiate **odontoblasts** (cells that secrete dentin) and other structures of the dental pulp (Fig 16–8D). Mesenchyme also condenses around the enamel organ and will eventually differentiate into **cementoblasts** (cells that form cementum) and the **periodontal ligament.**

The enamel organ continues to enlarge and assumes a bell shape at about 8 weeks of gestation. The **outer** (external) **enamel epithelium,** which is continuous with the dental lamina, is indented by numerous capillary vessels. Cells immediately adjacent

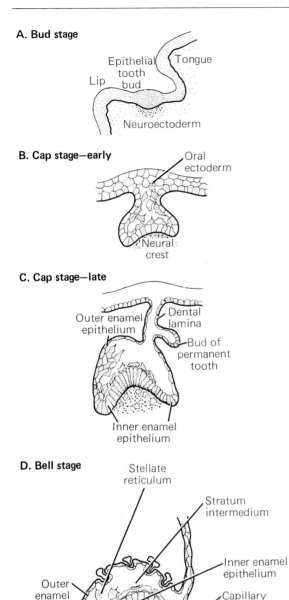

A. Bud stage

Epithelial tooth bud
Tongue
Lip
Neuroectoderm

B. Cap stage—early

Oral ectoderm
Neural crest

C. Cap stage—late

Outer enamel epithelium
Dental lamina
Bud of permanent tooth
Inner enamel epithelium

D. Bell stage

Stellate reticulum
Stratum intermedium
Inner enamel epithelium
Outer enamel epithelium
Capillary
Odontoblasts
Basal lamina
Cervical loop

Figure 16–8. The epithelium of a tooth bud (A) proliferates and invades the underlying mesenchyme to form a cap-shaped structure (B) and (C). In the cap stage, the epithelium differentiates into the inner enamel epithelium, which will give rise to ameloblasts. In the bell stage (D), neural crest cells differentiate into odontoblasts. (Modified and reproduced, with permission, from Warshawsky H: The teeth. In: *Histology: Cell and Tissue Biology,* 5th ed. Weiss L (editor). Elsevier, 1983.)

to the dental papilla assume a columnar shape and form the **inner** (internal) **enamel epithelium.** These cells differentiate into **ameloblasts** (cells that will secrete enamel). Other epithelial cells between the outer and inner layers form the **stellate reticulum** and the **stratum intermedium;** the functions of these layers are not well defined (Fig 16–8D).

It should be noted that a continuous basal lamina separates the outer enamel epithelium from the surrounding connective tissues. This basal lamina then curves around and separates the inner enamel epithelium from ectomesenchymal cells of the dental papilla. The point (a circle in 3 dimensions) where the outer enamel epithelium meets the inner enamel epithelium is termed the **cervical loop** (Fig 16–8D).

Ameloblast differentiation is induced by ectomesenchymal cells of the dental papilla. Before ameloblasts begin to secrete enamel, they cause a superficial layer of cells of the dental papilla to elongate and differentiate into odontoblasts. Odontoblasts begin to secrete predentin, which in turn stimulates the secretion of enamel by ameloblasts. Thus, a wave of reciprocal inductions passes from the future occlusal surface of the crown toward the neck of the tooth.

A. Formation of Dentin: Odontoblasts secrete procollagen, which becomes organized into the collagen fibrils of **predentin.** These cells also mediate the mineralization of collagen fibrils, leading to the formation of dentin. The cell bodies of odontoblasts retreat into the pulp cavity as dentin accumulates, but their processes remain in **dentinal tubules** that span the entire thickness of the dentin.

B. Formation of Enamel: Ameloblasts are unusual epithelial cells in that their bases, adjacent to the basal lamina, become their secretory surfaces. Tight junctions are found around both the histologic apex (functional base) and the histologic base (functional apex) of each cell. Rough endoplasmic reticulum and an elaborate Golgi complex are found in the cytoplasm between the nucleus and the functional apex of these cells. Ameloblasts are responsible for the breakdown of the basal lamina that separates these cells from odontoblasts and dentin. Short, conical extensions of ameloblasts **(Tomes processes)** are the sites of secretion of enamel matrix. The lateral surfaces of Tomes processes secrete the organic matrix of the **interrod enamel,** while the apical surface is responsible for deposition of the matrix of **enamel rods** (prisms). The role of ameloblasts in mineralization is controversial, but hydroxyapatite crystals are formed on the organic matrix. This matrix is later almost completely removed, probably by the ameloblasts. After enamel formation is completed, the enamel organ consists of a stratified squamous epithelium that is rapidly eroded when the tooth erupts into the oral cavity.

C. Root Development: After crown development is complete and just prior to its eruption, the cervical loop grows apically to envelop the dental papilla and forms **Hertwig's root sheath,** which is composed of the fused outer and inner enamel epithelia. The inner layer induces formation of odontoblasts that produce the dentin of the tooth root. When dentin has been formed, the root sheath breaks up, and newly formed dentin induces differentiation of **cementoblasts** from mesenchymal cells of the surrounding dental sac. Cementoblasts form the bonelike tissue **(cementum)** covering the roots of teeth.

D. Permanent Teeth: On the labial side of each dental lamina, a mass of ectodermal cells pushes out to form the **successional lamina** (Fig 16–8C). Here too, 20 regions of intensified mitotic activity are found, one corresponding to each of the permanent counterparts of the deciduous teeth. In addition, dental lamina cells burrow backward, and the tooth germs of the 3 permanent molars are budded off in succession. The tooth germs for the second and third molars are not formed until after birth.

ESOPHAGUS

This part of the gastrointestinal tract is a muscular tube whose function is to transport foodstuffs from the mouth to the stomach. It is covered by nonkeratinized stratified squamous epithelium (Fig 16–9). In

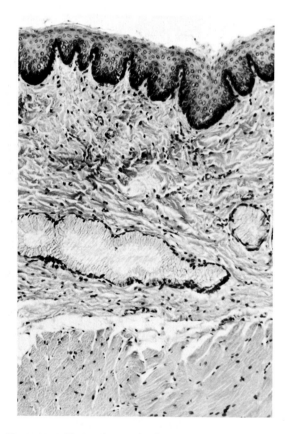

Figure 16–9. Photomicrograph of a section of the upper region of the esophagus. Mucous glands are in the submucosa; striated muscle in the muscularis externa. H&E stain, × 20.

general, it has the same layers as the rest of the digestive tract. In the submucosa are groups of small mucus-secreting glands, the **esophageal glands.** In the lamina propria of the region near the stomach are groups of glands called **esophageal cardiac glands** that also secrete mucus. At the distal end of the esophagus, the muscular layer consists of only smooth muscle cells; in the mid portion, a mixture of striated and smooth muscle cells; and at the proximal end, only striated muscle cells. The muscularis mucosae appears at the level of the cricoid cartilage and consists of longitudinally oriented smooth muscle fibers. Above this level, it is replaced by a layer of elastic fibers. Only that portion of the esophagus in the peritoneal cavity is covered by serosa. The rest is covered by a layer of loose connective tissue called the adventitia, which blends into the surrounding tissue.

STOMACH

The stomach is a dilated segment of the digestive tract whose main functions are to add an acidic fluid to the ingested food, transform it by muscular activity into a viscous mass (chyme), and continue the digestive process begun in the oral cavity by secreting the proteolytic enzyme **pepsin.** Gross inspection reveals 4 regions: **cardia, fundus, body,** and **pylorus** (Fig 16–10). The fundus and body are identical in microscopic structure, so that only 3 histologic regions are recognized. The mucosa and submucosa of the undistended stomach are thrown into longitudinally directed folds known as **rugae.** When the stomach is filled with food, these folds are flattened out.

Mucosa

The gastric mucosa consists of a **surface epithelium** that invaginates to varying extents into the lamina propria, forming **gastric pits.** Emptying into gastric pits are branched, tubular **glands** (cardiac, gastric, and pyloric) characteristic of each region of the stomach. The **lamina propria** of the stomach is composed of loose connective tissue interspersed with smooth muscle and lymphoid cells. Separating the mucosa from the underlying submucosa is a layer of smooth muscle, the **muscularis mucosae.** This layer is composed of an outer group of longitudinal fibers and circular fibers closer to the lumen.

When the luminal surface of the stomach is viewed under low magnification, numerous small circular or ovoid invaginations of the lining epithelium are observed. These are the openings of the gastric pits, or **foveolae gastricae** (Figs 16–10 and 16–11). The epithelium covering the surface and lining the pits is a simple columnar epithelium, and all the cells secrete mucus. The epithelial cells are 20–40 μm in height, have a round or oval nucleus near their base, and contain numerous mucous granules. These membrane-limited granules contain carbohydrate-rich proteins formed in the extensive, supranuclear Golgi complex of the surface and pit cells. When released from these

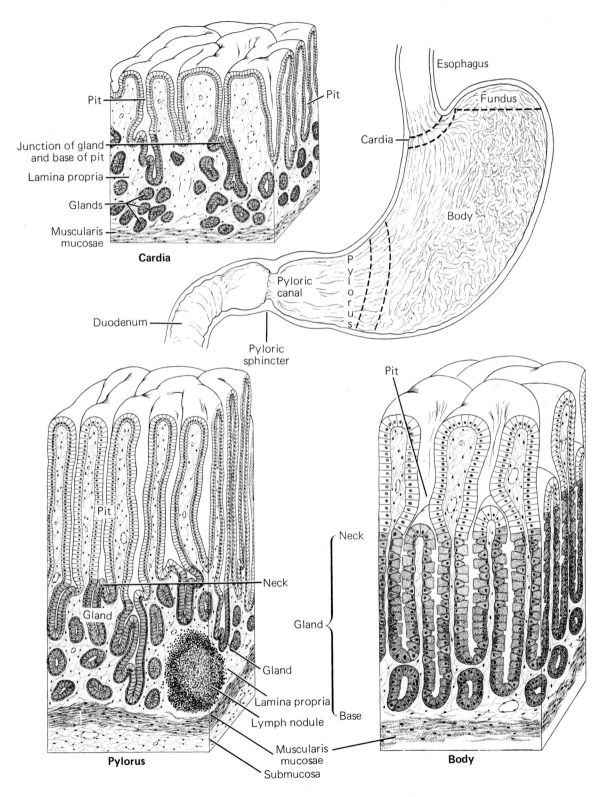

Figure 16–10. Regions of the stomach and their histologic structure.

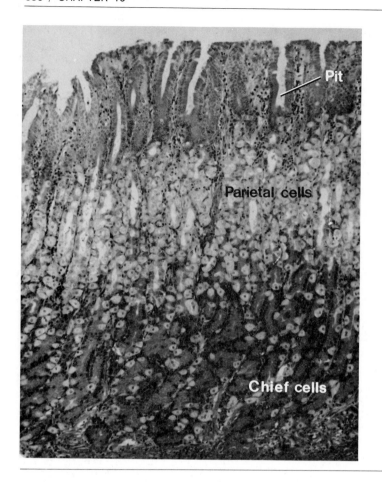

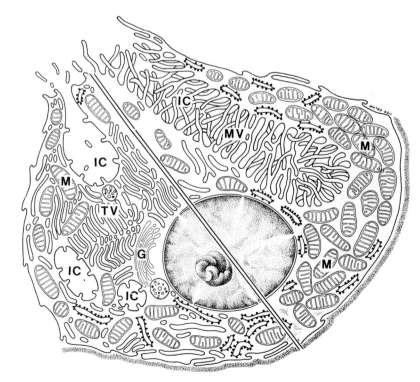

Figure 16–11 (at left). Photomicrograph of a section of a gastric gland in the fundus of the stomach. Parietal (light) cells predominate in the upper region of the gland; chief (dark) cells (zymogenic cells) predominate in the lower region. H&E stain, × 100.

Figure 16–12 (at right). The parietal cell. Composite diagram showing the ultrastructural differences between a resting *(left)* and active *(right)* cell. Observe that the tubulovesicles (TV) present in the cytoplasm of the resting cell fuse to form microvilli that fill up the intracellular canaliculi (IC). Golgi complex (G), mitochondria (M), microvilli (MV). (Based on the work of Ito S, Schofield GC: Studies on the depletion and accumulation of microvilli and changes in the tubovesicular compartment of mouse parietal cells in relation to gastric acid secretion. *J Cell Biol* 1974;**63**:364.)

cells, the mucus forms a thick layer that protects these cells from the effects of the strong acid secreted by the stomach. Recent evidence suggests that tight junctions around surface and pit cells also form a part of the barrier to acid. Substances that cause gastric irritation, such as aspirin, can disrupt this layer and lead to ulceration.

Cardiac Region

The cardia is a narrow circular band, 1.5–3 cm in width, at the transition between the esophagus and stomach (Fig 16–10). Its lamina propria contains simple or branched tubular cardiac glands. The terminal portion of these glands is frequently coiled and often has a large lumen. Most of the secretory cells produce mucus and lysozyme, but a few parietal cells (which secrete HCl) can be found. These glands are similar in structure to the cardiac glands of the terminal portion of the esophagus.

Fundus & Body

The lamina propria of these regions is filled with branched, tubular **gastric** (fundic) **glands,** 3–7 of which open into the bottom of each gastric pit. The distribution of epithelial cells in gastric glands is not uniform (Figs 16–10 and 16–11). The **neck** consists of undifferentiated cells and mucous neck cells, while the **base** (or body) of the glands contains parietal (oxyntic) cells, chief (zymogenic) cells, and enteroendocrine cells.

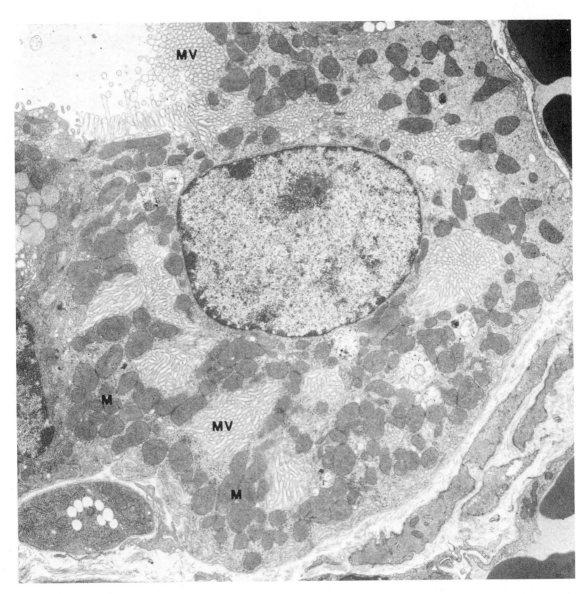

Figure 16–13. Electron micrograph of an active parietal cell. Observe the microvilli (MV) protruding into the intracellular canaliculi and the abundant mitochondria (M). × 10,200. (Courtesy of S Ito.)

(1) Undifferentiated cells are found in the neck region but are few in number. They are low columnar cells with oval nuclei near the bases of the cells. Few or no mucous granules are seen in their cytoplasm. Many free ribosomes and polyribosomes are present, but rough endoplasmic reticulum is scant. Mitochondria are scarce, but a prominent Golgi complex is seen in a supranuclear position. The nucleolus is well developed. Undifferentiated cells are located where uptake of ^{3}H-thymidine has been seen, using autoradiography, and where mitoses have been observed. These cells differentiate and move upward to replace the pit and surface mucous cells, which have a turnover time of 3–7 days. Other undifferentiated cells migrate deeper into the glands and differentiate into mucous neck cells, parietal cells, chief cells, and enteroendocrine cells. These cells are replaced much more slowly than surface mucous cells.

(2) Mucous neck cells are present in clusters or as single cells between parietal cells in the necks of gastric glands. Despite being mucous cells, they have morphologic and histochemical characteristics that make their mucous secretion quite different from that of the surface epithelial mucous cells. They are irregular in shape, having their nuclei at the base of the cell. In the electron microscope, they show a large supranuclear Golgi complex and numerous single profiles of rough endoplasmic reticulum, each of which is wrapped around a mitochondrion. Their ovoid or spherical granules are near the apical surface and are stained intensely with PAS or mucicarmine. Unlike the neutral mucous secretions of the surface cells, mucous neck cells secrete an acidic mucus.

(3) Parietal (oxyntic) cells are present mainly in the upper half of gastric glands and are intercalated between mucous neck cells (Figs 16–10 and 16–11). They are scarcer in the gland's base. They are rounded or pyramidal cells, 20–35 μm in diameter, with one or sometimes 2 centrally placed spherical nuclei and an intensely eosinophilic cytoplasm. Upon observation in the electron microscope, the most striking feature is a deep, circular invagination of the apical plasma membrane forming the **intracellular canaliculus.** In the resting cell, a number of tubulovesicular structures can be seen in the apical region of the cell just below its plasmalemma (Fig 16–12, left side). When stimulated to produce hydrochloric acid, tubulovesicles fuse with the cell membrane and form more microvilli (Fig 16–12, right side). Actin filaments, present between tubulovesicles, probably play a role in the interaction of these structures. The eosinophilic cytoplasm possesses a great number of mitochondria with abundant cristae, a discrete Golgi complex near the cell base, and no secretory granules (Figs 16–12 and 16–13).

Parietal cells produce the hydrochloric acid present in gastric juice. In human disease, the number of parietal cells is correlated with the acid-producing capacity of the stomach. In cases of atrophic gastritis, both parietal and chief cells are much less numerous, and the gastric juice has little or no acid or pepsin activity.

Parietal cells secrete hydrochloric acid, 0.16 mol/L; potassium chloride, 0.07 mol/L; traces of other electrolytes; and gastric intrinsic factor (see below). There is evidence that the acid secreted originates from chlorides present in the blood plus a cation (H^+) resulting from the action of an enzyme—**carbonic anhydrase.** Carbonic anhydrase acts on CO_2 to produce carbonic acid, which dissociates into bicarbonate and H^+. Both the cation and the chloride ion are actively transported across the cell membrane, whereas water diffuses passively along the osmotic gradient (Fig 16–14). The presence of abundant mitochondria in the parietal cells indicates that their metabolic processes are highly energy-consuming. As a matter of fact, this cell type presents histochemical peculiarities that characterize it as one of the cells with the highest observable energy metabolism.

Radioautographic studies performed with labeled vitamin B_{12} suggest that the parietal cells are, in humans, the site of production of **intrinsic factor,** a glycoprotein that binds avidly to vitamin B_{12}. In other species, however, this substance may be present in other cells.

The presence of intrinsic factor is normally required for vitamin B_{12} absorption, and this vitamin binds strongly to intrinsic factor in the lumen of the stomach. This complex is absorbed by the cells in the

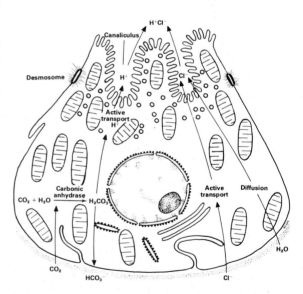

Figure 16–14. Diagram of a parietal cell, showing the main steps in the synthesis of hydrochloric acid. Blood CO_2 under the action of carbonic anhydrase produces carbonic acid, which dissociates into bicarbonate ion and a proton, H^+, which reacts with the chloride ion to produce hydrochloric acid. The tubulovesicles of the cell apex seem to be related to hydrochloric acid secretion, since they decrease in number after parietal cell stimulation. The bicarbonate ion returns to the blood and is responsible for a measurable increase in blood pH during digestion.

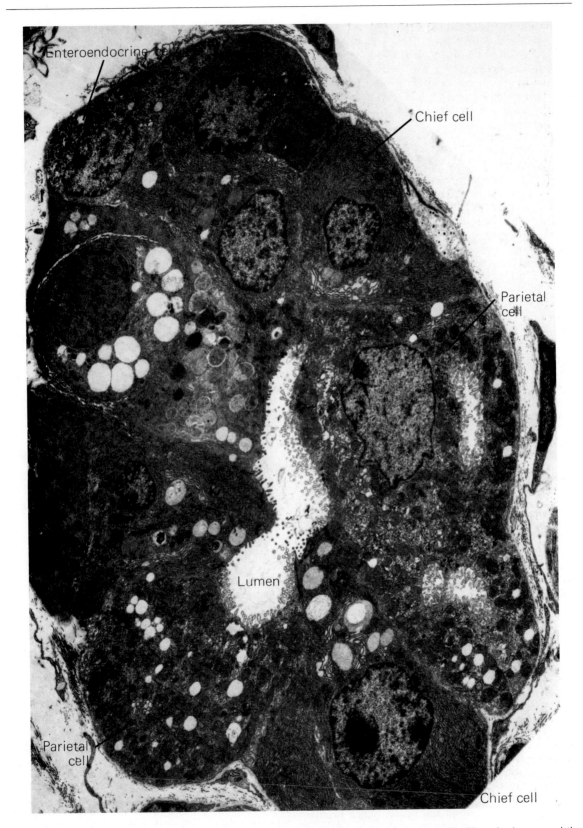

Figure 16–15. Electron micrograph of a section of gastric gland in the fundus of the stomach. Note the lumen and the parietal (containing abundant mitochondria), chief (extensive rough endoplasmic reticulum), and enteroendocrine (with secretory granules) cells. × 5300.

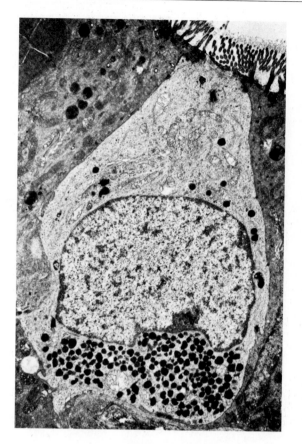

Figure 16–16. Electron micrograph of an enteroendocrine cell of human duodenum. × 6900. (Courtesy of AGE Pearse.)

tivity of gastric lipase is weak and of doubtful physiologic importance.

(5) Enteroendocrine cells of the digestive tract are discussed more extensively below. These cells are found near the bases of gastric glands (Figs 16–15 and 16–16). In the fundus and body of the stomach, **5-hydroxytryptamine** (serotonin) has been shown to be one of the principal secretory products. Tumors called **carcinoids** arise from these cells.

Pylorus

The pylorus has deep gastric pits into which open branched, tubular glands, the **pyloric glands,** which are similar to the glands of the cardiac region. In the pyloric region, one finds long pits and short coiled glands—the reverse of the situation in the cardiac region (Fig 16–17). These glands secrete mucus as well as appreciable amounts of the enzyme lysozyme. **Gastrin (G) cells** are intercalated among the mucous cells of pyloric glands. These cells release **gastrin,** which stimulates the secretion of acid by the parietal cells of gastric glands. Other enteroendocrine cells **(D cells)** secrete **somatostatin,** which inhibits the release of other hormones, including gastrin.

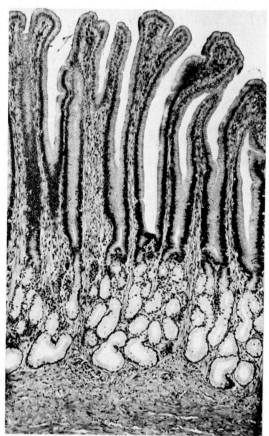

Figure 16–17. Photomicrograph of a section of the pyloric region of the stomach. Observe the deep gastric pits with short pyloric glands in the lamina propria. H&E stain, × 40.

ileum. This explains why lack of intrinsic factor can lead to vitamin B_{12} deficiency—a disease that results in a disorder of the red blood cell–forming mechanism known as **pernicious anemia** and is usually caused by **atrophic gastritis.** In a high percentage of cases, pernicious anemia seems to be an autoimmune disease, since antibodies against parietal cell proteins are often detected in the blood of patients with the disease.

The secretory activity of parietal cells is instigated by different mechanisms. One is through cholinergic nerve endings. Histamine and a polypeptide called **gastrin,** both secreted in the gastric mucosa, act strongly to stimulate the production of hydrochloric acid.

(4) Chief (zymogenic) cells (Fig 16–15) predominate in the lower region of the tubular glands and have all the characteristics of a protein-synthesizing and exporting cell. The granules present in their cytoplasm contain the inactive enzyme pepsinogen. Their basophilia is due to the abundant rough endoplasmic reticulum (see Chapter 4). In humans, these cells produce the enzymes pepsin and lipase. When inactive pepsinogen is released into the acid environment of the stomach, the proenzyme is converted into the highly active proteolytic enzyme **pepsin.** The lipolytic ac-

Other Layers of the Stomach

The **submucosa** is composed of loose connective tissue and blood and lymph vessels and is infiltrated by lymphoid cells and mast cells. The **muscularis externa** is composed of smooth muscle fibers oriented in 3 main directions. The external layer is longitudinal; the middle layer is circular; and the internal layer is oblique. At the pylorus, the middle circular layer is greatly thickened to form the **pyloric sphincter.** The **serosa** is thin and covered by mesothelium.

THE SMALL INTESTINE

In the small intestine, the processes of digestion are completed and the products of digestion are absorbed. The small intestine is relatively long—approximately 5 m—and this permits prolonged contact between food and digestive enzymes, as well as between the digested products and the absorptive cells of the epithelial lining. The small intestine consists of 3 segments: **duodenum, jejunum,** and **ileum.** The 3 segments have many characteristics in common and will be discussed together.

Mucous Membrane of the Small Intestine

Grossly, the lining of the small intestine shows a

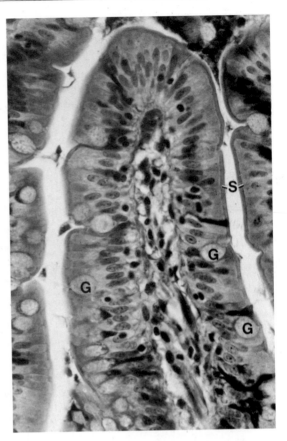

Figure 16–19. Photomicrograph of the tip of a villus of the human ileum. Observe the connective tissue core with blood and lymph vessels surrounded by the epithelial layer, in which goblet cells (G) frequently occur. At right, the striated border (S) formed by microvilli present on the surface of the cell is clearly visible. H&E stain, × 450.

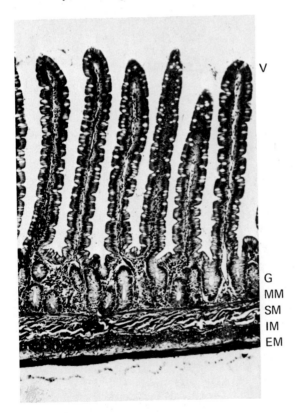

Figure 16–18. Photomicrograph of the small intestine. Observe the villi (V), the intestinal glands (G), muscularis mucosae (MM), submucosa (SM), and the external and internal muscle layers (EM and IM). H&E stain, × 40.

series of permanent folds, **plicae circulares** or **valves of Kerckring,** consisting of mucosa and submucosa and having a semilunar, circular, or spiral form. The plicae are most developed in, and consequently a characteristic of, the jejunum. Although frequently present, they do not constitute a significant feature of the duodenum and ileum. Under magnification, **intestinal villi** are seen. These structures, 0.5–1.5 mm long, are outgrowths of the mucosa (epithelium plus lamina propria) projecting into the lumen of the small intestine. In the duodenum they are leaf-shaped, gradually assuming the form of a finger as the ileum is reached (Figs 16–18 and 16–22).

Between the villi are small openings of simple tubular glands called **intestinal glands (crypts** or **glands of Lieberkühn)** (Figs 16–18 and 16–22).

The epithelium of the villi is continuous with that of the glands. In the crypts of Lieberkühn, one finds undifferentiated cells, some **absorptive cells** and **goblet cells, Paneth cells,** and **enteroendocrine cells.** The undifferentiated cells of the crypts give rise to

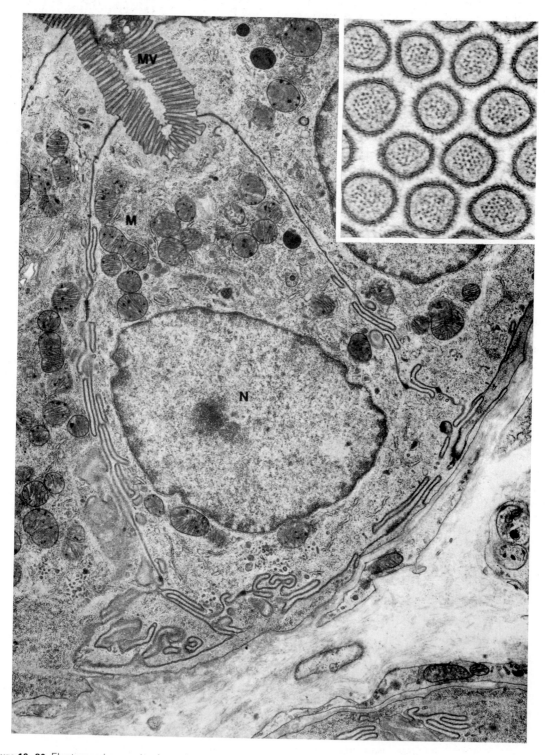

Figure 16–20. Electron micrograph of an absorptive epithelial cell of the small intestine. Observe the accumulation of mitochondria (M) in their apexes. The luminal surface is covered with microvilli (MV) (shown in transverse section in the inset). Actin filaments, sectioned transversely, constitute the principal structural feature in the core of the microvilli. N, nucleus. × 6300. (Courtesy of KR Porter.)

the columnar absorptive cells and the mucus-secreting goblet cells of the villus epithelium. Enteroendocrine cells are also present here.

The **absorptive cells** are tall, columnar cells, about 25 μm high × 8–10 μm wide, each with an oval nucleus in the basal half of the cell. At the apex of each cell is a homogeneous layer called the **striated (brush) border** (Fig 16–19). With the aid of the electron microscope, the striated border is seen to be a layer of densely packed **microvilli** (Figs 16–20 and 16–23). Each microvillus is a cylindric protrusion of the apical cytoplasm and consists of a cell membrane enclosing a core of filaments, mostly actin filaments. Each microvillus is approximately 1 μm tall × 0.1 μm in diameter. It is estimated that each absorptive cell has an average of about 3000 microvilli and that 1 mm² of mucosa contains about 200 million of these structures. Microvilli have the important physiologic function of considerably increasing the area of contact between the intestinal surface and food. Studies performed by isolating the striated border of these cells by differential centrifugation and then applying immunofluorescence techniques suggest that the striated border is the site of activity of the disaccharidases of the small intestine. These enzymes, bound to microvilli, hydrolyze the disaccharides into monosaccharides, which are easily absorbed. Deficiencies of these disaccharidases have been described in human diseases characterized by digestive disturbances. Some of these enzymatic deficiencies seem to be of genetic origin. An analogous localization has been postulated for dipeptidases that hydrolyze dipeptides into their component amino acids.

A more important function of the columnar intestinal cells is to absorb the metabolites that result from the digestive process. This is discussed further below.

Goblet cells are interspersed between the absorptive cells (Figs 16–19 and 16–22). They are less abundant in the duodenum and increase in number as the ileum is approached. They produce acid glycoproteins whose main function is to protect and lubricate the lining of the intestine.

Paneth cells in the basal portion of the intestinal glands are exocrine serous cells that synthesize a complex of protein and polysaccharide. They have a well-developed rough endoplasmic reticulum and Golgi complex. Researchers utilizing immunocytochemical methods have detected lysozyme—an enzyme that digests the cell wall of some bacteria—in the large, eosinophilic secretory granules of these cells (Figs 16–21 and 16–22). Lysozyme possesses antibacterial activity and may play a role in controlling the intestinal flora.

M (membranous epithelial) cells are specialized epithelial cells overlying the lymphoid follicles of Peyer's patches. They are relatively flat cells whose apical surface is thrown into small folds rather than microvilli. M cells can endocytose antigens and transport them to the underlying lymphoid cells where immune responses to foreign antigens can be initiated.

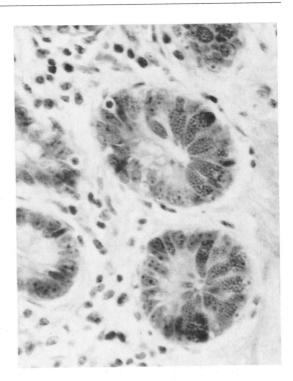

Figure 16–21. Section of the basal portion of the intestinal glands showing the Paneth cells with their typical large secretory granules. × 600.

Endocrine Cells of the Gastrointestinal Tract

In addition to the cells discussed above, the gastrointestinal tract contains a series of widely distributed **enteroendocrine cells.** They have the characteristics of APUD cells (see Chapter 4). A variety of histochemical methods have been utilized to study these cells, and a large number of names have been given to what is now believed to be a single class of hormone- and amine-secreting cells. Thus, argyrophil, argentaffin, and enterochromaffin are names that describe the techniques used to study enteroendocrine cells. These cells have a pale-staining cytoplasm, and their secretory granules are at the pole of the cell in contact with the basal lamina (Figs 16–23 and 16–24). Their apical cytoplasm may (the open type) or may not (the closed type) reach the lumen of the organ. It has been postulated that the apical cytoplasm of the open type of enteroendocrine cell constitutes a type of sensory receptor that monitors the luminal contents. Depending on the contents, the enteroendocrine cell would either be stimulated or inhibited. The original APUD concept advanced by Pearse postulated that all these cells arise from the neural crest. This has been challenged by several authors who maintain that enteroendocrine cells arise locally from undifferentiated cells of the digestive tract epithelium.

For the purpose of simplification, all of these cells will be considered at one time, without regard to location in the gastrointestinal tract. This subject is

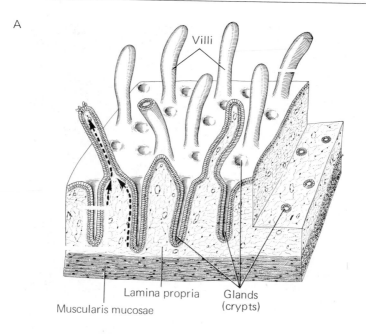

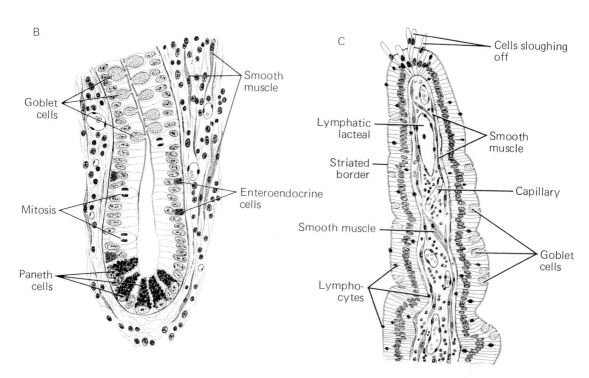

Figure 16–22. Schematic diagrams illustrating the structure of the small intestine. *A:* The small intestine under low magnification. In the villus to the left, observe the desquamation of epithelial cells. Because of constant mitotic activity of the cells from the blind end of the glands and the upward migration of these cells (dotted arrows), the intestinal epithelium is continuously renewed. Observe the glands of Lieberkühn. *B:* The intestinal glands have a lining of intestinal epithelium and goblet cells (upper portion). At a lower level, the immature epithelial cells are frequently seen in mitosis; note also the presence of Paneth and enteroendocrine cells. As the immature cells progress upward, they differentiate and develop microvilli seen as a striated border in the light microscope. Thus, in the blind end of these glands, cell proliferation and cell differentiation occur simultaneously. *C:* A villus tip showing the columnar covering epithelium with its striated border and a moderate number of goblet cells. In the connective tissue core of the villus, capillaries, a lymphatic lacteal, smooth muscle cells, and leukocytes can be seen. Lymphocytes are in the epithelial layer in great numbers. (Redrawn and reproduced, with permission, from Ham AW: *Histology,* 6th ed. Lippincott, 1969.)

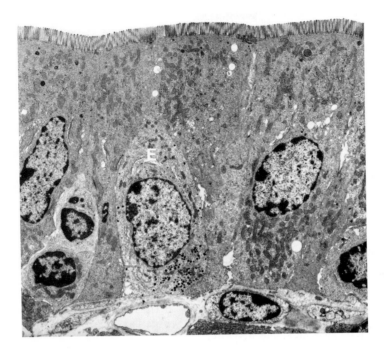

Figure 16–23. Electron micrograph of epithelium of the small intestine. When viewed with the light microscope, abundant microvilli at the cell apex can be seen to form the striated border. At left are 2 lymphocytes migrating in the epithelium. In the center is shown an enteroendocrine cell (E) with its basal secretory granules. × 1850.

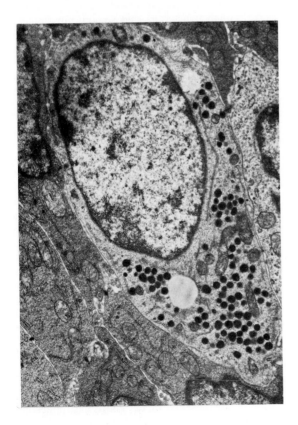

Figure 16–24 (at left). A secretin-producing cell from dog duodenum. × 10,250. (Courtesy of AGE Pearse.)

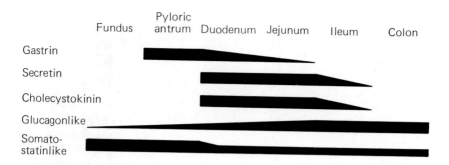

Figure 16–25. Distribution of gastrointestinal endocrine cells along the digestive tract. (Based on Grossman MI: Distribution of gastrointestinal APUD cells along the digestive tract. *Proc Int Cong Endocrinol* 1976;**2**:1.)

being actively studied at present. Better localization of several cell types will undoubtedly be achieved and new cell types discovered. The experimental results are summarized in Fig 16–25 and Table 16–1. It is apparent that cells having the characteristics of the APUD series and producing glucagon can be found throughout the mucosal lining of the stomach, whereas gastrin-producing cells are restricted to the pylorus. Although the picture of gastrointestinal endocrinology is still incomplete, it is clear that the activity of the digestive system is controlled by the nervous system

Table 16–1. Principal enteroendocrine cells in the gastrointestinal tract.

Cell type and Location	Hormone Produced	Major Action
A—stomach	Glucagon	Hepatic glycogenolysis
G—pylorus	Gastrin	Stimulation of gastric acid secretion
S—small intestine	Secretin	Pancreatic and biliary bicarbonate and water secretion
K—small intestine	Gastric inhibitory polypeptide (GIP)	Inhibition of gastric acid secretion
L—small intestine	Glucagonlike substance (glicentin)	Hepatic glycogenolysis
I—small intestine	Cholecystokinin	Pancreatic enzyme secretion, gallbladder contraction
D—pylorus, duodenum	Somatostatin	Local inhibition of other endocrine cells
Mo—small intestine	Motilin	Increased gut motility
EC—digestive tract	Serotonin, substance P	Increased gut motility
D_1—digestive tract	Vasoactive intestinal polypeptide (VIP)	Ion and water secretion, increased gut motility

and modulated by a complex and efficient system of peptide hormones produced locally.

Lamina Propria Through Serosa

The lamina propria of the small intestine is composed of loose connective tissue with blood and lymph vessels, nerve fibers, and smooth muscle cells. Just below the basal lamina, a layer of antibody-producing lymphoid cells and macrophages exists, forming an immunologic barrier at this region.

The lamina propria penetrates the core of the intestinal villi, taking along blood and lymph vessels, nerves, connective tissue, and smooth muscle cells. The latter cell type is responsible for the rhythmic movements of the villi, which are important for absorption.

The **muscularis mucosae** does not present any peculiarities in this organ. The **submucosa** contains, in the initial portion of the duodenum, clusters of ramified, coiled tubular glands that open into the intestinal glands. These are the **duodenal** (or **Brunner) glands** (Figs 16–26 and 16–27). Their cells are of the mucous type. The product of secretion of the glands is distinctly alkaline (pH 8.1–9.3), and it acts to protect the duodenal mucous membrane against the effects of the acid gastric juice and to bring the intestinal contents to the optimum pH for pancreatic enzyme action.

The lamina propria and the submucosa of the small intestine contain aggregates of lymphoid nodules known as **Peyer's patches.** Each patch consists of 10–200 nodules and is visible to the naked eye as an oval area on the antimesenteric side of the intestine. There are about 30 patches in the human, most of which are found in the ileum. When viewed from the luminal surface, each Peyer patch appears as a dome-shaped area devoid of villi. Instead, the covering epithelium consists of flattened **M cells** (see above).

Cell Renewal in the Gastrointestinal Tract

The epithelial cells of the entire gastrointestinal tract respond to certain stimuli (hormones, cholinergic neural activity) by the production of new cells. Cells of the basal layer of the esophageal epithelium, of the

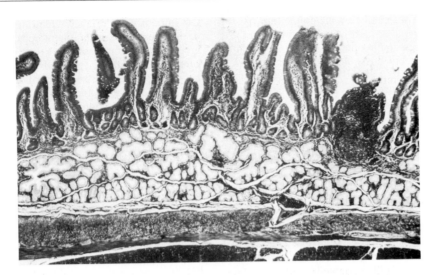

Figure 16–26. Photomicrograph of the duodenum, showing villi and duodenal glands (of Brunner) in the submucosa. The dark structure at the right is a lymphoid nodule; at the bottom are 2 smooth muscle layers of the muscularis externa. H&E stain, × 30.

neck of gastric glands, of the lower half of the glands of Lieberkühn, and of the lower third of the crypts of the large intestine are rapidly labeled with ³H-thymidine and consequently identified as proliferating cells. From this proliferative zone in each region, cells move to the maturation area where they undergo structural and enzymic maturation, providing the functional cell population of each region.

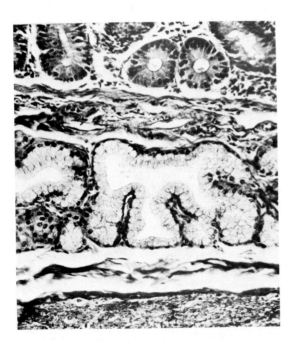

Figure 16–27. Details of the submucosal duodenal glands under higher magnification than that shown in Fig 16–26. H&E stain, × 300.

In humans, replacement of the esophageal epithelium occurs every 2–3 days. In the gastric epithelium, mitotic activity is found only in the neck region of gastric glands. Most of the new cells migrate upward to form pit and surface mucous cells. These cells live only 4–6 days before they are sloughed off. Other new cells differentiate into mucous neck, parietal, chief, or enteroendocrine cells. These cells turn over at a much slower rate.

The lower half of the crypt of Lieberkühn is the site of undifferentiated cell proliferation in the small intestine (Fig 16–22). Most of these cells migrate upward and differentiate into absorptive cells. Others become goblet cells or enteroendocrine cells. All 3 cell types live only 3–6 days. This high replacement rate explains why the intestine is promptly affected by the administration of antimitotic drugs, as in cancer chemotherapy. Owing to effects of these drugs, the epithelial cells continue to be lost at the tips of villi, but cell proliferation is inhibited. This atrophy of the epithelium results in defective absorption of nutrients, excessive fluid loss, and diarrhea. Paneth cells of the crypts turn over much more slowly, living about 30 days before being replaced.

Epithelial cells of the large intestine are replaced about every 6 days by the proliferation and differentiation of cells in the lower third of the glands.

Vessels & Nerves of the Small Intestine

The blood vessels that nourish the intestine and serve to remove absorbed products of digestion penetrate the muscularis externa and form a large plexus in the submucosa (Fig 16–28). From the submucosa, branches extend through the muscularis mucosae and lamina propria and into the villi. Each villus receives, according to its size, one or more branches that form a capillary network just below its epithelium. At the tips of the villi, one or more venules arise from these capillaries and run in the opposite direction, reaching the veins of the submucosal plexus. The lymph vessels of the intestine begin as blind tubes in the core of the villi. These structures, despite being larger than the blood capillaries, are difficult to observe because their walls are usually collapsed. These vessels **(lacteals)** run to the region of lamina propria above the muscularis mucosae, where they form a plexus. From there they are directed to the submucosa, where they surround lymph nodules. These vessels anastomose repeatedly and leave the intestine along with the blood vessels.

The innervation of the intestines is formed by an intrinsic and an extrinsic component. The intrinsic component is constituted by groups of neurons that form the **myenteric (Auerbach's) plexus,** present between the outer longitudinal and the inner circular layers of the muscularis externa, and the **submucosal (Meissner's) plexus** in the submucosa. The plexuses contain some sensory neurons that receive information from nerve endings near the epithelial layer and in the smooth muscle layer regarding the composition of the intestinal content (chemoreceptors) and the degree of expansion of the intestinal wall (mechanoreceptors). The other nerve cells are effectors and innervate the muscle layers and hormone-secreting cells. The intrinsic innervation formed by these plexuses is responsible for the intestinal contractions that occur in the total absence of the extrinsic innervation. The extrinsic innervation is formed by parasympathetic cholinergic nerve fibers that stimulate the activity of the intestinal smooth muscle and by sympathetic adrenergic nerve fibers that depress intestinal smooth muscle activity.

Histophysiology of the Small Intestine

The presence of plicae, villi, and microvilli greatly increases the surface of the intestinal lining—an important characteristic in an organ where absorption occurs so intensely. It has been calculated that the presence of plicae increases the intestinal surface 3-fold and the villi increase it 10-fold, whereas the microvilli increase it 20-fold. Together these processes are thus responsible for a 600-fold increase in

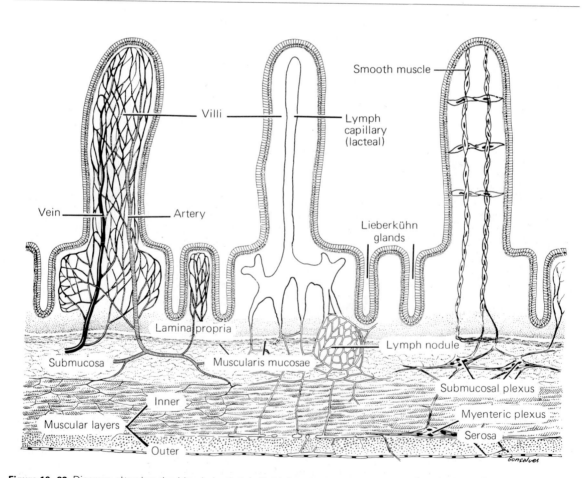

Figure 16–28. Diagram showing the blood circulation *(left),* lymphatic circulation *(center),* and innervation *(right)* of the small intestine. The smooth muscle system for contracting the villi is illustrated in the villus on the right.

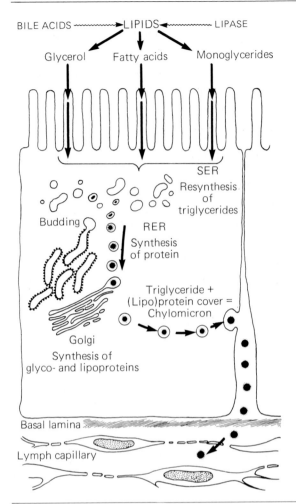

BILE ACIDS ------→ LIPIDS ←------ LIPASE

Glycerol   Fatty acids   Monoglycerides

SER
Resynthesis of triglycerides

Budding

RER
Synthesis of protein

Triglyceride + (Lipo)protein cover = Chylomicron

Golgi
Synthesis of glyco- and lipoproteins

Basal lamina

Lymph capillary

Figure 16–29. Lipid absorption in the small intestine. Lipase promotes the hydrolysis of lipids to monoglycerides and fatty acids in the intestinal lumen. These compounds are stabilized in an emulsion by the action of bile acids. The products of hydrolysis cross the microvilli membranes passively and are collected in the cisternae of the smooth endoplasmic reticulum, where they are resynthesized to triglycerides. These triglycerides are surrounded by a thin layer of proteins forming particles called chylomicrons (0.2–1 μm in diameter). Chylomicrons are transferred to the Golgi complex, and from there they migrate to the lateral membrane, cross it by a process of membrane fusion (exocytosis), and flow in the extracellular space in the direction of the blood and lymph vessels. Most chylomicrons go to the lymph and a few to the blood vessels. The long-chain lipids ($> C_{12}$) go mainly to the lymph vessels. Fatty acids of less than 10–12 carbon atoms are not reesterified to triglycerides but leave the cell directly and enter the blood vessels. RER, rough endoplasmic reticulum; SER, smooth endoplasmic reticulum. (Based on results published by Friedman HI, Cardell RR Jr in: Alterations in the endoplasmic reticulum and Golgi complex of intestinal epithelial cells during fat absorption and after termination of this process: A morphological and morphometric study. *Anat Rec* 1977;**188**:77.)

the intestinal surface, resulting in a total area of 200 m².

In the small intestine, the digestive process is completed and its products are absorbed. Lipid digestion occurs mainly as a result of the action of pancreatic lipase and bile. In humans, most of the lipid absorption occurs in the duodenum and upper jejunum. Figs 16–29 and 16–30 illustrate present concepts of this process of absorption.

The amino acids and monosaccharides derived from digestion of proteins and carbohydrates are absorbed by the epithelial cells by active transport without visible morphologic correlates. In newborn animals, but apparently not in humans, transfer of undigested proteins from colostrum occurs as a result of pinocytotic processes in the cell apex. In this way, antibodies secreted into the colostrum can be transferred to the young animal—an important aspect of the immune defense mechanism. This capacity to transfer proteins is almost completely lost after a few days and is minimal in adults. In diseases marked by severe damage to epithelial cells, the transfer of undigested proteins to the blood increases considerably.

Another process that is probably of importance for intestinal function is the rhythmic movement of the villi. This is the result of the contraction of smooth muscle cells running vertically between the muscularis mucosae and the tip of the villi (see villus at right in Fig 16–28). These movements occur at the rate of several strokes per minute. During digestion, their rate increases; in fasting animals, the rate is much lower. These contractions also tend to empty the lymph vessels and propel the lymph and absorbed metabolites to the mesenteric lymphatics.

The microfilaments found in the microvilli (Figs 16–23 and 16–31) are composed of actin. Movement of the microvilli is thought to play an important role in mixing the microenvironment—an important event in the process of metabolite absorption.

In disorders marked by atrophy of the intestinal mucosa due to infections or nutritional deficiencies, the absorption of metabolites is greatly hindered, producing the **malabsorption syndrome.**

Frequently, lymphocytes are seen between the intestinal epithelial cells. The widely held view that these cells migrate to the intestinal lumen where they

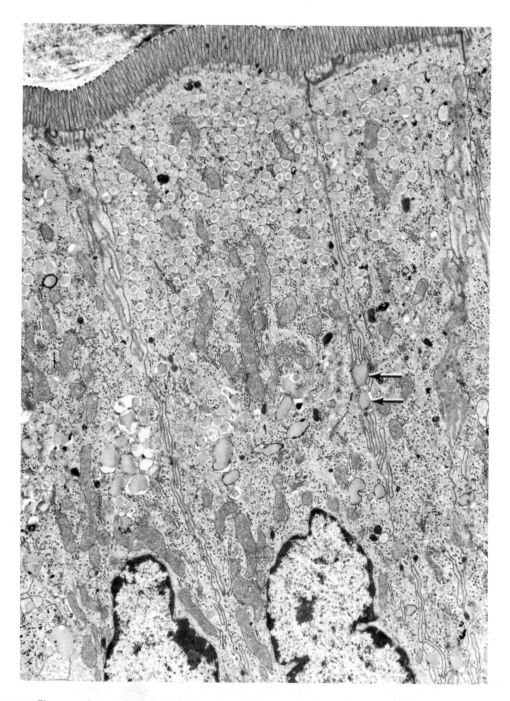

Figure 16–30. Electron micrograph of the intestinal epithelium in the lipid absorption phase. Observe the accumulation of lipid droplets in vesicles of the smooth endoplasmic reticulum. (Compare with Fig 16–20.) These vesicles fuse near the nucleus, forming larger lipid droplets that migrate laterally and cross the cell membranes to the extracellular space (arrows). × 5000. (Courtesy of HI Friedman.)

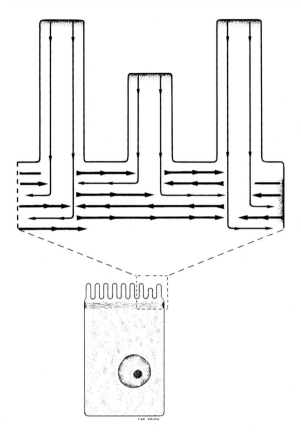

Figure 16–31. Diagram explaining the movements of micro-villi. Upper drawing is an enlargement of part of the surface of an intestinal cell. The microvilli contain actin filaments (thin arrows) that interact with myosin filament (thick arrows) in the cell apex. The dense regions in the tips of the microvilli are the probable sites of insertion of the actin filaments. The localization of these proteins was identified by using immunofluorescence cytochemistry. Compare this figure with Fig 4–12. (Based on studies by Rodewald R, Newman SB, Karnovsky MJ: Contraction of isolated brush borders from the intestinal epithelium. *J Cell Biol* 1976;**70**:541.)

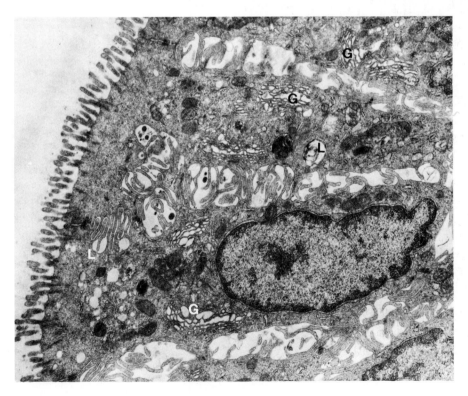

Figure 16–32. Electron micrograph of epithelial cells of the large intestine. Observe the microvilli at the luminal surface, the well-developed Golgi complex (G), lysosomes (L), and dilated intercellular spaces filled by microvilli. × 3900.

are digested has been challenged, and some authors think that the lymphocytes in the intestinal epithelium migrate back to the lamina propria and from there return to the lymph vessels.

THE LARGE INTESTINE

The large intestine consists of a mucosal membrane with no folds except in its distal (rectal) portion. No villi are present in this portion of the intestine. The epithelial lining is columnar, and the cells have short, irregular microvilli, suggesting an absorptive function for these cells (Fig 16–32). The **intestinal glands of Lieberkühn** are long and characterized by a great abundance of goblet cells and a small number of enteroendocrine cells (Figs 16–33 and 16–34). This organ is well suited to its main functions: water absorption and formation of the fecal mass plus production of mucus, a highly hydrated gel that not only lubricates the intestinal surface but also covers bacteria and particulate matter. The absorption of water occurs passively following the active transport of sodium out of the basal surfaces of these epithelial cells.

The lamina propria is rich in lymphoid cells and nodules. The nodules frequently extend into the submucosa. This richness in lymphoid tissue is probably

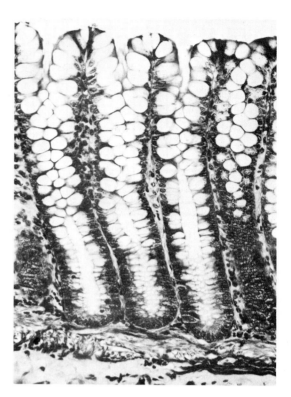

Figure 16–34. Photomicrograph of a section of large intestine. Observe the intestinal glands with abundant goblet cells. H&E stain, × 95.

due to the extremely abundant bacterial population present in the large intestine. The muscularis externa is composed of longitudinal and circular strands. This layer differs from the small intestine, since fibers of the outer longitudinal layer congregate in 3 thick longitudinal bands called **teniae coli.** In the intraperitoneal portions of the colon, the serous layer is characterized by small pendulous protuberances composed of adipose tissue—the **appendices epiploicae** (Fig 16–35).

In the anal region, the mucous membrane forms a series of longitudinal folds, the **rectal columns of Morgagni.** About 2 cm above the anal opening, the intestinal mucosa is replaced by stratified squamous epithelium. In this region, the lamina propria contains a plexus of large veins that, when excessively dilated and varicose, produce hemorrhoids.

THE APPENDIX

The appendix is an evagination of the cecum characterized by a relatively small, narrow, and irregular lumen due to the presence of abundant lymphoid follicles in its wall. Its general structure is similar to that of the large intestine. However, it contains fewer and shorter intestinal glands and has no teniae coli (Fig 16–36).

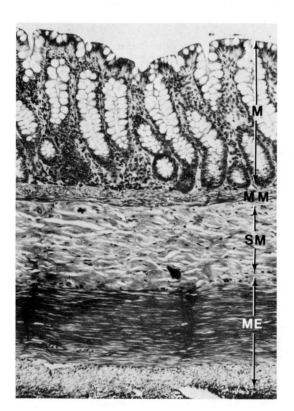

Figure 16–33. Photomicrograph of a section of large intestine with its various layers. Observe the absence of villi. M, mucosa; MM, muscularis mucosa; SM, submucosa; ME, muscularis externa. H&E stain, × 30.

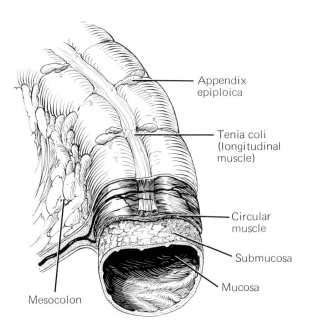

Figure 16–35. Cross section of colon. (Reproduced, with permission, from Way LW [editor]: *Current Surgical Diagnosis & Treatment,* 7th ed. Lange, 1985.)

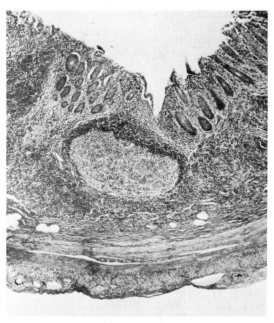

Figure 16–36. Photomicrograph of a section of appendix. There are few glands and numerous lymphoid nodules. H&E stain, × 20.

REFERENCES

Andrew A: The APUD concept: Where has it led us? *Br Med Bull* 1982;**38**:221.

Cheng H, Leblond CP: Origin, differentiation and renewal of the four main epithelial cell types in the mouse small intestine. 5. Unitarian theory of the origin of the four epithelial cell types. *Am J Anat* 1974;**141**:537.

Creamer B: Variations in small-intestinal villous shape and mucosal dynamics. *Br Med J* 1964;**2**:1371.

Davenport HW: Why the stomach does not digest itself. *Sci Am* (Jan) 1972;**226**:87.

Forte JG: Mechanism of gastric H^+ and Cl^- transport. *Annu Rev Physiol* 1980;**42**:111.

Freeman JA: Goblet cell fine structure. *Anat Rec* 1966;**154**:121.

Friedman HI, Cardell RR Jr: Alterations in the endoplasmic reticulum and Golgi complex of intestinal epithelial cells during fat absorption and after termination of this process: A morphological and morphometric study. *Anat Rec* 1977;**188**:77.

Fujita T, Kobayashi S: Structure and function of gut endocrine cells. *Int Rev Cytol [Suppl]* 1977; No. 6:187.

Gabella G: Innervation of the gastrointestinal tract. *Int Rev Cytol* 1979;**59**:130.

Gray GM: Carbohydrate digestion and absorption: Role of the small intestine. *N Engl J Med* 1975;**292**:1225.

Grube D, Forssmann WG: Morphology and function of the entero-endocrine cells. *Horm Metab Res* 1979;**11**:589.

Hoedemseker PJ et al: Further investigations about the site of production of Castle's gastric intrinsic factor. *Lab Invest* 1966;**15**:1163.

Ito S, Schofield GC: Studies on the depletion and accumulation of microvilli and changes in the tubulovesicular compartment of the mouse parietal cells in relation to gastric acid secretion. *J Cell Biol* 1974;**63**:364.

Ito S, Winchester RJ: The fine structure of the gastric mucosa in the rat. *J Cell Biol* 1963;**16**:541.

Klockars M, Reitamo S: Tissue distribution of lysozyme in man. *J Histochem Cytochem* 1975;**23**:932.

Larsson LI: Peptide secretory pathways in GI tract: Cytochemical contributions to regulatory physiology of the gut. *Am J Physiol* 1981;**239**:237.

Leeson TS, Leeson CR: The fine structure of Brunner's glands in man. *J Anat* 1968;**103**:263.

Marsh MN: Studies of intestinal lymphoid tissue. (2 parts.) *Gut* 1975;**16**:665, 675.

Mjör IA, Fejerskov O: *Histology of the Human Tooth,* 2nd ed. Munksgaard, 1979.

Moog F: The lining of the small intestine. *Sci Am* (Nov) 1981;**245**:154.

Mooseker MS, Tilney LG: Organization of an actin filament-membrane complex: Filament polarity and membrane attachment in the microvilli of intestinal epithelial cells. *J Cell Biol* 1975;**67**:725.

Owen RL, Jones AL: Epithelial cell specialization within human Peyer's patches: An ultrastructural study of intestinal lymphoid follicles. *Gastroenterology* 1974;**66**:189.

Peeters T, Vantrappen G: The Paneth cell: A source of intestinal lysozyme. *Gut* 1975;**16**:553.

Pfeiffer CJ, Rowden G, Weibel J: *Gastrointestinal Ultrastructure.* Academic Press, 1974.

Rubin W et al: The normal human gastric epithelia: A fine structural study. *Lab Invest* 1968;**19**:598.

Tagaki T et al: Scanning electron microscopy on the human gastric mucosa: Fetal, normal and various pathological conditions. *Acta Pathol Jpn* 1974;**24**:233.

Toskes PP, Deren JJ: Vitamin B_{12} absorption and malabsorption. *Gastroenterology* 1973;**65**:662.

17

Glands Associated With the Digestive Tract

The subjects of this chapter are the salivary glands, pancreas, liver, and gallbladder. The functions of the salivary glands are to wet and lubricate the oral cavity and its contents; to initiate the digestion of carbohydrates; to secrete certain substances such as IgA, lysozyme, lactoferrin, iodide, urea, thiocyanate, and potassium; and to reabsorb sodium. The main functions of the pancreas are to produce digestive enzymes that act in the small intestine and to secrete the hormones insulin and glucagon into the bloodstream. The liver produces bile, an important fluid in the digestion of fats; plays a major role in lipid, carbohydrate, and protein metabolism; inactivates and metabolizes many toxic substances and drugs; and participates in iron metabolism and the synthesis of blood proteins and factors necessary for blood coagulation. The gall-

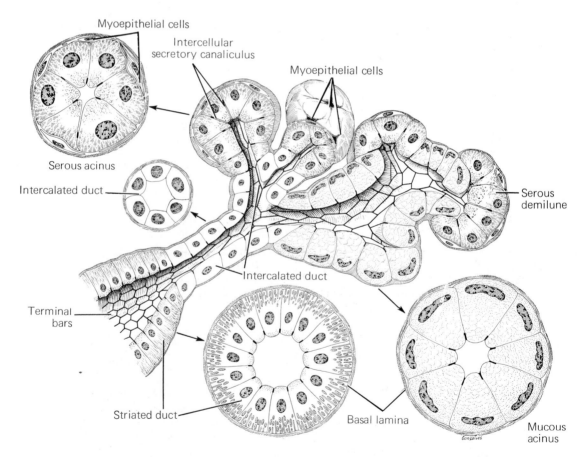

Figure 17–1. The structure of the submandibular (submaxillary) gland. In the secretory portion, acini are composed of pyramidal serous and mucous cells and tubules of mucous cells. In serous cells, the nuclei are euchromatic and rounded, and in the basal third of the cell an accumulation of rough endoplasmic reticulum is evident. The cellular apex is filled with protein-rich secretory granules. The nuclei of mucous cells are flattened with condensed chromatin and located near the bases of the cells. Mucous cells have little rough endoplasmic reticulum and contain distinct secretory granules. The intercalated ducts are short and are lined by cuboidal epithelium. The striated ducts are composed of columnar cells with characteristics of ion-transporting cells (see Fig 17–6 and Chapter 4), such as basal membrane invaginations and mitochondrial accumulation. (After Braus.)

bladder reabsorbs water from the bile and stores the bile in a concentrated form.

THE SALIVARY GLANDS

Besides the small glands scattered throughout the oral cavity described in the previous chapter, 3 pairs of large salivary glands are present: the **parotid, submandibular (submaxillary),** and **sublingual glands.**

These glands consist of cells that produce the primary saliva, containing enzymes, IgA, mucus, electrolytes, water, etc. Collections of secretory cells are called **secretory end-pieces (adenomeres),** and they are of 2 general types—serous and mucous (Fig 17–1).

Serous cells are usually pyramidal in shape with a broad base resting on the basal lamina and a narrow apical surface furnished with short, irregular microvilli facing the lumen (Figs 17–2 and 17–3). Serous cells have a spherical, euchromatic nucleus located in the basal third of the cell and surrounded by numerous profiles of rough endoplasmic reticulum. With appropriate stains, the basal cytoplasm is basophilic owing to the numerous ribosomes. The cytoplasm between the nucleus and the lumen contains an extensive Golgi complex and numerous membrane-limited **secretion granules,** which are usually eosinophilic. Mitochondria, lysosomes, occasional lipid droplets, microfilaments, and microtubules are also present. Adjacent secretory cells are joined together by junctional complexes consisting of zonulae occludentes (tight junctions), zonulae adherentes (adhering junctions), desmosomes, and gap junctions. These

junctional complexes may be located well below the apical margin, in which case **intercellular secretory canaliculi** (Fig 17–1) are formed. These canaliculi increase the area available for discharge of serous secretions. Serous cells usually form a spherical mass of cells called an **acinus** (alveolus) with a lumen in the center. This structure can be likened to a grape attached to its stem. The stem corresponds to the duct system, which is described below.

Mucous cells are usually cuboidal to columnar in shape; their nuclei are heterochromatic, oval, and pressed toward the bases of the cells (Figs 17–4 and 17–5). In the light microscope, their apical cytoplasm is foamy and lightly stained owing to the solubility of mucinogens (mucus-forming substances) in ordinary fixatives. Seen with the electron microscope, mucous cells have the organelles usually associated with glycoprotein synthesis (extensive rough endoplasmic reticulum and Golgi complex). Mucinogen granules are surrounded by a membrane, but their contents are less electron-dense than seromucous granules. Mucous cells are most often organized as **tubules,** consisting of cylindric arrays of secretory cells surrounding a lumen.

In the **submandibular gland** of humans, serous and mucous cells are arranged in a characteristic pattern. Mucous cells form tubules, but their ends are capped by serous cells, which constitute the **serous demilunes.**

Myoepithelial cells are found within the basal lamina of glandular and ductal epithelia of salivary glands. Myoepithelial cells surrounding serous acini are highly branched cells (sometimes called **basket**

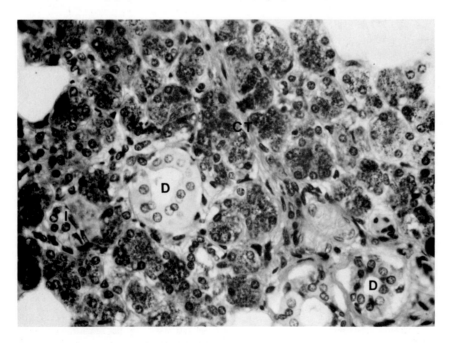

Figure 17–2. Photomicrograph of a human parotid gland, showing serous acini and striated ducts (D). An intercalated duct (I) consisting of pale-staining cuboidal cells is present in the lower left of the section. A connective tissue septum (CT) separates the lobules. H&E stain, × 360.

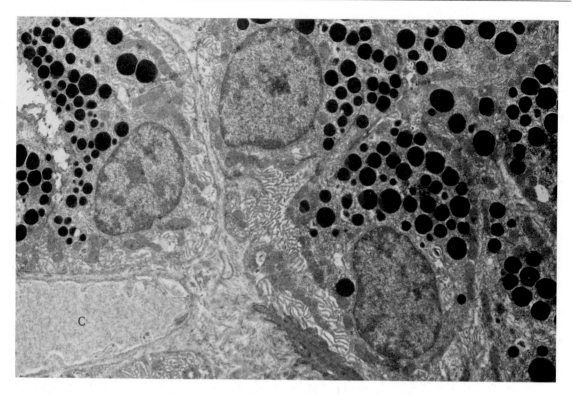

Figure 17–3. Section of a parotid gland showing 3 nuclei of serous cells and their characteristic secretory granules. At lower left is a fenestrated capillary (C). × 3000. (Courtesy of LL George.)

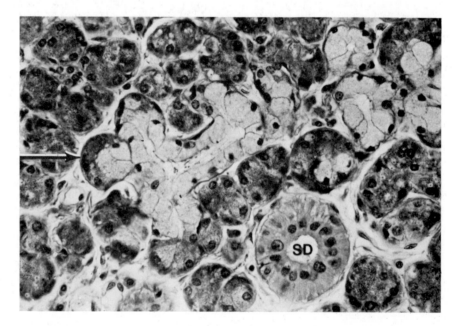

Figure 17–4. Photomicrograph of a section of human submandibular gland. Observe the presence of dense serous and pale-staining mucous cells. In the lower right region is a striated duct (SD). The arrow indicates a demilune where serous cells are eccentrically displaced, assuming the form of a crescent. H&E stain, × 360.

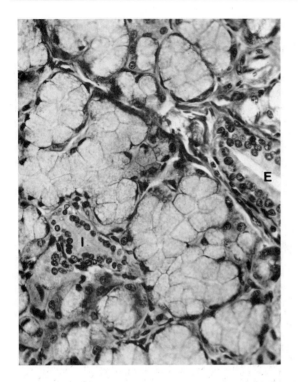

Figure 17–5. Photomicrograph of a human sublingual gland showing the predominance of mucous cells. Examples of an intralobular (I) and connective tissue –ensheathed interlobular (E) duct are also present. H&E stain, × 600.

cells), whereas those associated with mucous tubules and intercalated ducts are spindle-shaped and lie parallel to the length of the duct. Both types of myoepithelial cell possess large quantities of actin-containing microfilaments, and myosin has been demonstrated using labeled antimyosin antibodies.

Secretory end-pieces empty into **intercalated ducts** lined by cuboidal epithelial cells. Several of these ducts then join to form another type of **intralobular duct,** the **striated duct.**

Striated ducts are characterized by radial striations that extend from the bases of the cells to the level of the nuclei. When viewed in the electron microscope, these striations are seen to consist of infoldings of the basal plasma membrane as well as numerous mitochondria aligned parallel to the infolded membranes (Figs 17–4 and 17–6). (See Chapter 4 for further discussion.)

Striated ducts of each lobule converge and drain into ducts in the connective tissue septae separating the lobules. At these points, they become **interlobular ducts** or **excretory ducts.** Their lining epithelium is initially stratified cuboidal, but more distal parts of excretory ducts are lined by stratified columnar epithelium. Ultimately, the main duct of each major salivary gland empties into the oral cavity and is lined by nonkeratinized stratified squamous epithelium.

The large salivary glands are not mere collections of epithelial cells but contain other components such as connective tissue, blood and lymph vessels, and

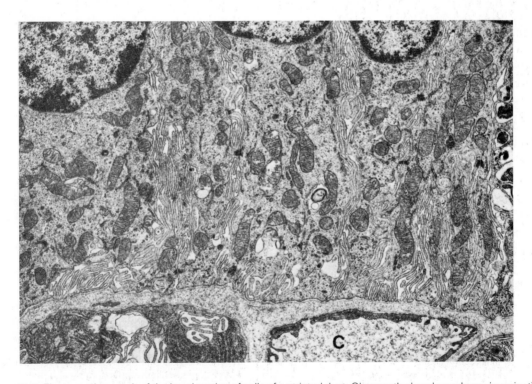

Figure 17–6. Electron micrograph of the basal portion of cells of a striated duct. Observe the basal membrane invaginations and mitochondria disposed in palisades, characteristics of ion-transporting cells. At the lower right is a fenestrated capillary (C) × 6000. (Courtesy of LL George.)

nerves, organized in a definite pattern. These glands are surrounded by a capsule of connective tissue, rich in collagen fibers. From this capsule, septa of connective tissue penetrate the gland, dividing it into lobules. Vessels and nerves enter the gland at the hilum and gradually branch into the lobules. A rich vascular and nervous plexus surrounds the secretory and ductal components of each lobule.

The specific characteristics of each of the major salivary glands will now be described.

Parotid Glands

The parotid gland is a branched acinar gland. Its secretory portion is composed almost exclusively of serous cells (Fig 17–2). These cells have a moderate number of ribosomes in their basal regions as compared to the pancreatic exocrine cell. In humans, in addition to having the characteristics of a serous cell, the secretory granules of these cells exhibit a positive periodic acid–Schiff (PAS) reaction indicating the presence of polysaccharides (sialomucin and sulfomucin) in these granules. The secretory granules (Fig 17–3) are rich in proteins and have a high amylase activity. The other components of this gland are similar to the general description just given. In humans, secretory cells represent about 90% of the gland's cell volume; striated ducts account for about 5%; and the remainder consists of excretory ducts, connective tissue, vessels, nerves, etc. The encapsulating connective tissue contains many plasma cells and lymphocytes. The plasma cells secrete an immunoglobulin, IgA, which complexes with a **secretory piece,** synthesized by the serous acinar, intercalated duct, and striated duct cells. The IgA–secretory piece complex released into the saliva is resistant to enzymatic digestion and constitutes an immunologic defense mechanism against orally introduced pathogens.

Submandibular (Submaxillary) Glands

The submandibular gland is a branched tubuloacinar gland (Fig 17–4). Its secretory portion contains both mucous and serous cells. The serous cells contain protein secretory granules that are PAS-positive owing to the presence of carbohydrate moieties (sialomucin

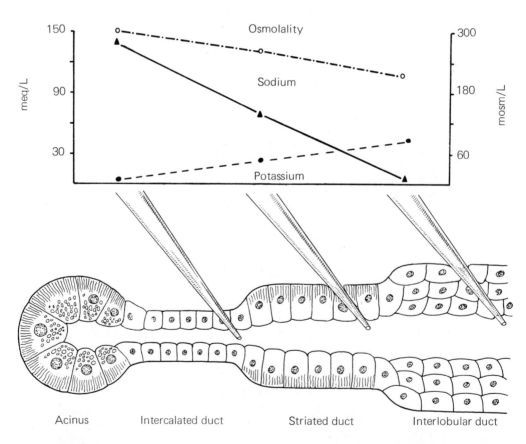

Figure 17–7. Diagram illustrating the results obtained from micropuncture experiments in the salivary gland. When the puncture is close to the secretory portion in the intercalated duct, the sodium and potassium content and the osmolality of the saliva are equal to that observed in the blood. With gradual movement away from the intercalated ducts, the potassium content increases and sodium content and osmolality decrease. This strongly suggests that these changes are mediated by the epithelial lining of the ducts.

and sulfomucin). The serous cells are the main component and are easily distinguished from pure mucous cells by their rounded nuclei and basophilic, PAS-positive cytoplasm. The presence of extensive lateral and basal membrane infoldings toward the vascular bed increases the ion-transporting surface area 60 times, thus facilitating electrolyte and water transport during primary secretion. As a consequence of these folds, the cell boundaries are indistinct. These cells are responsible for the weak amylolytic activity present in this gland and its saliva. The cells that form the demilunes in both the submandibular and sublingual glands contain and secrete the enzyme **lysozyme**, whose main activity is to hydrolyze the walls of certain bacteria. In humans, this gland consists of 80% serous cells, 5% mucous cells, and 5% striated ducts; the remainder consists of vessels, nerves, and other ducts (Fig 17–4).

Sublingual Gland

The sublingual gland is (like the submandibular gland) a branched tubuloacinar gland. It contains, however, no acini formed exclusively by serous cells, and mucous cells predominate in the sublingual gland. Serous cells form demilunes on mucous acini. This gland consists of 60% mucous cells, 30% serous cells, and 3% striated ducts (Fig 17–5); the remainder consists of vessels, nerves, and other ducts.

Histophysiology of the Salivary Glands

Moistening and lubricating functions of the salivary glands are performed by the water and glycoproteins of saliva. The latter are synthesized mainly by the mucous cells and to a lesser degree by the serous cells of the glands. These fluids also provide solvents for substances that stimulate the taste buds. Human saliva consists of secretions from the parotid glands (25%), the submandibular glands (70%), and the sublingual gland (5%).

Another important function of these glands is the digestion of carbohydrates. The major part of the hydrolysis of ingested carbohydrates is due to salivary

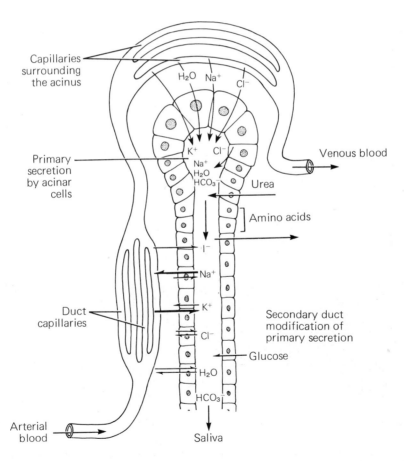

Figure 17–8. Schematic illustration of the characteristic blood vessel organization that provides for 2 capillary nets around the ducts and acini in the parotid gland. Primary saliva secretion occurs in the acini and subsequently becomes modified as it passes through the duct system. Note the presence of a countercurrent flow between blood and saliva in the ducts. (From Davenport HW: *Physiology of the Digestive Tract.* Year Book, 1977.)

amylase activity. This digestion begins in the mouth but takes place also in the stomach before the gastric juice acidifies the food, thereby decreasing considerably amylase activity.

As mentioned above, serous acinar, intercalated duct, and striated duct cells synthesize the secretory piece necessary for the transport of secretory IgA from the connective tissues, across the acinar and ductal cells, and into the saliva. Lactoferrin and lysozyme are also secreted by acinar and intercalated duct cells. Lactoferrin binds iron, a nutrient necessary for bacterial growth, while lysozyme hydrolyzes the cell wall of certain bacteria. Thus, saliva is important in defending the oral cavity against pathogens.

Studies performed by inserting micropipettes into the striated and excretory ducts strongly suggest that the saliva produced by the secretory cells—called **primary saliva**—has the same ionic composition as and is therefore isosmotic with blood. As it progresses through the striated and excretory ducts, the duct cells actively reabsorb sodium and secrete potassium (Fig 17–7). The ionic modification of saliva is facilitated by the double capillary network associated with the secretory and duct portions of the gland (Fig 17–8). This explains why saliva is hypotonic and has a higher concentration of potassium and a lower concentration of sodium than blood. The striated ducts show morphologic and functional similarities to the renal tubules (Figs 17–6 and 20–12). Both have cells with char-

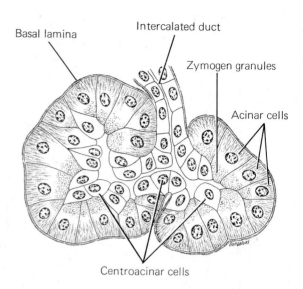

Figure 17–10. Schematic drawing of the structure of pancreatic acini. Acinar cells are pyramidal, with granules at their apex and rough endoplasmic reticulum at the cell base. The intercalated duct partially penetrates the acini. These duct cells are known as centroacinar cells. Note the absence of myoepithelial cells.

acteristics of ion-transporting cells, and both are sensitive to aldosterone.

Parasympathetic stimulation provokes a copious, watery secretion with relatively little organic content. Sympathetic nerve stimulation produces small amounts of viscous saliva, rich in organic material.

THE PANCREAS

The pancreas is a mixed exocrine and endocrine gland. The endocrine portion is composed of the **islets of Langerhans** (see Chapter 22). The exocrine portion is a compound acinar gland (Fig 17–9), similar in structure to the parotid gland. In histologic sections, a differential diagnosis can be made based on the absence of striated ducts and the presence of the islets of Langerhans in the pancreas. Another characteristic detail is that the initial portions of intercalated ducts penetrate the lumens of the acini. Nuclei, surrounded by a pale cytoplasm, belong to **centroacinar cells** that constitute the intra-acinar portion of the intercalated duct (Figs 17–10 and 17–11). Such cells are found only in pancreatic acini. Intercalated ducts are tributaries of larger interlobular ducts lined by columnar epithelium in which goblet cells can be observed. Striated ducts are not present in the pancreatic duct system.

The exocrine pancreatic acinus is composed of several serous cells surrounding a lumen (Fig 17–12). These cells are highly polarized, with a large amount of basally located rough endoplasmic reticulum sur-

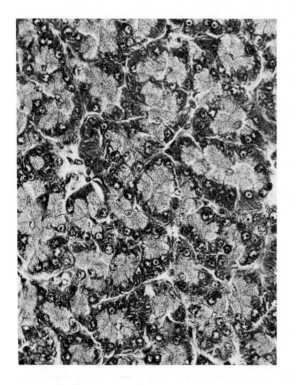

Figure 17–9. Photomicrograph showing the appearance of the acinar portion of the pancreas with its secretory cells. H&E stain, × 400.

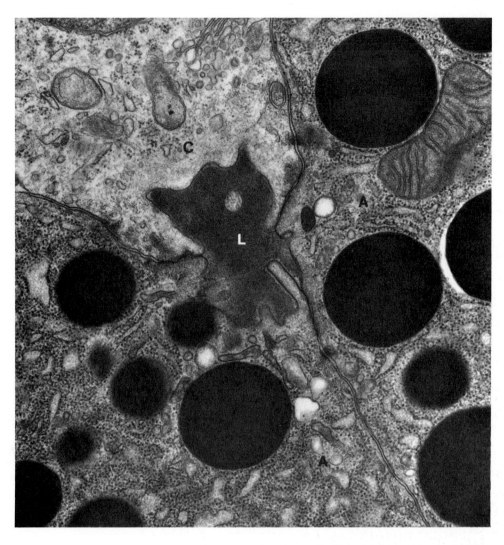

Figure 17–11. Electron micrograph of the apex of 2 pancreatic acinar cells (A) and a centroacinar cell (C) from the rat pancreas. Observe the lack of secretory granules and the very scant rough endoplasmic reticulum in the centroacinar cell as compared with the acinar cell. L, acinar lumen. × 30,000.

rounding a spherical nucleus (Figs 17–9 and 17–13). The rough endoplasmic reticulum is the site of synthesis and segregation of digestive enzymes and proteins destined for lysosomes and for insertion into the plasma membrane. The digestive enzymes are transferred to the Golgi complex, where they are packaged, concentrated (Figs 3–15 and 4–23), and finally stored as mature secretory (**zymogen**) granules near the apex of the cell (Figs 17–11, 17–12, and 17–13). In the rat, under conditions of maximal stimulation, the pancreas can secrete up to 1.5% of its total protein content in 1 hour. The number of zymogen granules present in each cell is variable and depends on the digestive phase, attaining its maximum in fasted animals.

The pancreas is covered by a thin capsule of connective tissue that sends septa into it, separating the pancreatic lobules. The acini are surrounded by a basal lamina supported by a delicate sheath of reticular fibers. It has a rich capillary network.

The human exocrine pancreas secretes, besides water and ions, the following enzymes and proenzymes: trypsinogen, chymotrypsinogen, carboxypeptidase, ribonuclease, deoxyribonuclease, triacylglycerol lipase, phospholipase A_2, elastase, and amylase.

The control of pancreatic secretion is performed mainly through 2 hormones—**secretin** and **cholecystokinin** (previously called pancreozymin)—produced by enteroendocrine cells of the duodenal mucosa. Stimulation of the vagus nerve will also produce pancreatic secretion.

Secretin promotes secretion of an abundant fluid, poor in protein and enzyme activity and rich in bicarbonate. Its function is mainly to promote water and ion transport, which probably occurs in the duct cells

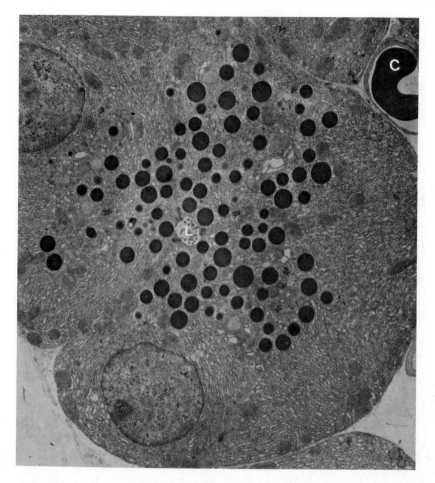

Figure 17–12. Low-magnification electron micrograph of an exocrine pancreatic acinus. The lumen (L) is near the center of the picture. Note the polarization of the cells—rough endoplasmic reticulum is located closest to the connective tissue and capillaries (C), while the mature secretory (zymogen) granules congregate near the lumen of the acinus. × 4500.

and not in the acinar cells. This secretion serves to neutralize the acidic **chyme** (partially digested food) so that pancreatic enzymes can function at their optimal neutral pH range. Cholecystokinin promotes secretion of a less abundant but protein- and enzyme-rich fluid. This hormone acts mainly in the process of extrusion of the zymogen granules. The integrated action of both of these hormones provides for a heavy secretion of enzyme-rich pancreatic juices. In conditions of extreme malnutrition such as kwashiorkor, pancreatic acinar cells undergo atrophy and lose much of their rough endoplasmic reticulum, and the production of digestive enzymes is hindered.

THE LIVER

With the exception of the skin, the liver is the largest organ of the body and is the largest gland, weighing about 1.5 kg. It is situated in the abdominal cavity beneath the diaphragm. Most of its blood

(70–80%) comes from the portal vein; the smaller percentage is supplied by the hepatic artery. Through the portal vein, all the materials absorbed via the intestines reach the liver except the complex lipids (chylomicrons), which are transported mainly by lymph vessels. The position of the liver in the circulatory system is optimal for gathering, transforming, and accumulating metabolites and for neutralizing and eliminating toxic substances. This elimination occurs in the bile, an exocrine secretion of the liver of importance in lipid digestion.

In addition to these main functions, other important functions of the liver will be discussed later.

Stroma

The liver is covered by a thin connective tissue capsule (**Glisson's capsule**) that becomes thicker at the **hilum,** where the portal vein and hepatic artery enter the liver and the right and left hepatic ducts and lymphatics exit. These vessels and ducts are surrounded by connective tissue fibers and cells all the

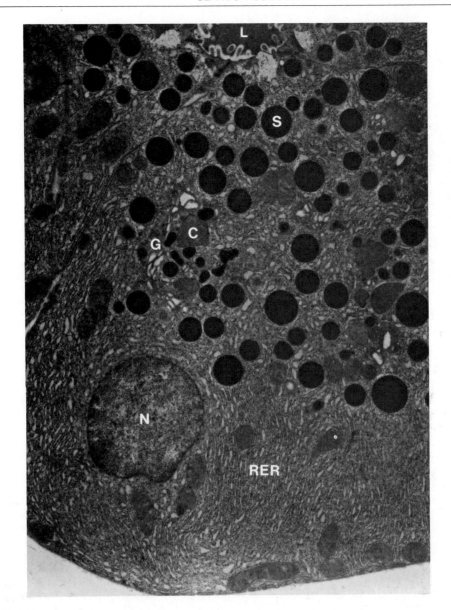

Figure 17–13. Electron micrograph of an acinar cell from the rat pancreas. Note the nucleus (N) surrounded by numerous cisternae of rough endoplasmic reticulum (RER) near the base of the cell. The Golgi complex (G) is situated at the apical pole of the nucleus and is associated with several condensing vacuoles (C) and numerous mature secretory (zymogen) granules (S). The lumen (L) contains proteins recently released from the cell by exocytosis. × 8000.

way to their termination (or origin) in the portal spaces between classic liver lobules. At this point, a delicate reticular fiber network is formed that supports the hepatocytes and sinusoidal endothelial cells of the liver lobules.

The Liver Lobule

The main structural component of the liver is the liver cell or **hepatocyte.** These epithelial cells are grouped in plates that are interconnected in such a way as to show, in light microscope sections, struc-

tural units called **classic liver lobules** (Fig 17–14). The liver lobule is formed of a polygonal mass of tissue about 0.7 × 2 mm in size (Figs 17–14 and 17–15). In certain animals (eg, the pig), lobules are separated from each other by a layer of connective tissue. This does not occur in humans, where the lobules are in close contact along most of their extent, making it difficult to establish precisely the exact limits between different lobules. In some regions, however, the lobules are demarcated by connective tissue containing bile ducts, lymphatics, nerves, and

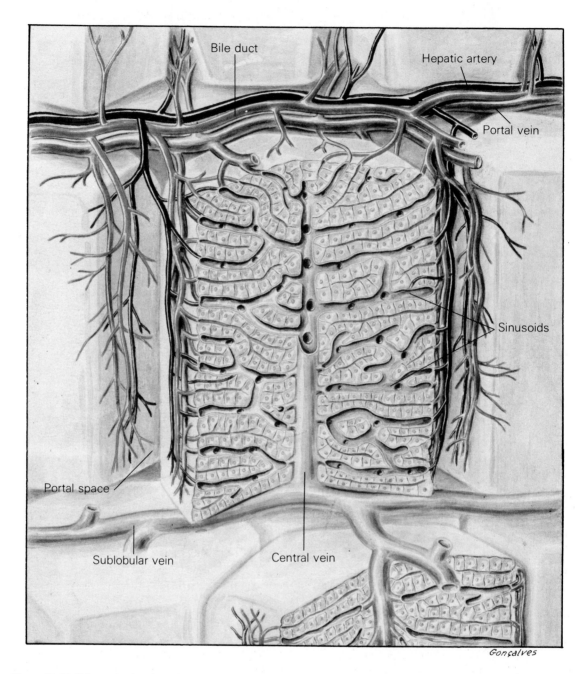

Figure 17–14. Schematic drawing of the structure of the liver. In the center, the liver lobule is surrounded by the portal space. The portal spaces are shown dilated here for the sake of clarity; in the human liver, these spaces are much smaller and in some places nonexistent. Arteries, veins, and bile ducts occupy the portal spaces. Lymph vessels, nerves, and connective tissue are also present but are not shown in this illustration. Observe in the lobule the radial disposition of the plates formed by liver cells. The sinusoid capillaries separate plates of liver cells. The bile canaliculi can be seen between the liver cells. The sublobular (intercalated) veins drain blood from the lobules. (Redrawn and reproduced, with permission, from Bourne G: *An Introduction to Functional Histology*. Churchill, 1953.)

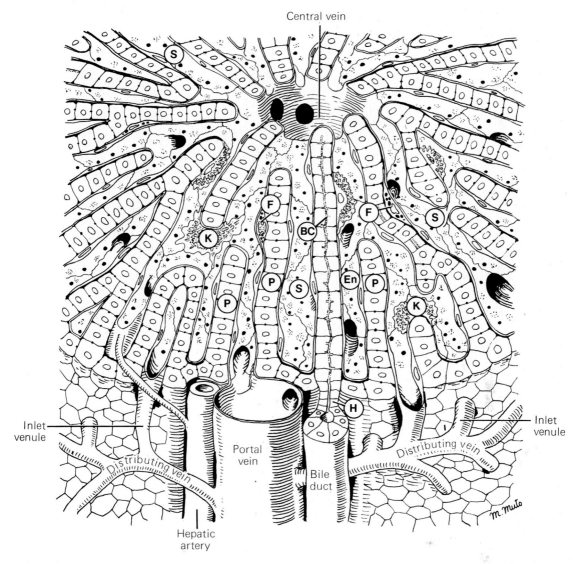

Figure 17–15. Three-dimensional aspect of the normal liver. In the upper center, the central vein; in the lower center, the portal vein. BC, bile canaliculi; P, liver plates; H, Hering canal; K, Kupffer cells; S, sinusoid; F, fat-storing cell; En, sinusoid endothelial cell. (Courtesy of M Muto.)

blood vessels. These regions, the **portal spaces,** are present at the corners of the lobules and are occupied by the **portal triads.** The human liver contains 3–6 portal triads per lobule, each containing a venule (a branch of the portal vein); an arteriole (a branch of the hepatic artery); a duct (part of the bile duct system); and lymphatic vessels. The venule is usually the largest of these structures, containing blood coming from the superior and inferior mesenteric and splenic veins. The arteriole contains blood from the celiac trunk of the abdominal aorta. The duct, lined by cuboidal epithelium, carries bile from the parenchymal cells (hepatocytes) and eventually empties into the hepatic duct. One or more lymphatics carry lymph that eventually enters the blood circulation. All of these struc-

tures are embedded in a sheath of connective tissue (Fig 17–16).

The hepatocytes are radially disposed in the liver lobule. They form a layer one or 2 cells thick in a fashion similar to the bricks of a wall. These cellular plates are directed from the periphery of the lobule to its center and anastomose freely, forming a labyrinthine and spongelike structure (Fig 17–15). The space between these plates contains capillaries, the **liver sinusoids** (Figs 17–14, 17–15, and 17–16). As seen in Chapter 12, sinusoids are irregularly dilated vessels composed only of a discontinuous layer of fenestrated endothelial cells. No basal lamina is present, and diaphragms are not present across the fenestrae. The fenestrae are about 100 nm in diameter

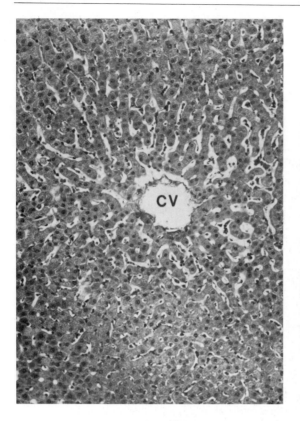

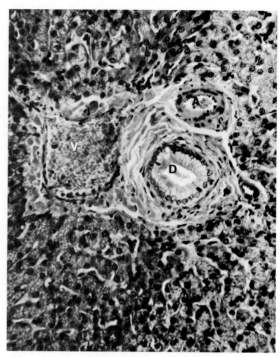

Figure 17–16. Photomicrograph of the liver. *Left:* A central vein (CV). Observe the liver plates that anastomose freely, limiting the space occupied by the sinusoids. H&E stain, × 200. *Right:* A portal space with its characteristic artery (A), vein (V), and bile duct (D) surrounded by connective tissue. Masson's stain, × 300.

and are grouped in clusters forming "sieve plates" (Fig 17–17A).

The endothelial cells are separated from the underlying hepatocytes by a subendothelial space known as the **space of Disse,** which contains some reticular fibers and microvilli of the hepatocytes (Figs 17–18 and 17–21). Consequently, blood fluids readily percolate through the endothelial wall and make intimate contact with the hepatocyte surface (Fig 17–17A). In addition to the endothelial cells, the sinusoids also contain phagocytic cells of the mononuclear phagocyte series known as **Kupffer cells.** These cells are found on the luminal surface of the endothelial cells. Kupffer cells have cytologic characteristics such as clear vacuoles, lysosomes, and rough endoplasmic reticulum scattered throughout the cytoplasm that distinguish them from the endothelial cells. Evidence shows that these cells derive from bone marrow, as do other macrophages. The **fat-storing cells** (Ito cells) (Fig 17–15) are stellate cells located in the spaces of Disse. They have the capacity to accumulate exogenously administered vitamin A as retinyl esters in lipid droplets, but the role of these cells in vitamin A metabolism and transport remains obscure.

The liver sinusoidal capillaries have large openings—the "sieve plates" mentioned above (Fig 17–17A)—which permit easy exchange of macromolecules from the sinusoidal lumen to the liver cell and vice versa (Fig 17–18). This is physiologically important because of the large number of macromolecules secreted into the blood by hepatocytes such as lipoproteins, albumin, fibrinogen, etc, and because the liver also takes up and catabolizes many of these large molecules. The sinusoid is surrounded and supported by a delicate sheath of reticular fibers important in maintaining its form. The sinusoids arise in the periphery of the lobule, fed by the inlet venules, terminal branches of the portal veins, and hepatic arterioles, and they run in the direction of its center, where they drain into the **central vein** (Figs 17–14 and 17–15).

Liver Blood Supply

The liver is unusual in that it receives blood from 2 sources: (1) the **portal vein** that carries oxygen-poor, nutrient-rich blood from the abdominal viscera, and (2) the **hepatic artery** that supplies oxygen-rich blood (Figs 17–14 and 17–15).

A. Portal Vein System: The portal vein branches repeatedly and sends small venules, the **portal venules,** to portal triads. These are sometimes called the **interlobular branches.** The portal venules branch

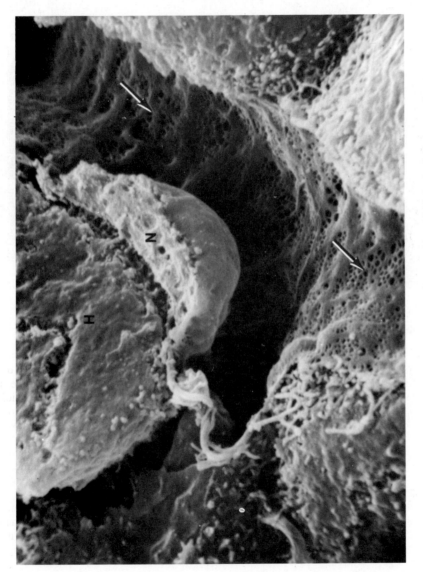

Figure 17–17A. Scanning electron micrograph of a liver sinusoidal lining cell. Numerous fenestrations (arrows) allow exchange of large particles such as lipoproteins between the hepatocyte (H) and the sinusoidal lumen. N, nucleus of sinusoidal lining cell. × 7100. (Courtesy of R Hamilton.)

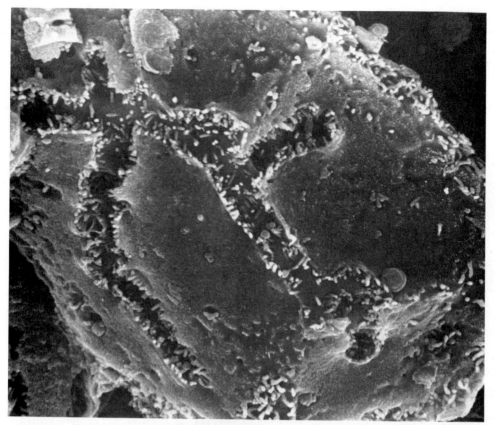

Figure 17–17C. Branching bile canaliculi observed in the liver by scanning electron microscopy. Observe the microvilli lining its internal surface. (Reproduced, with permission, from Motta P, Muto M, Fujita T: *The Liver: An Atlas of Scanning Electron Microscopy.* Igaku-Shoin, 1978.)

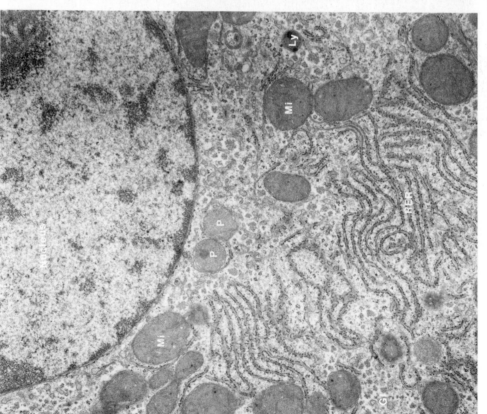

Figure 17–17B. Electron micrograph of a hepatocyte. In the cytoplasm, below the nucleus, are mitochondria (Mi), rough endoplasmic reticulum (RER), glycogen (Gl), lysosomes (Ly), and peroxisomes (P). × 6600.

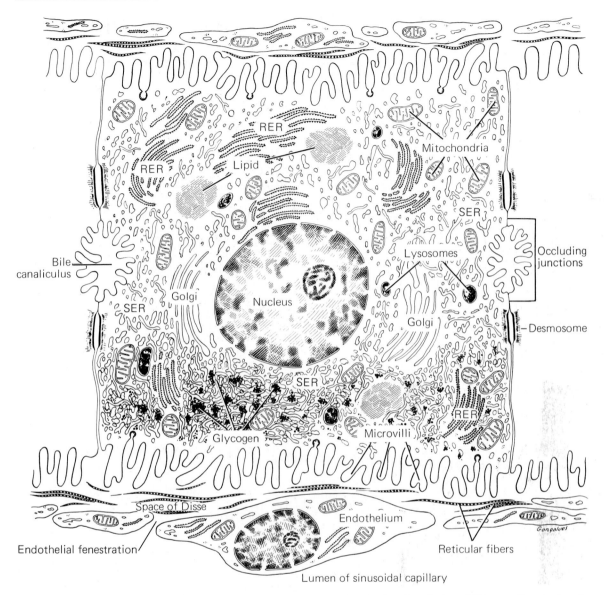

Figure 17–18. Diagram of the ultrastructure of a hepatocyte. RER, rough endoplasmic reticulum; SER, smooth endoplasmic reticulum. × 10,000.

into **distributing veins** that run around the periphery of the lobule. From the distributing veins, small **inlet venules** empty into the **sinusoids.** The sinusoids run radially and converge in the center of the lobule to form the **central,** or **centrolobular, vein.** This vessel has thin walls consisting of only endothelial cells supported by a sparse population of collagen fibers. As the central vein progresses along the lobule, it receives more and more sinusoids and gradually increases in diameter. At its end, it leaves the lobule at its base by merging with the larger **sublobular vein** (Fig 17–14). The sublobular veins gradually converge and fuse, forming the 2 or more large **hepatic veins** that empty into the inferior vena cava.

B. Arterial System: The hepatic artery branches repeatedly and forms the **interlobular arteries;** some irrigate the structures of the portal canals and others end directly in the sinusoids at varying distances from the portal spaces, thus providing a mixture of arterial and portal venous blood in the sinusoids (Fig 17–15).

Blood flows from the periphery to the center of the **classic hepatic lobule.** Consequently, oxygen and metabolites, as well as all other toxic or nontoxic substances absorbed in the intestines, reach first the peripheral cells and then the central cells of the lobule. This partly explains why the cytologic and physiologic behavior of the perilobular cells is different from that of the centrolobular cells. This duality of behavior of

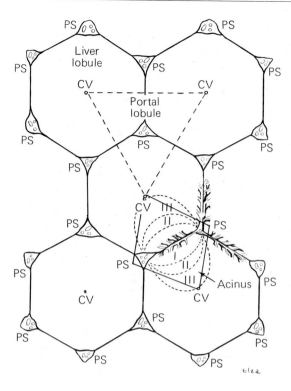

Figure 17–19. Schematic drawing illustrating the territories of the classic liver lobules, hepatic acini, and portal lobules. The classic lobule has a central vein (CV) and is outlined by lines that connect the portal spaces (PS) (solid lines). The portal lobules have their center in the portal space and are outlined by lines that connect the central veins (upper triangle). They comprise the portion of the liver from which bile flows to a portal space. Finally, the hepatic acinus comprises the region irrigated by one distributing vein (diamond-shaped figure). Zonation of the hepatic acinus is indicated by Roman numerals I, II, and III. (Redrawn and reproduced, with permission, from Leeson TS, Leeson CR: *Histology,* 2nd ed. Saunders, 1970.)

the hepatocyte is particularly evident in pathologic specimens, where certain changes occur preferentially either in the central or in the peripheral cells of the lobule.

The description just given of the liver lobule with its blood supply corresponds to the classic concept of this subject in which the centrolobular vein constitutes the axis of the lobule. (See the hexagons limited by portal spaces [PS] with the central vein [CV] in the center in Fig 17– 19.)

Other points of reference may be used in analyzing possible functional units of the liver's structure. Thus, another unit can be visualized, the **portal lobule,** which has at its center the portal triad and at its periphery the regions of adjoining hepatic lobules, all of which drain bile into the bile duct of the central portal triad. A portal lobule would be triangular, as opposed to the polygonal appearance of the classic liver lobule; it would have a central vein at the tip of

each of its angles; and it would contain parts of 3 adjoining liver lobules. (See the dashed triangle in Fig 17– 19 with the portal space [PS] at its center.)

Another way of subdividing the liver into functional lobules is to regard as a unit of liver parenchyma that region which is irrigated by a terminal branch of the distributing veins. This unit is called the **hepatic acinus** (of Rappaport). These appear diamond-shaped in section (see area CV, PS, CV, PS in Fig 17– 19). In addition to the terminal branches of the portal vein, an arterial branch and a bile ductule are in the center of this subdivision of hepatic parenchyma, which is situated in adjacent areas of 2 different classic hepatic lobules (Fig 17– 19).

In relation to their proximity to the distributing veins, cells in the hepatic acinus can be subdivided into zones (Fig 17– 19). Cells in zone I would be those closest to the vessel and consequently the first to be affected by or to alter the incoming blood. Cells in zone II would be second to respond to the blood, while those in zone III would see portal vein blood that had been previously altered by cells in both zones I and II. For example, after feeding, cells in zone I would be the first to receive incoming glucose and subsequently store it as glycogen. Any glucose passing the cells in zone I would likely be picked up by cells in zone II. In the event of fasting, cells in zone I would be the first to respond to glucose-poor blood by breaking down glycogen and releasing it as glucose. In this event, the cells in zones II and III would not respond to the fasting condition until glycogen was depleted from zone I cells. This zonal arrangement would account for some of the differences in the selective damage of hepatocytes by various noxious agents or in different disease conditions.

The Hepatocyte

Liver cells are polyhedral, with 6 or more surfaces, and have a diameter of approximately 20– 30 μm. In sections stained with hematoxylin and eosin, the cytoplasm of the hepatocyte is eosinophilic, mainly because of the presence of large numbers of mitochondria and to some extent smooth endoplasmic reticulum. Hepatocytes located at different distances from the portal triads show variations in structural, histochemical, and biochemical characteristics. The surface of each liver cell is in contact with the wall of the sinusoids, through the space of Disse, and with the surfaces of other hepatocytes. Wherever 2 hepatocytes abut, they delimit a tubular space between them known as the **bile canaliculus** (Figs 17–17C, 17–18, 17–20, and 17–21).

These canaliculi are the first portions of the bile duct system. They are tubular spaces, 1– 2 μm in diameter, limited by only the plasma membranes of 2 hepatocytes and have a small number of microvilli in their interior (Figs 17– 18, 17– 20, and 17– 21). The cell membranes near these canaliculi are firmly joined by occluding junctions as described in Chapter 4. Gap junctions are frequent between hepatocytes and are sites of intercellular communication, an im-

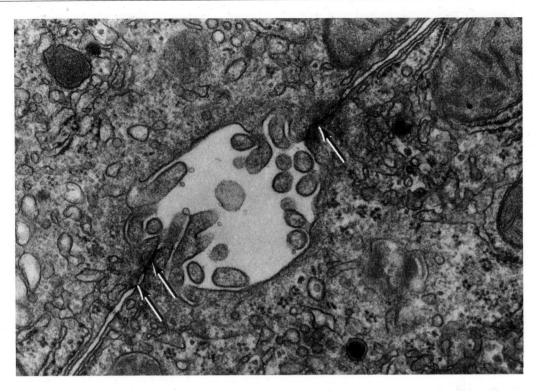

Figure 17–20. Electron micrograph of a rat liver bile canaliculus showing the microvilli in its lumen and the junctional complexes (arrows) that seal off this space from the remaining extracellular space. × 54,000. (Courtesy of SL Wissig.)

portant process for the coordination of the physiologic activities of these cells. The bile canaliculi form a complex anastomosing network progressing along the plates of the liver lobule and terminating in the region of the portal canals (Fig 17–15). The bile flow therefore progresses in a direction opposite to that of the blood, ie, from the center of the classic lobule to its periphery. At the periphery, bile enters the **bile ductules,** or **Hering's canals** (Fig 17–22). These are composed of cuboidal cells with a clear cytoplasm and few organelles. After a short distance, these bile ductules cross the limiting hepatocytes of the lobule and end in the **bile ducts** in the portal triads (Figs 17–15 and 17–16). Bile ducts are lined by a cuboidal or columnar epithelium and have a distinct connective tissue sheath. They gradually enlarge and fuse, forming the right and left **hepatic ducts** that subsequently leave the liver.

The surface of the hepatocyte which faces the space of Disse bears many microvilli protruding in that space but always leaving a space between them and the cells of the sinusoidal wall (Figs 17–18 and 17–21). The liver cell has one or 2 rounded nuclei with one or 2 typical nucleoli. Some of the nuclei are polyploid; ie, they contain some even multiples of the haploid number of chromosomes. Polyploid nuclei are characterized by their greater size, which is proportionate to their ploidy. The hepatocyte has an abundant endoplasmic reticulum in both its smooth and rough

varieties (Figs 17–17B and 17–18). In the hepatocyte, the rough endoplasmic reticulum forms aggregates dispersed in the cytoplasm, called **basophilic bodies** by classic microscopists. Several proteins— eg, blood albumin and fibrinogen—are synthesized on ribosomes in these structures. Various important processes occur in the smooth endoplasmic reticulum that is distributed diffusely throughout the cytoplasm. This organelle is responsible for the process of conjugation in which various substances are bound to sulfate or glucuronide during their inactivation or detoxification before excretion from the body. The smooth endoplasmic reticulum of the hepatocyte is a labile system that reacts promptly to changes in the environment. Administration of certain drugs, such as barbiturates, to laboratory animals causes a rapid increase in the smooth endoplasmic reticulum of the liver cell, with a parallel increase in the activity of enzymes responsible for conjugation of these drugs. This reaction of the smooth endoplasmic reticulum has led to the use of barbiturates, such as phenobarbital, in the treatment of **neonatal hyperbilirubinemia.** This state is due to the underdeveloped smooth endoplasmic reticulum in livers of infants and the consequent lower levels of glucuronyltransferase, an enzyme necessary for the conjugation of bilirubin and glucuronic acid. This conjugation product is more water-soluble and thus more easily excreted by the kidneys. If bile pigments, such as bilirubin, reach high

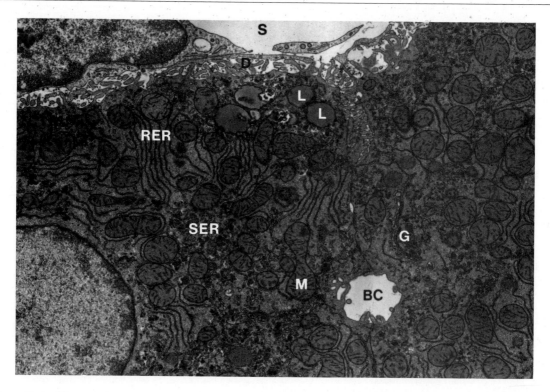

Figure 17–21. Electron micrograph of the liver of a rat. Note the 2 adjacent hepatocytes with a bile canaliculus (BC) between them. The hepatocytes contain numerous mitochondria (M) and smooth (SER) and rough (RER) endoplasmic reticulum. A prominent Golgi complex (G) is near the bile canaliculus. The sinusoid (S) is lined by endothelial cells with large open fenestrae. The space of Disse (D) is occupied by numerous microvilli projecting from the hepatocytes. L, lipid droplet. × 9200. (Courtesy of D Schmucker.)

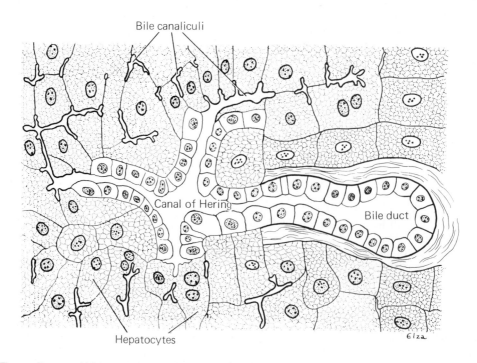

Figure 17–22. The confluence of bile canaliculi with Hering's canals, which are lined by cuboidal epithelium. Hering's canals merge with bile ducts in the portal spaces.

levels in infants, damage to the basal ganglia of the brain can occur. At present, the preferred treatment for neonatal hyperbilirubinemia is phototherapy, wherein the infant is exposed to blue light from ordinary fluorescent tubes. Unconjugated bilirubin is converted to water-soluble photoisomers that can be excreted by the kidneys without prior conjugation.

Another typical component of the liver cell is glycogen. This polysaccharide appears in the electron microscope as coarse, electron-dense granules that frequently collect within accumulations of smooth endoplasmic reticulum (Figs 3–21, 17–18, and 17–23). The amount of glycogen present in the liver conforms to a diurnal rhythm and depends also upon the nutritional state of the animal. Liver glycogen is a depot of glucose and is mobilized if the blood glucose level falls below normal. In this way, hepatocytes maintain a steady level of blood glucose, the main metabolite used by the body.

Each liver cell has many mitochondria (approxi-

mately 2000) with a spherical or ovoid form. Their cristae are not so numerous or closely packed as mitochondria of the muscle cell, a characteristic consistent with the moderate oxygen consumption observed in the liver. Similar to what occurs in most cellular components, the proteins of the liver mitochondria are constantly being renewed. The average life span of the structural proteins of this organelle is calculated to be about 10 days. Another common cellular component is the lipid droplet, whose quantity varies greatly (Fig 17–21). Hepatocyte lysosomes are important in the turnover and degradation of intracellular organelles. They also play a fundamental role in the process of receptor-mediated endocytosis of many macromolecular ligands. These macromolecules are first transported to endosomes that later fuse with lysosomes. In these secondary lysosomes, catabolism of asialoglycoproteins, lipoproteins, etc, occurs. Peroxisomes are abundant in hepatocytes, although their exact function in this cell is still a subject

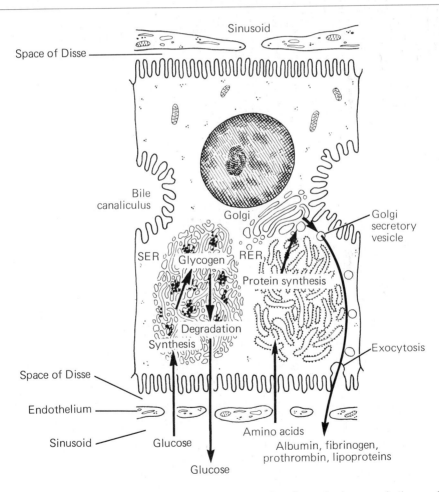

Figure 17–23. Protein synthesis and carbohydrate storage in the liver. Protein synthesis occurs in the rough endoplasmic reticulum, which explains why liver cell lesions lead to a decrease in the amounts of albumin, fibrinogen, and prothrombin in a patient's blood. In several diseases, glycogen degradation is depressed with abnormal intracellular accumulation of this compound. SER, smooth endoplasmic reticulum; RER, rough endoplasmic reticulum.

of speculation. Administration of the pancreatic hormone glucagon promotes the appearance of many autophagosomes in the liver cell. They might be related to turnover of hepatocyte organelles. Golgi complexes in the liver are numerous—up to 50 per cell. Each complex consists of flattened cisternae, small vesicles, and larger vacuoles lying near the bile canaliculi. The functions of this organelle include formation of lysosomes and secretion of plasma proteins (eg, albumin), glycoproteins (eg, transferrin), and lipoproteins (eg, very low density lipoproteins [VLDL]).

HISTOPHYSIOLOGY & LIVER FUNCTION

The liver cell probably is the most versatile cell in the body. It is at the same time a cell with endocrine and exocrine functions, and it synthesizes and accumulates certain substances, detoxifies others, and transports still others. We shall now examine the main activities of this cell.

Protein Synthesis

Besides synthesizing the proteins for its own maintenance, the liver cell produces various plasma proteins for export—among them albumin, prothrombin, fibrinogen, and lipoproteins. These proteins are synthesized on ribosomes attached to the rough endoplasmic reticulum. Contrary to what is observed in other glandular cells, the hepatocyte does not store proteins in its cytoplasm as secretory granules but continuously releases proteins into the bloodstream. Thus, it functions as an endocrine gland during this activity (Fig 17–23).

Radioautographic studies using the electron microscope show that protein is synthesized in the rough endoplasmic reticulum of the hepatocyte. The protein migrates to the Golgi complex and is subsequently extruded into the blood. About 5% of the protein exported by the liver is produced by the cells of the macrophage system (Kupffer cells); the remainder is synthesized in the hepatocytes.

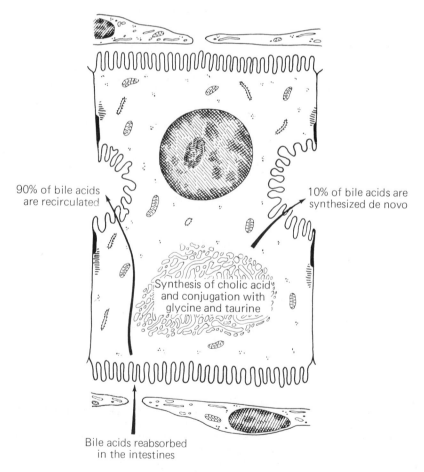

90% of bile acids are recirculated

10% of bile acids are synthesized de novo

Synthesis of cholic acid and conjugation with glycine and taurine

Bile acids reabsorbed in the intestines

Figure 17–24. Mechanism of secretion of bile acids. About 90% of these compounds derive from bile acids reabsorbed in the intestinal epithelium and recirculated to the liver. The remainder are synthesized in the liver by conjugating cholic acid with the amino acids glycine and taurine. This process occurs in the smooth endoplasmic reticulum.

Bile Secretion

Bile production is an exocrine secretion in the sense that the hepatocytes transform and transport blood components into the bile canaliculi. Besides water and electrolytes, bile has several other essential components: bile acids, phospholipids, cholesterol, and bilirubin. The secretion of bile acids is illustrated in Fig 17–24. About 90% of these substances are derived by reabsorption from the distal intestinal epithelium, being transported as such by the hepatocyte from the blood to bile canaliculi (enterohepatic recirculation). About 10% of these compounds are synthesized in the smooth endoplasmic reticulum of the hepatocyte by conjugation of cholic acid with the amino acid glycine or taurine. Thus, glycocholic and taurocholic acids are produced. Cholic acid is also synthesized by the liver from cholesterol. Bile acids have an important function in emulsifying the lipids in the digestive tract, promoting easier digestion by lipase and subsequent absorption. Bile acids, along with biliary phospholipids, serve to solubilize cholesterol and facilitate its excretion from the body. Abnormal proportions of these constituents may lead to the formation of gallstones (cholelithiasis). Gallstones can block bile flow and cause jaundice—bile pigments in blood—owing to rupture of tight junctions around bile canaliculi.

Bilirubin, most of which results from breakdown of hemoglobin, is formed in the mononuclear phagocyte system (this includes the Kupffer cells of the liver

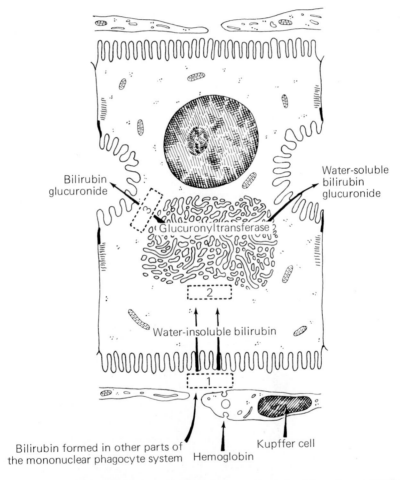

Figure 17–25. The secretion of bilirubin. This water-insoluble compound is derived from the metabolism of hemoglobin in macrophages of the mononuclear phagocyte system, including the Kupffer cells of the liver sinusoids. In hepatocytes, by means of glucuronyltransferase activity, bilirubin is conjugated in the smooth endoplasmic reticulum with glucuronide, forming a water-soluble compound. When bile secretion is blocked by one of several possible mechanisms, the yellow bilirubin glucuronide accumulates in the blood and jaundice results. Several mechanisms can produce jaundice: (1) a defect in the capacity of the cell to trap and absorb bilirubin (rectangle 1); (2) inability of the cell to conjugate bilirubin because of deficiency in the enzyme glucuronyltransferase (rectangle 2); or (3) problems in the transfer and excretion of bilirubin into the biliary canaliculi (rectangle 3). One of the most frequent causes of jaundice, however, is obstruction of bile flow, which often results from gallstones or tumors of the pancreas.

sinusoids) and is transported to hepatocytes. In the smooth endoplasmic reticulum of the hepatocyte, hydrophobic (water-insoluble) bilirubin is conjugated to glucuronic acid, forming a water-soluble **bilirubin glucuronide** (Fig 17–25). In a further step, bilirubin glucuronide is secreted into the bile canaliculi.

The hepatocyte also has the ability to actively transport several dyes. This ability to eliminate dyes is used as a test of liver function. One of the dyes most often used for this purpose is sulfobromophthalein (Bromsulphalein, BSP).

Storage of Metabolites

Lipids and carbohydrates are stored in the liver in the form of triglycerides and glycogen (Figs 17–21 and 17–23). This capacity to store energetic metabolites is important because it supplies the body with energy between meals. Figure 17–23 shows how this is done for the carbohydrates. The liver also serves as the major storage compartment for vitamins, especially vitamin A.

Metabolic Functions

The hepatocyte is responsible for converting lipids and amino acids into glucose by means of a complex enzymatic process called **gluconeogenesis.** It is also the main site of amino acid deamination, resulting in the production of urea. This compound is transported in the blood to the kidney and excreted by that organ.

Detoxification & Inactivation

Various drugs and substances can be inactivated by oxidation, methylation, or conjugation. The enzymes participating in these processes are located mainly in the smooth endoplasmic reticulum. Glucuronyltransferase, an enzyme that conjugates glucuronic acid to bilirubin, also causes conjugation of several other compounds such as steroids, barbiturates, antihistamines, and anticonvulsants.

Liver Regeneration

Despite being an organ whose cells are renewed at a slow rate, the liver has an extraordinary capacity for regeneration. The loss of hepatic tissue due to the action of toxic substances or surgical removal triggers a mechanism by which liver cells begin to divide, and this continues until restoration of the original mass of tissue is achieved. In rats, the liver can regenerate a loss of 75% of its weight in 1 month. In humans, this capacity is considerably restricted. The process of regeneration is probably controlled by circulating substances called **chalones,** which inhibit the mitotic division of a certain cell type. When a tissue is injured or partially removed, the amount of chalones it produces decreases; consequently, a burst of mitotic activity occurs in this tissue. As regeneration proceeds, the amount of chalones produced is increased and mitotic activity decreases. This is a self-regulating process.

The regenerated liver tissue is usually similar to the removed tissue. However, in the case of continuous or repeated damage to this organ, an abundant production of connective tissue occurs simultaneously with liver cell regeneration. This excess of connective tissue results in disorganization of liver structure, a condition known as **cirrhosis.** Liver function is impaired in this condition, since scar tissue (collagen) replaces functional hepatocytes.

THE BILIARY TRACT

The bile produced by the liver cell flows through the **bile canaliculi, bile ductules,** and **bile ducts.**

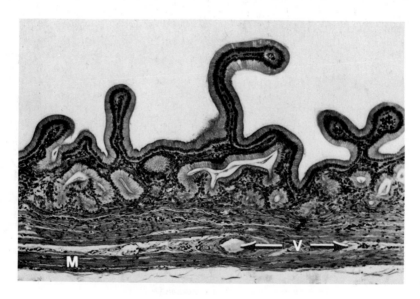

Figure 17–26. Photomicrograph of a section of gallbladder. Observe the lining columnar epithelium, the smooth muscle layer (M), and the blood vessels (V). H&E stain, × 30.

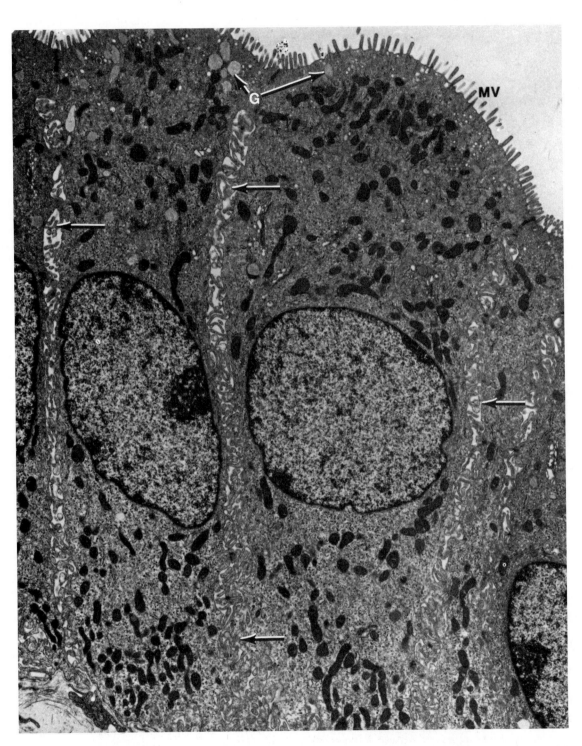

Figure 17–27. Electron micrograph of the gallbladder of the guinea pig. Observe the microvilli (MV) on the surface of the cell and the secretory granules (G) containing glycosaminoglycans. Arrows indicate the intercellular spaces. These cells transport sodium chloride from the lumen to the subjacent connective tissue. Water follows passively, and bile is thereby concentrated. These cells also secrete mucus into the bile. × 5600.

These structures gradually merge, forming a network that converges to form the **hepatic duct.** The hepatic duct, after receiving the **cystic duct** from the gallbladder, continues to the duodenum as the **common bile duct** (or **ductus choledochus**).

The hepatic, cystic, and common bile ducts are lined by a mucous membrane that consists of simple columnar epithelium. The lamina propria is thin and surrounded by an inconspicuous layer of smooth muscle. This muscle layer becomes thicker near the duodenum and finally forms, in the intramural portion, a sphincter that regulates bile flow (sphincter of Oddi).

THE GALLBLADDER

The gallbladder is a hollow, pear-shaped organ attached to the lower surface of the liver. It can store 30–50 mL of bile. It communicates with the hepatic duct through the cystic duct. The wall of the gallbladder consists of the following layers (Fig 17–26): (1) a mucosa composed of simple columnar epithelium and lamina propria, (2) a layer of smooth muscle, (3) a well-developed perimuscular connective tissue layer, and (4) a serous membrane.

The mucosa has abundant folds that are particularly evident in the empty bladder. The epithelial cells are rich in mitochondria and have their nuclei in their basal third (Fig 17–27). All these cells are capable of secreting small amounts of mucus. Microvilli are frequent at the apical surface. Near the cystic duct, the epithelium invaginates into the lamina propria, forming tubuloacinar glands with a wide lumen. Cells of these glands have characteristics of mucus-secreting cells and are responsible for production of most of the mucus present in bile.

The muscular layer is thin, with most of the smooth muscle cells oriented around the circumference of the gallbladder. A thick connective tissue layer binds the superior surface of the gallbladder to the liver. The opposite surface is covered by a typical serous layer, the peritoneum.

The main function of the gallbladder is to store bile and concentrate it by reabsorbing its water. This process depends upon an active sodium-transporting mechanism in its epithelium. Water reabsorption is an osmotic consequence of the sodium pump. Contraction of the smooth muscle of the gallbladder is induced by **cholecystokinin,** a hormone produced by enteroendocrine cells (I-cells) located in the epithelial lining of the small intestine. Release of cholecystokinin is, in turn, stimulated by the presence of dietary fats in the small intestine.

REFERENCES

Pancreas & Salivary Glands

Castle JD, Jamieson JD, Palade GE: Radioautographic analysis of the secretory process in the parotid acinar cell of the rabbit. *J Cell Biol* 1972;**53**:290.

Junqueira LCU: Control of cell secretion. In: *Secretory Mechanisms of Salivary Glands.* Schneyer LH, Schneyer CA (editors). Academic Press, 1967.

Junqueira LCU, de Moraes FF: Comparative aspects of the vertebrate major salivary glands' biology. In: *Functionelle und Morphologische Organization der Zelle: Sekretion und Exkretion.* Wohlfarth-Buttermann KE (editor). Springer, 1965.

Korsrud FR, Brandtzaeg P: Characterization of epithelial elements in human major salivary glands by functional markers: Localization of amylase, lactoferrin, lysozyme, secretory component, and secretory immunoglobulin by paired immunofluorescence staining. *J Histochem Cytochem* 1982; **30**:657.

Tomasi TB, Bienenstock J: Secretory immunoglobins. *Adv Immunol* 1968;**9**:11.

Young JA, Van Lennep EW: *The Morphology of Salivary Glands.* Academic Press, 1978.

Young JA et al: A microperfusion investigation of sodium resorption and potassium secretion by the main excretory duct of the rat submaxillary gland. *Pfluegers Arch* 1967;**295**:157.

Liver & Biliary Tract

Brown MS, Goldstein JL: How LDL receptors influence cholesterol and atherosclerosis. *Sci Am* (Nov) 1984;**251**:58.

Bruni C, Porter KR: The fine structure of the parenchymal cell of the normal rat liver. 1. General considerations. *Am J Pathol* 1965;**46**:691.

Diamond JM, Tormey JM: Studies on the structural basis of water transport across epithelial membranes. *Fed Proc* 1966;**25**:1458.

Elias H, Sherrick JC: *Morphology of the Liver.* Academic Press, 1969.

Howard JG: The origin and immunological significance of the Kupffer cells. In: *Mononuclear Phagocytes.* Van Furth R (editor). Blackwell, 1970.

Ito T, Shibasaki S: Electron microscopic study on the hepatic sinusoidal wall and the fat-storing cells in the human normal liver. *Arch Histol Jpn* 1968;**29**:137.

Jones AL, Fawcett DW: Hypertrophy of the agranular endoplasmic reticulum in hamster liver induced by phenobarbital. *J Histochem Cytochem* 1966;**14**:215.

Mueller JC, Jones AL, Long JA: Topographical and subcellular anatomy of the guinea pig gallbladder. *Gastroenterology* 1972;**63**:856.

Rouiller C (editor): *The Liver: Morphology, Biochemistry, Physiology.* 2 vols. Academic Press, 1963, 1964.

Wisse E, Knook DL (editors): *Kupffer Cells and Other Sinusoidal Cells.* Elsevier/North-Holland, 1977.

Respiratory System

18

The respiratory system includes the **lungs** and a system of tubes that link the sites of gas exchange with the external environment. In addition, a **ventilation mechanism,** consisting of the thoracic cage, intercostal muscles, diaphragm, and elastic tissues of the lung, is important in the movement of air through the conducting and respiratory parts of the lungs. It is customary to divide the lungs into 2 principal regions (Fig 18–1): a **conducting portion,** consisting of the nasal cavity, nasopharynx, larynx, trachea, bronchi, bronchioles, and terminal bronchioles; and a **respiratory portion,** consisting of respiratory bronchioles, alveolar ducts, and alveoli. **Alveoli** are specialized saclike structures that make up the greater part of the lungs. It is here that oxygen and carbon dioxide are exchanged between inspired air and blood—the principal function of the lungs.

The conducting portion serves 2 main functions: (1) to provide a conduit through which air can travel to and from the lungs, and (2) to condition the inspired air. To carry out these functions, each subdivision of the conducting portion exhibits several structural features in common with the others. In order to ensure an uninterrupted supply of air, a combination of cartilage, elastic fibers, and smooth muscle provide the conducting portion with a rigid structural support and a necessary flexibility and extensibility. The cartilages, primarily hyaline (with some elastic cartilage in the larynx), are found in the periphery of the lamina propria, and they have various forms ranging from small plaques to irregular rings and, in the trachea, C-shaped cartilages. The cartilages generally serve to support the walls of the conducting portion, preventing collapse of the lumen and thereby ensuring continuous access of air to the lungs. Both the conducting and respiratory portions are richly endowed with elastic fibers that provide these structures with flexibility and allow them to "spring back" after distention. In the conducting portion, the elastic fibers are found in the lamina propria and are mainly longitudinally oriented. Elastic fiber concentration is inversely proportionate to the diameter of the conducting tubule (ie, the smallest bronchioles have the highest proportion of elastic fibers). Bundles of smooth muscle are found encircling the tubes from the trachea to the alveolar ducts (a subdivision of the respiratory portion). Constriction of the smooth muscle serves to reduce the diameter of the conducting tubules and thereby regulates air flow during inspiration and expiration.

Conditioning of Air

A major function of the conducting portion is to "condition" the inspired air. Before it enters the lungs, inspired air is cleansed, moistened, and warmed. To carry out these functions, the mucosa of the conducting portions is lined by a specialized respiratory epithelium (described below), and there are numerous mucous and serous glands as well as a rich superficial vascular network in the lamina propria.

As the air enters the nose, large vibrissae (specialized hairs) serve to remove coarse particles of dust and other substances. Once the air reaches the nasal fossae, particulate and gaseous impurities are trapped in a layer of mucus. This mucus, in conjunction with serous secretions, also serves to moisten the incoming air, which protects the delicate alveolar lining from

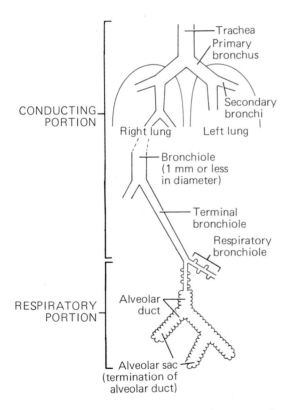

Figure 18–1. The main divisions of the respiratory tract. For instructional purposes, the natural proportions of these structures have been altered; thus, for example, the respiratory bronchiole is in reality a short transitional structure.

Table 18–1. Structural changes in the conducting portions of the respiratory tract.

	Nasal Fossae	Naso-pharynx	Larynx	Trachea	Bronchi		Bronchioles		
					Large	Small	Regular	Terminal	Respiratory
Epithelium	Pseudostratified columnar ciliated*†						⟶ Transition ⟶		
							Pseudo-stratified columnar ciliated →	Simple columnar ciliated →	Simple cuboidal ciliated
Goblet cells	Abundant				Present	Few	Scattered	None	
Glands	Abundant			Present		Few	None		
Cartilage			Complex (hyaline and elastic)	C-shaped rings	Irregular rings	Plates and islands	None		
Smooth muscle	None			Spanning open ends of C-shaped rings	Crisscrossing spiral bundles				
Elastic fibers	None	Present			Abundant				

*Stratified squamous in regions of direct air flow or abrasion.
†Vestibule of nose shows transition from keratinized stratified squamous to pseudostratified columnar ciliated epithelium.

desiccation. In addition, the incoming air is warmed by a rich superficial vascular network.

Respiratory Epithelium

Most of the conducting portion is lined by pseudostratified columnar ciliated epithelium containing a rich population of goblet cells. Deeper in the bronchial tree, this epithelial cell population is modified as the epithelium undergoes a transition to simple squamous epithelium. As the bronchi subdivide into the bronchioles, the pseudostratified organization gives way to a simple columnar epithelium, which is further reduced to a simple cuboidal layer in the smallest (terminal) bronchioles. The rich goblet cell population tapers off in the smaller bronchi and is totally absent from the epithelium in the terminal bronchioles. It is important to note that ciliated cells, which accompany the goblet cells, continue through the finer bronchioles in the absence of goblet cells. The continuation of the ciliated cells beyond the goblet cells serves to prevent mucus from accumulating in the respiratory portion of the system. The superficial mucus, which entraps particulate matter and absorbs water-soluble gases (eg, SO_2 and ozone), floats on a subjacent "sol" phase secreted by serous glands located in the lamina propria. Cilia of these epithelia move the more fluid "sol" phase, together with the overlying mucous layer, toward the oral cavity. Here, the mucous layer is either swallowed or expectorated. In addition to removing particulate and soluble pollutants, the mucous and serous layers also serve to saturate the inspired air with water vapor.

Typical respiratory epithelium consists of 6 cell types as seen in the electron microscope. **Ciliated columnar cells** constitute the most abundant type. Each cell possesses about 300 cilia on its apical surface (Figs 18–2, 18–3, and 18–4), while beneath the cilia, in addition to basal bodies, there are numerous small mitochondria. From experimental studies, it has been demonstrated that adenosine triphosphate (ATP) is required for ciliary beating, an observation that is consistent with the apical localization of mitochondria. Evidence has been presented that a disorder characterized by infertility in males and chronic respiratory tract infection—**Kartagener's syndrome**—is due to immobility of cilia and flagella induced by deficiency of a protein called **dynein,** normally present in the cilia. This protein is responsible for sliding of the microtubules, a process necessary for ciliary movement.

The next most abundant cells are the **mucous goblet cells** (Fig 18–4). The apical portion of these cells (described in Chapter 4) contains the polysaccharide-rich mucous droplets. The remaining columnar cells are known as "**brush cells**" (Figs 18–3 and 18–4) owing to the numerous microvilli present on their apical surface. Two types of brush cells are present. One has the cytologic characteristics of an immature cell and most likely represents replacements for dead or dying ciliated or goblet cells. The other brush cells have afferent nerve endings on their basal surfaces and are considered to be sensory receptors. **Basal (short) cells** are small rounded cells that lie on the basal lamina but do not extend to the luminal surface of the epithelium. These cells are believed to be the generative cells that undergo mitoses and subsequently differentiate into the other cell types. The remaining cell type is the **small granule cell,** which resembles a basal cell except that it possesses numerous granules 100–300 nm in diameter with dense cores. Histochemical studies reveal that these cells constitute a population of APUD cells (see Chapter 4). These endocrinelike granule cells may act as effectors in the integration of the mucous and serous secretory processes. All cells of the pseudostratified columnar ciliated epithelium touch the basal layer, and the epithelium is adherent to a prominent basal lamina (Fig 18–4, bottom).

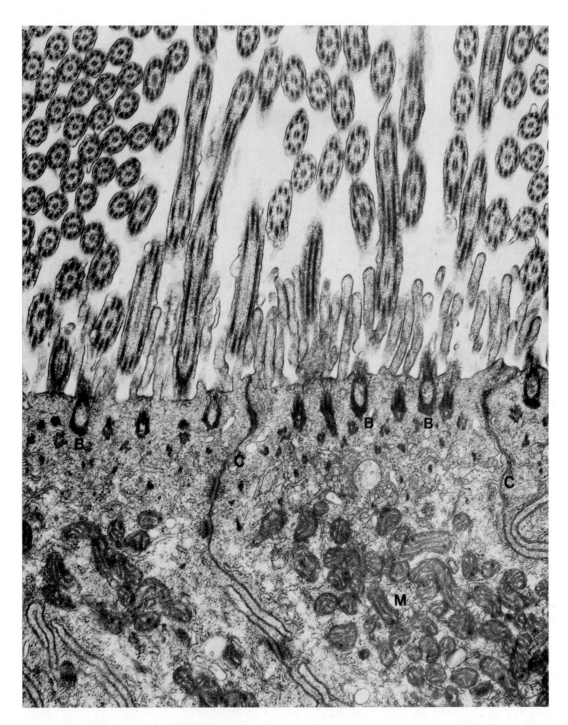

Figure 18–2. Electron micrograph of ciliated columnar epithelium. Observe the ciliary microtubules in transverse and oblique section. In the cell apex are the U-shaped basal bodies (B) that serve as the source and anchoring sites for the ciliary axonemes. At (M), the local accumulation of mitochondria is related to energy production for ciliary movement. At (C), observe junctional complexes. Note the emergence of microvilli between the ciliary roots. × 9200.

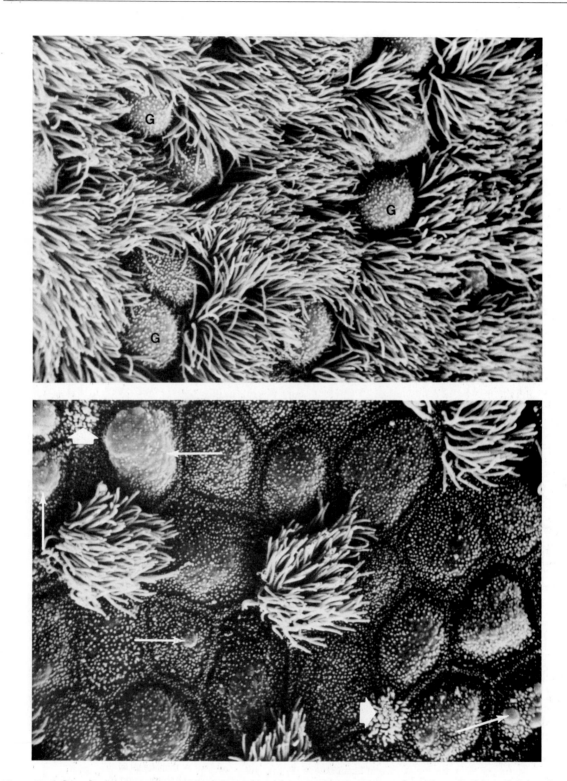

Figure 18–3. Scanning electron micrograph of the surface of rat respiratory mucosa. G, goblet cells. Most of the surface is covered by the cilia. In the lower micrograph, subsurface accumulations of mucus are evident in the goblet cells (thin arrows). Examples of brush cells are indicated by the thick arrows. Above, × 2500. Below, × 3000. (Reproduced, with permission, from Andrews P: A scanning electron microscopic study of the extrapulmonary respiratory tract. *Am J Anat* 1974;**139**:421.)

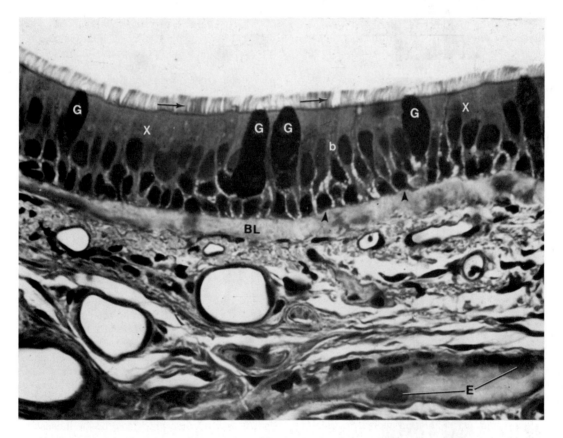

Figure 18–4. *Top:* Section of monkey trachea showing typical respiratory epithelium, thick basal lamina, richly vascularized connective tissue of the lamina propria, and the presence of glands containing both serous and mucous cells. Beneath the glands lies the dense connective tissue of the perichondrium, which surrounds the supporting hyaline cartilage (not visible). × 200. *Bottom:* Enlargement of the rectangular area shown above. The tracheal lumen is lined by typical pseudostratified columnar ciliated epithelium with goblet cells. This epithelium plays a significant role in conditioning the inspired air. Beneath the unusually thick basal lamina (BM) lies the lamina propria, whose rich vascularity aids in warming the incoming air. G, goblet cells containing mucous secretion; X, ciliated columnar cells; b, nonciliated brush cell; arrowheads, rounded basal cell; →, cilia; E, en face view of venule endothelial cells. × 500.

From the nasal cavity through the larynx, portions of the epithelium are stratified squamous. This type of epithelium is evident in regions exposed to direct air flow or physical abrasion (eg, oropharynx, epiglottis, vocal folds), since it provides more protection from attrition than typical respiratory epithelium. If air flow currents are altered or new abrasive sites develop, the affected areas can convert from typical pseudostratified columnar ciliated epithelium to stratified squamous epithelium. Similarly, in smokers, the proportion of ciliated cells to goblet cells is altered in order to aid in clearing the increased particulate and gaseous (eg, CO, SO_2) pollutants. Although the greater number of goblet cells in a smoker's epithelium provide for a more rapid clearance of pollutants, the reduction of ciliated cells due to excessive CO results in a decrease in the movement of the mucous layer and frequently leads to congestion of the smaller airways. These *reversible* changes in cellular organization are referred to as **metaplasia.**

NASAL CAVITY

The nasal cavity consists of 2 different structures: the external **vestibule** and the internal **nasal fossae;** the latter are separated by the nasal septum.

Vestibule

The vestibule is the most anterior and dilated portion of the nasal cavity. The outer integument of the nose enters the **nares** (nostrils) and continues part way up the vestibule. Around the inner surface of the nares are numerous sebaceous and sweat glands in addition to the thick short hairs or **vibrissae** that serve to filter out large particles from the inspired air. Within the vestibule, the epithelium loses its keratinized nature and then undergoes a transition into typical respiratory epithelium before entering the nasal fossae.

Nasal Fossae

Within the skull lie 2 cavernous chambers separated by the osseous **nasal septum.** Extending from each lateral wall are 3 bony shelflike projections known as **conchae.** Of the superior, middle, and inferior conchae, only the middle and inferior projections are covered by respiratory epithelium. The superior conchae are covered by a specialized olfactory epithelium. The structure and function of olfactory epithelium is discussed in Chapter 10. The narrow ribbonlike passages created by the conchae improve the conditioning of the inspired air (1) by increasing the surface area containing respiratory epithelium and (2) by creating turbulence in the air flow that results in increased contact between air streams and the mucous layer. Within the lamina propria of the conchae are large venous plexuses known as **swell bodies.** Every 20–30 minutes, the swell bodies on one side of the nasal fossae become engorged with blood, which results in distention of the conchal mucosa and a concomitant decrease in the flow of air. During this time, most of the air is directed through the other nasal fossa. These periodic intervals of occlusion reduce air flow, so that the respiratory epithelium can recover from desiccation. Allergic reactions can cause abnormal engorgement of swell bodies in both fossae and result in severely restricted air flow.

In addition to swell bodies, the nasal cavity has a rich and complexly organized vascular system. Large vessels form a close-meshed latticework next to the periosteum, from which arcading branches lead toward the surface. Smaller vessels branch from the arcading vessels and run perpendicular to the surface. These smaller vessels form a rich capillary bed beneath the epithelium. Blood flows forward from the rear to each fossa. In each arcading loop, the flow of blood counters the flow of inspired air. As a result, the incoming air is efficiently warmed by a countercurrent system.

PARANASAL SINUSES

The paranasal sinuses are cavities in the frontal, maxillary, ethmoid, and sphenoid bones that are lined with a thinner respiratory epithelium containing few goblet cells. The lamina propria contains only a few small glands and is continuous with the underlying periosteum. The mucus produced in these cavities drains into the nasal passages as a result of the activity of its ciliated epithelial cells.

NASOPHARYNX

The nasopharynx is the first part of the pharynx, continuing caudally with the oral portion of this organ, the **oropharynx.** It is lined with respiratory-type epithelium in the portion that is in contact with the soft palate.

LARYNX

The larynx is an irregular tube that connects the pharynx to the trachea. Within the lamina propria lie a number of laryngeal cartilages, structurally the most complex in the respiratory tree. The larger cartilages (thyroid, cricoid, and most of the arytenoids) are hyaline cartilage, and some are subject to calcification in old people. The smaller cartilages (epiglottis, cuneiform, corniculate, and the tips of the arytenoids) are elastic cartilage. Ligaments bind the cartilages together, and most are articulated by the intrinsic muscles of the larynx, which in themselves are unusual in that they are striated skeletal muscle. In addition to their supporting role (maintenance of an open airway), these cartilages serve as a valve to prevent swallowed food or fluid from entering the trachea. They also serve as a means of producing tone for phonation.

The **epiglottis,** which projects from the rim of the

larynx, extends into the pharynx and therefore has both a lingual and laryngeal surface. The entire lingual surface and the apical portion of the laryngeal side are covered by stratified squamous epithelium. Toward the base of the epiglottis on the laryngeal side, the epithelium undergoes a transition into pseudostratified columnar ciliated epithelium. Mixed mucous and serous glands, found beneath the epithelium, make deep excursions that create characteristic pockmarks in the underlying elastic cartilage.

Below the epiglottis, the mucosa forms 2 pairs of folds that extend into the lumen of the larynx. The upper pair constitute the **false vocal cords** (or vestibular folds), and they are covered by typical respiratory epithelium beneath which lie numerous serous glands within the lamina propria. The lower pair of folds constitute the **true vocal cords.** Within the vocal folds, which are covered by a stratified squamous epithelium, lie large bundles of parallel elastic fibers that compose the **vocal ligament.** Parallel to the ligaments are bundles of skeletal muscle, the **vocalis muscles,** which regulate the tension of the fold and its ligaments and consequently, as air is forced between the folds, provide for production of sounds of different frequencies.

TRACHEA

The trachea is a thin-walled tube, about 10 cm long, that extends from the base of the larynx (the cricoid cartilage) to the point at which it bifurcates

into the 2 primary bronchi. The trachea is lined with a typical respiratory mucosa (Figs 18–4 and 18–5). Sixteen to 20 C-shaped rings of hyaline cartilage, found in the lamina propria, serve to keep the tracheal lumen patent. The open ends of the C-shaped rings are located on the posterior surface of the trachea. A fibroelastic ligament and bundle of smooth muscle (trachealis muscle) bind to the perichondrium and bridge the open ends of these C-shaped cartilages. The ligament prevents overdistention of the lumen, while the muscle allows the lumen to close down. Contraction of the muscle and the concomitant narrowing of the tracheal lumen are used in the cough reflex. Following contraction, the resulting smaller bore of the trachea will provide for increased velocity of expired air, which aids in clearing the air passage.

BRONCHIAL TREE

The trachea divides into 2 **primary bronchi,** which enter the lungs at the hilum (Fig 18–7). In addition, at each hilum, arteries enter and veins and lymphatic vessels leave the lungs. These structures are surrounded by dense connective tissue and form a unit called the **pulmonary root.**

After entering the lungs, the primary bronchi course downward and outward, giving rise to 3 bronchi in the right lung and 2 in the left lung, each of which supplies a pulmonary lobe (Fig 18–1). These **lobar bronchi** divide repeatedly, giving rise to smaller bronchi, the terminal branches of which are called **bron-**

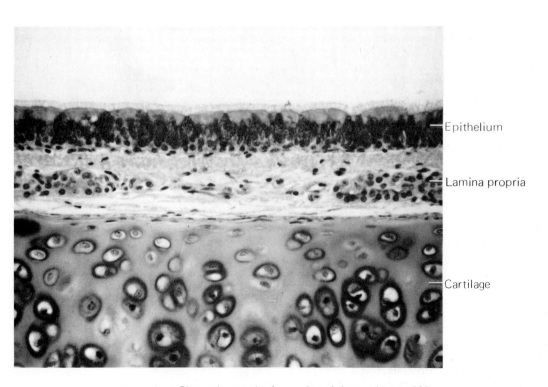

Figure 18–5. Photomicrograph of a section of dog trachea. × 200.

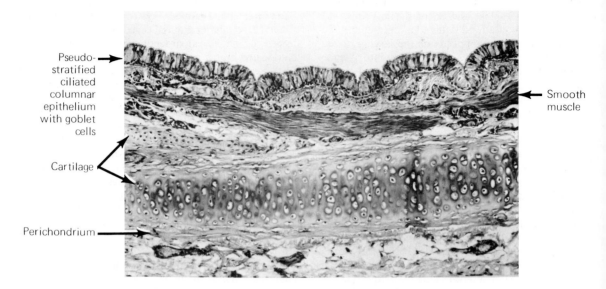

Pseudo-
stratified
ciliated
columnar
epithelium
with goblet
cells

Smooth
muscle

Cartilage

Perichondrium

Figure 18-6. Photomicrograph of a large bronchus. Observe the ciliated pseudostratified epithelium with many goblet cells, 2 cartilaginous plates, and smooth muscle. H&E stain, × 180.

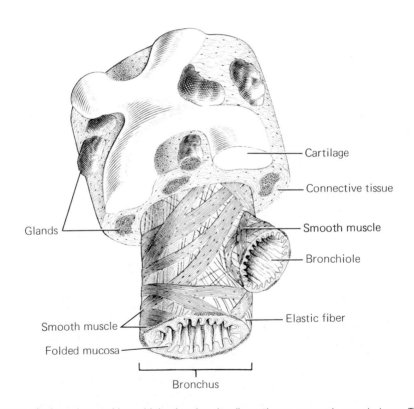

Cartilage

Connective tissue

Smooth muscle

Bronchiole

Glands

Elastic fiber

Smooth muscle

Folded mucosa

Bronchus

Figure 18-7. Diagram of a bronchus and bronchiole showing the discontinuous smooth muscle layer. The contraction of this muscle induces folding of the mucosa. Smooth muscle is present in all of the bronchiolar tree, up through the respiratory bronchiole. The elastic fibers present in the bronchus continue into the bronchiole. An irregular cartilaginous plate sectioned in 2 regions is shown in white. The adventitia is not represented in this drawing.

chioles. Each bronchiole enters a pulmonary lobule, where it branches to form 5 – 7 **terminal bronchioles.**

The pulmonary lobules are pyramid-shaped, with the apex directed toward the pulmonary hilum. Each lobule is delimited by a thin connective tissue septum, best seen in the fetus. In adults, these septa are frequently incomplete, resulting in a poor delineation of the lobules. Lobules nearest the **pleura** (the outer covering of the lungs) are frequently delineated as a result of the accumulation of carbon and dust particles deposited in the connective tissue of the interlobular septa.

The primary bronchi generally have the same histologic appearance as the trachea. As we proceed toward the respiratory portion, we can observe a simplification of the histologic organization of both the epithelium and underlying lamina propria. It must be stressed, however, that this simplification is gradual, and no abrupt transition can be observed between the bronchi and bronchioles. For this reason, the division of the bronchial tree into bronchi, bronchioles, etc, is to some extent artificial despite the fact that it has teaching and practical value.

Bronchi

Each primary bronchus branches dichotomously 9 – 12 times, each branch becoming progressively smaller until a diameter of about 5 mm is reached. With 2 exceptions, the mucosa of the bronchi is structurally similar to that in the trachea (Figs 18 – 6 and 18 – 7). Unlike those found in the trachea, the bronchial cartilages are more irregular in shape; in the larger portions of the bronchi, the cartilage rings completely encircle the lumen. As bronchial diameter decreases, the cartilage rings are replaced by isolated plates or islands of hyaline cartilage. Beneath the epithelium, in the bronchial lamina propria, one can observe the presence of a smooth muscle layer consisting of crisscrossing bundles of spirally arranged smooth muscle (Fig 18 – 7). Bundles of smooth muscle become a more prominent feature in the walls of the conducting portion as one approaches the respiratory zone. In histologic sections, this muscular layer may appear to be discontinuous. The contraction of this muscle after death is responsible for the folded appearance of the bronchial mucosa observed in histologic section. The lamina propria is rich in elastic fibers and contains an abundance of mucous and serous glands whose ducts open into the bronchial lumen. Numerous lymphocytes are found both within the lamina propria and among the epithelial cells. Lymphatic nodules are present and are particularly numerous at the branching points of the bronchial tree.

Bronchioles

Bronchioles are intralobular airways with diameters of 5 mm or less (Fig 18 – 7). Bronchioles have neither cartilage nor glands in their mucosa and have only scattered goblet cells within the epithelium of the initial segments. In the larger bronchioles, the epithelium is pseudostratified ciliated columnar, which decreases in height and complexity to become simple ciliated columnar or cuboidal epithelium in the smaller **terminal bronchioles.** The epithelium of terminal bronchioles also contains **Clara cells** (Fig 18 – 8) with dome-shaped apical surfaces that project into the lumen. This appearance may be a fixation artifact. In humans, Clara cells are about 10 μm tall $\times$ 5.5 μm wide. They do not have cilia at their apical surfaces, hence the alternative name of **nonciliated bronchiolar epithelial cells.** The nucleus is basally located and usually has a prominent indentation. The cytoplasm contains long cisternae of rough endoplasmic reticulum on all sides of the nucleus; smooth endoplasmic reticulum is sparse or absent. Elongated mitochondria are scattered throughout the cell, and the Golgi complex is found at the apical or lateral sides of the nucleus. Small accumulations of glycogen can be seen in the basal cytoplasm of some cells. A few membrane-bound granules (0.3 μm in diameter) are seen in the apical cytoplasm.

Clara cells appear to be secretory cells, and they take the place of goblet cells found in more proximal bronchioles. The composition of the Clara cell's secretion remains unknown. These cells have high concentrations of cytochrome P-450, which may signify a role in the inactivation of harmful substances in inspired air.

The lamina propria is largely composed of smooth muscle and elastic fibers. The musculature of both the bronchi and bronchioles is under the control of the vagus nerve and the sympathetic nervous system. Stimulation of the vagus nerve decreases the diameter of these structures, whereas sympathetic stimulation produces the opposite effect. This explains why epinephrine and other sympathomimetic drugs are frequently employed to relax smooth muscle during asthmatic attacks. When the thicknesses of the bronchial and bronchiolar walls are compared, it can be seen that the bronchiolar muscle layer is proportionately better developed than that of the bronchi. Increased airway resistance in asthma is believed to be due mainly to contraction of bronchiolar smooth muscle.

Respiratory Bronchioles

Each terminal bronchiole subdivides into 2 or more respiratory bronchioles that serve as regions of transition between the conducting and respiratory portions of the respiratory system (Figs 18 – 9 and 18 – 10). The respiratory bronchiolar mucosa is structurally identical to that of the terminal bronchioles except that their walls are interrupted by numerous saccular **alveoli** (Figs 18 – 1 and 18 – 9). Portions of the respiratory bronchioles are lined with ciliated cuboidal epithelial cells and Clara cells, but at the rim of the alveolar openings the bronchiolar epithelium becomes continuous with the squamous alveolar lining cells (type I epithelial cells). Proceeding distally along these bronchioles, the number of alveoli increases greatly, and the distance between them is markedly reduced. Between alveoli, the bronchiolar epithelium consists of ciliated cuboidal epithelium; however, in more distal

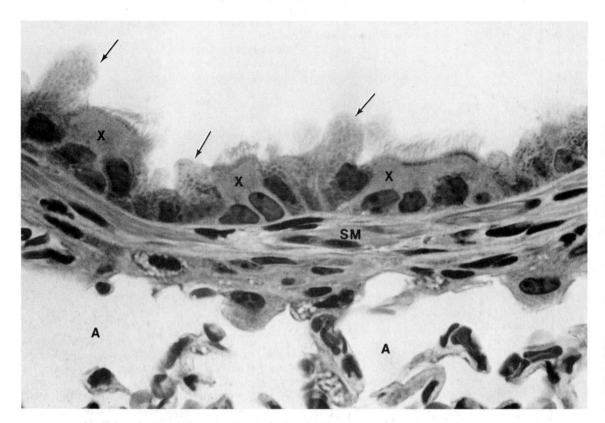

Figure 18–8. Portion of a terminal bronchiole in mouse lung. In addition to the ciliated cuboidal cells (X), there are larger secretory Clara cells (arrows). Bundles of smooth muscle (SM) cells lie beneath the epithelium. Surrounding the terminal bronchiole are alveoli (A). × 800.

Terminal bronchiole

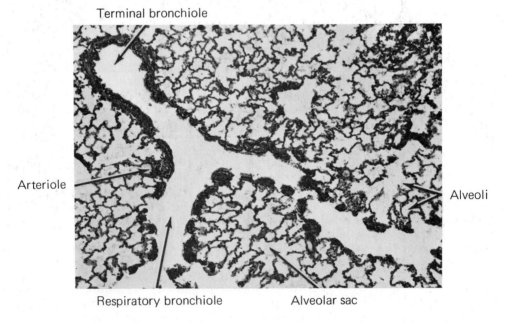

Arteriole

Alveoli

Respiratory bronchiole   Alveolar sac

Figure 18–9. Photomicrograph of a thick section of lung showing a terminal bronchiole dividing into 2 respiratory bronchioles in which alveoli appear. The spongelike appearance of the lung is due to the abundance of alveoli and alveolar sacs. H&E stain, × 80.

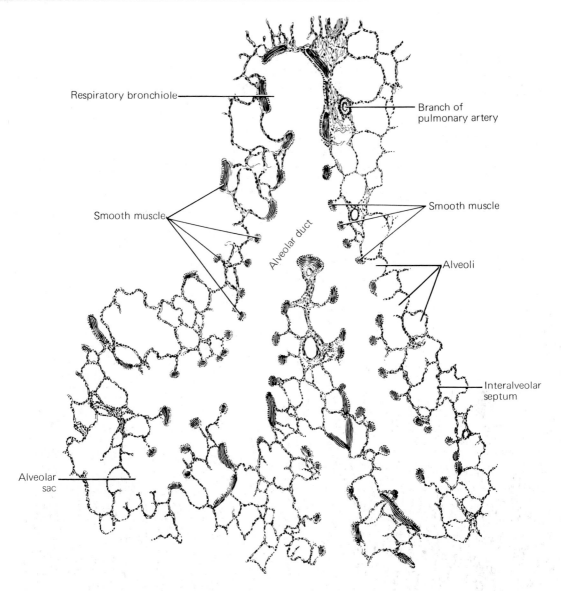

Figure 18–10. Diagram of a portion of the bronchial tree. Observe that smooth muscle present in the alveolar ducts disappears in the alveoli. (Redrawn from Baltisberger.)

portions, the cilia may be absent. Smooth muscle and elastic connective tissue lie beneath the epithelium of respiratory bronchioles. Since the alveoli are sites of gas exchange, the term "respiratory bronchiole" aptly describes the dual function of this segment of the respiratory tree.

Alveolar Ducts

Proceeding distally along the respiratory bronchioles, the number of alveolar openings into the bronchiolar wall becomes ever greater until the wall consists of nothing else, and the tube is now termed an alveolar duct (Fig 18–10). Both the alveolar ducts and alveoli are lined by extremely attenuated squamous epithelial cells. In the lamina propria surrounding the rim of the alveoli is a network of smooth muscle cells. These sphincterlike smooth muscle bundles appear as knobs between adjacent alveoli. Smooth muscle disappears at the distal ends of alveolar ducts. A rich matrix of elastic and collagen fibrils provides the only support for the duct and its alveoli.

Alveolar ducts open into **atria,** which communicate with **alveolar sacs.** Two or more alveolar sacs arise from each atrium. A heavy investment of elastic and reticular fibers forms a complex network encircling the openings of atria, alveolar sacs, and alveoli. The elastic fibers enable the alveoli to expand upon inspiration and to passively contract during expiration.

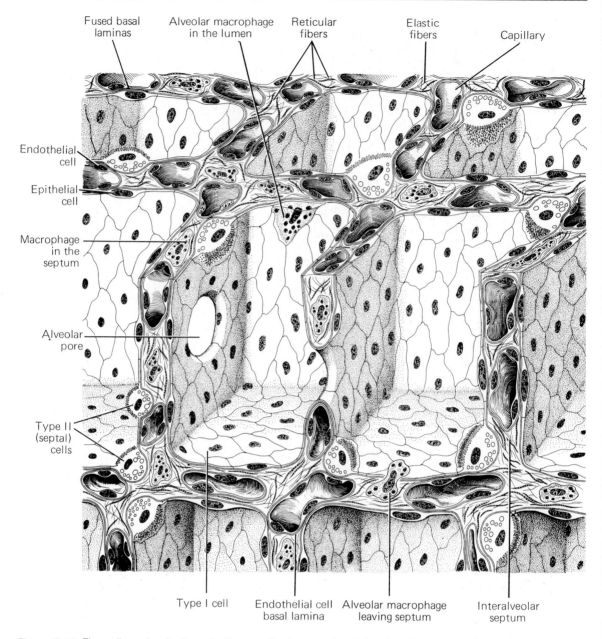

Figure 18-11. Three-dimensional schematic diagram of pulmonary alveoli showing the interalveolar septum and its structure. Observe the capillaries, connective tissue, and macrophages. These cells can also be seen in the alveolar lumens or passing into them. Alveolar pores are numerous. Type II cells are identified by their abundant apical microvilli. The alveoli are lined by a continuous epithelial layer.

The reticular fibers serve as a support that prevents overdistention and damage to the delicate capillaries and thin alveolar septa.

Alveoli

Alveoli are saclike evaginations, about 200 μm in diameter, of the respiratory bronchioles, alveolar ducts, and alveolar sacs. Alveoli are the terminal portions of the bronchial tree and are responsible for the spongy structure of the lungs. Structurally, alveoli resemble small pockets open on one side, similar to the honeycombs of a beehive. Within these cuplike structures, oxygen and CO_2 are exchanged between the air and the blood. The structure of the alveolar walls is specialized for enhancing diffusion between the external and internal environments. Generally, each wall lies between 2 neighboring alveoli and is thus termed an **interalveolar septum** or **wall.** An

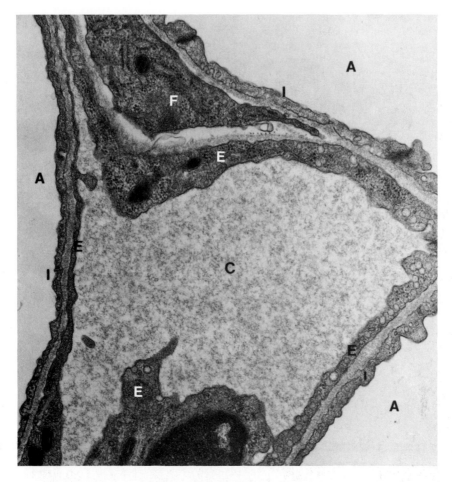

Figure 18–12. Electron micrograph of the alveolar wall. Note the capillary lumen (C), alveolar spaces (A), the alveolar type I epithelial cells (I), the capillary endothelial cells (E), and a fibroblast (F). × 30,000. (Courtesy of MC Williams.)

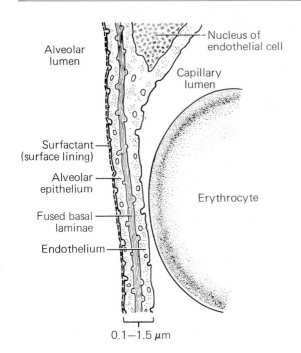

Alveolar lumen

Nucleus of endothelial cell

Capillary lumen

Surfactant (surface lining)

Alveolar epithelium

Erythrocyte

Fused basal laminae

Endothelium

0.1–1.5 μm

alveolar septum consists of 2 thin squamous epithelial layers between which lie capillaries, elastic and collagen fibers, and fibroblasts. The capillaries and connective tissue matrix constitute the **interstitium.** Within the interstitium of the alveolar septa is found the richest capillary network in the body (Fig 18–11).

Air in the alveoli is separated from capillary blood by 3 components referred to collectively as the **blood-air barrier:** (1) the cytoplasm of the epithelial cells; (2) the fused basal laminas of the closely apposed epithelial and endothelial cells; and (3) the cytoplasm of the endothelial cells (Figs 18–12 and 18–13). The

Figure 18–13 (at left). Portion of the alveolar septum showing the blood-air barrier. To reach the red cell, O_2 traverses the surface lining, the alveolar epithelial cytoplasm, the basal laminae, the endothelial cell cytoplasm, and the plasma. In some locations, there is loose interstitial tissue between the epithelium and the endothelium. (Approximate magnification × 20,000.) (Modified and reproduced, with permission, from Ganong WF: *Review of Medical Physiology,* 8th ed. Lange, 1977.)

total thickness of these layers varies from 0.1 to 1.5 μm. Within the interalveolar septa, anastomosing pulmonary capillaries are supported by a meshwork of reticular and elastic fibers. These fibers, which are arranged to permit expansion and contraction of alveolar walls, are the primary means of structural support of the alveoli. Within the interstitium of the septa, leukocytes, macrophages, and fibroblasts can also be found (Fig 18–11).

Oxygen of the alveolar air passes into the capillary blood through the above-mentioned layers (Fig 18–13); CO_2 diffuses in the opposite direction. Liberation of CO_2 from H_2CO_3 is catalyzed by the enzyme carbonic anhydrase present in red blood cells. It is not surprising, therefore, that the erythrocyte contains more of this enzyme than any other cell in the body. The lungs contain approximately 300 million alveoli, thus increasing considerably their internal exchange surface, which has been calculated to be approximately 140 m². The number of alveoli and therefore the total area are known to vary directly with height.

The interalveolar septum is composed of 5 main cell types: capillary endothelial cells (30%); type I (squamous) epithelial cells (8%); type II (septal, great

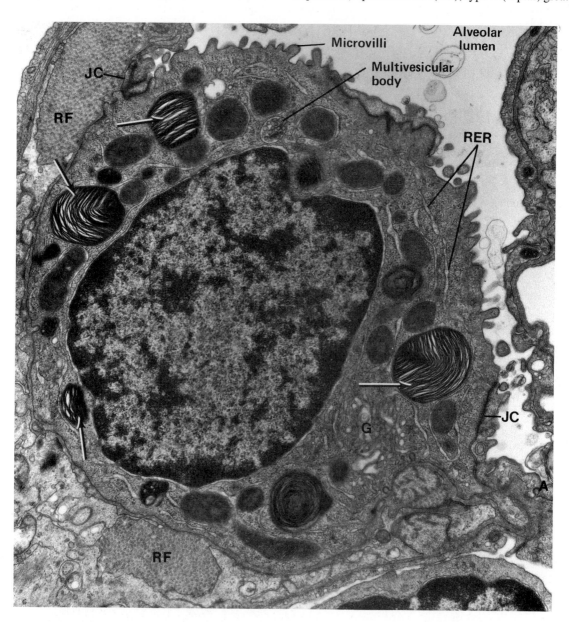

Figure 18–14. Type II cell from rat lung protruding into the alveolar lumen. Arrows point to lamellar bodies containing newly synthesized pulmonary surfactant. RER, rough endoplasmic reticulum; G, Golgi complex. At A, the cytoplasm of a type I epithelial cell is seen. Note the microvilli of the type II cell and the junctional complexes (JC) with the type I epithelial cell. RF, reticular fibers. × 17,000. (Courtesy of MC Williams.)

alveolar) cells (16%); interstitial cells including fibroblasts and mast cells (36%); and alveolar macrophages (10%) (Figs 18–12 and 18–14).

Endothelial cells of the capillaries are extremely thin and have a smaller, more elongated nucleus than the type I epithelial cells with which they are frequently confused. The endothelial lining of the capillaries is continuous and not fenestrated (Fig 18–12). The nuclei and other organelles are clustered to allow the remaining areas of the cell to become extremely thin in order to increase the efficiency of gas exchange. The most prominent feature of the cytoplasm in the flattened portions of the cell are numerous pinocytotic vesicles.

Type I cells, also called squamous alveolar cells, are extremely attenuated cells that line the alveolar surfaces. Type I cells make up 97% of the alveolar surface, while type II cells make up the remaining 3%. These cells are so thin, sometimes only 25 nm in thickness, that electron microscopic analysis was needed to prove that all capillaries are covered by an epithelial lining (Figs 18–9 and 18–12). To reduce the thickness of the blood-air barrier, organelles such as the Golgi complex, endoplasmic reticulum, and mitochondria are grouped around the nucleus, leaving large areas of cytoplasm virtually free of organelles. The cytoplasm in the thin portion contains abundant pinocytotic vesicles, which may play a role in the turnover of surfactant (described below) and the removal of small particulate contaminants from the outer surface. In addition to desmosomes, all type I epithelial cells have occluding junctions that serve to prevent the leakage of tissue fluid into the alveolar air space (Fig 18–15). The main role of this cell is to provide a barrier of minimal thickness that is readily permeable to gases.

Type II cells, or **great alveolar cells** (also called **septal cells**), are found interspersed among the type I epithelial cells with which they have occluding and desmosomal junctions (Figs 18–11 and 18–14). Type II cells are roughly cuboidal cells that are usually found in groups of 2 or 3 along the alveolar surface at points where the alveolar walls unite and form angles. These cells, which rest on the basal lamina, are part of the epithelium, for they have the same origin as the squamous epithelial cells that line the alveolar walls. Cytologically, these cells resemble typical secretory cells. They have mitochondria, rough endoplasmic reticulum, a well-developed Golgi complex, and microvilli on their free apical surface. In histologic sections, they exhibit a characteristic vesicular or foamy cytoplasm. The vacuoles are due to the presence of **lamellar bodies** (Fig 18–14) that are preserved and evident in tissue prepared for electron microscopy. The lamellar bodies, which average about 0.2 μm in diameter, contain concentric or parallel lamellae limited by a unit membrane. Histochemical studies reveal that these bodies, which contain phospholipids, glycosaminoglycans, and proteins, are continuously synthesized and released at the apical surface of the cell. The lamellar bodies give rise to a material that spreads over the alveolar surfaces, providing an

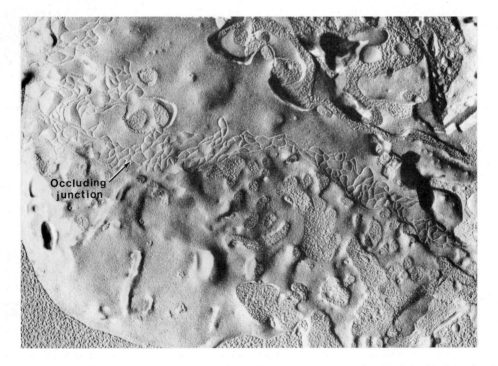

Figure 18–15. Cryofracture preparation showing an occluding junction between 2 type I epithelial cells of the alveolar lining. × 25,000. (Reproduced, with permission, from Schneeberger EE: *Lung Liquids.* Ciba Foundation Symposium No. 38. Elsevier/North-Holland, 1976.)

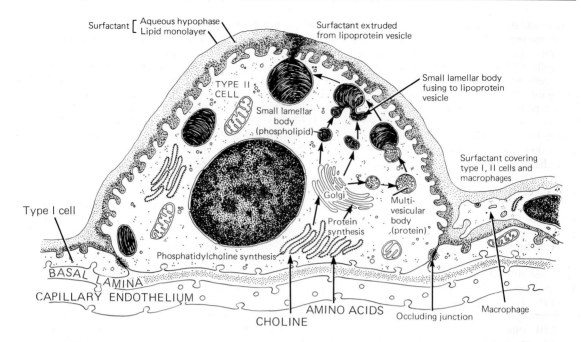

Figure 18–16. The physiology of surfactant secretion by the type II cell. The surfactant consists of an overlying monomolecular film of lipid and an underlying aqueous hypophase. When present in the alveolar lumen, macrophages lie outside the epithelium but within the surfactant layer. Occluding junctions around the margins of the epithelial cells prevent leakage of tissue fluid into the alveolar lumen.

extracellular coating, **pulmonary surfactant,** that lowers alveolar surface tension. The secretion of pulmonary surfactant by type II cells has been elucidated with the aid of electron microscopy and radioautography and is summarized in Fig 18–16.

The surfactant layer consists of an aqueous, protein-containing hypophase covered by a monomolecular phospholipid film, primarily composed of **dipalmitoyl lecithin.** Pulmonary surfactant serves several major functions in the economy of the lung. Primarily, it aids in reducing the surface tension of the alveolar cells. Without surfactant, alveoli would tend to collapse during expiration. Reduction of surface tension means that less inspiratory force is needed to inflate the alveoli, thus reducing the work of breathing. In fetal development, surfactant appears in the last weeks of gestation and coincides with the appearance of lamellar bodies in the type II cells. In cases of premature birth, infants frequently exhibit labored breathing that results in respiratory distress. **Hyaline membrane disease** in newborns has been shown to be the result of insufficient surfactant production, so that the infant has difficulty in expanding the alveoli. Fortunately, surfactant synthesis can be induced by administration of glucocorticoids, so that the respiratory distress syndrome usually represents a short-term management problem. Recently, surfactant has also been suggested to have a bactericidal effect, aiding in the removal of potentially dangerous bacteria that reach the alveoli.

The surfactant layer is not static but is constantly being turned over. The lipoproteins are gradually removed from the surface by the pinocytotic vesicles of the squamous epithelial cells, by macrophages, and by type II epithelial cells. These substances therefore undergo a continuous cycle of secretion and reabsorption.

Alveolar lining fluids are also removed via the conducting passages as a result of ciliary activity. As the secretions pass up through the airways, they combine with bronchial mucus, forming a **bronchoalveolar fluid.** This fluid aids in the removal of particulate and noxious components from the inspired air. Within the fluids are several lytic enzymes (eg, lysozyme, collagenase, and β-glucuronidase) that are probably derived from the alveolar macrophages.

Alveolar Macrophages

The thinnest barrier between blood plasma and inspired air is reduced to an alveolar epithelium, a fused basal lamina, and the capillary endothelium. Although seemingly susceptible to bacterial and viral infection, chronic inflammation does not exist, since a barrier to infection is provided by the alveolar macrophage (Fig 18–11). These macrophages, also called **dust cells,** are derived from monocytes that originate in bone marrow. They are found in the interior of the alveolar septum and are often seen on the surface of the alveolus. Recent evidence suggests that macrophages do not recross the alveolar wall. Numerous carbon- and dust-laden macrophages in the connective tissue around major blood vessels or in the pleura probably represent cells that have never passed through the epithelial lining. The phagocytized debris within these cells was most likely passed from the alveolar lumen into the interstitium by the pinocytotic activity of the type I epithelial cells. The alveolar macrophages that scavenge the outer surface of the epithelium, within the surfactant layer, are carried to the pharynx where they are swallowed.

In heart failure, the lungs become congested with blood and red blood cells pass into alveoli, where they are phagocytized by alveolar macrophages. In such cases, these macrophages are called **heart failure cells** and are identified by a positive histochemical reaction for iron pigment (hemosiderin).

In addition to the cells discussed above, the alveolar septum also contains fibroblasts, mast cells, and a recently identified contractile cell. Interstitial fibroblasts synthesize collagen, elastic fibers, and glycosaminoglycans. Collagen constitutes 15–20% of the parenchymal mass and consists primarily of types I and III collagen. Type III fibers correspond to the alveolar reticular fibers (Fig 18–11), whereas type I collagen is concentrated in the walls of the conducting passages and in the pleura. Lung collagen proliferation is common, and more than 100 disease entities are known to be associated with lung fibrosis.

Contractile interstitial cells in the septum are found bound to the basal surface of the alveolar epithelium and not to the endothelial cells. These cells, which react with antiactin and antimyosin antibodies, contract and reduce the volume of the alveolar lumen. In vitro, it has been demonstrated that lung parenchymal tissue will contract when exposed to pharmacologic agents such as epinephrine and histamine.

Alveolar Pores

The interalveolar septum may contain one or more pores, 10–15 μm in diameter, connecting neighboring alveoli (Figs 18–11 and 18–17). They may equalize pressure in the alveoli or make possible collateral circulation of air when a bronchiole is obstructed.

Alveolar Lining Regeneration

It has been observed that inhalation of NO_2 promotes destruction of most of the cells lining the alveoli (type I and type II cells). The action of this compound or other toxic substances with the same effect is followed by a drastic increase in the mitotic activity of

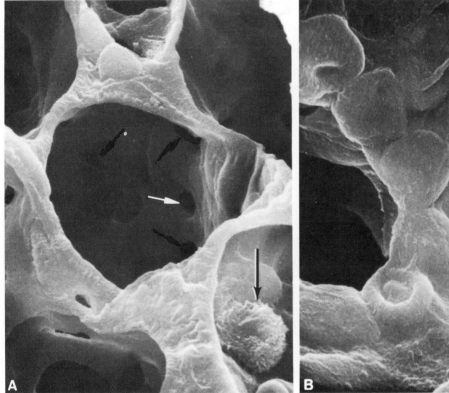
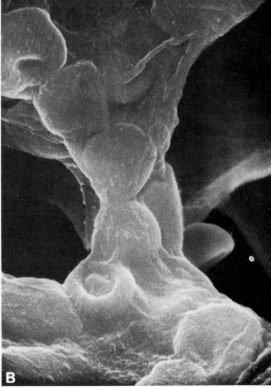

Figure 18–17. Scanning electron micrograph of mouse lung. Observe in *(A)* the thin septa and an alveolar pore (white arrow). At the black arrow, a macrophage with its typical ruffled membrane. × 3200. In *(B),* the alveolar wall is so thin that one can see the shape of the red blood cells in a capillary. × 6700. (Courtesy of Greenwood MF, Holland P: The mammalian respiratory tract surface: A scanning electron microscope study. *Lab Invest* 1972;27:296.)

the remaining type II cells. In the second step of alveolar lining regeneration, most of the type II cells are transformed into type I cells, and the alveolar lining regains its normal appearance. The normal turnover rate of type II cells is estimated to be 1% per day, maintaining a continuous renewal of its own type and also of type I cells.

PULMONARY BLOOD VESSELS

Circulation in the lungs includes both nutrient (systemic) and functional (pulmonary) vessels.

The functional circulation is represented by pulmonary arteries and veins. Pulmonary arteries are thin-walled owing to the low pressures (25 mm Hg systolic, 5 mm Hg diastolic) encountered in the pulmonary circuit. These arteries contain more smooth muscle cells and elastic fibers than do pulmonary veins. The arteries have an internal elastic membrane, whereas this structure is absent in pulmonary veins. Within the lung the pulmonary artery branches, accompanying the bronchial tree (Fig 18–18). Its branches are surrounded by adventitia of the bronchi and bronchioles. At the level of the alveolar duct, the branches

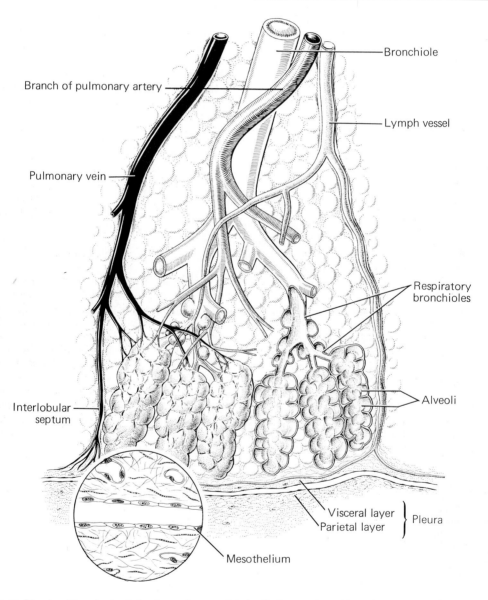

Figure 18–18. Blood and lymph circulation in a pulmonary lobule. Both vessels and bronchi are enlarged out of proportion in this drawing. In the interlobular septa, only the vein (left) or lymph vessel (right) has been represented, although both actually coexist in this region. At lower left, an enlargement of the pleura showing its mesothelial lining. (Based partially on Ham AW: *Histology,* 6th ed. Lippincott, 1969.)

of this artery form a capillary network in the interalveolar septa and in close contact with the alveolar epithelium. The lung has the best-developed capillary network in the body. The capillaries occur between all alveoli, including those present in the respiratory bronchioles.

Venules that originate in the capillary network occur singly in the parenchyma and somewhat removed from the airways; they are supported by a thin covering of connective tissue and enter the interlobular septa (Fig 18–18). After veins leave a lobule, they follow the bronchial tree toward the hilum.

Nutrient vessels include bronchial arteries and veins, which are smaller than the pulmonary artery and veins. The branches of the bronchial arteries also accompany or follow the bronchial tree, but only to the respiratory bronchioles, at which point they anastomose with the pulmonary artery.

PULMONARY LYMPHATIC VESSELS

The lymphatic vessels (Fig 18–18) follow the bronchi and the pulmonary vessels; they also occur in the interlobular septa, and all drain into lymph nodes in the region of the hilum. This lymphatic network is called the deep network to distinguish it from the superficial network, which includes lymphatic vessels present in the visceral pleura. The lymphatic vessels of the superficial network drain toward the hilum. They either follow the entire length of the pleura or penetrate the lung tissue via the interlobular septa.

In the terminal portions of the bronchial tree and beyond the alveolar ducts, lymphatic vessels do not occur.

NERVES

Both parasympathetic and sympathetic efferent fibers innervate the lungs, and general visceral afferent fibers, carrying poorly localized pain sensations, are also present. Most of the nerves are found in the connective tissues surrounding the larger airways. Parasympathetic stimulation, via the vagus nerves, results in bronchial constriction, while sympathetic stimulation causes bronchial dilatation. Drugs that mimic sympathetic neurotransmitters, such as isoproterenol, are used to cause bronchial dilation during asthmatic attacks.

PLEURA

The pleura (Fig 18–18) is the serous membrane covering the lung. It consists of 2 layers, parietal and visceral, which are continuous in the region of the hilum. Both membranes are composed of mesothelial cells resting on a fine connective tissue layer containing collagen and elastic fibers. The elastic fibers of the visceral pleura are continuous with those of the pulmonary parenchyma.

These 2 layers, therefore, delimit a cavity entirely lined by squamous mesothelial cells. Under normal conditions, this pleural cavity contains only a film of liquid that acts as a lubricating agent, permitting the smooth sliding of one surface over the other during respiratory movements. In certain pathologic states, the pleural cavity can become a real cavity, containing liquid or air in its interior. The walls of the pleural cavity, like all serosal cavities (peritoneal and pericardial), are quite permeable to water and other substances—thus the high frequency of fluid accumulation in this cavity in pathologic conditions. This fluid is derived from the blood plasma by exudation. Conversely, under certain conditions, liquids or gases present in the pleural cavity can be rapidly reabsorbed.

RESPIRATORY MOVEMENTS

During inhalation, contraction of the intercostal muscles elevates the ribs and contraction of the diaphragm lowers the bottom of the thoracic cavity, increasing its diameter and resulting in pulmonary expansion. The bronchi and bronchioles increase in diameter and length during inhalation. The respiratory portion also enlarges, mainly as a result of expansion of the alveolar ducts; the alveoli enlarge only slightly. The elastic fibers of the pulmonary parenchyma are stretched by this expansion, so that during exhalation caused by muscle relaxation the retraction of the lungs is passive, mainly because of the elastic fibers, which were under tension.

REFERENCES

Allen A: Mucus: A protective secretion of complexity. *Trends in Biochemical Science* 1983;**8**:169.

Andrews PM: A scanning electron microscopic study of the extrapulmonary respiratory tract. *Am J Anat* 1974;**139**:399.

Bouhuy SA: *Lung Cells in Disease.* Elsevier/North-Holland, 1976.

Breeze RG, Wheeldon EB: The cells of the pulmonary airways. *Am Rev Respir Dis* 1977;**116**:705.

Camner P, Mossberg B, Afzelius BA: Evidence for congenital nonfunctional cilia in the tracheobronchial tract in two subjects. *Am Rev Respir Dis* 1975;**112**:807.

Evans MJ: Transformation of type II cells to type I cells following exposure to NO_2. *Exp Mol Pathol* 1975;**22**:142.

Gehr P, Bachofen M, Weibel ER: The normal human lung: Ultrastructure and morphometric estimation of diffusion capacity. *Respir Physiol* 1978;**32**:121.

Goerke J: Lung surfactant. *Biochim Biophys Acta* 1979;**344**:241.

Greenwood M, Holland P: The mammalian respiratory tract surface: A scanning electron microscope study. *Lab Invest* 1972;**27**:296.

Heineman HO, Fishmann AP: Nonrespiratory functions of mammalian lungs. *Physiol Rev* 1969;**49**:1.

Kuhn C III: The cells of the lung and their organelles. In: *The Biochemical Basis of Pulmonary Function.* Crystal RG (editor). Marcel Dekker, 1976.

Nagaishi C: *Functional Anatomy and Histology of the Lung.* University Park Press, 1972.

Nugent J, O'Connor M (editors): Mucus and mucosa. Ciba Foundation Symposium No. 109. Pitman, 1984.

Plopper CG, Hill LH, Mariassy AT: Ultrastructure of the nonciliated bronchiolar epithelial (Clara) cell of mammalian lung. 3. A study of man with comparison of 15 mammalian species. *Exp Lung Res* 1980;**1**:171.

Thurlbeck WM, Abell MR (editors): *The Lung: Structure, Function, and Disease.* Williams & Wilkins, 1978.

Weibel ER: Morphological basis of alveolar-capillary gas exchange. *Physiol Rev* 1973;**53**:419.

Weibel ER: *The Pathway for Oxygen.* Harvard Univ Press, 1984.

Widdicombe JG, Pack RJ: The Clara cell. *Eur J Respir Dis* 1982;**63**:202.

Skin

19

The skin is the heaviest single organ of the body, accounting for about 16% of total body weight and displaying, in adults, 1.2–2.3 m² of surface to the external environment. It is composed of an epithelial layer of ectodermal origin, **epidermis,** and a layer of connective tissue of mesodermal origin, **dermis** (or **corium.** The junction of dermis and epidermis is irregular, and projections of the dermis called **papillae** interdigitate with evaginations of the epidermis called **epidermal ridges** (Fig 19–1). In 3 dimensions, these interdigitations may be of the peg-and-socket variety (thin skin) or formed of ridges and grooves (thick skin). Beneath the dermis lies the **hypodermis,** or **subcutaneous tissue,** a loose connective tissue that may contain a pad of adipose cells, the **panniculus adiposus.** The hypodermis, not considered part of the

skin, binds skin loosely to the subjacent tissues and corresponds to the superficial fascia of gross anatomy. Epidermal derivatives include hairs, nails, and sebaceous and sweat glands.

The external layer of the skin is relatively impermeable to water, which prevents extreme water loss by evaporation and allows for terrestrial life. The skin functions as a receptor organ in continuous communication with the environment (see Chapter 10) and protects the organism from impact and friction injuries. A pigment called **melanin,** produced and stored in the cells of the epidermis, provides further protective action against the sun's ultraviolet rays. Glands of the skin, blood vessels, and adipose tissue participate in thermoregulation, body metabolism, and excretion of various substances. Vitamin D₃ is formed,

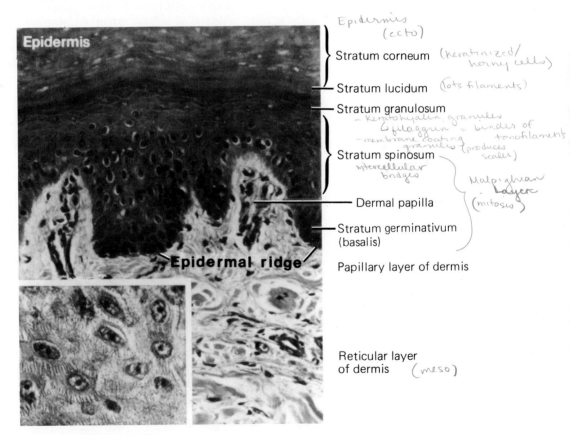

Figure 19–1. Photomicrographs of a section of human thick skin from the sole of the foot. Observe the papillae of the papillary layer and the thickness of the stratum corneum. The inset, at higher magnification, shows cells of the stratum spinosum with characteristic "spiny" intercellular bridges. H&E stain, × 100 and × 600.

under the action of sunlight, from precursors synthesized by the skin. Because skin is endowed with elasticity, it can expand to cover large areas in conditions associated with swelling, such as edema and pregnancy.

Upon close observation, certain portions of human skin show ridges and grooves arranged in distinctive patterns. These ridges appear first during intrauterine life at 13 weeks in the tips of the digits (fingerprints) and later in the volar surfaces of the hands and feet. The patterns assumed by the ridges and the intervening sulci are known as **dermatoglyphics.** They are unique for each individual and are used for personal identification, appearing as loops, arches, whorls, or combinations of these forms. These configurations are probably determined by multiple genes, and dermatoglyphics (fingerprints) is a field that has come to be of considerable medical and anthropologic as well as legal interest.

EPIDERMIS

The epidermis consists mainly of a stratified squamous keratinized epithelium, but it contains 3 less abundant cell types: **melanocytes, Langerhans cells, and Merkel cells.** The keratinizing epidermal cells are called **keratinocytes.** It is customary to distinguish between **thick skin** (glabrous, ie, smooth, nonhairy), found on the palms and soles; and **thin skin** (hairy), found elsewhere on the body. The designations thick and thin refer to the thickness of the epidermal layer, which varies between 75 and 150 μm for thin skin (Fig 19–2) and 400 and 600 μm for thick skin (Fig 19–1). Total skin thickness (epidermis plus dermis) also varies according to site. For example, skin on the back is about 4 mm thick, while that of the scalp is about 1.5 mm thick.

From the dermis outward, the epidermis consists of 5 layers of keratin-producing cells (keratinocytes) disposed as follows:

(1) The **stratum basale (stratum germinativum)** consists of a single layer of basophilic columnar or cuboidal cells which rest on the basal lamina at the dermal-epidermal junction that separates the dermis from the epidermis. Their long axes are perpendicular to the basal lamina. Desmosomes in great quantity bind the cells of this layer in their lateral and upper surfaces. Hemidesmosomes, found in the basal plasmalemma, help bind these cells to the basal lamina (Fig 4–4B). The stratum basale is characterized by intense mitotic activity and is responsible, in conjunction with the initial portion of the next layer, for constant renewal of epidermal cells. The human epidermis is renewed about every 15–30 days depending on the region of the body, age, and other factors. All cells in the stratum basale contain filaments about 10 nm in diameter (cytokeratins; see Intermediate Filaments in Chapter 3). As the cells progress upward, the number of filaments increases until they represent, in the stratum corneum, half of its total protein.

(2) The **stratum spinosum** consists of cuboidal, polygonal, or slightly flattened cells with a central nucleus and a cytoplasm with processes filled with bundles of filaments. These bundles converge into many small cellular extensions, terminating with desmosomes located at the tips of these spiny projections (Figs 19–1 and 19–3). The cells of this layer are firmly bound together by this system of filament-filled cytoplasmic spines and desmosomes that punctuate the cell surface, giving a prickle-studded appearance in the light microscope (Figs 19–1 and 19–4). These tonofilament bundles, visible under the light microscope, are called **tonofibrils.** At one time they were believed to cross the intercellular bridges that unite cell to cell; however, they are now known to end and

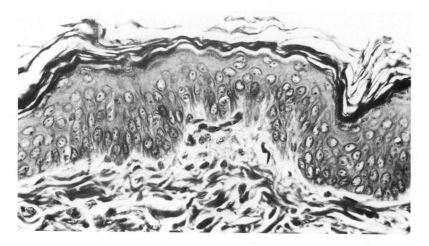

Figure 19–2. Photomicrograph of a section of human abdominal (thin) skin. Compare with Fig 19–1 and note the thinness of the whole epidermis and, specifically, the stratum corneum. The strata are not as clearly seen as in Fig 19–1. H&E stain, × 310.

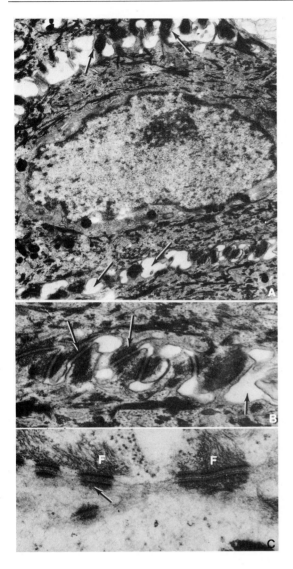

Figure 19–3. Electron micrograph of the stratum spinosum of human skin. *A:* A cell of the stratum spinosum with its cytoplasm full of tonofibrils and with melanin granules. The arrows show the spines, or "intercellular bridges," with their desmosomes. × 8400. *B* and *C:* Desmosomes in greater detail. Observe that a dense substance appears between the cell membranes and that bundles of cytoplasmic filaments (F) (tonofibrils) insert themselves on the desmosomes. × 36,000 and × 45,000. (Courtesy of C Barros.)

malpighian layer, which consists of both the stratum basale and stratum spinosum.

(3) The **stratum granulosum** is characterized by 3–5 layers of flattened polygonal cells containing centrally located nuclei and cytoplasm filled with coarse basophilic granules called **keratohyalin granules.** Biochemical studies show that keratohyalin granules contain a histidine-rich protein as well as cystine-containing proteins. The histidine-rich protein is a highly phosphorylated precursor of a protein called filaggrin. The numerous phosphate groups account for the intense basophilia of keratohyalin granules. The function of filaggrin appears to be to bind together the tonofilaments to form the densely packed aggregates seen in cells of succeeding layers. Keratohyalin granules are not surrounded by a membrane.

Another characteristic structure found with the electron microscope in the cells of the granular layer of epidermis is the **membrane-coating granule,** ovoid or rodlike in appearance and about 0.1–0.3 μm in diameter. These granules, formed in the Golgi complex, move to the upper part of the cell near its plasma membrane. They fuse with the membrane and discharge their contents into the intercellular spaces of the granular layer. In the electron microscope these granules have a lamellar appearance. Histochemical reactions indicate that they contain glycosaminoglycans and phospholipids. The function of this extruded material is similar to that of an intercellular cement substance which acts as a barrier to penetration by foreign materials and provides in the skin a very important sealing effect. Studies made in keratinized and nonkeratinized human oral epithelium show that penetration by peroxidase and lanthanum tracers does not occur in the regions where this material fills the extracellular space. Formation of this barrier, which appeared first in reptiles, was one of the important evolutionary events that permitted development of terrestrial life.

A final feature of cells of the stratum granulosum and the uppermost cells of the stratum spinosum is the appearance, at the inner surface of the plasma membrane, of a submembranous protein envelope of electron-dense material. The envelope is about 10 nm thick and closely applied to the plasma membrane, making the cell membrane appear to be thickened. It has been learned that the submembranous envelope is composed of several highly cross-linked polypeptides including involucrin (MW 140,000) and keratolinin (MW 36,000) that bestow on the membrane great resistance to breakdown. The cross-linking is carried out by a transglutaminase found in suprabasal keratinocytes.

(4) The **stratum lucidum,** which is more apparent in thick skin, is translucent and composed of a thin layer of extremely flattened eosinophilic cells (Fig 19–1). The organelles and nuclei are no longer evident, and the cytoplasm consists primarily of densely packed filaments embedded in an electron-dense matrix. Desmosomes are still evident between adjacent cells.

insert in the cytoplasmic densities of the desmosomes. It is believed that the filaments play an important role in maintaining cohesion among cells and in resisting the effects of abrasion. The epidermis of areas subject to continuous friction and pressure (such as the soles of the feet) has a thicker stratum spinosum with more abundant tonofibrils and desmosomes.

All mitoses are confined to what is termed the

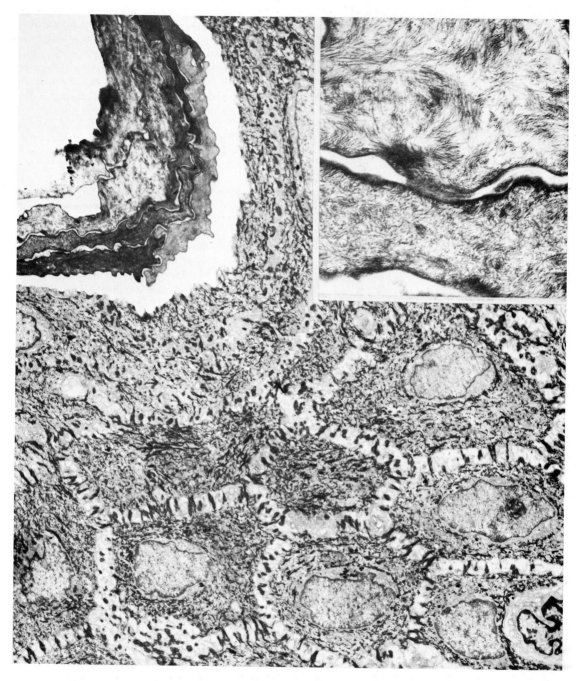

Figure 19–4. Electron micrograph of a section of human skin at the transition between the stratum spinosum and stratum corneum. Observe the cells with their typical cytoplasmic extensions, "intercellular bridges," and cytoplasmic tonofibrils. At upper left is the stratum corneum, seen in detail in the inset at upper right. Observe that these cells are packed with 10-nm intermediate filaments. × 5500 and × 36,000. (Courtesy of C Barros.)

(5) The **stratum corneum** consists of 15–20 layers of flattened nonnucleated keratinized cells whose cytoplasm is filled with a birefringent filamentous scleroprotein, **keratin** (Figs 19–1 and 19–4). Keratin contains at least 6 different polypeptides with molecular weights ranging from 40,000 to 70,000. Three polypeptide chains coil around one another to form subunits (~ 47 nm long) of the tonofilament. At least one of the polypeptides is different from the others in the subunit. Thus, great diversity in composition is possible. Nine of the 3-chain subunits coil around each other, forming a filament about 10 nm in diameter. End-to-end aggregation of 3-chain subunits leads to growth in length of the tonofilment. The composition of tonofilaments changes as epidermal cells differentiate. Basal cells contain polypeptides of lower molecular weight, whereas more differentiated cells synthesize the higher-molecular-weight polypeptides. Tonofilaments are packed together in a matrix contributed by the keratohyalin granules.

After keratinization, the cells consist of only fibrillar and amorphous proteins and thickened plasma membranes and are called **horny cells.** Lysosomal hydrolytic enzymes play a role in the disappearance of the cytoplasmic organelles. At the surface of the stratum corneum, cells are continuously shed.

This description of the epidermis corresponds to its most complex structure in areas where it is very thick, as on the soles of the feet. In thin skin, the stratum granulosum and stratum lucidum are often less well developed, and the stratum corneum may be quite thin.

Renewal of the epidermis under normal conditions occurs every 15–30 days and is due to mitotic activity in the germinativum and spinosum layers. In **psoriasis,** a common skin disease, there is an increase in the number of proliferating cells in the stratum basale and stratum spinosum as well as an increase in the rate of proliferation of these cells. This results in greater epidermal thickness and more rapid renewal of the epidermis—7 days instead of 15–30 days.

Melanocytes

The color of the skin results from several factors, but the most important are its content of melanin and carotene, the number of blood vessels in the dermis, and the color of the blood flowing in them.

Eumelanin is a dark brown pigment produced by a specialized cell of the epidermis, the melanocyte, found beneath or between the cells of the stratum basale and in the hair follicles. The pigment found in red hair is called pheomelanin and contains cysteine as part of its structure. Melanocytes are derived from neural crest cells. They have rounded cell bodies from which long irregular extensions branch into the epidermis, running between the cells of the germinativum and spinosum layers. Tips of these extensions terminate in invaginations of the cells present in the 2 layers. The electron microscope reveals a pale-staining cell containing numerous small mitochondria, a well-developed Golgi complex, and short cisternae of rough endoplasmic reticulum. Intermediate filaments, about 10 nm in diameter, are also present (Figs 19–5 and 19–6). Melanocytes are not attached to adjacent keratinocytes by desmosomes, but hemidesmosomes are present that bind melanocytes to the basal lamina. Synthesis of melanin occurs in the interior of the melanocyte, and tyrosinase plays an important role in this process. As a result of tyrosinase activity, tyrosine is transformed first into 3,4-dihydroxyphenylalanine **(dopa)** and then into dopaquinone, which is converted, after a series of transformations, into melanin. Tyrosinase is synthesized on ribosomes, transported in the lumen of the rough endoplasmic reticulum of melanocytes, and accumulated in vesicles formed at the Golgi zone (Fig 19–7). In the development of the mature melanin granule, 4 stages can be distinguished:

Stage I: A vesicle surrounded by a membrane, showing beginning of tyrosinase activity and formation of fine granular material; at its periphery, electron-dense strands show an orderly arrangement of tyrosinase molecules on a protein matrix.

Stage II: The vesicle is ovoid now and shows, in its interior, parallel filaments with a periodicity of about 10 nm or cross-striations of about the same periodicity. Melanin is deposited on the protein matrix.

Stage III: As a result of increased melanin formation, the internal periodic fine structure is less visible.

Stage IV: The mature melanin granule is visible in the light microscope, and melanin completely fills the vesicle. No ultrastructure is visible. The mature granules are ellipsoid in shape with a length of 1 μm and a diameter of 0.4 μm.

The absence of tyrosinase activity or other defects in melanin synthesis lead to a condition called **albinism** in which no pigment is produced even though the melanocytes still possess granules through stage II of their development.

Once formed, the melanin granules migrate within cytoplasmic extensions of the melanocyte and are transferred to cells of the germinativum and spinosum layers of the epidermis. This transfer process has been viewed, with the aid of cinematography, in skin tissue culture. Melanin granules are essentially "injected" into keratinocytes in a process called **cytocrine secretion.** Once inside the keratinocyte, melanin granules accumulate in the supranuclear region of the cytoplasm, thus protecting the nuclei of dividing cells from the deleterious effects of solar radiation. Whereas melanocytes synthesize melanin, epithelial cells act as a depot and contain more of this pigment than melanocytes. Inside keratinocytes, melanin granules fuse with lysosomes—the reason that melanin disappears in upper epithelial cells. In this interaction between keratinocytes and melanocytes, which results in the pigmentation of the skin, the important factors

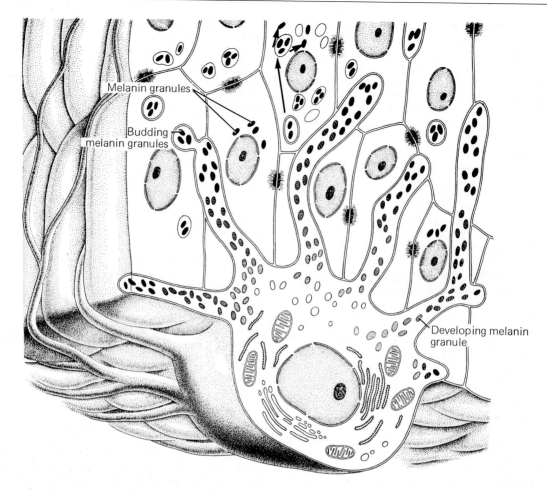

Figure 19–5. Diagram of a melanocyte. Its arms extend upward into the interstices between keratinocytes. The melanin granules are synthesized in these cells, migrate to its arms, and are transferred into the cytoplasm of keratinocytes. Ribosomes, Golgi complex, rough endoplasmic reticulum, and mitochondria are also present. (Based on the work of Fitzpatrick and Szabó, 1959.)

are the rate of formation of melanin granules within the melanocyte, their transfer into the keratinocytes, and the ultimate disposition of the granules by the keratinocytes. A feedback mechanism may exist between melanocytes and keratinocytes.

Melanocytes can be easily visualized by incubating fragments of epidermis in dopa. This compound is converted to dark brown deposits of melanin in melanocytes, a reaction catalyzed by the enzyme tyrosinase. Using this method, it is possible to count the number of melanocytes of the epidermis per unit area. Such studies show that these cells are not distributed at random among keratinocytes; rather, there is a pattern in their distribution called the epidermal-melanin unit. In humans, the ratio of dopa-positive melanocytes to keratinocytes in the stratum basale is constant for each area of the body but varies from one region to another. For example, there are about 1000 melanocytes/mm^2 in thigh skin, whereas 2000/mm^2 are present in skin of the scrotum. The number of

melanocytes per unit area is not influenced by sex or race, and skin color differences are due mainly to differences in the number of melanin granules in keratinocytes.

Darkening of the skin after exposure to ultraviolet rays (wavelength = 290–320 nm) of sunlight (tanning) is the result of a 2-step process. A physicochemical reaction occurs first, darkening the preexistent melanin and releasing it rapidly into the keratinocytes. In a second stage, the rate of melanin synthesis in the melanocytes accelerates, resulting in an increase in the amount of this pigment.

Melanocyte-stimulating hormone (α- and β-MSH), produced in the intermediate lobe of the pituitary, has a marked influence on melanophores of amphibia, promoting centrifugal migration of pigment in their long cytoplasmic processes and an increase in the number of melanin granules in keratinocytes. These hormones do not exist in a free form in humans. In humans, lack of cortisol from the adrenal cortex causes overproduction of ACTH, which increases the pigmentation of the skin, as in **Addison's disease** (a disease due to dysfunction of the adrenal glands). ACTH contains a peptide sequence identical to the amino sequence of α-MSH of other mammals. Excess ACTH production in patients with Addison's disease is thought to be responsible for the hyperpigmentation seen in these individuals.

Langerhans Cells

These star-shaped cells are found mainly in the stratum spinosum of the epidermis. After impregnation with gold chloride, they are delineated sharply against an unstained background. In the electron microscope they have an indented nucleus and a clear cytoplasm with no tonofilaments in their cytoplasm and no desmosomes in the plasma membrane. They contain characteristic rodlike or racket-shaped inclusions (**Birbeck's granules**) in their cytoplasm. There are between 400 and 1000 Langerhans cells per square millimeter of skin surface. These cells are believed to be responsible for processing and presenting cutaneous antigens to lymphoid cells present in the epidermis. Langerhans cells are also found in the epithelium of the oral mucosa and the vagina as well as in the thymus. Langerhans cells have been shown to arise from bone marrow precursors and are usually included in the mononuclear phagocyte system (see Chapter 5).

Merkel Cells

The Merkel cells, generally present in the thick skin of palms and soles, somewhat resemble the epidermal epithelial cells but have small dense granules in their cytoplasm. The composition of these granules is not known. Free nerve endings forming an expanded terminal disk are present at the base of the Merkel cells. Merkel cells may serve as sensory mechanoreceptors, although they have also been implicated as having APUD cell–like activity.

DERMIS

The dermis is composed of the connective tissue that supports the epidermis and binds it to the subjacent layer, the subcutaneous tissue (hypodermis). The thickness of the dermis varies depending upon the region of the body, reaching its maximum of 4 mm on the back. The superficial surface of the dermis is very irregular and has many projections (dermal papillae) that interdigitate with projections (epidermal pegs or ridges) of the epidermis (Fig 19–1). These structures are more numerous in skin subject to frequent pressure and are believed to increase and reinforce the dermo-epidermal junction. During embryonic development, dermis determines the developmental pattern of the overlying epidermis. Dermis obtained from the sole always induces the formation of a heavily keratinized epidermis irrespective of the site of origin of the epithelial cells.

The distinctive dermo-epidermal junction is seen in histologic sections of the human skin, and this understructure of the epidermis is unique in each part of the body. A basal lamina is always found between the stratum germinativum and the papillary layer of the dermis and follows the contour of the interdigitations between these layers. Underlying the basal lamina is a delicate net of reticular fibers called the lamina reticularis. When viewed with the light microscope, this composite structure is called the basement membrane.

Two layers with rather indistinct boundaries have been described in the dermis. They are the outermost papillary layer and the deeper reticular layer (Fig 19–1). The **papillary layer** is thin and is composed of loose connective tissue. Besides fibroblasts, other connective tissue cells are present, the most abundant being mast cells and macrophages. Extravasated leukocytes are also seen. The papillary layer is so called because it constitutes the major part of the dermal papillae. From this layer, special collagen fibrils insert into the basal lamina and extend into the dermis. They are thought to have a special function, binding the dermis to the epidermis, and are called **anchoring fibrils** (Fig 4–4). The **reticular layer** is thicker, composed of irregular dense connective tissue (mainly type I collagen), and therefore has more fibers and fewer cells than the papillary layer. The glycosaminoglycan content of the dermis varies in different regions. The principal glycosaminoglycan in the skin is dermatan sulfate. The dermis contains a network of elastic fibers (Fig 19–8) in which the thicker fibers are characteristically found in the reticular layer. From this region emerge fibers that become gradually thinner and end by inserting in the basal lamina. As these fibers progress toward the basal lamina, they gradually lose their amorphous elastin component and only the microfibrillar component inserts into the basal lamina. This elastic network is responsible for the elasticity of the skin.

Age-related changes in the dermis can be observed histologically and biochemically. Collagen fibers thicken and collagen synthesis decreases with age. Elastic fibers steadily increase in number and thickness, so that the elastin content of human skin increases approximately 5-fold from fetal to adult life. In old age, extensive cross-linking of the collagen and loss of elastic fibers cause the skin to become more fragile, lose its suppleness, and assume many wrinkles. Several disorders are characterized by a considerable increase in skin and ligament extensibility due to defective collagen fibril processing. Examples are cutis laxa and Ehlers-Danlos syndrome (Table 5–3).

The dermis has a rich network of blood and lymph vessels. In certain areas of the skin, blood can pass directly from arteries to veins through arteriovenous anastomoses or shunts. These play a very important role in temperature and blood pressure regulation, since dermal vessels can accommodate about 4.5% of the blood volume. A rich capillary network in the papillary layer surrounds the epidermal ridges and

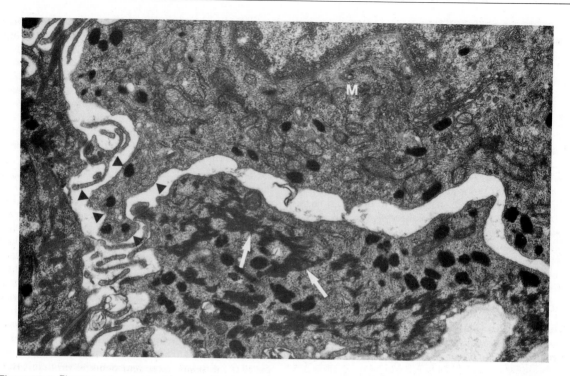

Figure 19–6. Electron micrograph of human skin showing part of a melanocyte (M) in the upper portion. Note the dense melanosomes in this cell. The lower half of the picture is occupied by a keratinocyte with its cytoplasm containing numerous melanosomes and tonofibrils (arrows). The arrowheads outline a cytoplasmic extension of the melanocyte between keratinocytes. Compare with Fig 19–5. × 6000.

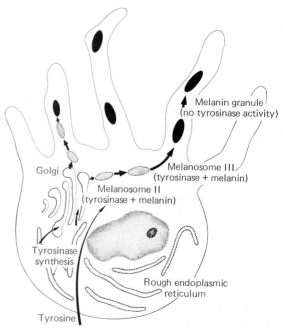

Figure 19–7 (at right). Diagram of a melanocyte, illustrating the principal process occurring during melaninogenesis. Tyrosinase is synthesized in the rough endoplasmic reticulum and is accumulated in vesicles of the Golgi complex. The free vesicles are now called melanosomes. Melanin synthesis begins in the stage II melanosomes, where this compound is accumulated and forms stage III melanosomes. Later, this structure loses its tyrosinase activity and becomes a melanin granule. Melanin granules migrate to arm tips and are then transferred to the keratinocytes of the malpighian layer.

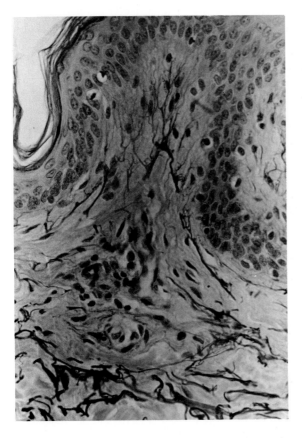

Figure 19–8. Photomicrograph of a section of human abdominal skin stained for elastic fibers. Note the gradual decrease in the diameter of fibers as they approach the epidermis. The very thin superficial fibers are formed only by microfibrils that insert into the basal lamina. × 600.

functions in regulating body core temperature and nourishing the overlying epidermis, which contains no blood vessels of its own.

Besides these components, the dermis also contains some epidermal derivatives, the hair follicles and the sweat and sebaceous glands. A rich supply of nerves is found in the dermis, and the effector nerves to the skin are postganglionic fibers of sympathetic ganglia of the paravertebral chain. No parasympathetic innervation is present. The afferent nerve endings form a superficial dermal network with free nerve endings, a hair follicle network, and the innervation of encapsulated sensory organs (Meissner's and pacinian corpuscles).

SUBCUTANEOUS TISSUE

This layer consists of loose connective tissue that binds the skin loosely to the subjacent organs, making it possible for the skin to slide over them. The hypodermis often contains fat cells, varying in number

according to the area of the body and in size according to the nutritional status of the individual. This layer is also referred to as the superficial fascia and, where thick enough, the panniculus adiposus.

HAIRS

Hairs are elongated keratinized structures derived from an invagination of the epidermal epithelium. Their color, size, and disposition are variable according to race, age, sex, and the region of the body. Hairs are found everywhere on the body except on the palms, soles, lips, glans penis, clitoris, and labia minora. The face has about 600 hairs/cm², while the remainder of the body has about 60/cm². Hairs grow discontinuously and have periods of growth followed by periods of rest. This growth does not occur synchronously in all regions of the body or even in the same area; it tends rather to occur in patches. The duration of the growth and rest periods also varies according to the region of the body. Thus, in the scalp, the growth periods (anagen) may last for several years, whereas the rest periods (catagen and telogen) average 3 months. Hair growth of certain regions of the body such as the scalp, face, and pubis is strongly influenced not only by sex hormones—especially androgens—but also by adrenal and thyroid hormones. Hair growth is not affected by frequency of cutting or shaving.

Each hair arises from an epidermal invagination, the **hair follicle,** which has during its growth period a terminal dilatation called the **hair bulb.** At the base of the hair bulb, a **dermal papilla** can be observed (Figs 19–9 and 19–10). The dermal papilla contains a capillary network, which is vital in sustaining the hair follicle. The loss of blood flow or vitality of dermal papilla will result in death of the follicle. The epidermal cells covering this dermal papilla form the hair root that produces and is continuous with the hair shaft which protrudes beyond the skin.

During periods of growth, the epithelial cells that make up the bulb are equivalent to those in the stratum germinativum of the skin. They divide constantly and differentiate into the following cell types:

(1) In certain types of thick hairs, the cells of the central region of the root at the apex of the dermal papilla produce large vacuolated and moderately keratinized cells that form the **medulla** of the hair (A in Fig 19–9).

(2) The cells located around the central region of the root (B in Fig 19–9) multiply and differentiate into heavily keratinized, compactly grouped fusiform cells forming the **hair cortex.**

(3) Farther peripherally are the cells (C in Fig 19–9) that produce the **hair cuticle,** a layer composed of cells that, midway up the bulb, are cuboidal, then become tall and columnar, and, higher up, change from horizontal to vertical, at which point they form a layer of flattened, heavily keratinized cells disposed as shingles covering the cortex. These cuticle cells

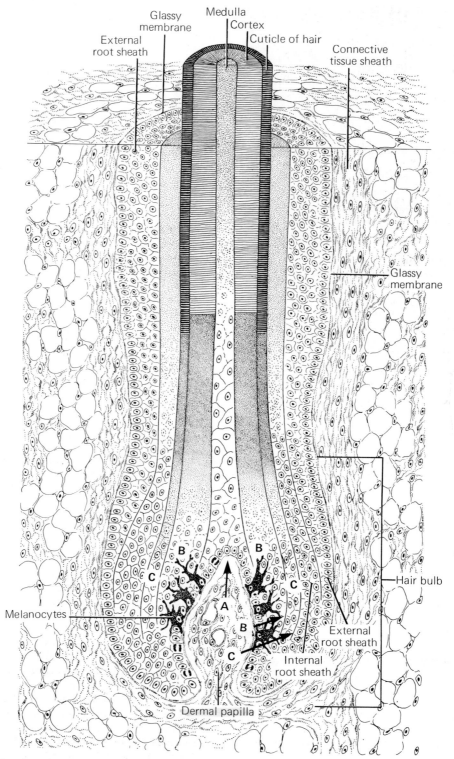

Figure 19–9. Drawing of a hair and its follicle. The follicle has a bulbous terminal expansion that contains a dermal papilla, which contains capillaries and is covered by cells that form the hair root and develop into the hair shaft. The central cells (A) indicated by the arrow produce large, vacuolated, poorly cornified cells that form the medulla of the hair. The cells that produce the cortex of the hair are located laterally (B). Cells forming the hair cuticle originate in the next layer (C). The peripheral epithelial cells develop into the internal and external root sheaths. The external root sheath is continuous with the epidermis, while the cells of the internal root sheath disappear at the level of the openings of the sebaceous gland ducts.

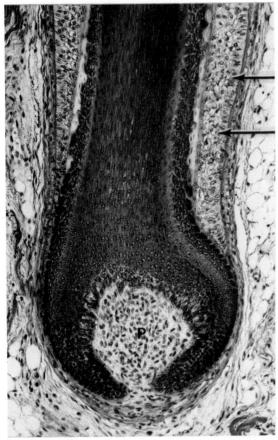

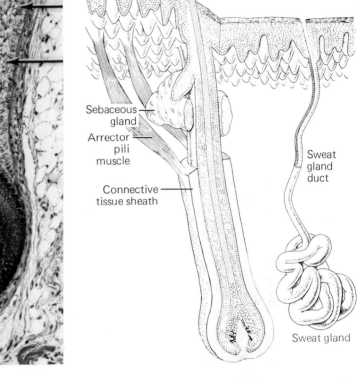

Figure 19–10. Photomicrograph of a section of hair follicle from a human lip. Observe the papilla (P) and the outer root sheath (arrows), surrounded by a connective tissue sheath. H&E stain, × 118.

Figure 19–11. Diagram of the relationships between the skin, hair follicle, arrector pili muscle, and sebaceous and sweat glands. The arrector pili muscle has its origin in the connective tissue sheath of the hair follicle and its insertion in the papillary layer of the dermis.

are the last cell line in the hair follicle to differentiate.

(4) Finally, the most peripheral cells give rise to the **internal root sheath,** which completely surrounds the initial part of the hair shaft. The internal sheath is a transient structure whose cells degenerate and disappear above the level of the sebaceous glands. The **external root sheath** is continuous with epidermal cells, and near the surface it shows all the layers of epidermis. Near the dermal papilla it is thinner and is composed of cells corresponding to the stratum germinativum of the epidermis.

Separating the hair follicle from the dermis is a noncellular hyaline layer, the **glassy membrane** (Fig 19–9), which represents a thickening of the basal lamina. The dermis that surrounds the follicle is denser, forming a special sheath of connective tissue. Bound to this sheath and connecting it to the papillary layer of the dermis are bundles of smooth muscle cells, the **arrector pili** muscles (Fig 19–11). They are disposed in an oblique direction, and their contraction results

in the erection of the hair shaft to a more upright position. Contraction of arrector pili muscles also causes a depression of the skin where the muscles attach to the dermis. This produces the "gooseflesh" of common parlance.

Hair color is due to the activity of melanocytes located between the papilla and the epithelial cells of the hair root that produce the pigment present in the medullary and cortical cells of the hair shaft (Fig 19–9). These melanocytes produce and transfer melanin to the epithelial cells by a mechanism similar to that described for the epidermis.

Although the keratinization processes in the epidermis and hair appear to be similar, they differ in the following ways:

(1) The epidermis produces relatively soft, keratinized outer layers of dead cells that adhere slightly to the skin and desquamate continuously. In the hair the opposite occurs, with the production of a hard and compact keratinized structure.

(2) Whereas in the epidermis keratinization occurs continuously and over the entire surface, in the hair it is intermittent and present only in the hair root. The hair papilla has an inductive action on the covering epithelial cells, promoting their proliferation and differentiation. Thus, injuries to the dermal papillae result in the loss of hair.

(3) Contrary to what happens in the epidermis, where all cells differentiate in the same direction, giving rise to the final keratinized layer, in the hair root, cells differentiate into various cell types that differ in ultrastructure, histochemistry, and function. Mitotic activity in hair follicles is under the influence of androgens.

NAILS

Nails are plates of keratinized epithelial cells on the dorsal surface of each distal phalanx (Fig 19–12). The proximal part of the nail, hidden in the nail groove, is the **nail root.** The epithelium of the fold of skin covering the nail root consists of the usual layers of cells. The stratum corneum of this epithelium forms the **eponychium,** or **cuticle.** The **nail plate** rests on a bed of epidermis termed the **nail bed.** Only the stratum basale and the stratum spinosum are present in the nail bed. The nail plate corresponds to the stratum corneum of skin. The epithelium of the nail bed arises from the **nail matrix.** The proximal end of the matrix lies deep to the nail root, while its distal end extends to the outer edge of the **lunula,** which is the white, opaque crescent at the proximal end of the nail. Cells of the matrix divide, move distally, and eventually cornify, forming the proximal part of the nail plate. The nail plate then slides forward over the nail bed, which makes no contribution to the formation of the plate. The distal end of the plate becomes free of the nail bed and is worn away or cut off. The nearly transparent nail plate and the thin epithelium of the nail bed provide a useful window on the amount of oxygen in the blood by allowing a view of the color of blood in the dermal vessels.

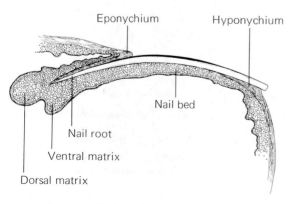

Figure 19–12. The nail and its components.

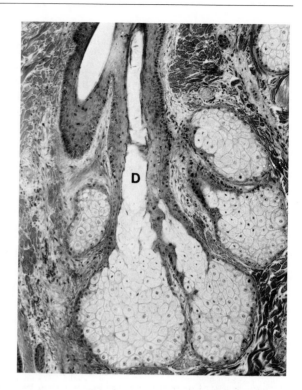

Figure 19–13. Photomicrograph of a sebaceous gland. It consists of several acini, which are limited externally by proliferating, flattened epithelial cells that give rise to the fat-filled cells of the acinar center. D, duct. H&E stain, × 100.

GLANDS OF THE SKIN

Sebaceous Glands

Sebaceous glands are embedded in the dermis over most of the body surface. There are about 100 of these glands per square centimeter over most of the body, but the frequency increases to 400–900/cm² on the face, forehead, and scalp. Sebaceous glands are not found in glabrous skin of the palms and soles. They are acinar glands that usually have several acini opening into a short duct. This duct usually ends in the upper portion of a hair follicle (Fig 19–11), but in certain regions, such as the glans penis, glans clitoridis, and lips, it opens directly onto the epidermal surface. The acini consist of a basal layer of undifferentiated flattened epithelial cells that rest on the basal lamina. These cells proliferate and differentiate, filling the acini with rounded cells containing abundant fat droplets in their cytoplasm (Fig 19–13). Their nuclei gradually shrink, and the cells simultaneously become filled with fat droplets and burst. The product of this process is the secretion of the sebaceous gland, which is gradually moved to the surface of the skin. This is an example of a holocrine gland, for its product of secretion, **sebum,** is released with remnants of dead cells. This product is composed of a complex mixture of lipids that contains triglycerides, waxes, squalene, and cholesterol and its esters. Sebaceous glands begin to function at puberty. The primary controlling factor of sebaceous gland secretion in men is testicular testosterone; in women, it is a combination of ovarian and adrenal androgens. The flow of sebum is continuous, and a disturbance in the normal secretion and flow of sebum is one of the reasons for the development of acne. The functions of sebum in humans are largely unknown. It may have weak antibacterial and antifungal properties. Sebum does not have any importance in preventing water loss.

Sweat Glands

Sweat glands are widely distributed in the skin. Certain regions such as the glans penis are exceptions.

The **eccrine (merocrine)** sweat glands are simple, coiled, tubular glands whose ducts open at the skin surface (Fig 19–11). Their ducts do not divide and are thinner in diameter than the secretory portion (Fig 19–14). The secretory part of the gland is embedded in the dermis, measures approximately 0.4 mm in diameter, and is surrounded by myoepithelial cells (described in Chapter 4). Contraction of these cells is believed to help to discharge the secretion. A fairly thick basal lamina lies outside the secretory portion of the glands. Two types of cells have been described in the secretory portion of eccrine sweat glands. **Dark cells** (mucoid cells) are pyramidal cells that line most of the luminal surface of the secretory portion of the gland. Their basal surface does not touch the basal lamina. The cytoplasm of dark cells contains rod-shaped mitochondria, a well-developed Golgi complex, cisternae of rough endoplasmic reticulum, and numerous free ribosomes. Secretory granules con-

taining glycoproteins are abundant in the apical cytoplasm. **Clear cells** are devoid of secretory granules but contain an abundance of glycogen particles. The basal plasmalemma has numerous invaginations characteristic of cells involved in transepithelial salt reabsorption and fluid transport.

The ducts are lined by stratified cuboidal epithelium (Fig 19–14). The peripheral cells have large nuclei and numerous mitochondria, but other organelles are poorly developed. The cells bordering the lumen are characterized by a prominent terminal web that is intensely eosinophilic.

The fluid secreted by these glands is not viscous and contains little protein. Its main components are water, sodium chloride, urea, ammonia, and uric acid. Its sodium content of 85 meq/L is distinctly below that of blood (144 meq/L), and the cells present in the sweat ducts are responsible for sodium reabsorption. The fluid in the lumen of the secretory portion of the gland is an ultrafiltrate of the blood plasma. This ultrafiltrate is derived from a network of capillaries that intimately envelop the secretory region of each gland. Following its release on the surface of the skin, sweat evaporates, cooling the surface. In the underlying dermis, blood in the extensive capillary loops encircling the dermal papillae is subsequently cooled as its heat is conducted into the overlying epidermis. The elimination of catabolites suggests that the sweat glands also have an excretory function.

In addition to eccrine sweat glands, another type of sweat gland—the **apocrine** gland—is present in the axillary, areolar, and anal regions. The term apocrine implies that a portion of the apical cytoplasm is shed in the process of secretion. Most investigators now agree that this apparent shedding is an artifact

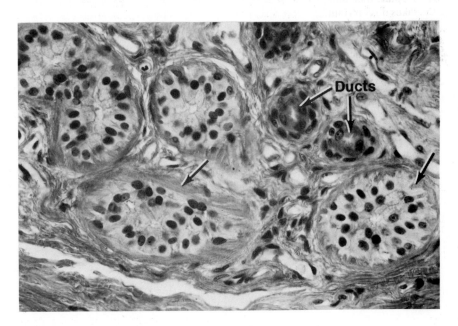

Figure 19–14. Photomicrograph of a human eccrine sweat gland. At upper right are 2 ducts transversely sectioned. Observe the myoepithelial cells, which form a sheath around the gland (arrows). H&E stain, × 360.

of fixation and that secretion occurs by exocytosis (merocrine secretion). Apocrine glands are much larger (3–5 mm in diameter) than eccrine sweat glands. They are embedded in the subcutaneous tissue, and their ducts open into hair follicles. These glands produce a viscous secretion which is initially odorless but which acquires its distinctive odor by bacterial decomposition. It has been postulated that the secretions of apocrine and sebaceous glands are pheromones, hormones that act at distant sites and serve as sexual attractants in many animal species. Evidence for this postulate is controversial and not very convincing for humans. Apocrine glands are innervated by adrenergic nerve endings, whereas eccrine glands receive cholinergic fibers.

The glands of Moll in the margins of the eyelids and the ceruminous glands of the ear are modified sweat glands.

VESSELS & NERVES OF THE SKIN

The arterial vessels that nourish the skin form 2 plexuses, one located between the papillary and reticular layers and one between the dermis and the subcutaneous tissue. Thin branches leave these plexuses and vascularize the dermal papillae. Each papilla has only one arterial ascending and one venous descending branch. Veins are disposed in 3 plexuses, 2 of them in the position described for the arterial vessels and the third in the middle of the dermis. Arteriovenous anastomoses with glomera (see Chapter 12) are frequent in the skin. Lymphatic vessels begin as blind sacs in the papillae of the dermis and converge to form 2 plexuses as described for the arterial vessels.

One of the most important functions of the skin is to receive stimuli from the environment, and it has an abundant sensory innervation. Besides free nerve endings in the epidermis and cutaneous glands, receptors are present in the dermis and subcutaneous tissue, being more frequently found in the dermal papillae (see Chapter 10). The hair follicles possess a rich network of nerve endings essential in the processing of tactile impressions from the environment.

REFERENCES

Cohen J, Szabó G: Study of pigment donation in vitro. *Exp Cell Res* 1968;**50**:418.

Edelson RL, Fink JM: The immunologic function of the skin. *Sci Am* (June) 1985;**252**:46.

Epstein WL, Maibach HI: Cell renewal in human epidermis. *Arch Dermatol* 1965;**92**:462.

Goldsmith LA (editor): *Biochemistry and Physiology of the Skin.* Vols 1 and 2. Oxford Univ Press, 1983.

Guevedo WC Jr: Epidermal melanin units: Melanocyte-keratinocyte interactions. *Am Zool* 1972;**12**:35.

Halprin KM: Epidermal "turnover time": A reexamination. *J Invest Dermatol* 1972;**86**:14.

Hayward AF: Membrane coating granules. *Int Rev Cytol* 1979;**59**:97.

Millington PF, Wilkinson R: *Skin.* Cambridge Univ Press, 1983.

Montagna W: *The Structure and Function of Skin,* 3rd ed. Academic Press, 1974.

Munger BL: The cytology of apocrine sweat glands. 2. Human. *Z Zellforsch Mikrosk Anat* 1965;**68**:837.

Shelley WB, Lennart J: The Langerhans cell: Its origin, nature and function. *Acta Derm Venereol (Stockh)* 1978;**79**:7.

Stenn KS: Collagen heterogeneity of skin. *Am J Dermatopathol* 1979;**1**:87.

Strauss JS, Fochi PE, Downing DT: The sebaceous glands: Twenty-five years of progress. *J Invest Dermatol* 1976;**67**:90.

Terzakis JA: The ultrastructure of monkey eccrine sweat glands. *Z Zellforsch Mikrosk Anat* 1964;**64**:493.

Winkelmann RK: The Merkel cell system and a comparison between it and the neurosecretory or APUD cell system. *J Invest Dermatol* 1977;**69**:41.

Zelickson AS: *Ultrastructure of Normal and Abnormal Skin.* Lea & Febiger, 1967.

Urinary System

20

The urinary system consists of the paired kidneys and ureters and the unpaired bladder and urethra. This system contributes to the maintenance of homeostasis by producing urine, in which various metabolic waste products are eliminated. The kidneys also regulate the fluid and electrolyte balance of the body and are the site of production of the hormones renin and erythropoietin. Urine produced in the kidneys passes through the ureters to the bladder, where it is temporarily stored, and is then released to the exterior through the urethra.

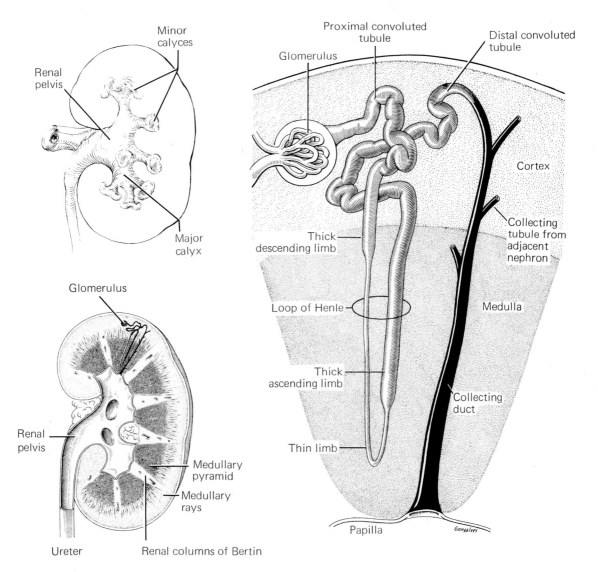

Figure 20–1. *Left:* The general organization of the kidney. *Right:* Parts of a juxtamedullary nephron and its collecting tubule (the latter shown in black).

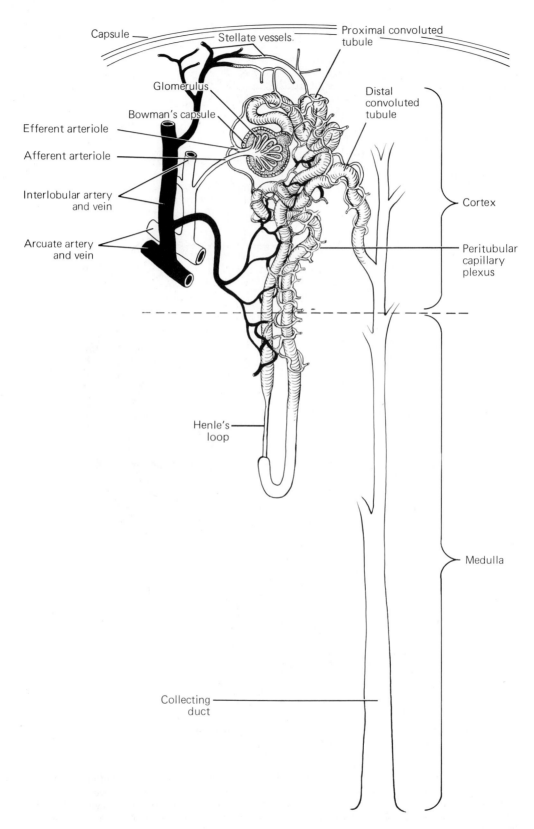

Figure 20–2. Schematic diagram of the vascular supply of a nephron in the outer part of the cortex. Arteries and capillaries are white; veins are black.

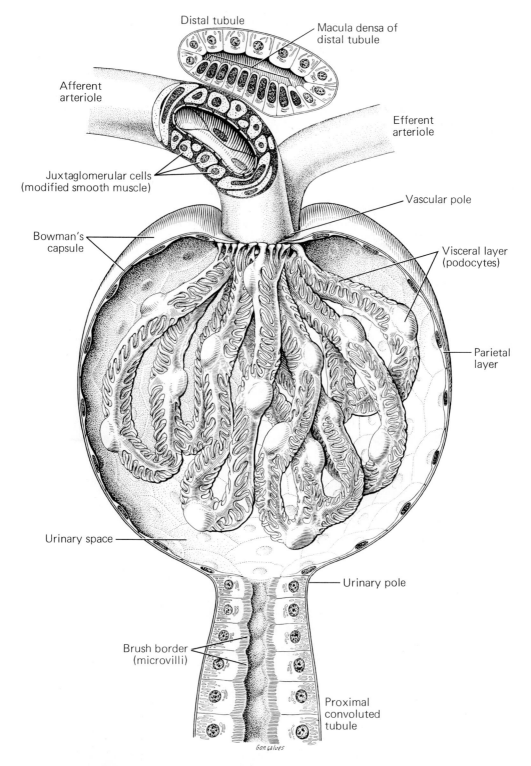

Distal tubule

Macula densa of
distal tubule

Afferent
arteriole

Efferent
arteriole

Juxtaglomerular cells
(modified smooth muscle)

Vascular pole

Bowman's
capsule

Visceral layer
(podocytes)

Parietal
layer

Urinary space

Urinary pole

Brush border
(microvilli)

Proximal
convoluted
tubule

Gonçalves

Figure 20–3. The renal corpuscle. The upper part shows the vascular pole, with afferent and efferent arterioles and the macula densa. Note the juxtaglomerular cells in the wall of the afferent arteriole. Podocytes cover glomerular capillaries. The part of the podocyte containing the nucleus protrudes into the urinary space, while podocyte processes cover the outer surfaces of the glomerular capillaries. Note the flattened cells of the parietal layer of Bowman's capsule. The lower part of the drawing shows the urinary pole and the proximal convoluted tubule.

THE KIDNEYS

Each kidney is about 11 cm long, 6 cm wide, and 3 cm thick and weighs about 150 g. A kidney resembles a bean with a concave medial border, the **hilum**—where nerves enter, blood and lymph vessels enter and exit, and the ureter exits—and a convex lateral surface (Fig 20–1). Kidney tissue surrounds a cavity, the **renal sinus,** that contains the **renal pelvis.** The renal pelvis is the expanded upper end of the ureter and is divided into 2 or 3 **major calyces.** Several smaller branches, the **minor calyces,** arise from each major calyx (Fig 20–1). The kidney is contained within a thin, collagenous **renal capsule** and is surrounded by a mass of perirenal adipose tissue.

The kidney can be divided into an outer, granular-appearing **cortex** and an inner, striated-appearing **me-**dulla (Figs 20–1 and 20–2). In humans, the renal medulla is composed of 10–18 conical or pyramidal structures, the **medullary pyramids,** whose bases form the corticomedullary junction and whose vertices protrude into the minor calyces (Fig 20–1). The tips of the pyramids are called **renal papillae** and are perforated by 10–25 orifices, the openings of the **collecting ducts,** forming the **area cribrosa.**

From the base of each medullary pyramid, parallel arrays of tubules, called **medullary rays,** penetrate the cortex (Fig 20–1). Each medullary ray consists of one or more collecting tubules together with the straight portions of several **nephrons,** the functional units of the kidney. Surrounding each medullary ray is the **cortical labyrinth,** consisting of renal corpuscles and convoluted portions of the nephron. The mass of cortical tissue surmounting each medullary pyramid

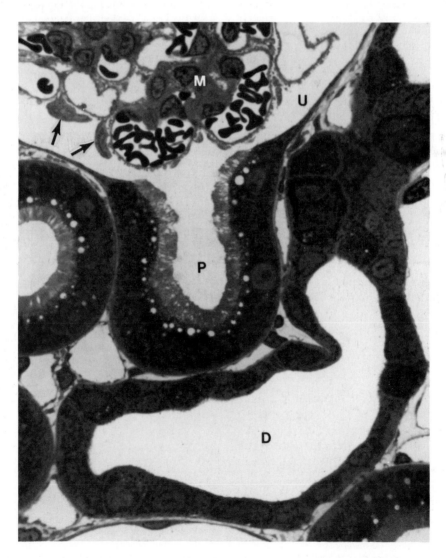

Figure 20–4. Section of rat kidney cortex showing the urinary pole of a renal corpuscle. Arrows point to 2 podocytes that encompass the capillaries of the renal glomerulus. P, proximal convoluted tubule; D, distal convoluted tubule; U, urinary space; M, mesangial cells. × 950. (Courtesy of SL Wissig.)

forms a **renal lobe,** and each medullary ray forms the center of a conical **renal lobule** (Fig 20–20). Cortical tissue is also found between medullary pyramids, and these structures are termed **columns of Bertin** (Fig 20–1).

Nephrons

Each kidney is composed of 1–4 million functional filtering units called nephrons. Each nephron consists of (1) a dilated portion, the **renal corpuscle;** (2) the **proximal convoluted tubule;** (3) the thin and thick limbs of the **loop of Henle;** and (4) the **distal convoluted tubule** (Fig 20–1). The **collecting tubules** and **ducts,** which are of different embryologic origin from the nephron, collect the urine produced by nephrons and conduct it to the renal pelvis. The nephron and the collecting duct into which it empties constitute a **uriniferous tubule.**

Each renal corpuscle is about 200 μm in diameter and consists of a tuft of capillaries, the **glomerulus,** surrounded by a double-walled epithelial capsule called **Bowman's capsule** (Figs 20–1, 20–2, 20–3, and 20–18). The internal layer of the capsule envelops the capillaries of the glomerulus and is called the **visceral layer,** whereas the external layer forms the outer limit of the renal corpuscle and is called the

parietal layer of Bowman's capsule (Figs 20–2 and 20–3). Between the 2 layers of Bowman's capsule is the **urinary space,** which receives the fluid filtered through the capillary wall and the visceral layer. Each renal corpuscle has a **vascular pole,** where the **afferent arteriole** enters and the **efferent arteriole** leaves (Fig 20–18), and a **urinary pole,** where the proximal convoluted tubule begins (Fig 20–3 and 20–4). After entering the renal corpuscle, the afferent arteriole usually divides into 2–5 primary branches, each of which subdivides into capillaries, forming the renal glomerulus.

The parietal layer of Bowman's capsule consists of a simple squamous epithelium supported by a basal lamina and a thin layer of reticular fibers (Figs 20–3 and 20–5). At the urinary pole, the epithelium changes to the simple columnar epithelium characteristic of the proximal tubule (Figs 20–3 and 20–4).

While the epithelium of the parietal layer remains relatively unchanged, the internal or visceral layer is greatly modified during embryonic development. The cells of this internal layer, called **podocytes** (Figs 20–3, 20–6, 20–7, and 20–8), have a cell body from which arise several **primary processes.** Each primary process gives rise to numerous **secondary processes** (Figs 20–6, 20–7, and 20–8) that embrace

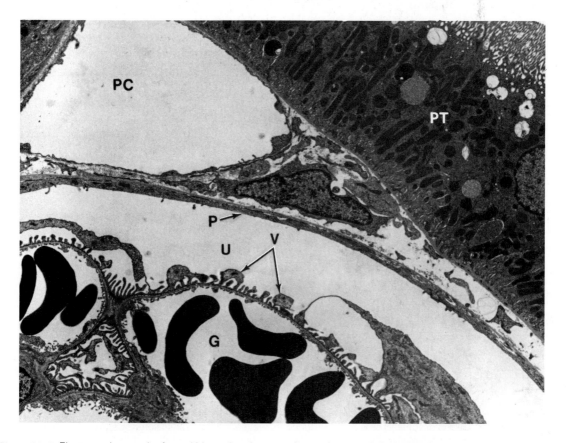

Figure 20–5. Electron micrograph of a rat kidney showing part of a renal corpuscle including the parietal layer of Bowman's capsule (P), the urinary space (U), glomerular capillaries (G) containing erythrocytes, and the visceral layer of Bowman's capsule (V). PC, peritubular capillary; PT, proximal tubule. × 2850. (Courtesy of SL Wissig.)

the capillaries of the glomerulus. At a regular distance of 25 nm, the secondary processes (**pedicels**) are in direct contact with the basal lamina, which is formed jointly by capillary endothelial cells and podocytes. However, the cell bodies of podocytes and their primary processes do not touch the basal lamina (Figs 20–6 and 20–8). The pedicels from one podocyte embrace more than one capillary, and on a single capillary, the pedicels of 2 podocytes alternate in position next to the basal lamina (Fig 20–8). Pedicels contain few or no organelles, but microfilaments and microtubules are numerous.

The secondary processes of podocytes interdigitate, delimiting elongated spaces, about 25 nm wide— the **filtration slits.** Spanning adjacent processes (and, therefore, bridging the filtration slits), a thin diaphragm has been described that is about 6 nm thick and is comparable to the diaphragm encountered in fenestrated endothelial cells. The cytoplasm of podocytes contains numerous free ribosomes, a few cisternae of rough endoplasmic reticulum, infrequent mitochondria, and a prominent Golgi complex, as well as vesicles and microfilaments (Figs 20–8 and 20–9).

Between the fenestrated endothelial cells of the glomerular capillaries and the podocytes that cover their external surfaces is a thick (~ 0.1 μm) basal lamina. This layer is believed to be the filtration barrier separating blood contained in the capillaries from the urinary space. This basal lamina is derived from the fusion of capillary- and podocyte-produced basal laminae. With the aid of the electron microscope, one can distinguish a central electron-dense layer (lamina densa) and, on each side, a more electron-lucent layer (lamina rara; Fig 20–9). Histochemical methods are

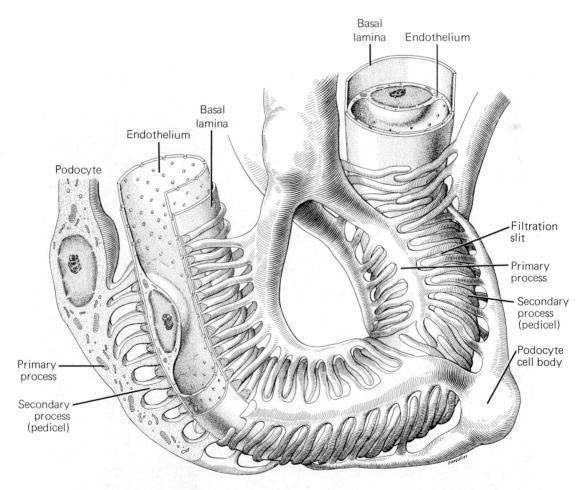

Figure 20–6. Schematic representation of a glomerular capillary, with the visceral layer of Bowman's capsule (formed by podocytes). In this capillary, endothelial cells are fenestrated; however, the basal lamina on which they rest is continuous. At left is a podocyte shown in partial section. As viewed from the outside, the part of the podocyte containing the nucleus protrudes into Bowman's space. Each podocyte has many primary processes from which arise an even greater number of secondary processes. The secondary processes are in contact with the basal lamina. (Redrawn and modified after Gordon. Reproduced, with permission, from Ham AW: *Histology,* 6th ed. Lippincott, 1969.)

providing evidence that the 2 electron-lucent zones have biochemical compositions different from those of the denser central zone. Heparan sulfate, which is a polyanionic molecule, has been detected in the electron-lucent zones, where it could impede the passage of negatively charged proteins across the basal lamina. Thus, the glomerular basal lamina is a selective macromolecular filter in which the collagen (type IV) present in the lamina densa acts as a physical filter, while the anionic sites in the laminae rarae act as a charge barrier. Particles greater than 10 nm in diameter do not readily cross the basal lamina, and negatively charged proteins with molecular weights greater than that of albumin (MW 69,000) pass across only sparingly. In diseases such as diabetes mellitus, the glomerular filter becomes much more permeable to proteins.

The endothelial cells of glomerular capillaries have a thin cytoplasm that is thicker around the nucleus, where most of the organelles are clustered. The fenestrae of these cells are larger (70–90 nm in diameter) and more numerous than in the fenestrated capillaries of other organs, and they lack the thin diaphragm commonly observed spanning the openings of other fenestrated capillaries.

Besides endothelial cells and podocytes, the glomerular capillaries have **mesangial cells** adhering to their walls in places where the basal lamina forms a sheath that is shared by 2 or more capillaries (Figs 20–4 and 20–10). Mesangial cells possess short cytoplasmic extensions and are covered by a layer of amorphous material resembling the lamina densa of basal laminae. Little is known about their function, but they may be supporting elements for the capillaries and constitute a pericytelike population of cells. After the injection of ferritin (an electron-scattering, iron-containing protein easily identified with the electron microscope), the cytoplasm of mesangial cells appears to be engorged with this protein. These cells may act as macrophages and serve to clean the basal lamina of particulate material that accumulates during the filtration process.

Proximal Convoluted Tubule

At the urinary pole of the renal corpuscle, the squamous epithelium of the parietal layer of Bow-

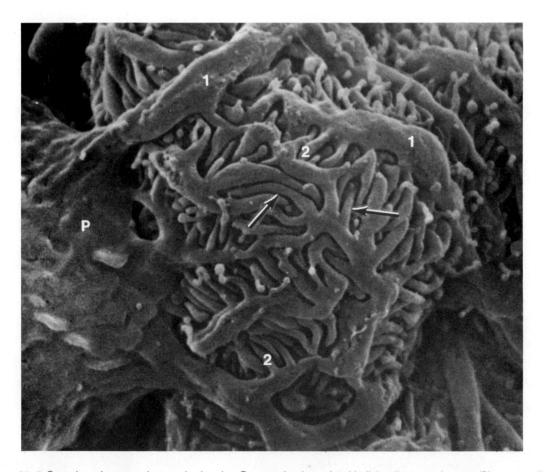

Figure 20–7. Scanning electron micrograph showing Bowman's visceral epithelial cells, or podocytes (P), surrounding capillaries of the renal glomerulus. Two orders of branching of the podocyte processes are apparent: the primary processes (1) and the secondary processes, or pedicels (2). The small spaces between adjacent processes constitute the filtration slits (arrows). × 10,700.

man's capsule is continuous with the columnar epithelium of the proximal convoluted tubule (Figs 20–1, 20–2, and 20–4). It is longer than the distal convoluted tubule and is therefore more frequently seen near renal corpuscles in the cortical labyrinth.

The proximal convoluted tubule is lined by simple cuboidal or columnar epithelium (Figs 20–4, 20–11, and 20–12). The cells of this epithelium have an acidophilic cytoplasm owing to the presence of numerous elongated mitochondria. The cell apex possesses abundant microvilli about 1 μm in length which form a **brush border** (Figs 20–3, 20–11, 20–12, and 20–13). Because the cells are large, each transverse section of a proximal tubule contains only 3–5 spherical nuclei, usually located in the center of the cell (Fig 20–11).

In the living animal, proximal convoluted tubules have a wide lumen and are surrounded by peritubular capillaries. In routine histologic preparations, the brush border is usually disorganized and the peritubular capillary lumens are greatly reduced in size or collapsed.

Related to the capacity of proximal tubule cells for reabsorbing macromolecules, the apical cytoplasm of these cells has numerous canaliculi between the bases of the microvilli. Pinocytotic vesicles are formed by evaginations of the canalicular membranes (Fig 20–14). These vesicles contain macromolecules (mainly proteins with molecular weights less than 70,000) that have passed across the glomerular filter. The pinocytotic vesicles fuse with lysosomes where degradation of macromolecules occurs, and monomers are returned to the circulation. The basal portions of these cells have abundant membrane invaginations and lateral interdigitations with neighboring cells. The Na$^+$/K$^+$-ATPase (''sodium pump'') responsible for actively transporting sodium ions out of these cells is localized in these basolateral membranes. Mitochondria are concentrated at the base of the cell (Figs 20–12, 20–13, and 20–14) and arranged parallel to the long axis of the cell. This mitochondrial location and the increase in the area of the cell membrane at the base of the cell are characteristics of cells engaged in active ion transport (see Chapter 4). Because of the extensive interdigitation of the lateral membranes, no discrete cell margins can be observed with the light microscope between cells of the proximal tubule.

Loop of Henle

The loop of Henle is a U-shaped structure consisting of (1) a **thick descending limb,** very similar in structure to the proximal convoluted tubule; (2) a **thin descending limb;** (3) a **thin ascending limb;**

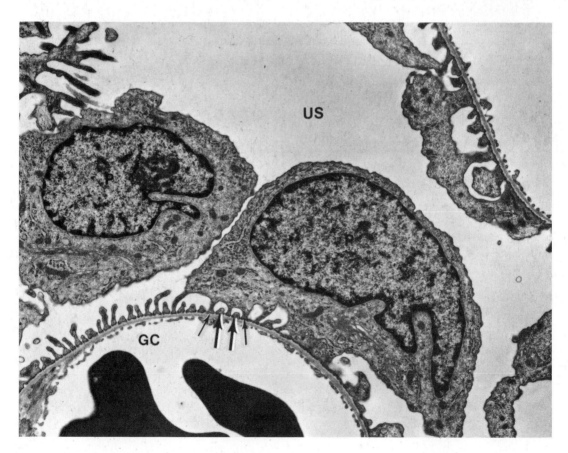

Figure 20–8. Electron micrograph showing the cell bodies of 2 podocytes (P) and the alternation of secondary processes from 2 different cells (arrows). US, urinary space; GC, glomerular capillary. × 9000. (Courtesy of SL Wissig.)

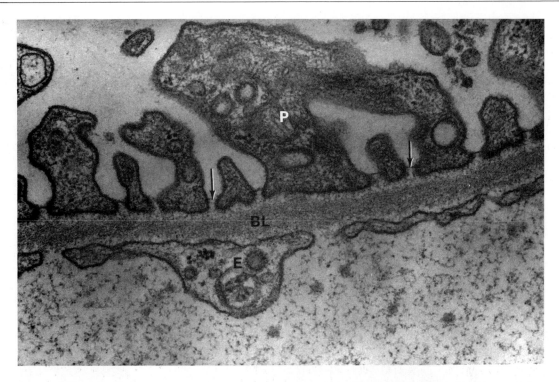

Figure 20–9. Electron micrograph of the filtration barrier in a renal corpuscle. Note the endothelium (E) with open fenestrae, the fused basal laminae of epithelial and endothelial cells (BL), and the processes of podocytes (P). The basal lamina consists of a central lamina densa bounded on both sides by a light-staining lamina rara. Arrows indicate the thin diaphragms crossing the filtration slits. × 45,750. (Courtesy of SL Wissig.)

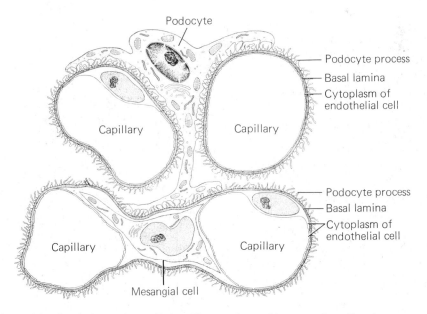

Figure 20–10. Mesangial cells of glomerular capillaries. They are located between 2 capillary lumens, enveloped by the basal lamina.

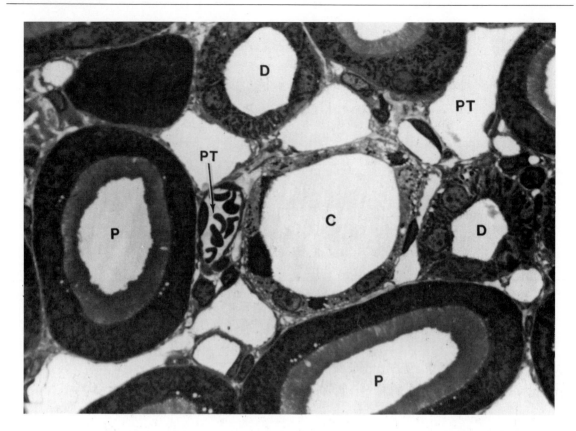

Figure 20–11. Section of rat kidney showing cross sections of proximal convoluted tubules (P) with a prominent brush border, distal convoluted tubules (D), a collecting duct (C), and numerous peritubular capillaries (PT), only one of which contains erythrocytes. × 1130. (Courtesy of SL Wissig.)

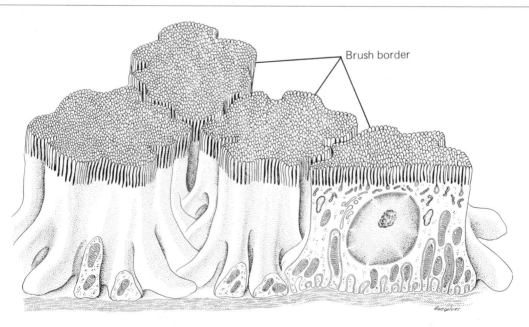

Figure 20–12. Schematic drawing of proximal convoluted tubule cells. These cuboidal cells have abundant microvilli constituting the brush border on their apical surfaces. They have 2 types of lateral processes: some along the whole side of the cell and others only in the basal half of the cell. The latter are longer than the former and penetrate deeply among the neighboring cells. In order to make the drawing more easily understandable, artificial spaces have been shown among the cells. (Modified from a figure [5] by Bulger R: *Am J Anat* 1965;**116**:237.)

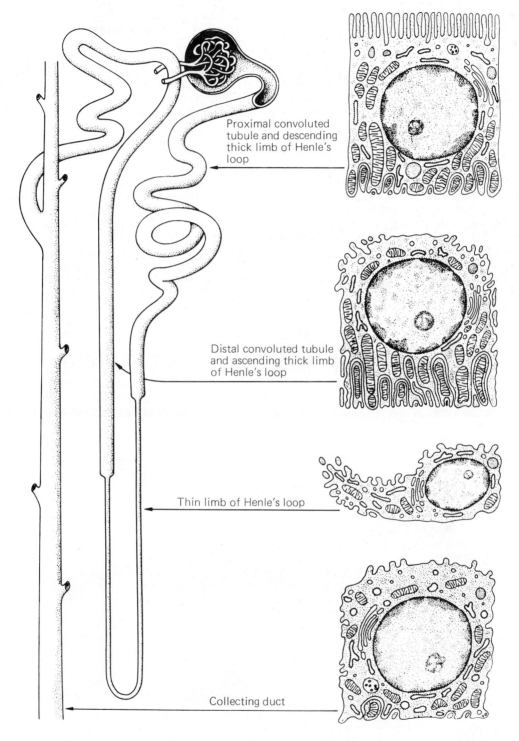

Figure 20–13. Cellular ultrastructure of the nephron represented schematically. Cells of the ascending thick limb of Henle's loop and the distal tubule are similar in their ultrastructure, but they differ in function.

and (4) a **thick ascending limb,** which closely resembles the distal convoluted tubule in structure. In the outer medulla, the thick descending limb, with an outer diameter of about 60 μm, suddenly narrows to about 12 μm and continues as the thin descending limb. The lumen of this segment of the nephron is wide because the wall consists of squamous epithelial cells whose nuclei protrude only slightly into the lumen (Figs 20–15 and 20–16). A brush border is absent, but short, irregularly spaced microvilli are present. There is some variation in cell structure along the length of the thin limb. Until recently, the thin ascending limb was believed to actively transport Na^+ from the lumen into the renal interstitium. However, these cells do not have the ultrastructural characteristics of ion-transporting cells. The thin limbs resemble blood capillaries, with which they may be confused; differences in content, appearance of nuclei, and thickness of the wall are the main criteria used for differentiation.

Approximately one-seventh of all nephrons are located near the corticomedullary junction and are therefore called **juxtamedullary nephrons.** The other nephrons are called **cortical nephrons.** All nephrons participate in the processes of filtration, reabsorption,

and secretion. However, juxtamedullary nephrons are of prime importance in establishing the gradient of hypertonicity in the medullary interstitium, which is the basis of the kidney's ability to produce a hypertonic urine. Juxtamedullary nephrons have very long loops of Henle, extending deep into the medulla. These loops consist of a short thick descending limb, long thin descending and ascending limbs, and a thick ascending limb (Fig 20–13). Cortical nephrons have very short descending thin limbs and no thin ascending limbs (Fig 20–2). The thin limbs of juxtamedullary nephrons are responsible for producing the hypertonic environment of the medullary interstitium.

Distal Convoluted Tubule

When the thick ascending limb of the loop of Henle penetrates the cortex, it preserves its histologic structure (Fig 20–13) but becomes tortuous and is called the distal convoluted tubule, which is the last segment of the nephron (Fig 20–1). This tubule is lined by simple cuboidal epithelium.

In histologic sections, the distinction between the proximal and distal convoluted tubules, both found in the cortex, is based on the following characteristics. Cells of proximal tubules are larger, have brush bor-

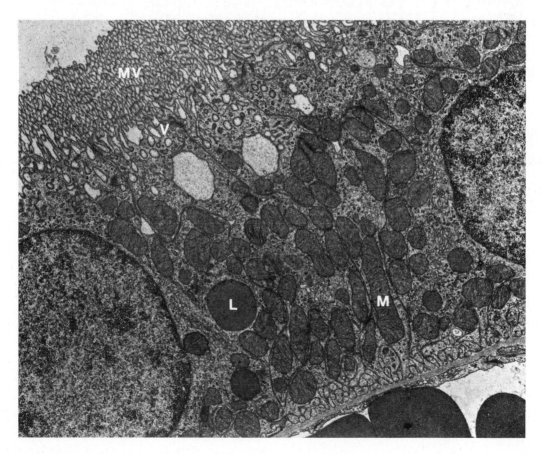

Figure 20–14. Electron micrograph of a proximal convoluted tubule. Note the obliquely sectioned microvilli (MV), the pinocytotic (apical) vesicles (V), a lysosome (L), and the mitochondria (M). A peritubular capillary appears in the lower right corner. × 9500. (Courtesy of SL Wissig.)

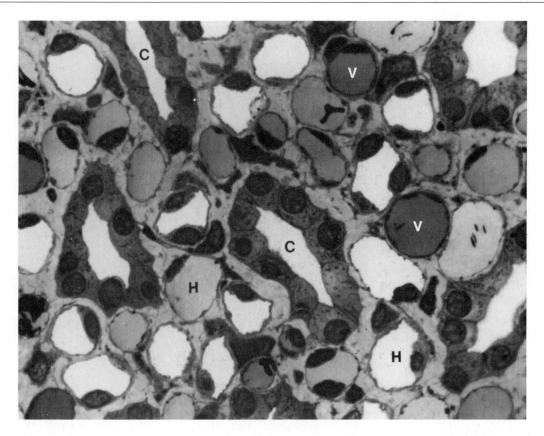

Figure 20–15. Cross section through the medulla of a rat kidney showing collecting tubules (C), capillary vessels of the vasa recta (V), and thin limbs of Henle's loop (H). × 1100. (Courtesy of SL Wissig.)

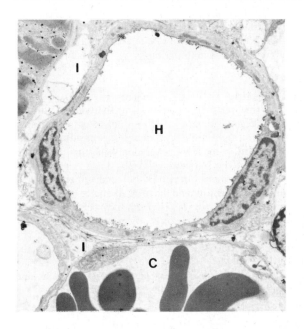

Figure 20–16. Electron micrograph of the thin part of Henle's loop (H) composed entirely of squamous cells. Note fenestrated capillaries with red blood cells (C) and the interstitium (I) with bundles of collagen fibrils. × 3300. (Courtesy of J Rhodin.)

ders, and are more acidophilic because of the abundance of mitochondria (Figs 20–11 and 20–14). The lumens of the distal tubules are larger, and because distal tubule cells are flatter and smaller than those of the proximal tubule, more cells and more nuclei are seen in the distal tubule wall than in the proximal tubule wall in the same histologic section. Distal tubule cells are less acidophilic than proximal tubule cells, and they do not have the prominent brush borders found on proximal tubule cells. The apical canaliculi and vesicles that characterize the proximal tubule are absent in distal tubule cells. Lateral boundaries between these cells are not observed with the light microscope because of the interdigitations between adjacent cells. Cells of the distal convoluted tubule have elaborate basal membrane invaginations and associated mitochondria indicative of their ion transport function (Fig 20–17).

Along its path in the cortex, the distal convoluted tubule establishes contact with the vascular pole of the renal corpuscle of its parent nephron. At this point of close contact, the distal tubule is modified, as is the afferent arteriole. In this juxtaglomerular region, cells of the distal convoluted tubule usually become columnar, and their nuclei are closely packed together. Most of the cells have a Golgi complex in the basal region. This modified segment of the wall of the distal

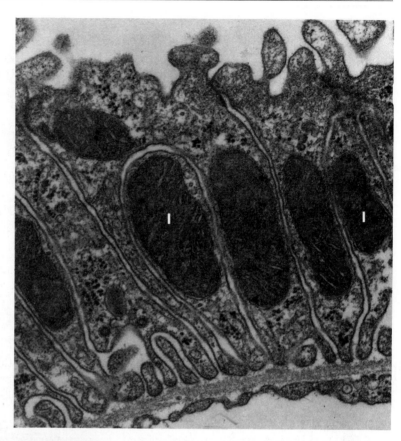

Figure 20–17 (at right). Electron micrograph of a distal convoluted tubule showing the numerous invaginations of the basal plasma membrane and associated mitochondria. Regions labeled I are interdigitations of adjacent distal tubule cells. × 30,600. (Courtesy of SL Wissig.)

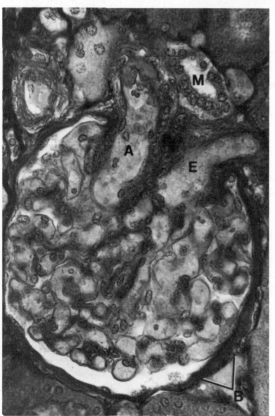

tubule, which appears darker in microscopic preparations (because of the close proximity of its nuclei), is called the **macula densa** (Figs 20–3 and 20–18). The functional significance of the macula densa, although not certain, may be to transfer to the afferent arteriole data on the osmolarity of the fluid in the distal tubule.

Collecting Tubules & Ducts

Urine passes from the distal convoluted tubules to collecting tubules, which join each other, forming larger, straight collecting ducts, the **papillary ducts of Bellini,** which widen gradually as they approach the tips of the pyramids (Fig 20–1).

The smaller collecting tubules are lined with cuboidal epithelium and have a diameter of approximately 40 μm (Fig 20–11). As they penetrate deeper into the medulla, their cells become taller (Fig 20–15) until they are columnar cells. The diameter of the collecting duct reaches 200 μm near the tips of the pyramids.

Along their entire extent, collecting tubules and ducts are composed of cells that stain weakly with the

Figure 20–18 (at left). Section of a human renal corpuscle showing the afferent arteriole (A), the efferent arteriole (E), and the macula densa (M). B, Bowman's capsule. × 325.

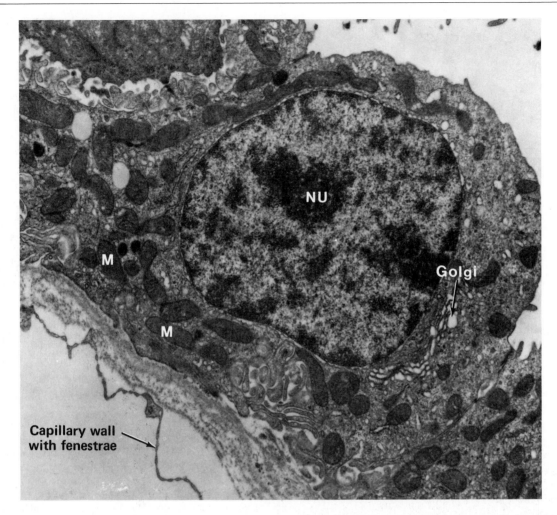

Figure 20–19. Electron micrograph of a collecting tubule wall. Note the mitochondria (M), Golgi complex, and the nucleolus (Nu). × 15,000.

usual stains. They have an electron-lucent cytoplasm with few organelles (Figs 20–13 and 20–19) and almost no invaginations of the basal cell membrane. In collecting tubules and cortical collecting ducts, a dark-staining cell, the intercalated cell, is also seen (Fig 20–11). Its significance is not understood. The intercellular limits of collecting tubule and duct cells are clearly visible under the light microscope, since there are no interdigitations between the lateral margins of adjacent cells (Fig 20–15). Cortical collecting ducts are joined at right angles by several generations of smaller collecting tubules draining each medullary ray. In the medulla, collecting ducts are a major component of the urine-concentrating mechanism.

Juxtaglomerular Apparatus

Adjacent to the renal corpuscle, the media of the afferent arteriole consists of modified smooth muscle cells. These cells, called **juxtaglomerular (JG) cells** (Fig 20–3), have ellipsoid nuclei and a cytoplasm full

of granules that stain with the PAS technique. The macula densa of the distal convoluted tubule is usually located close to the region of the afferent arteriole containing the juxtaglomerular cells, forming, with this portion of the arteriole, the juxtaglomerular apparatus (Figs 20–3 and 20–18). Also a part of the juxtaglomerular apparatus are some lightly staining cells whose functions are not well understood. They are variously called extraglomerular mesangial cells, lacis cells, or polkissen ("pole cushions"). In the area of the juxtaglomerular cells, the internal elastic membrane of the afferent arteriole disappears.

When examined with the electron microscope, juxtaglomerular cells have characteristics of protein-secreting cells, including an abundant rough endoplasmic reticulum, a highly developed Golgi complex, and secretory granules measuring approximately 10–40 nm in diameter. Juxtaglomerular cells produce the enzyme **renin,** and the amount of renin present in a kidney is proportionate to the number of secretory

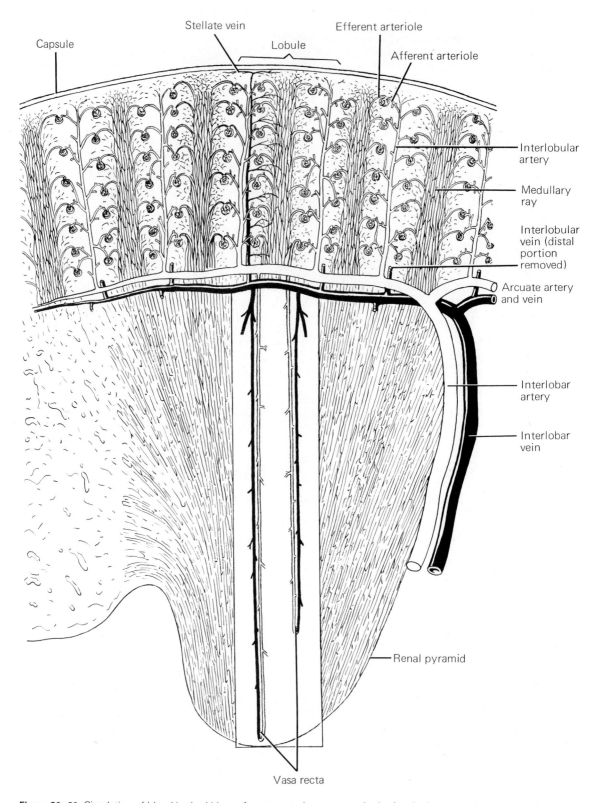

Figure 20–20. Circulation of blood in the kidney. Arcuate arteries are seen in the border between the cortex and medulla.

granules in these cells; furthermore, fluorescent antibodies (antirenin) have been shown to react specifically with the juxtaglomerular cells. Renin acts on a plasma protein called **angiotensinogen,** producing an inactive decapeptide called **angiotensin I.** This substance, as a result of the action of a converting enzyme present in high concentration in lung endothelial cells, loses 2 amino acids, becoming an octapeptide called **angiotensin II.**

After a significant blood loss, renin secretion increases. This is probably detected by decreased tension in the juxtaglomerular cells in the wall of the afferent arteriole. Angiotensin II is produced, and its main physiologic effect is to enhance secretion of the adrenocortical hormone **aldosterone.** Aldosterone acts on cells of the renal tubules (mostly the distal tubules) to increase the reabsorption of sodium and chloride ions. This, in turn, expands the extravascular fluid volume, leading to an increase in blood pressure. Increased blood pressure distends the juxtaglomerular cells and inhibits renin secretion, thus completing the negative feedback loop. Sodium deficiency can initiate a similar reaction. Angiotensin II is also a potent vasoconstrictor.

Blood Circulation

Each kidney receives blood from its **renal artery,** which, before entering this organ, usually divides into 2 branches: one to the anterior part of the kidney and the other to the posterior part. While still in the hilum, these branches give rise to arteries that further branch to form the **interlobar arteries** located between the renal pyramids (Figs 20–1 and 20–20). At the level of the corticomedullary junction, the interlobar arteries form the **arcuate arteries.** From the arcuate arteries, **interlobular arteries** branch off at right angles and follow a course in the cortex perpendicular to the renal capsule. Interlobular arteries form the boundaries of renal lobules, which consist of a medullary ray and the adjacent cortical labyrinth (Fig 20–20). From the interlobular arteries arise the **afferent arterioles,** which supply blood to the capillaries of the glomeruli. From these capillaries blood passes into the **efferent arterioles,** which at once branch again to form a **peritubular capillary network** that will nourish the proximal and distal tubules and carry away reabsorbed ions and low-molecular-weight materials. The efferent arterioles that are associated with juxtamedullary nephrons form long, thin capillary vessels which follow a straight path into the medulla and then loop back toward the corticomedullary boundary (Fig 20–15). These vessels are called **vasa recta,** or straight vessels. The descending vessel is a continuous-type capillary, while the ascending vessel has a fenestrated endothelium. These vessels, containing blood that has been filtered through the glomeruli, provide nourishment and oxygen to the medulla. Because of their looped structure, these vessels do not carry away the high osmotic gradient set up in the interstitium by the thin limbs of Henle's loop (Fig 20–22).

The capillaries of the outer cortex and of the capsule of the kidney converge to form the **stellate veins** (so called because of the configuration when seen from the surface of the kidney), which empty into the interlobular veins.

Veins follow the same course as arteries. Blood from interlobular veins flows into arcuate veins and from there to the interlobar veins. Interlobar veins converge to form the renal vein through which blood leaves the kidney (Fig 20–20).

Renal Interstitium

Both the cortex and the medulla contain specialized cells in the spaces between uriniferous tubules and the blood and lymph vessels. Some of these **interstitial cells** resemble fibroblasts, and others are probably lymphocytes. In the medulla, some interstitial cells have numerous small lipid droplets in their cytoplasm. These cells may produce a hormone that lowers blood pressure.

HISTOPHYSIOLOGY OF THE KIDNEY

The kidney regulates the chemical composition of the internal environment by a complex process that involves **filtration, active absorption, passive absorption,** and **secretion.** Filtration takes place in the glomerulus, where an ultrafiltrate of blood plasma is formed. The tubules of the nephron, primarily the proximal convoluted tubules, reabsorb from this filtrate the substances that are useful for body metabolism, thus maintaining the homeostasis of the internal environment. They also transfer from blood to the tubular lumen certain waste products that are eliminated with the urine. Under certain circumstances, the collecting ducts are permeable to water, thus contributing to the concentration of urine, which usually is hypertonic in relation to blood plasma. In this way, the organism controls its water, intercellular fluid, and osmotic balance.

The 2 kidneys produce about 125 mL of filtrate per minute; of this amount, 124 mL is absorbed and only 1 mL is released into the calyces as urine. Every 24 hours, about 1500 mL of urine is formed.

Filtration

The blood flow in the 2 kidneys of an adult amounts to 1.2–1.3 L of blood per minute, which means that all of the circulating blood in the body passes through the kidneys every 4–5 minutes. The glomeruli are composed of arterial capillaries in which the hydrostatic pressure is higher than that found in other capillaries. This pressure is about 45 mm Hg in rats and squirrel monkeys and is presumed to be similar in humans.

The glomerular filtrate is formed in response to the hydrostatic pressure of blood, which is opposed by the following forces: (1) osmotic ("oncotic") pressure of plasma colloids (20 mm Hg), and (2) hydrostatic pressure of the fluids in Bowman's capsule (10 mm Hg). The net filtration pressure at the afferent end of glomerular capillaries is thus 15 mm Hg.

The glomerular filtrate has a chemical composition similar to that of blood plasma but contains almost no protein, since macromolecules do not readily cross the glomerular wall. The largest protein molecules that succeed in crossing the glomerular filter have a molecular weight of about 70,000, and small amounts of plasma albumin appear in the filtrate.

Endothelial cells of glomerular capillaries are fenestrated with numerous openings (70- to 90-nm in diameter) without diaphragms, so that the endothelium is easily permeated. According to most authors, filtration occurs in the basal lamina. Electron microscopic examination of a kidney after injection of large molecules (eg, ferritin; MW 650,000) reveals that they pass through the endothelial cell fenestrae but are held up at the basal lamina. The basal lamina not only constitutes a size barrier but also a charge barrier. The presence of polyanions such as heparan sulfate and chondroitin sulfate proteoglycans will repel negatively charged molecules, including most serum proteins. The filtration slits between the secondary processes of podocytes also play a role in retaining molecules that pass through both the openings of endothelial cells and the matrix of the basal lamina.

Proximal Convoluted Tubule

The glomerular filtrate formed in the renal corpuscle passes into the proximal convoluted tubule, and the processes of reabsorption and excretion begin here. The site of reabsorption of diverse substances can be precisely identified, and the points of reabsorption of various substances are different. The proximal convoluted tubule reabsorbs all of the glucose and amino acids and about 85% of the sodium chloride and water contained in the filtrate. Glucose, amino acids, and sodium are absorbed by the tubular cells through an active process involving Na^+/K^+-ATPase located in the basolateral cell membranes. Water diffuses passively, following the osmotic gradient. When the amount of glucose in the filtrate exceeds the absorbing capacity of the proximal tubule, urine becomes more abundant and contains glucose.

Reabsorption of the small amount of protein present in the filtrate takes place by pinocytosis. Proteins first appear in the pinocytotic vesicles located at the bases of the microvilli. These vesicles then fuse with lysosomes, where the proteins are digested. Small peptides are hydrolyzed to amino acids by enzymes present in brush border membranes. The amino acids resulting from both of these processes are reutilized

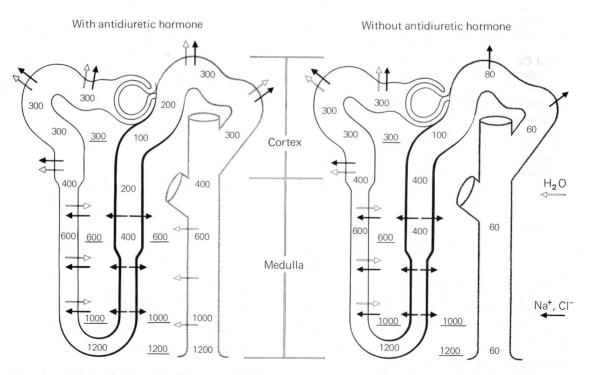

Figure 20–21. Countercurrent multiplier system formed by the loop of Henle. The segment of Henle's loop impermeable to water is represented by thick lines. The collecting tubules and ducts, which are sensitive to antidiuretic hormone (ADH), are indicated by serrated lines. *Left:* Under the influence of ADH, the urine formed is hypertonic. *Right:* With very low levels of ADH or none at all, a great quantity of hypotonic urine is formed. The numbers in the tubules and interstitial spaces indicate the local concentration in mosm/L. (Redrawn and reproduced, with permission, from Pitts RF: *Physiology of the Kidney and Body Fluids,* 2nd ed. Year Book, 1968.)

by the tubular cells or returned to the blood to be used by other cells.

In addition to these activities, the proximal convoluted tubule secretes creatinine and substances foreign to the organism such as para-aminohippuric acid, phenol red, and iodopyracet (an iodinated organic compound used as an x-ray contrast medium) from the interstitial plasma into the filtrate. This is an active process referred to as tubular secretion. Study of the rates of secretion of these substances is useful in the clinical evaluation of kidney function.

Loop of Henle

Although the filtrate that leaves the loop of Henle is hypotonic, this segment of the nephron is necessary for the formation of a final hypertonic urine, and only animals with a loop of Henle in their kidneys are capable of producing hypertonic urine. The loop of Henle creates a gradient of hypertonicity in the medullary interstitium that influences the concentration of the urine as it flows through the collecting ducts (Fig 20–21).

The descending thin limb of the loop of Henle is freely permeable to water, but the entire ascending limb is impermeable to water. In the thick ascending limb, chloride is actively transported out of the tubule, with sodium following passively, to establish the gradient of hypertonicity in the medullary interstitium necessary for urine concentration. The osmolarity of the interstitium at the tips of the pyramids is about 4 times that of blood (Fig 20–21).

Distal Convoluted Tubule

In the distal convoluted tubule, there is an ion exchange site at which, if aldosterone is present in high enough concentration, sodium is reabsorbed and potassium ions are secreted—ie, it is the site of the mechanism controlling the total salt and water in the body mentioned above in the discussion of the juxtaglomerular apparatus. The distal tubule also secretes hydrogen and ammonium ions into tubular urine. This activity is essential for maintenance of the acid-base balance in the blood.

Collecting Ducts

The epithelium of collecting ducts is responsive to antidiuretic hormone (ADH), secreted by the posterior pituitary. If water intake is limited, ADH is secreted, and the epithelium of the collecting ducts becomes permeable to water. In the presence of ADH, intramembrane particles in the luminal membrane aggregate to form what may be channels for water reabsorption.

Formation of Hypotonic or Hypertonic Urine

The loop of Henle forms a countercurrent multiplier system that generates an osmotic gradient in the medullary interstitium by repetitive transfer of relatively small amounts of sodium and chloride along the length of the loop (Fig 20–21).

Hypotonic or isotonic urine present in the collecting ducts of the medulla (the interstitial fluid of the cortex is isotonic) will lose water into the interstitium if there is enough ADH present to make the ducts permeable to water, and hypertonic urine will be formed. When ADH is lacking, the walls of the collecting ducts are impermeable to water, so that concentration of urine does not occur and the kidneys produce abundant hypotonic urine (Fig 20–21).

The vasa recta, or straight vessels, of the medullary region are situated so that blood circulation does not disturb the osmotic gradient created by the ion pump of the loop of Henle. This countercurrent exchange system is shown in Fig 20–22. The vasa recta are very thin-walled vessels, similar in structure to capillaries found in other organs. Each straight vessel forms a loop whose branches run side by side (Figs 20–15 and 20–21). While passing through the vasa

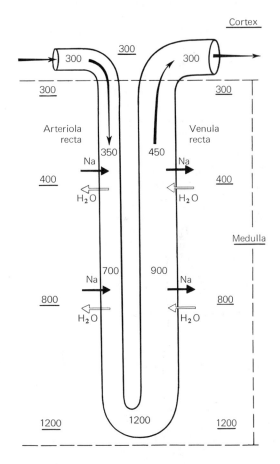

Figure 20–22. The countercurrent exchange system formed by the straight vessels of the kidney. The number 300 in the cortical segment of the arteriole and venule represents blood osmolarity (more precisely, 285–295 mosm/L). The sodium and water exchanges between these straight vessels and the interstitium are passive, depending on the osmotic gradient formed by the loop of Henle.

recta toward the inner medulla, blood loses water and gains sodium because, in the medulla, the interstitial fluid gradually becomes more and more hypertonic. Returning in the opposite direction, blood is again exposed to the same gradient—now decreasing—and therefore loses sodium and gains water. The water lost by the descending vessel is gained by the ascending one, and the sodium that enters the descending vessel is released by the ascending one. These movements of water and sodium are passive, taking place without utilization of energy. Thus, no net change in interstitial osmolarity is produced by this system, but the blood can supply oxygen and nutrients to medullary cells and carry away water that passed out of collecting ducts under the influence of ADH.

Hormonal Effects

As explained above, water balance is controlled in part by the posterior lobe of the pituitary, which secretes ADH. When there is a high intake of water, production of ADH is inhibited, the walls of the collecting ducts become impermeable to water, and water is not reabsorbed. The result is the formation of large amounts of hypotonic urine with water eliminated, while the ions necessary for osmotic balance are retained. When small amounts of water are ingested or when a great loss of water occurs (eg, owing to excessive sweating or diarrhea), the walls of collecting ducts become permeable to water, which is reabsorbed, and the urine is hypertonic.

Steroid hormones of the adrenal cortex, mainly **aldosterone,** increase distal tubular reabsorption of sodium from the filtrate and thus decrease sodium loss in the urine. Aldosterone also facilitates the elimination of potassium and hydrogen ions. This hormone is critical in maintaining electrolyte balance in the body. Aldosterone deficiency in adrenalectomized animals and in humans with **Addison's disease** results in an excessive loss of sodium in the urine.

BLADDER & URINARY PASSAGES

The bladder and the urinary passages store the urine formed in the kidneys and conduct it to the exterior. The calyces, pelvis, ureter, and bladder have the same basic histologic structure. The walls of the ureters become gradually thicker with increasing proximity to the bladder.

The mucosa of these organs consists of **transitional epithelium** and a lamina propria of loose to dense connective tissue. Surrounding the lamina propria of these organs is a dense, woven sheath of smooth muscle (Fig 20–23).

The transitional epithelium of the bladder in the undistended state is 5–6 cells in thickness; the superficial cells are rounded and bulge into the lumen. These cells are frequently polyploid or binucleate. When the epithelium is stretched, as when the bladder is full of urine, the epithelium is only 3–4 cells in thickness and the superficial cells become squamous.

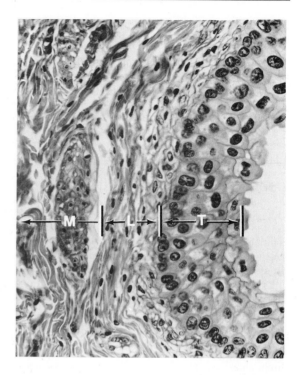

Figure 20–23. Photomicrograph of the urinary bladder wall. The transitional epithelium (T) lies on a thin lamina propria (L). A thick, woven muscularis consists of helically wound bundles of smooth muscle (M). H&E stain, reduced from × 320.

The superficial cells of the transitional epithelium are responsible for the osmotic barrier between urine and tissue fluids. They have a special membrane of thick plates separated by narrow bands of thinner membrane. When the bladder contracts, the membrane folds along the thinner regions, and the thicker plates invaginate to form fusiform cytoplasmic vesicles that represent a reservoir of these thick plates (Fig 20–24). This luminal membrane is assembled in the Golgi complex and has an unusual chemical composition; cerebroside is the major component of the polar lipid fraction.

The muscular layers in the calyces, renal pelvis, and ureters have a helical arrangement. As the ureteral muscle cells reach the bladder, they become longitudinal; therefore, the intravesical part of the ureter is composed of longitudinal fibers which then fan out distally to form the superficial trigone whose muscles continue dorsally to the verumontanum in the male and the external urethral meatus in the female.

Beginning 2–3 cm proximal to the bladder, Waldeyer's sheath of muscle is found on the outer surface of the ureter. It extends to the ureteral meatus, below which it fans out to form the deep trigone, which ends at the bladder neck.

The muscle fibers of the bladder run in every direction (without distinct layers) until they approach

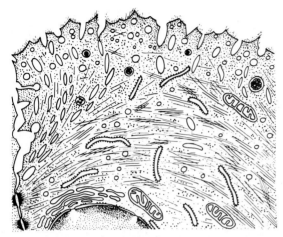

Contracted bladder

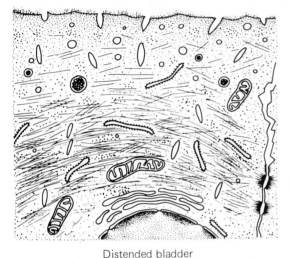

Distended bladder

Figure 20–24. Ultrastructure of superficial cells of the bladder transitional epithelium. *Top:* When the bladder is contracted. *Bottom:* When the bladder is distended by a large volume of urine.

the bladder neck, where 3 distinct layers can be identified: (1) The internal longitudinal layer, which, distal to the bladder neck, becomes circular around the prostatic urethra and the prostatic parenchyma in the male. It extends to the external meatus in the female. Its fibers form the true involuntary urethral sphincter. (2) The middle layer, which ends at the bladder neck. (3) The outer longitudinal layer, which continues to the end of the prostate and to the external urethral meatus in the female.

The ureters pass through the wall of the bladder obliquely, so that a valve is formed that prevents the backflow of urine. The intravesical ureter has only longitudinal muscle fibers.

The urinary passages are covered externally by an adventitial membrane—except for the upper part of the bladder, which is covered by (serous) peritoneum.

Urethra

The urethra is a tube that carries the urine from the bladder to the exterior. In the male, sperm also pass through it during ejaculation. In the female, the urethra is exclusively a urinary organ.

A. Male Urethra: The male urethra consists of 4 parts: a **prostatic part,** a **membranous part,** a **bulbous part,** and a **pendulous part.**

The prostate (see Chapter 23) is situated very close to the bladder, and the initial part of the urethra passes through it. Ducts that transport the secretions of the prostate open into the prostatic urethra.

In the dorsal and distal part of the prostatic urethra, there is an elevation, the **verumontanum,** which protrudes into its interior. In the tip of the verumontanum opens a blind tube called the prostatic utricle, which has no known function. On the sides of the verumontanum open the ejaculatory ducts through which the seminal fluid enters the proximal urethra to be stored just prior to ejaculation. The prostatic urethra is lined by transitional epithelium.

The membranous urethra extends for only 1 cm and is lined with pseudostratified columnar epithelium. Surrounding this part of the urethra there is a sphincter of striated muscle, the **external sphincter** of the urethra. The voluntary external striated sphincter adds further closing pressure to that exerted by the involuntary urethral sphincter formed by the continuation of the internal longitudinal muscle of the bladder.

The bulbous and pendulous parts of the urethra are located in the **corpus spongiosum** of the penis. Distally, the urethral lumen dilates, forming the **fossa navicularis.** The epithelium of this portion of the urethra is mostly pseudostratified and columnar, with areas that are squamous and stratified.

The glands of Littre are mucous glands found along the entire length of the urethra but mostly in the pendulous part. The secretory portions of some of these glands are directly linked to the epithelial lining of the urethra; others possess excretory ducts.

B. Female Urethra: The female urethra is a tube 4–5 cm long, lined with stratified squamous epithelium with areas of pseudostratified columnar epithelium. The mid part of the female urethra is surrounded by an external striated voluntary sphincter.

REFERENCES

Arakawa M, Tokunaga J: Further scanning electron microscope studies of the human glomerulus. *Lab Invest* 1974;**31:**436.

Barajas L: The ultrastructure of the juxtaglomerular apparatus as disclosed by 3-dimensional reconstruction from serial sections. *J Ultrastruct Res* 1970;**33:**116.

Barger AC, Herd JA: The renal circulation. *N Engl J Med* 1971;**284:**482.

Bing J, Karimierczac J: Renin content of different parts of the juxtaglomerular apparatus. *Acta Pathol Microbiol Scand* 1962;**54:**80.

Brenner BM, Rector FC Jr (editors): *The Kidney,* 2nd ed. Vol 1. Saunders, 1981.

Bulger RE, Dobyan DC: Recent advances in renal morphology. *Annu Rev Physiol* 1982;**44:**147.

Bulger RE et al: Human renal ultrastructure. 2. The thin limb of Henle's loop and the interstitium in healthy individuals. *Lab Invest* 1967;**16:**124.

Farquhar MG: The glomerular basement membrane: A selective macromolecular filter. In: *Cell Biology of Extracellular Matrix.* Hay E (editor). Plenum Press, 1981.

Ganong WF: Formation and excretion of urine. In: *Review of Medical Physiology,* 12th ed. Lange, 1985.

Harmanci MC et al: Antidiuretic hormone-induced intramembranous alterations in mammalian collecting ducts. *Am J Physiol* 1978;**235:**F440.

Hicks RM: The mammalian urinary bladder: An accommodating organ. *Biol Rev* 1975;**50:**215.

Jamison RL, Maffly RH: The urinary concentrating mechanism. *N Engl J Med* 1976;**295:**1059.

Kanwar YS, Farquhar MG: Presence of heparan sulfate in the glomerular basement membrane. *Proc Natl Acad Sci USA* 1979;**76:**1303.

Kanwar YS, Rosenzweig LJ: Clogging of the glomerular basement membrane. *J Cell Biol* 1982;**93:**489.

Kriz W, Lever AF: Renal countercurrent mechanisms: Structure and function. *Am Heart J* 1969;**78:**101.

Michielsen P, Creemers J: The structure and function of the glomerular mesangium. In: *Ultrastructure of the Kidney.* Dalton AJ, Haguenau F (editors). Academic Press, 1967.

Miller F, Palade GE: Lytic activities in renal protein absorption droplets: An electron microscopical cytochemical study. *J Cell Biol* 1964;**23:**519.

Muller J et al: Evidence that ADH-stimulated intramembrane particle aggregates are transferred from cytoplasmic to luminal membranes in toad bladder epithelial cells. *J Cell Biol* 1980;**85:**83.

Osvaldo L, Latta H: The thin limb of the loop of Henle. *J Ultrastruct Res* 1966;**15:**144.

Spinelli F: Structure and development of the renal glomerulus as revealed by scanning electron microscopy. *Int Rev Cytol* 1974;**39:**345.

Staehelin LA, Chlapowski FJ, Bonneville MA: Luminal plasma membrane of the urinary bladder. 1. Three-dimensional reconstruction from freeze-etch images. *J Cell Biol* 1972;**53:**73.

Venkatachalam MA et al: Structural and functional effects of glomerular polyanion. In: *Biology and Chemistry of Basement Membranes.* Kefalides NA (editor). Academic Press, 1978.

Pituitary & Hypothalamus

21

In the evolutionary development of the metazoans, multicellularity led to a division of labor wherein cells carrying out particular functions assembled into coherent associations known as tissues. The integration and coordination of the activities of various tissues are under the control of chemical messengers, the **hormones,** synthesized and released by cells of the **endocrine system.** The products of endocrine glands are not secreted through ducts but are released directly into the connective tissue or vascular network.

A hormone is an organic chemical liberated at a specific time in small amounts by endocrine cells into the tissue fluids or vascular system. In general, hormones exert their effects at a distance from the site of their secretion. The tissues and organs that hormones act on are called **target organs.** The endocrine and nervous systems, both of which have the function of integrating the activities of diverse parts of the organism, are clearly coordinated in function. Hormones of many endocrine glands have an effect on the nervous system, and several endocrine organs are stimulated or inhibited by neural mechanisms. Fig 21–1 illustrates several situations in which endocrine function is controlled by the nervous system. Most biologic phenomena are under the overlapping control of both systems. This interlocking mechanism is so remarkable that its nervous and endocrine elements are regarded as constituting a single **neuroendocrine system.**

The structure, histophysiology, and cytophysiology of the endocrine glands comprise the subject matter of this and the following chapters.

PITUITARY (Hypophysis)

The **pituitary gland,** or **hypophysis,** weighs about 0.5 g, and its normal dimensions in humans are about $10 \times 13 \times 6$ mm. It lies in a bony cavity of the sphenoid bone called the **sella turcica,** an important radiologic landmark. The pituitary gland is connected to the hypothalamus at the base of the brain, with which it has important anatomic and functional relationships.

During embryogenesis, the pituitary develops partly from oral ectoderm and partly from nerve tissue. The neural component arises as an evagination from the floor of the diencephalon and grows caudally as a stalk, without detaching itself from the brain. The oral component arises as an outpocketing of ectoderm from the roof of the primitive mouth of the embryo and grows cranially, forming a structure called **Rathke's pouch.** Later, a constriction at the base of this pouch separates it from the oral cavity. Its anterior wall thickens at the same time, so that the lumen of Rathke's pouch is reduced to a small fissure (Fig 21–2).

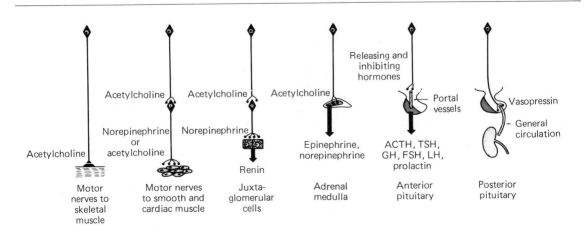

Figure 21–1. Diagrammatic representation of 6 situations in which humoral substances are released by neurons. The last 2 are examples of neurosecretion. (Reproduced, with permission, from Ganong WF: *Review of Medical Physiology,* 12th ed. Lange, 1985.)

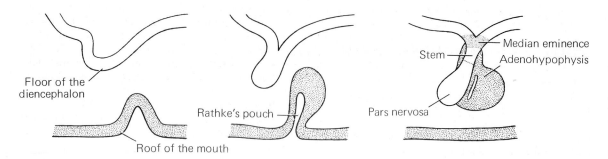

Figure 21–2. Diagram of the development of the adenohypophysis and neurohypophysis. The ectoderm of the roof of the mouth and its derivatives is stippled (lower portion). In the upper portion is the neural ectoderm from the floor of the diencephalon.

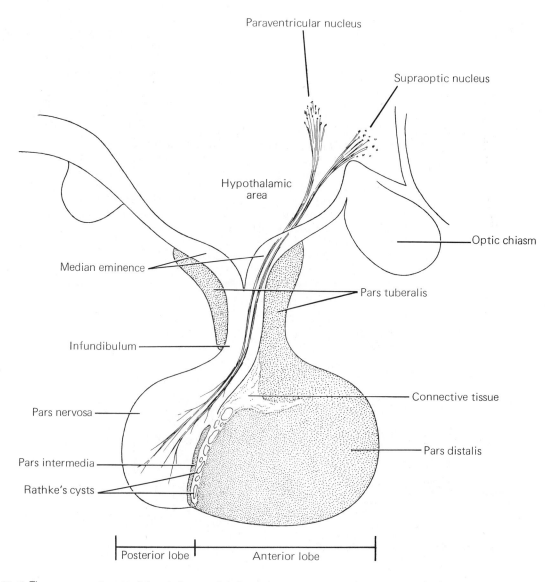

Figure 21–3. The component parts of the pituitary and their relation to the hypothalamus. The pars tuberalis, pars distalis, and pars intermedia form the adenohypophysis. The infundibulum and pars nervosa form the neurohypophysis. (Modified, redrawn, and reproduced, with permission, from the *Ciba Collection of Medical Illustrations,* by Frank H. Netter, MD.)

The part of the pituitary that develops from nerve tissue is the **neurohypophysis.** It consists of a large portion, the **pars nervosa,** or **infundibular process,** and the smaller **infundibulum,** or **neural stalk** (Fig 21–3). The infundibulum is composed of the **stem** and **median eminence.** The infundibulum is continuous with the hypothalamus and connects the pituitary with the central nervous system. Through the infundibulum pass important nerve tracts destined for the pars nervosa, as well as substances that act upon the anterior lobe of the pituitary.

The part of the pituitary that arises from oral ectoderm is known as the **adenohypophysis** and is subdivided into 3 portions: a large part, the **pars distalis** or **anterior lobe;** a cranial part, the **pars tuberalis,** which surrounds the infundibulum; and the **pars intermedia,** which lies between the neurohypophysis and the pars distalis, separated from the latter by the remaining cavity of Rathke's pouch, the residual cleft (Fig 21–3). The **posterior lobe** of the pituitary consists of the pars nervosa and the pars intermedia.

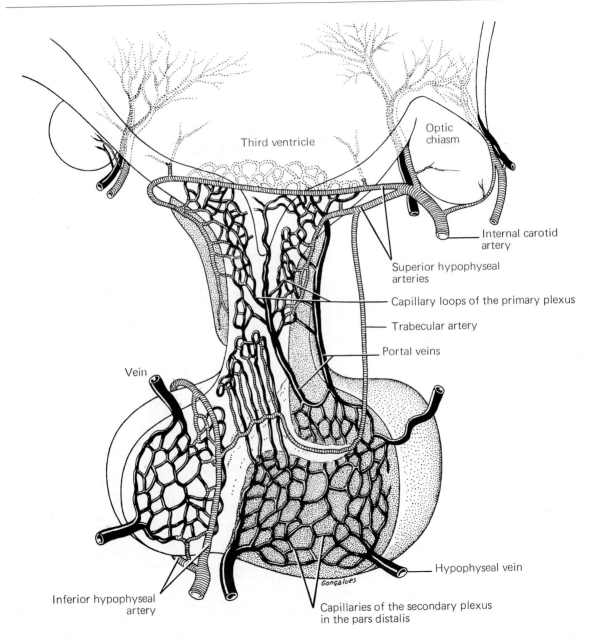

Figure 21–4. Diagram of the blood circulation in the pituitary, including the portal system. (Redrawn and reproduced, with permission, from the *Ciba Collection of Medical Illustrations,* by Frank H. Netter, MD.)

Blood Supply

The blood supply of the pituitary derives from 2 groups of blood vessels: from above, the right and left **superior hypophyseal arteries** supply the median eminence and the infundibulum; from below, the right and left **inferior hypophyseal arteries** mainly provide for the neurohypophysis and a small supply to the stalk. Both groups of arteries arise from the internal carotid arteries. The superior hypophyseal arteries supply blood to the proximal portion of the pituitary stalk (median eminence). Here these arteries break up into a **primary capillary plexus** consisting of fenestrated capillaries. Neurosecretory neurons, containing releasing or inhibitory hormones (factors) affecting adenohypophyseal function, end in close proximity to the basal lamina surrounding these capillaries (Fig 21–2). The capillaries of the primary plexus rejoin to form the long **portal veins** that traverse the pituitary stalk and ultimately break up into a **secondary capillary plexus** in close relationship to cells of the adenohypophysis (Fig 21–4). This **hypophyseal portal system** is of the utmost importance in regulating anterior pituitary function. Blood from both pituitary lobes drains into the cavernous sinuses through a number of venous channels (Fig 21–4).

The nerve supply of the anterior lobe is derived from the carotid plexus, which accompanies the arteriolar branches. These nerves appear to have a vaso-

motor function and do not directly affect the cells of the anterior lobe.

ADENOHYPOPHYSIS

Pars Distalis

The part of the pituitary arising from oral ectoderm, the pars distalis, is composed of several types of secretory cells arranged as cords or follicles. Other types of cells present include numerous capillary endothelial cells as well as relatively few fibroblasts that produce the reticular fibers which support the cords of hormone-secreting cells. The pars distalis comprises 75% of the mass of the pituitary gland.

Two classes of epithelial cells have been described in the pars distalis: chromophobe and chromophil cells. **Chromophobe cells** make up about 50% of the epithelial cells in the anterior lobe. They are so named because they do not stain intensely with the usual dyes used in studying pituitary cytology (Figs 21–5 and 21–9). When observed with the light microscope, chromophobes tend to occur in clusters, show no visible secretory granules, and have a small amount of pale-staining cytoplasm. Electron microscopic examination reveals that some chromophobes have a few secretory granules, and it is now believed that they are degranulated representatives of the several chro-

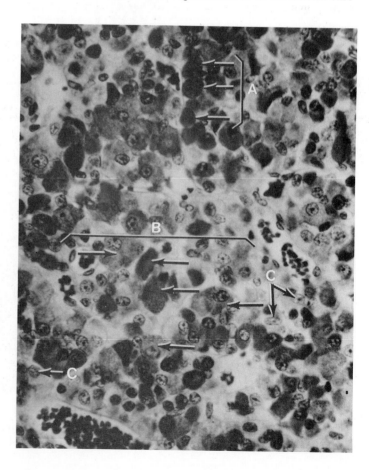

Figure 21–5 (at right). Photomicrograph of a section of the pars distalis of the pituitary. At (A), acidophilic cells stain orange-red; at (B), basophilic cells (lower arrows) stain blue. At left and right, note unstained chromophobe (C) cells. Mallory's stain, × 185.

mophil cell types. Most chromophobes belong to a class of cells called **follicular cells.** These cells have long, branching processes that seem to form a supporting network for the other parenchymal cells of the anterior pituitary.

Using a variety of dyes, **chromophil cells** can be differentiated into **acidophils** (40%), which bind acid dyes such as orange G, and **basophils** (10%), which are stained by several basic dyes including aniline blue. Basophils can also be demonstrated using the periodic acid–Schiff (PAS) technique. It should be understood that these dyes interact with the contents of the hormone-containing secretory granules in the cells. Chromophil cells secrete either simple proteins (acidophils) or glycoproteins (basophils) and will have the characteristics described in Chapter 4 of such cells. Anterior pituitary cells have a prominent rough endoplasmic reticulum, a large Golgi complex, and numerous membrane-limited granules containing the hormonal secretory product (Fig 21–6). In the glycoprotein-producing cells (gonadotropic, corticotropic, and thyrotropic cells), the carbohydrate portion of the hormone molecule is added to the protein moiety both in the endoplasmic reticulum and the Golgi complex. After appropriate stimulation, the hormone is released by exocytosis and can enter capillary vessels for delivery to the target organ or organs.

Chromophil cells are generally 12–15 μm in diameter, although their size as well as their number can vary in response to such factors as age, pregnancy, and functional status of the target organs. The distribution of various cell types within the pituitary is not homogeneous. Acidophils predominate at the periphery, whereas chromophobes and basophils show a preference for the more central part of the gland.

Numerous histologic staining techniques have been applied to the study of pituitary chromophil cells, resulting in numerous classifications, often conflicting. At present, immunohistochemical methods (Fig 21–7) applied at both the light and electron microscopic levels are most useful in distinguishing the several cell types.

Secretory Cells of the Pituitary Gland

The secretory cells of the pituitary can be classified on the basis of the hormone secreted and staining characteristics (Table 21–1).

A. Somatotropic Cells: The association of acidophilic tumors of the pituitary with acromegaly or gigantism has linked these cells with **growth hormone (somatotropin)** production and secretion in the normal pituitary. Immunofluorescence studies of human pituitary tissue support this conclusion. The acidophilic granules are easily seen with the light microscope. Somatotropic cells are easily recognized with the electron microscope by their numerous round to oval (350- to 400-nm) secretory granules, central nuclei, and large Golgi complexes.

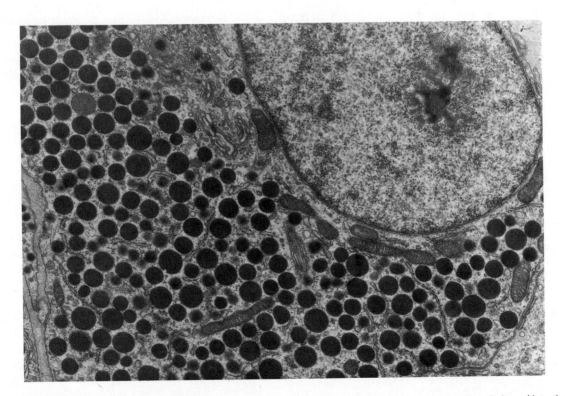

Figure 21–6. Electron micrograph of a somatotrope (growth hormone–secreting cell) of the cat anterior pituitary. Note the numerous secretory granules, long mitochondria, cisternae of rough endoplasmic reticulum, and prominent juxtanuclear Golgi complex. × 10,270.

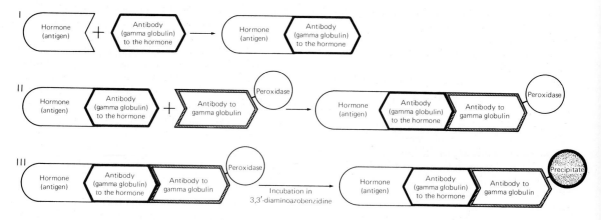

Figure 21–7. Intracellular detection of pituitary hormones by means of immunocytochemistry. *First stage:* The sections are treated by a solution containing an antibody to the hormone to be studied. The antibody binds to the hormone. *Second stage:* The section is incubated in a solution containing an antibody to the first antibody labeled by coupling it to peroxidase. This second antibody binds to the first antibody. *Third stage:* The section is incubated in a substrate (3,3'-diaminoazobenzidine plus H_2O_2) that forms a brown precipitate in the sites which contain the hormone.

B. Mammotropic Cells: These cells contain eosinophilic granules and can be distinguished from somatotropic cells, which also contain acidophilic granules, by their preferential affinity for erythrosin or carmine stains. These cells are small and irregular in shape except during pregnancy, when they enlarge considerably. They are located in a small zone in the lateral acidophilic wings of the pituitary and are present in both sexes but are more numerous in females. As seen with the electron microscope, the secretion granules, containing **prolactin,** are less than 200 nm in diameter in males and nonpregnant females. In pregnant and lactating females, the granules increase in size to over 600 nm in diameter. Lysosomes are more numerous when secretion is inhibited, and they are believed to function in the regulation of secretion by degrading the unused secretory granules (crinophagy).

C. Gonadotropic Cells: Although 2 gonadotropic hormones exist—**follicle-stimulating hormone (FSH)** and **luteinizing hormone (LH)**—only one type of gonadotropic cell can be demonstrated. These basophilic cells are generally larger than other cells of the adenohypophysis. By means of double labeling techniques, it can be shown that all the secretory granules (275–375 nm in diameter) contain both hormones.

D. Thyrotropic Cells: These cells produce **thyroid-stimulating hormone (TSH;** also called **thyrotropin)** and are located mainly in the central wedge of the adenohypophysis. They are large, polyhedral, and easily identified with the electron microscope, since their small granules, which are only 120–200 nm in diameter, line up just beneath the cell surface. Thyrotropic cells belong to the basophil subgroup. Thyrotropic cells and gonadotropic cells also show a positive PAS reaction because the hormones they produce are glycoproteins.

E. Corticotropic Cells: Corticotropic cells are polygonal in shape, with round eccentric nuclei, a well-developed Golgi complex, and rough endoplasmic reticulum that tends to be located at the periphery of the cytoplasm. Their granules are among the largest seen in the anterior pituitary, ranging from 375 to 550 nm in diameter, and thus readily visible with the light microscope. The cell is weakly basophilic and PAS-positive, since the precursor molecule of **adrenocorticotropin (ACTH),** called **pro-opiomelanocortin,** is glycosylated. In humans, ACTH itself is not glycosylated. Corticotropic cells are mostly found in the medial wedge of the pituitary, although some of them invade the neural lobe.

Histophysiology of the Pars Distalis

The hormones synthesized by this part of the pituitary are capable of exerting several kinds of effects. Some have a general metabolic action on the whole organism, whereas others act on specific structures known as target organs; the latter include nearly all of the other endocrine glands. Secretory granules appear in the human fetal pituitary at the end of the first

Table 21–1. Hormone-secreting cells in the human anterior pituitary. PAS, periodic acid–Schiff reaction. Courtesy of C Ezrin.)*

Cell Type	Hormone Secreted	Staining Reactions		
		General	Orange G	PAS
Somatotropic	Growth hormone	Acidophil	+	−
Mammotropic	Prolactin	Acidophil	+	−
Corticotropic	ACTH	Basophil	−	+
FSH gonadotropic	FSH	Basophil	−	+
LH gonadotropic	LH	Basophil	−	+
Thyrotropic	TSH	Basophil	−	+

*Reproduced, with permission, from Ganong WF: *Review of Medical Physiology,* 9th ed. Lange, 1979.

trimester of pregnancy. The time at which hormonal secretion is initiated and controlled by feedback mechanisms is unknown in humans. The following are the hormones synthesized by the pars distalis and their main effects (Fig 21–8):

A. Growth Hormone (Somatotropin): Human growth hormone is a protein that has a molecular weight of 21,500 and 191 amino acids in its straight chain structure. It influences many metabolic processes, but its most marked effect is to stimulate the growth of the epiphyseal cartilages of long bones. This is not a direct action, for somatotropin acts on the liver and kidney to elicit the production of several peptides called **somatomedins** that act on epiphyseal cartilages. An excess of somatotropin production in children and adolescents produces **gigantism.** If this excess occurs in adults, in whom no epiphyseal disks are present, only growth of the extremities of the body (mandible, nose, fingers, etc) takes place, producing the condition known as **acromegaly.** Deficient secretion of growth hormone during childhood causes **hypopituitary dwarfism,** mainly as a result of incomplete growth of the long bones.

B. Prolactin (Lactogenic Hormone): This protein hormone has a molecular weight of 22,000 and contains 198 amino acid residues. Prolactin has some structural similarity to growth hormone and human placental lactogen. Together with other hormones such as estrogens and progesterone, prolactin stimulates further breast development during pregnancy. After parturition, when estrogen and progesterone levels fall, prolactin can promote milk production (lactation). In addition to its effects on the mammary gland, prolactin also stimulates maternal behavior. The role of this hormone in males is not clear, although it is known that excessive secretion of prolactin can lead to hypogonadism.

C. Thyrotropin (Thyroid-Stimulating Hormone, TSH): This is a glycoprotein that contains 201 amino acid residues and has a molecular weight of 28,000. It consists of 2 noncovalently linked subunits referred to as α and β. The α subunit (MW 13,000) is similar to the corresponding subunits of FSH and LH, while the β subunit in each of these hormones is unique and is responsible for the specific biologic activity. Thyrotropin stimulates the synthesis and liberation of the thyroid hormones thyroxine (T_4) and triiodothyronine (T_3).

D. Follicle-Stimulating Hormone (FSH): FSH is a glycoprotein (MW 29,000) with 204 amino acids and is composed of α and β subunits. It stimulates spermatogenesis in the male and early follicular development in the ovary of the female.

E. Luteinizing Hormone (LH): The molecular weight of LH is about 29,000; it consists of an α chain (89 amino acids) and a β chain (115 amino acids). It is a glycoprotein containing 16% carbohydrate. LH is responsible for the final maturation of the graafian follicle, culminating in ovulation. This hormone is also responsible for the development of the corpus luteum and the secretion of progesterone by this gland.

LH helps to maintain the interstitial (Leydig) cells of the testis and stimulates their secretion of androgens, such as testosterone.

F. Adrenocorticotropic Hormone (ACTH; Corticotropin): ACTH has a molecular weight of 4500, contains 39 amino acids, and is not glycosylated. ACTH acts on cells of the inner zones of the adrenal cortex to stimulate synthesis and release of glucocorticoids and adrenal androgens. ACTH can also stimulate the secretion of aldosterone by zona glomerulosa cells. ACTH is derived from a larger precursor, **pro-opiomelanocortin** (MW $\sim 28,500$). In human corticotropic cells, this precursor is cleaved into ACTH and a carboxy-terminus peptide called β-lipotropin (β-LPH), which in very high doses causes lipolysis. The physiologic function of β-LPH is not known. β-LPH can be broken down further into fragments known as β–melanocyte-stimulating hormone (β-MSH) and β-endorphin, a peptide with opiatelike activity. It is doubtful whether these further cleavages occur in human corticotropic cells, although β-endorphin is secreted by certain neurons of the central nervous system.

Hypophysiotropic Hormones

It is now known that **releasing** and **inhibiting hormones** (factors) are synthesized by neurons in several regions of the preoptic and anterior parts of the hypothalamus and accumulate in endings adjacent to the primary capillary plexus of the median eminence. Upon appropriate stimulation, the releasing or inhibiting hormone is released from the axonal ending, passes into the hypophyseal portal system, and has its effect on the appropriate cells of the pars distalis. The following hormones are recognized at present:

A. Somatostatin, a 14-amino-acid peptide, inhibits growth hormone secretion. It arises from cell bodies in the suprachiasmatic nuclei. A peptide (44 amino acids) has been isolated that has growth hormone–releasing activity, but its site of origin is not yet known.

B. Prolactin secretion is inhibited by **dopamine,** which is synthesized by neurons of the arcuate nuclei. A prolactin-releasing factor (PRF) is present, but its chemical structure is uncertain.

C. Secretion of FSH and LH are both stimulated by a single **gonadotropin-releasing hormone (GnRH)** consisting of 10 amino acids and synthesized by neurons of the preoptic and arcuate nuclei.

D. A 41-amino-acid peptide has been isolated that appears to be the long-sought **corticotropin-releasing hormone (CRH).** This hormone appears to be synthesized by some of the neurons of the paraventricular nuclei. Others of these neurons synthesize vasopressin and oxytocin (see below).

Negative Feedback Control

In the cases of TRH, GnRH, and CRH, inhibitory control of the rate of secretion of these hormones is effected by secretory products of the target organs.

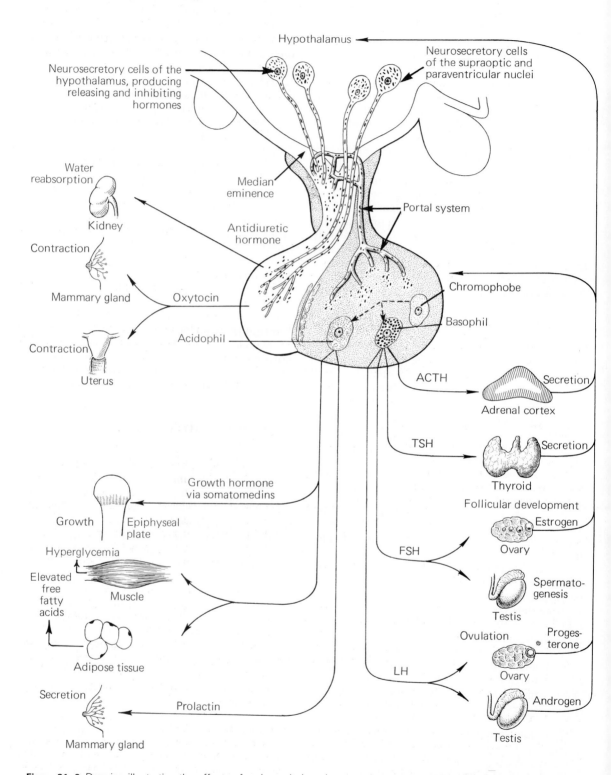

Figure 21–8. Drawing illustrating the effects of various pituitary hormones on target organs. Observe that several of the hormones produced by the target organs can act on the pituitary or hypothalamus to regulate their activity (negative feedback).

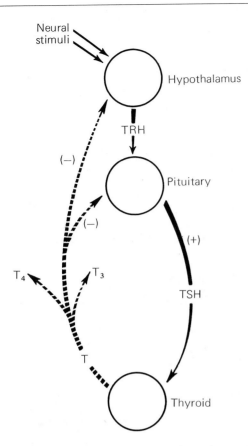

Figure 21–9. Relationships between the hypothalamus, the pituitary, and the thyroid. Thyrotropin-releasing hormone (TRH) promotes secretion of thyrotropin (TSH), which regulates the synthesis and secretion of the hormones T_3 and T_4. These hormones, besides their effect on peripheral tissues, regulate TSH and TRH secretion from the pituitary and the hypothalamus by a negative feedback mechanism. T, thyroglobulin. Solid arrows indicate stimulation; dashed arrows, inhibition.

An example of negative feedback control (Fig 21–9) is outlined below.

The pars distalis is known to synthesize **thyrotropin,** which acts on the thyroid gland, stimulating the production and secretion of thyroxine (T_4) and triiodothyronine (T_3). In addition to affecting the organism as a whole, thyroxine acts on the pituitary, inhibiting the cells that synthesize thyrotropin. Thyroxine may also act directly on the hypothalamus, inhibiting the nerve cells encountered there that produce TRH (thyrotropin-releasing hormone), which stimulates liberation of thyrotropin by the pituitary. In this way, a sensitive double control mechanism is established by which the concentration of a hormone in the blood regulates its own secretion through the secretory activity of the hypothalamus and pituitary (Fig 21–9). These control mechanisms play an important role in the adaptation of the organism to its environment. A great number of physical and psy-

chologic stimuli that reach the central nervous system are integrated at the level of the hypothalamus, which by means of the hypothalamic hormones modifies the secretion of the pituitary and consequently of the target organs, thus enabling them to respond efficiently to stimuli.

Pars Tuberalis

This funnel-shaped region surrounds the infundibulum of the neurohypophysis (Fig 21–3). Microscopically, it appears highly vascularized, for it is supplied by the superior hypophyseal arteries that terminate there as the primary capillary plexus of the hypophyseal portal system. Most of the cells of the pars tuberalis secrete gonadotropins (FSH and LH). They are arranged in cords alongside the blood vessels. Small follicles filled with an amorphous substance and lined with these cells are sometimes observed.

Pars Intermedia

In humans, the pars intermedia is a rudimentary region made up of cords of weakly basophilic cells that contain small secretory granules (200–300 nm) hardly visible with the light microscope. The function of these cells is not known. The lumen of Rathke's pouch is rarely found in adults, and follicles lined by cuboidal epithelium containing colloid and known as Rathke's cysts appear in its place (Fig 21–3).

NEUROHYPOPHYSIS

The neurohypophysis consists of the **pars nervosa** and the **infundibulum.** The latter connects the pituitary gland with the hypothalamus. As opposed to the adenohypophysis, which has epithelial characteristics, the neurohypophysis consists of about 100,000 unmyelinated axons of **neurosecretory cells.** The cell bodies of these neurons are not in the pituitary but are found in the **supraoptic** and **paraventricular nuclei** (Figs 21–3 and 21–8).

The fibers (unmyelinated axons) of the neurosecretory cells converge, forming the **hypothalamohypophyseal tract.** They enter the neurohypophysis, where they terminate blindly in close relation to the basal lamina of a rich capillary plexus. The neurosecretory material produced in the neuronal perikaryon moves along these axons into the neural lobe, where it is stored at the dilated blind endings of the axons and released as needed.

Neurosecretory Cells

The secretory neurons have all the characteristics of typical neurons, including the ability to conduct an action potential, but have more developed Nissl bodies related to the production of the neurosecretory material. In addition, the axons and the cell bodies contain granular inclusions that can be studied by specific techniques such as staining with Gomori's chrome hematoxylin stain. The hormones of the neurohypophysis are contained in these granules.

The electron microscope reveals that these neurosecretory granules have a diameter of 100–200 nm, are surrounded by a membrane, and are more numerous in the dilated terminal parts of the axons that are apposed to fenestrated blood capillaries. Here they form accumulations visible with the light microscope and known as **Herring bodies.**

In addition to the secretory granules, the terminal parts of the neurohypophyseal axons contain vesicles, 40–60 nm in diameter, that are morphologically similar to those found in cholinergic synapses. The function of these vesicles is still not known.

The **neurosecretory material** consists of hormones (either **oxytocin** or **vasopressin**), a binding protein (**neurophysin**) specific for each hormone, and **ATP.** The hormones are 9-amino-acid peptides having a ring structure formed by a disulfide bridge. Each has a slightly different composition, but this results in greatly different functions. The hormone-neurophysin complex is synthesized as a single, long peptide on ribosomes attached to membranes of Nissl bodies (rough endoplasmic reticulum). The peptide is partially glycosylated in the lumen of the endoplasmic reticulum and then passed on to the Golgi complex, where further glycosylation and packaging in secretory granules occur. As the granules pass down axons of the hypothalamohypophyseal tract, proteolysis of the precursor occurs to yield the hormone and its specific binding protein (neurophysin). Vasopressin and oxytocin are stored in the posterior pituitary and released into the blood by impulses in the nerve fibers from the hypothalamus. Although there is some overlap, the fibers from supraoptic nuclei are mainly concerned with vasopressin secretion, while most of those from the paraventricular nuclei are concerned with oxytocin secretion.

Neurohypophyseal Cells

The neurohypophysis consists mainly of axons from hypothalamic neurons. However, about 25% of the volume of this structure consists of a specific type of glial cell called a **pituicyte** (Fig 21–10). In addition, endothelial cells of capillaries are present.

Pituicytes are highly branched cells with processes that partially or completely surround neurosecretory cell axons. The cytoplasm of these cells may contain lipid droplets and pigment, but secretory granules are not seen. Numerous intermediate filaments, with a composition similar to the filaments found in astrocytes, are present.

Histophysiology

The neurohypophysis of all mammals except members of the pig family secretes 2 hormones, both cyclic peptides made up of 9 amino acids. These hormones are **arginine vasopressin**—also called **antidiuretic hormone (ADH)**—and **oxytocin.** These hormones are present in different secretory granules

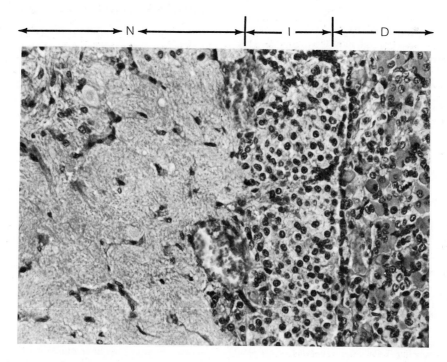

Figure 21–10. Section of the pituitary of a rat showing (from left to right) the neurohypophysis (N), the pars intermedia (I), and the pars distalis (D). Between the pars intermedia and the pars distalis is the pituitary cleft (C). Chromophilic and chromophobic cells are apparent in the pars distalis. The pars intermedia consists of cords of one cell type. In the neurohypophysis, nuclei of pituicytes are clearly visible. Mallory's stain, × 340.

and in different neurons. In large doses, vasopressin promotes the contraction of smooth muscle of blood vessels, raising the blood pressure. It acts mainly on the muscle layers of small arteries and arterioles. It is doubtful if endogenous vasopressin is secreted in an amount sufficient to exert any appreciable effect on blood pressure homeostasis. The main effect of vasopressin is to increase the permeability to water of the collecting tubules of the kidney. As a result, water is reabsorbed by these tubules and urine becomes hypertonic. Thus, vasopressin helps to regulate the osmotic balance of the internal milieu. This hormone is secreted whenever the osmotic pressure of the blood increases. In this case, the blood acts on osmoreceptor cells in the anterior hypothalamus, stimulating the secretion of this hormone from supraoptic neurons. Sections of the neurohypophysis of animals previously given injections of hypertonic solutions do not contain the neurosecretory material usually present in control animals. A variety of stimuli in addition to these increase vasopressin secretion, eg, pain, trauma, emotional upsets, and drugs such as morphine and nicotine. Circulating vasopressin is rapidly inactivated (its half-life in humans is about 18 minutes), mainly in the liver and kidneys, and acts on its target organ by increasing intracellular cyclic adenosine-3',5'-monophosphate (cyclic AMP, cAMP) levels.

Lesions of the hypothalamus, which destroy the neurosecretory cells, cause **diabetes insipidus,** a disease characterized by loss of renal capacity to concentrate urine. Consequently, an individual suffering from this disease may excrete up to 20 liters of urine per day (polyuria) and will drink enormous quantities of liquids.

Oxytocin stimulates contraction of the smooth muscle of the uterine wall during copulation and childbirth and contraction of myoepithelial cells that surround the alveoli and ducts of the mammary glands. The secretion of oxytocin is stimulated by distention of the vagina or of the uterine cervix and by nursing. This occurs via nerve tracts that act on the hypothalamus. The neurohormonal reflex triggered by nursing is called the **milk ejection reflex** (Fig 21 – 8).

REFERENCES

Bhatnagar AS (editor): *The Anterior Pituitary Gland.* Raven Press, 1983.

Brownstein MJ, Russell JT, Gainer H: Synthesis, transport, and release of posterior pituitary hormones. *Science* 1980; **207:**373.

Cross BA, Leng G (editors): The neurohypophysis: Structure, function and control. *Prog Brain Res* 1982;**60:**3.

Daniel PM: The blood supply of the hypothalamus and pituitary gland. *Br Med Bull* 1966;**22:**202.

Dierickx K, Vandesande F: Immunocytochemical localization of the vasopressinergic and oxytocinergic neurons in the human hypothalamus. *Cell Tissue Res* 1977;**184:**15.

Farquhar MG: Processing of secretory products by cells of the anterior pituitary gland. *Mem Soc Endocrinol (Cambridge)* 1971;**19:**79.

Ganong WF: *Review of Medical Physiology,* 12th ed. Lange, 1985.

Herlant M: The cells of the adenohypophysis and their functional significance. *Int Rev Cytol* 1974;**17:**299.

Krieger DT: Brain peptides: What, where, and why? *Science* 1983;**222:**975.

Kurosumi K: Functional classification of cell types of the anterior pituitary gland accomplished by electron microscopy. *Arch Histol Jpn* 1968;**29:**329.

Li JY, Dubois MP, Dubois PM: Ultrastructural localization of immunoreactive corticotropin, β-lipotropin, and α- and β-endorphin in cells of the human fetal anterior pituitary. *Cell Tissue Res* 1979;**204:**37.

Martin DW Jr et al: *Harper's Review of Biochemistry,* 20th ed. Lange, 1985.

Nakane PK: Classification of anterior pituitary cell types with immunoenzyme histochemistry. *J Histochem Cytochem* 1970;**18:**9.

Pantic VR: The specificity of pituitary cells and regulation of their activities. *Int Rev Cytol* 1975;**40:**153.

Pelletier G, Robert F, Hardy J: Identification of human anterior pituitary cells by immunoelectron microscopy. *J Clin Endocrinol Metab* 1978;**46:**534.

Phifer RF, Midgley AR, Spicer SS: Immunohistologic and histologic evidence that follicle-stimulating hormone and luteinizing hormone are present in the same cell type in the human pars distalis. *J Clin Endocrinol Metab* 1973;**36:**125.

Phifer RF, Spicer SS, Orth DN: Specific demonstration of the human hypophyseal cells which produce adrenocorticotropic hormone. *J Clin Endocrinol* 1970;**31:**347.

Reichlin S (editor): *The Neurohypophysis: Physiological and Clinical Aspects.* Plenum, 1984.

Seyama S, Pearl GS, Takei Y: Ultrastructural study of the human neurohypophysis. 1. Neurosecretory axons and their dilatations in the pars nervosa. *Cell Tissue Res* 1980;**205:**253.

Seyama S, Pearl GS, Takei Y: Ultrastructural study of the human neurohypophysis. 3. Vascular and perivascular structures. *Cell Tissue Res* 1980;**206:**291.

Smith RE, Farquhar MG: Lysosome function in the regulation of the secretory process in cells of the anterior pituitary gland. *J Cell Biol* 1966;**31:**319.

Takei Y et al: Ultrastructural study of the human neurohypophysis. 2. Cellular elements of neural parenchyma, the pituicytes. *Cell Tissue Res* 1980;**205:**273.

Tixier-Vidal A, Farquhar MG (editors): *The Anterior Pituitary.* Academic Press, 1975.

Adrenals, Islets of Langerhans, Thyroid, Parathyroids, & Pineal Body

THE ADRENAL (SUPRARENAL) GLANDS

The adrenal glands are paired organs that lie near the superior poles of the kidneys embedded in adipose tissue. They are flattened structures with a half-moon shape. In the human, they are about 4–6 cm long, 1–2 cm wide, and 4–6 mm thick, and together weigh about 8 g, but their weight and size vary depending upon the age and physiologic condition of the individual. Examination of a fresh section of adrenal gland shows it to be covered by a capsule of dense collagenous connective tissue and to consist of 2 concentric layers: a yellow peripheral layer, the **adrenal cortex;** and a reddish-brown central layer, the **adrenal medulla** (Figs 22–1 and 22–6). Cortical and medullary tissue sometimes occur at other sites as shown in Fig 22–2.

These 2 layers may be considered as 2 morphologically and functionally distinct organs that become united during embryonic development. They arise from different germ layers. The cortex arises from coelomic intermediate mesoderm, whereas the medulla consists of cells derived from the neural crest from which sympathetic ganglion cells also originate. In fact, one might consider the medulla to be a modified sympathetic ganglion whose postganglionic neurons lost their processes during development and became secretory cells. The general histologic appearance is typical of an endocrine gland wherein cells of both cortex and medulla are grouped in cords along capillaries (see Chapter 4).

The collagenous connective tissue capsule that covers the gland sends thin septa to the interior of the gland as trabeculae. The stroma consists mainly of a rich network of reticular fibers that supports the secretory cells.

Blood Supply

The adrenals are supplied by a number of arteries that enter at various points around their periphery (Fig

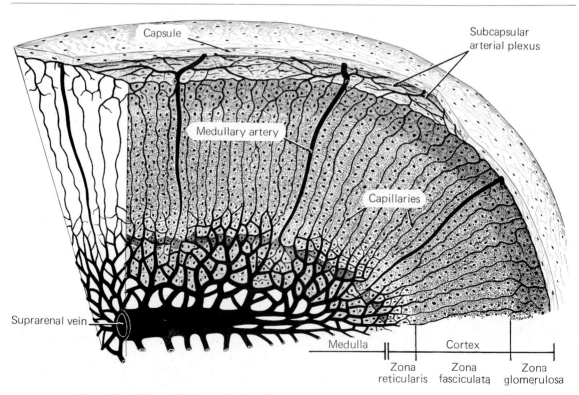

Figure 22–1. Diagram of the general architecture and blood circulation of the adrenal gland.

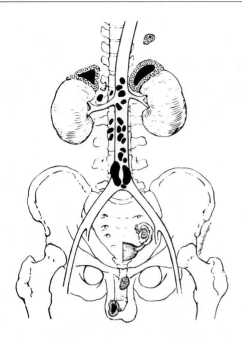

Figure 22–2. Human adrenal glands. Adrenocortical tissue is stippled; adrenal medullary tissue is black. Note location of adrenals at superior pole of each kidney. Also shown are extra-adrenal sites at which cortical and medullary tissue is sometimes found. (Reproduced, with permission, from Forsham in: *Textbook of Endocrinology,* 4th ed. Williams RH [editor]. Saunders, 1968.)

22– 1). The 3 main groups of arteries are the **superior suprarenal** artery, arising from the inferior phrenic artery; the **middle suprarenal** artery, arising from the aorta; and the **inferior suprarenal** artery, arising from the renal artery. The several arterial branches form a subcapsular plexus from which arise 3 groups of vessels: (1) arteries of the capsule; (2) arteries of the cortex, which branch repeatedly to form the capillary bed between the parenchymal cells (these capillaries drain into medullary capillaries); and (3) arteries of the medulla, which pass through the cortex before breaking up to form part of the extensive capillary network of the medulla.

This dual vascular supply provides the medulla with both arterial (via **medullary arteries**) and venous (via **cortical arteries**) blood. The endothelium of these capillaries is extremely attenuated and interrupted by small fenestrae, closed by thin diaphragms. A continuous basal lamina is present beneath the endothelium.

It was formerly believed that these endothelial cells were phagocytic and thus formed a part of the reticuloendothelial system. More recent studies with the electron microscope have failed to reveal evidence of phagocytosis by the endothelium. Macrophages present in the subendothelial space are the only cells participating in phagocytosis. In the adrenal glands of some animals, including humans, there is a sub-

endothelial space between endothelial cells of the capillaries and glandular cells, into which the microvilli of the latter protrude.

Capillaries of the medulla, together with those that supply the cortex, form the medullary veins, which join to constitute the **adrenal** or **suprarenal vein** (Fig 22– 1). The suprarenal vein is characterized by an incomplete sheath of longitudinally oriented smooth muscle cells in its media. In addition, the suprarenal vein is usually surrounded by a cuff of adrenocortical cells.

The Adrenal Cortex

Because of the different disposition and appearance of its cells, the adrenal cortex can be subdivided into 3 concentric layers which, in humans, are usually not sharply defined (Figs 22– 1 and 22– 3A): the **zona glomerulosa** (Fig 22– 3B), the **zona fasciculata** (Fig 22– 3C), and the **zona reticularis** (Fig 22– 3D). The zona glomerulosa secretes mineralocorticoids, primarily aldosterone, which are involved with maintenance of electrolyte (eg, sodium and potassium) and water balance. The zona fasciculata and probably the zona reticularis secrete the glucocorticoids cortisone and cortisol or, in some animals, corticosterone, which are concerned with the regulation of carbohydrate, protein, and fat metabolism. Androgens and perhaps estrogens are produced in small amounts in these 2 zones (Fig 22– 5).

The cells of the adrenal cortex have the characteristics of steroid-synthesizing cells described in Chapter 4. The glomerulosa, fasciculata, and reticularis zones occupy, respectively, 15%, 65%, and 7% of the total volume of the adrenals.

The layer immediately beneath the connective tissue capsule is the **zona glomerulosa,** in which the columnar or pyramidal cells are arranged in closely packed, rounded, or arched clusters surrounded by capillaries (Fig 22– 3A). Glomerulosa cells have a spherical nucleus, a well-developed nucleolus, and an acidophilic cytoplasm containing a few lipid droplets (Fig 22– 3B). The cell contour is smooth except near the subendothelial space, where the plasma membrane is thrown into folds and microvilli. A prominent feature of the cell is the extensive smooth endoplasmic reticulum that forms an anastomosing tubular network (Fig 22– 4). There are a few short segments of rough endoplasmic reticulum and some free ribosomes. The abundant mitochondria are ovoid and have tubular and lamellar cristae. The smooth endoplasmic reticulum sometimes occurs in close relationship to the lipid droplets. A well-developed Golgi complex is present. The localization of the enzymes participating in aldosterone synthesis has been determined by the differential centrifugation technique. The synthesis of cholesterol from acetate takes place in smooth endoplasmic reticulum, whereas the conversion of cholesterol to pregnenolone takes place in the mitochondria. The enzymes associated with the synthesis of progesterone and deoxycorticosterone from pregnenolone are found in smooth endoplasmic reticulum; those

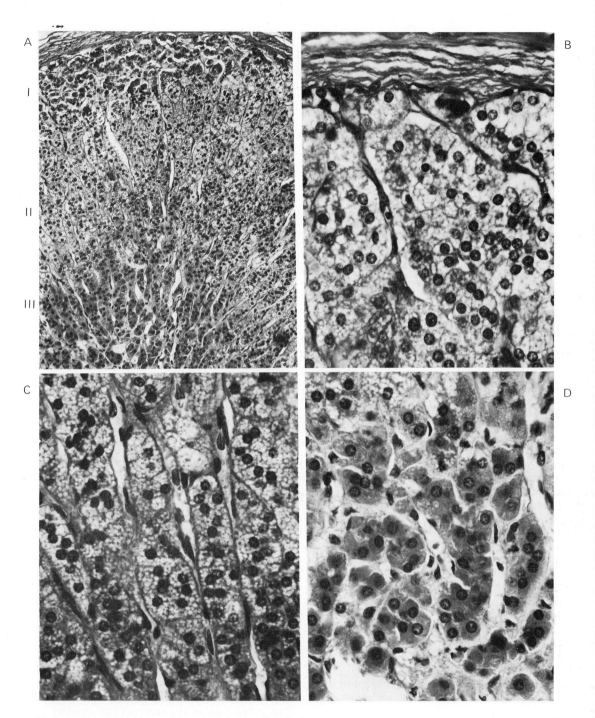

Figure 22–3. Photomicrographs of the adrenal cortex (H&E stain). *A:* A low-power general view. I, the glomerulosa; II, the fasciculata; III, the reticularis. × 80. *B:* The capsule and the zona glomerulosa. × 330. *C:* The zona fasciculata. × 330. *D:* The zona reticularis. × 330.

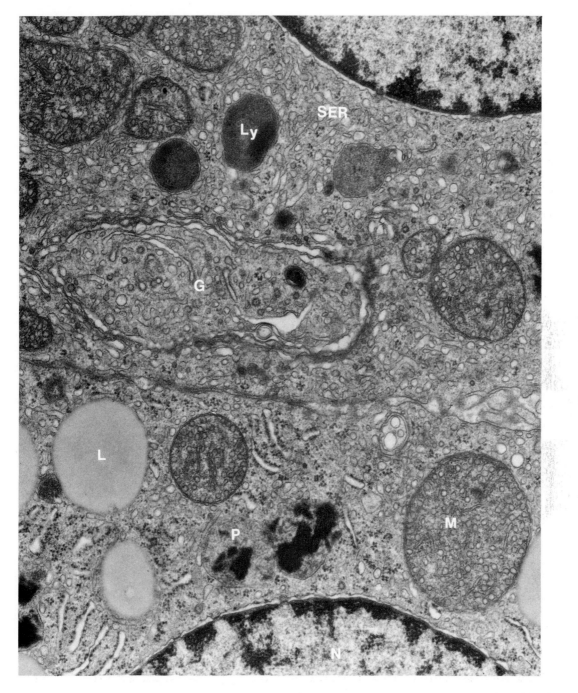

Figure 22–4. Fine structure of steroid-secreting cells from the zona fasciculata of the human adrenal cortex. L, lipid droplets containing cholesteryl esters; M, mitochondria with characteristic tubular and vesicular cristae; SER, smooth endoplasmic reticulum; N, nucleus; G, Golgi complex; Ly, lysosomes; P, lipofuscin pigment granules. × 25,700.

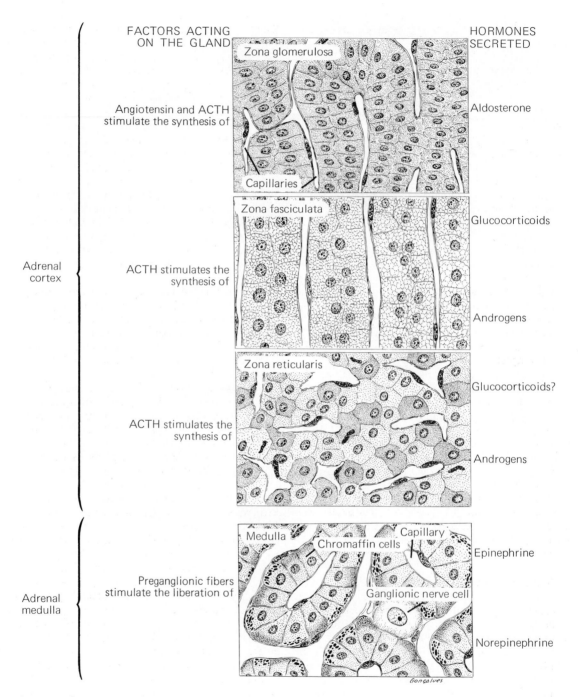

FACTORS ACTING
ON THE GLAND

HORMONES
SECRETED

Zona glomerulosa

Angiotensin and ACTH
stimulate the synthesis of

Aldosterone

Capillaries

Adrenal
cortex

Zona fasciculata

Glucocorticoids

ACTH stimulates the
synthesis of

Androgens

Zona reticularis

Glucocorticoids?

ACTH stimulates the
synthesis of

Androgens

Medulla

Capillary

Chromaffin cells

Epinephrine

Adrenal
medulla

Preganglionic fibers
stimulate the liberation of

Ganglionic nerve cell

Norepinephrine

Gonçalves

Figure 22–5. Structure and histophysiology of the adrenal gland. *Left:* Factors acting on the gland. *Right:* The hormones secreted.

enzymes that convert deoxycorticosterone → corticosterone → 18-hydroxycorticosterone → aldosterone are located in mitochondria.

The next layer of cells is known as the **zona fasciculata** because the cells are arranged in straight cords, one or 2 cells thick (Fig 22–3C), that run at right angles to the surface of the organ and have capillaries between them. The cells of the zona fasciculata are polyhedral, with a central nucleus, and their cytoplasm is slightly basophilic. Microvilli extend into the subendothelial space. The cells contain a great number of lipid droplets in their cytoplasm. As a result of dissolution of the lipids during the dehydration steps in tissue preparation, the fasciculata cells appear vacuolated in common histologic preparations (Fig 22–3C). The smooth endoplasmic reticulum is even more highly developed in the zona fasciculata than in the zona glomerulosa. The rough endoplasmic reticulum, which is more abundant in this zone, is responsible for the observed basophilia. The mitochondria are spherical in shape and contain short tubular or vesicular cristae.

The innermost layer of the cortex, between the zona fasciculata and the medulla, contains cells disposed in irregular cords forming an anastomosing network and is called the **zona reticularis** (Fig 22–3D). These cells are smaller than those of the other 2 layers. The cells have many of the features of the cells in the zona fasciculata, but they differ in the structure of the mitochondria, which are more often elongated. In addition, lipofuscin pigment granules in these cells are large and quite numerous. Their cytoplasm is acidophilic and contains a few lipid droplets and, at times, glycogen. Irregularly shaped cells with pyknotic nuclei—suggesting cellular degeneration—are often found in this layer (Fig 22–3D).

Cells of the adrenal cortex do not store their secretory products in granules; rather, they synthesize and secrete steroid hormones only upon demand. Steroids, being low-molecular-weight, lipid-soluble molecules, can freely diffuse through the plasma membrane and do not require the specialized process of exocytosis for their release.

Histophysiology

The function of the adrenal cortex is to produce steroids, lipids that contain the cyclopentanoperhydrophenanthrene nucleus. Chemical groups are added to or removed from this nucleus during the process of hormone biosynthesis, resulting in various substances with different physiologic activities. The steroids secreted by the cortex may be divided into 3 groups according to their main physiologic actions: **glucocorticoids, mineralocorticoids,** and **androgens** (Fig 22–5).

The **glucocorticoids,** mainly cortisol and corticosterone, exert a profound effect upon the metabolism of carbohydrates, as well as on that of proteins and lipids. In the liver, glucocorticoids promote the uptake and usage of fatty acids (energy source), amino acids (enzyme synthesis), and carbohydrates (glucose synthesis) that are utilized in gluconeogenesis and in glycogen assembly (glycogenesis). In fact, these hormones can stimulate the synthesis of so much glucose that the resulting high levels of this sugar that enter the blood produce a condition similar to diabetes mellitus. However, outside the liver, glucocorticoids induce an opposite, or catabolic, effect on peripheral organs (eg, skin, muscle, adipose tissue). In these structures, these steroid hormones not only decrease synthetic activity, but they also promote protein and lipid degradation. The by-products of degradation, amino and fatty acids, are removed from the blood and utilized by the synthetically active hepatocytes.

Glucocorticoids also suppress the immune response by decreasing the number of circulating eosinophils by accelerating their sequestration in the lungs and spleen. Circulating lymphocytes are reduced in number as a result of an increased destruction of these cells and inhibition of mitotic activity in lymph-forming organs. Patients receiving organ transplants are frequently given massive doses of these steroid hormones because of their ability to suppress the immune response.

The **mineralocorticoids,** of which aldosterone is the most important, act mainly on the distal renal tubules as well as the gastric mucosa and the salivary and sweat glands, stimulating the reabsorption of sodium. They may increase the concentration of potassium and decrease that of sodium in muscle and brain cells.

Dehydroepiandrosterone is the only sex hormone secreted in significant physiologic quantities by the adrenal cortex. It has masculinizing and anabolic effects, but it is less than one-fifth as potent as testicular androgens. For this reason, and because it is secreted in small quantities, it produces a negligible physiologic effect under normal conditions.

The basic function of the adrenal gland is to maintain essential homeostatic mechanisms, eg, the chemical constitution of the intercellular and extracellular fluids. This is easily understood when one considers the total effects of the hormones of this gland. A wide variety of physiologic stimuli as well as pathologic states—stress, fasting, temperature changes, infections, drugs, exercise, hemorrhage, etc—affect the central nervous system and, by stimulating hypothalamic secretion of corticotropin-releasing hormone, cause an increase in the production of ACTH by the pituitary (Fig 22–6). The increase in production of adrenal hormones permits the organism to counteract the effects of such stimuli. Since the organism is continuously receiving such stimuli, the adrenal gland and other homeostatic mechanisms are continually functioning, either in concert or in opposed balance, in order to maintain the equilibrium of the internal milieu.

In hypophysectomized animals, the effects of glucocorticoid deficiency can be observed while their ionic equilibrium is found to be essentially normal, so the secretion of aldosterone is not markedly affected. In the morphologic study of the adrenal glands

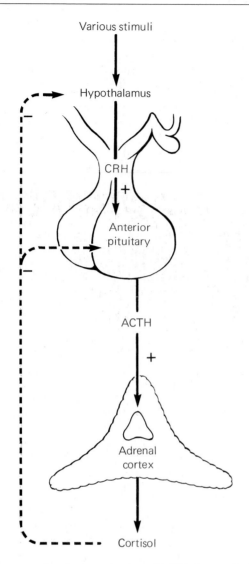

Figure 22–6. Feedback mechanism of ACTH-glucocorticoid secretion. Solid arrows indicate stimulation; dashed arrows, inhibition.

of these animals, cortical thinning is noticeable—mainly as a result of the atrophy of the zona fasciculata and zona reticularis—while the zona glomerulosa remains unaltered or may even be hypertrophic (Fig 22–7). Another argument in support of the theory that mineralocorticoid production occurs mainly in the glomerulosa is that in sodium deficiency the glomerulosa hypertrophies considerably, and this change is accompanied by a severalfold increase in aldosterone production. The presence only in the zona glomerulosa of the 18-hydroxylating enzyme necessary for the synthesis of aldosterone is another indication that synthesis of this hormone occurs in the zona glomerulosa.

The administration of ACTH to a hypophysectomized animal normalizes the secretion of glucocorticoids, demonstrating the dependence of these hormones on the pituitary hormones (Fig 22–5). The secretion of sex hormones is also controlled by ACTH. ACTH acts via the cAMP system, promoting an increase in the uptake of cholesterol and its conversion to pregnenolone by the mitochondria. It is now believed that ACTH does promote aldosterone secretion but that this secretion is regulated primarily via the renin-angiotensin system. Renin is produced by the juxtaglomerular cells that surround the renal afferent arterioles as they enter the glomeruli (see Chapter 20) and is liberated in response to several types of stimuli, eg, decrease of sodium concentration in the blood, decrease of the volume of circulating blood, and constriction of the renal artery. Once secreted, renin acts as an enzyme on a circulating α_2 globulin (angiotensinogen), causing the liberation of angiotensin I, a decapeptide that is converted by a "converting enzyme" present in abundant amounts in lung endothelial cells into angiotensin II, an octapeptide that in turn acts on the adrenal gland to stimulate the secretion of aldosterone.

The Fetal, or Provisional, Cortex

In humans and some other animals, the adrenal gland of the newborn is proportionately larger than that of the adult. At this early age, a layer known as

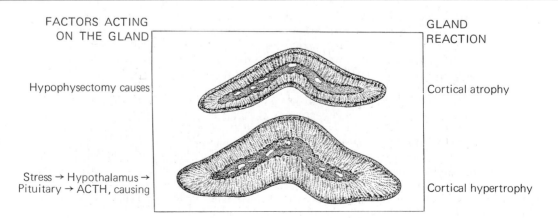

Figure 22–7. Effects of decreased and increased stimulation on the structure of the adrenal gland.

fetal cortex, or provisional cortex, is present between the thin permanent cortex and the medulla. This layer is fairly thick, and its cells are disposed in cords. After birth, the provisional cortex undergoes involution, while the permanent cortex—the initially thin layer—develops, differentiating into the 3 layers described above. A major function of the fetal adrenal is secretion of sulfate conjugates of androgens, which are converted in the placenta to active androgens and estrogens that enter the maternal circulation.

Adrenal Medulla

The adrenal medulla is composed of polyhedral parenchymal cells arranged in cords or clumps and supported by a reticular fiber network (Fig 22–8). A profuse capillary supply intervenes between adjacent cords. A few parasympathetic ganglion cells are also present. Medullary parenchymal cells arise from neural crest cells, as do the postganglionic neurons of sympathetic and parasympathetic ganglia. Parenchymal cells of the adrenal medulla may be regarded as modified sympathetic postganglionic neurons that have lost their axons and dendrites.

Medullary parenchymal cells contain a large nucleus, isolated cisternae of rough endoplasmic reticulum, numerous oval mitochondria, and a prominent Golgi complex. Microtubules and microfilaments are also present. The most distinctive organelles of these cells are membrane-limited, electron-dense secretory granules, 150–350 nm in diameter. These granules contain one or the other of the catecholamines, epinephrine or norepinephrine. When medullary cells are exposed to oxidizing agents (such as potassium bichromate), catecholamines are oxidized to a brown, melaninlike compound. Because of the affinity of these cells for chromium salts, the result is called the **chromaffin reaction,** and the cells and granules are termed **chromaffin cells** and **chromaffin granules.** Chromaffin granules also contain ATP, chromogranins (which may serve as binding proteins for catecholamines), dopamine β-hydroxylase (which converts dopamine to norepinephrine), and opiatelike peptides (including Leu- and Met-enkephalin) (Fig 22–9).

A large body of evidence shows that epinephrine and norepinephrine are secreted by 2 different types of cells in the medulla. Epinephrine-secreting cells have smaller, less electron-dense granules, and their contents fill the granule. On the other hand, norepinephrine-secreting cells have larger, more electron-dense granules; their contents are irregular in shape; and there is an electron-lucent layer beneath the surrounding membrane. About 80% of the catecholamine output of the adrenal vein is epinephrine. Dopamine is also detected in small quantities. The cell secreting this compound may be a rare medullary parenchymal cell with much smaller granules.

As noted previously, the adrenal medulla receives a dual blood supply consisting of (1) blood from the capillaries that traverse the cortex, and (2) arterial blood delivered directly to the medulla. In the former, high concentrations of glucocorticoids are found as a result of the secretory activity of cortical cells, while the direct arterial blood has much lower concentrations of these steroid hormones. Synthesis of the enzyme responsible for the conversion of norepinephrine to epinephrine, phenylethanolamine-N-methyltransferase (PNMT) is induced by high levels of glucocorticoids. Accordingly, clusters of epinephrine-secreting medullary cells are found around the terminations of cortical capillaries, while norepinephrine-secreting cells are found at the ends of medullary arteries.

All adrenal medullary cells are innervated by cholinergic endings of preganglionic sympathetic neurons. Unlike the cortex, which does not store steroids,

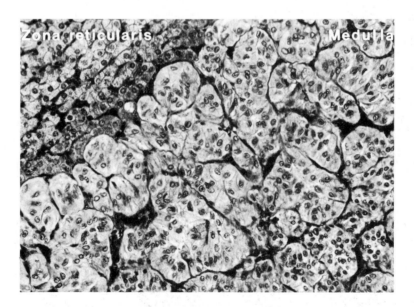

Figure 22–8. Photomicrograph of a section of adrenal medulla. H&E stain, × 200.

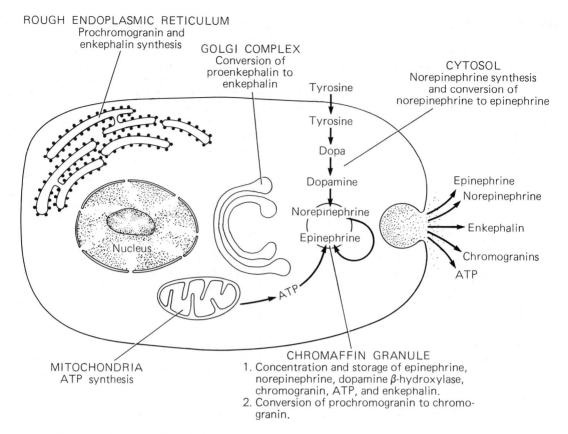

Figure 22–9. Diagram of a chromaffin cell showing the role of several organelles in the synthesis of constituents of the chromaffin granules.

cells of the medulla accumulate and store their hormones in granules. During normal activity, only small quantities are continuously secreted by the medulla. However, epinephrine and norepinephrine are secreted in large quantities in response to intense emotional reactions (eg, fright). Secretion of these substances is mediated by the preganglionic fibers that innervate chromaffin cells. Vasoconstriction, hypertension, changes in heart rate, and metabolic effects such as blood glucose elevation result from secretion of catecholamines into the bloodstream. These effects are part of the organism's defense reaction to stress (the "fight or flight" response).

Chromaffin cells are also found in the paraganglia (collections of catecholamine-secreting cells adjacent to autonomic ganglia) as well as in various viscera. Paraganglia are a diffuse source of catecholamines.

Adrenal Dysfunction

A common disorder of the adrenal medulla is a tumor of chromaffin cells known as **pheochromocytoma** that causes hyperglycemia and transient elevations of blood pressure. These tumors can also develop in extramedullary sites (Fig 22–2) as well as in the paraganglia.

Disorders of the adrenal cortex may be classified as **hyperfunction** or **hypofunction.** Tumors of the adrenal cortex can result in excessive production of glucocorticoids **(Cushing's syndrome)** or of aldosterone **(Conn's syndrome).** Increased secretion of aldosterone can also result from rare renin-secreting tumors of juxtaglomerular cells in the kidney. Cushing's syndrome is most often (90%) due to a pituitary adenoma resulting in excessive production of ACTH and rarely to adrenal hyperplasia or an adrenal tumor. Excessive production of adrenal androgens has little effect in mature males. In females, hirsutism (abnormal hair growth) is seen, while in prepubertal children, precocious puberty (males) and virilization (females) are encountered. These adrenogenital syndromes are due to several enzymatic defects in steroid metabolism leading to increased biosynthesis of androgens by the adrenal cortex.

Adrenocortical insufficiency **(Addison's disease)** is mainly due to autoimmune destruction of the adrenal cortex (80%) or is a complication of tuberculosis (20%). The signs and symptoms suggest failure of secretion of both glucocorticoids and mineralocorticoids by the adrenal cortex.

THE ISLETS OF LANGERHANS

The islets of Langerhans constitute the endocrine portion of the pancreas and appear as rounded clusters of cells embedded within exocrine pancreatic tissue.

Most islets are 100–200 μm in diameter and contain several hundred cells, but small islets of endocrine cells can be found interspersed among pancreatic exocrine cells. There may be over 1 million islets in the human pancreas, with a slight tendency for islets to be more abundant in the tail region.

Each islet consists of lightly stained polygonal or rounded cells arranged in cords separated by a network of fenestrated blood capillaries (Fig 22–10). The parenchymal cells as well as the blood vessels are innervated by autonomic nerve fibers. A fine capsule of reticular fibers surrounds each islet, separating it from the adjacent exocrine pancreatic tissue.

Using special staining methods, 4 different types of cells—A, B, D, and F—have been described in the islets. The B cells are most numerous and tend to be concentrated in the center of the islet (Fig 22–10); they constitute about 60–80% of the cells found in human pancreatic islets. These cells are small and contain in their cytoplasm granules that stain blue with Gomori's chrome hematoxylin and phloxine technique. The A cells are larger and less numerous (20%), are found usually at the periphery, and are characterized by the presence of secretory granules that stain red with the Gomori stain. The less numerous D and F cells are small and do not stain heavily.

The ultrastructure of these cells resembles that of cells synthesizing polypeptides, for they have a relatively diffuse rough endoplasmic reticulum, free polysomes, Golgi complex, and secretory granules (Fig 22–11). There is much less rough endoplasmic reticulum in these cells than in the acinar cells of the exocrine pancreas. This is in accord with the less intense protein synthesis that occurs in these cells as compared with this activity in the acinar cells.

A cells have numerous granules, about 300 nm in diameter, which contain the hormone **glucagon.** The granules are limited by a membrane and contain an extremely dense, eccentrically placed core surrounded by a less dense matrix.

The appearance of granules of **B cells** is species-specific. In humans, they are also about 300 nm in diameter, but the core consists of one or more angular crystals of **insulin** complexed with zinc. A clear zone intervenes between the crystals and the surrounding membrane.

D cells also contain membrane-bound granules; however, their contents differ from A and B cells in that they appear as homogeneous granules with moderate to low electron density. These granules store **somatostatin.**

Pancreatic polypeptide is stored in granules found in **F cells.** The membrane-limited granules are char-

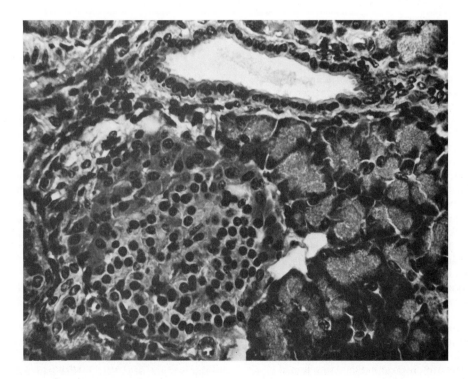

Figure 22–10. Photomicrograph of a section of the pancreas of a guinea pig. Observe the islet of Langerhans, where the A cells appear mainly in the periphery as large cells with a dark cytoplasm. The remaining cells are mostly B cells. Masson's stain, × 400.

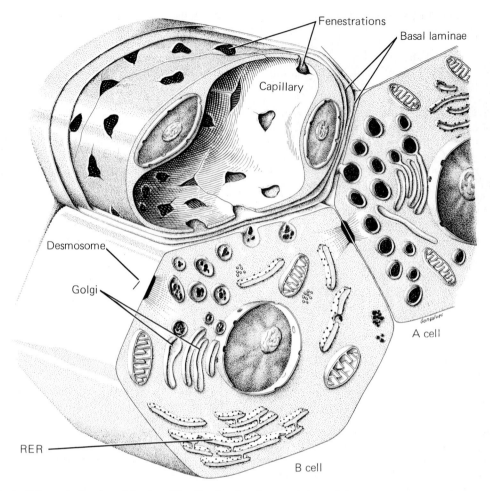

Figure 22–11. Schematic drawing of the A and B cells, showing the morphology of the secretory granules and their relation to blood vessels. The B cell has irregular granules, while the granules are round and uniform in the A cells. RER, rough endoplasmic reticulum.

acterized by a central, round dense area surrounded by a wide electron-lucent area.

Glucagon, a polypeptide with a molecular weight of 3485 and consisting of 29 amino acids, is produced by the A cells of pancreatic islets (Fig 22–12). Glucagon acts on several tissues to make energy available in the intervals between meals. In the liver, it causes breakdown of glycogen and promotes gluconeogenesis from amino acid precursors.

Insulin, in contrast, is the "hormone of plenty" because it causes the storage of excess nutrients arising during and shortly after a meal. The major target organs for insulin are the liver, muscle, and fat—organs specialized for storage of energy. Insulin is formed as a single polypeptide chain, **proinsulin,** containing 81–86 residues depending on the species. The conversion of proinsulin to insulin occurs by proteolytic cleavage, producing one molecule of insulin and one of C-peptide. Cleavage takes place at the time of transport of proinsulin to the Golgi complex, or

soon after, where it is packaged into granules (Fig 22–13). Since the granules contain insulin and C-peptide in the same amounts, packaging presumably occurs first, followed by cleavage. Insulin consists of an A chain (21 amino acids) and a B chain (30 amino acids) linked by 2 disulfide bridges and is stored as a zinc complex. The stimuli for insulin granule exocytosis include elevated blood glucose concentrations and increased levels of amino acids such as leucine and arginine.

Somatostatin was originally isolated from the hypothalamus and received its name because of its ability to inhibit growth hormone (somatotropin) secretion. Somatostatin is now known to be widely distributed in the gastrointestinal tract, including the pancreas. The hormone is a 14-amino-acid peptide with a molecular weight of 1640. In the pancreas, it acts to inhibit glucagon release and to decrease pancreatic exocrine secretion.

Pancreatic polypeptide has a molecular weight

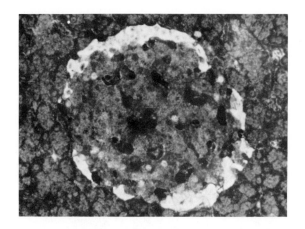

Figure 22–12. Photomicrograph of a preparation of a rat islet of Langerhans, stained with a fluorescent antibody against glucagon. Glucagon is produced by the A cells located in the periphery of the islet in this species. In this figure, the fluorescent A cells appear light against the dark background. × 50. (Courtesy of S Ito.)

of 4200 and contains 36 amino acids. This hormone inhibits pancreatic exocrine secretion of bicarbonate and enzymes, causes relaxation of the gallbladder, and decreases bile secretion.

Terminations of nerve fibers on islet cells can be observed by light or electron microscopy. Both sympathetic and parasympathetic nerve endings have been found in close (synaptic?) association with about 10% of the A, B, and D cells. Gap junctions presumably serve to transfer ionic· changes associated with autonomic discharge to the other cells. These nerves function as part of the insulin and glucagon control system.

THYROID

In early embryonic life, the thyroid is derived from the cephalic portion of the alimentary canal endoderm. Its function is to synthesize the hormones thyroxine (T_4) and triiodothyronine (T_3), which stimulate the rate of metabolism.

The thyroid gland is located in the cervical region, anterior to the larynx, and consists of 2 lobes united by an isthmus (Fig 22– 14). Thyroid tissue is composed of **follicles** consisting of a simple epithelial sphere whose lumen contains a gelatinous substance, the **colloid** (Fig 22– 15). In typical sections, follicle cells range from squamous to low columnar cells. Follicles may reach a diameter of 0.9 mm. The gland is covered by a loose connective tissue capsule that sends septa into the parenchyma. These septa become gradually thinner and reach all of the follicles, separating one from another by fine irregular connective tissue composed mainly of reticular fibers. The thyroid is an extremely vascularized organ, having an extensive blood and lymphatic capillary network surround-

ing the follicles. Endothelial cells of these capillaries are fenestrated, as in other endocrine glands. This configuration facilitates the passage of the hormones into the blood capillaries.

Innervation of the thyroid, via the sympathetic and parasympathetic systems, serves an essentially vasomotor function. Recent ultrastructural and radioautographic studies have shown a network of adrenergic fibers terminating near the basal lamina of the follicular cells. These findings, together with evidence that adrenergic and other amines influence thyroid iodine metabolism in isolated thyroid cells and in vivo, indicate that the neurogenic stimuli can influence thyroid function through a direct effect on the epithelial cells. However, thyroid-stimulating hormone (TSH; thyrotropin), which is secreted by the anterior pituitary, is the major regulator of the anatomic and functional state of the thyroid gland.

The morphologic appearance of thyroid follicles varies according to the region of the gland and its functional activity. In the same gland, larger follicles full of colloid and having a cuboidal or squamous epithelium are found alongside follicles lined by columnar epithelium. In spite of this variation, when the average composition of these follicles is squamous, the gland is considered hypoactive. When drugs capable of stimulating the synthesis of thyroid hormone are administered, a marked increase in the height of the follicular epithelium is observed. This phenomenon is accompanied by a decrease in quantity of the colloid and size of the follicles (Fig 22– 15).

The thyroid epithelium always rests on a basal lamina. The ultrastructure of the follicular epithelium exhibits all of the characteristics of a cell that simultaneously synthesizes, secretes, reabsorbs, and digests proteins (Fig 22– 19). The basal part of these cells is rich in rough endoplasmic reticulum. The nucleus is generally round and situated in the center of the cell. The apical pole has a discrete Golgi complex and small secretory granules with the staining characteristics of follicular colloid. Abundant lysosomes, 0.5– 0.6 μm in diameter, and some large phagosomes are found in this region. The cell membrane of the apical pole has a moderate number of microvilli. Mitochondria, distended cisternae of rough endoplasmic reticulum, and ribosomes are dispersed throughout the cytoplasm.

Another type of cell, the **parafollicular,** or **C, cell,** is found as part of the follicular epithelium or as isolated clusters between thyroid follicles (Fig 22– 16). When parafollicular cells are found inside the follicular basement membrane as part of the epithelium, their apical surfaces are never in contact with colloid. Rather, thin processes of thyroid follicular cells intervene between parafollicular cells and the colloid. Parafollicular cells are somewhat larger and stain less intensely than thyroid follicular cells. They contain an abundant rough endoplasmic reticulum, long mitochondria, and a large Golgi complex. The most striking feature of these cells is their numerous small (100– 180 nm in diameter), hormone-containing

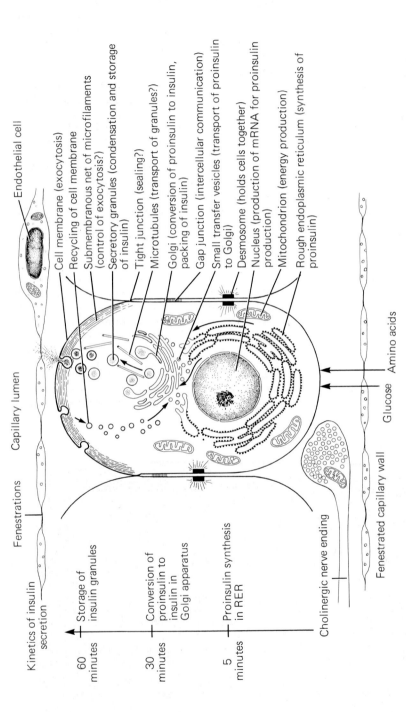

Endothelial cell

Cell membrane (exocytosis)

Recycling of cell membrane

Submembranous net of microfilaments (control of exocytosis?)

Secretory granules (condensation and storage of insulin)

Tight junction (sealing?)

Microtubules (transport of granules?)

Golgi (conversion of proinsulin to insulin, packing of insulin)

Gap junction (intercellular communication)

Small transfer vesicles (transport of proinsulin to Golgi)

Desmosome (holds cells together)

Nucleus (production of mRNA for proinsulin production)

Mitochondrion (energy production)

Rough endoplasmic reticulum (synthesis of proinsulin)

Capillary lumen

Fenestrations

Kinetics of insulin secretion

60 minutes — Storage of insulin granules

30 minutes — Conversion of proinsulin to insulin in Golgi apparatus

5 minutes — Proinsulin synthesis in RER

Cholinergic nerve ending

Fenestrated capillary wall

Amino acids

Glucose

Figure 22–13. The physiology of the B cell of the pancreatic islet. Note the complex secretory process, which has been simplified elsewhere in this book for teaching purposes. The process begins with the entrance of blood-borne amino acids into the cell, probably aided by an active amino acid pump present in the cell membrane. The amino acids are polymerized to proinsulin by the polysomes present on the surface of the rough endoplasmic reticulum, and the polypeptide chain is injected through the membrane of the RER into the lumen. The proinsulin is then transferred into small vesicles by a process of budding that occurs in the cisternae close to the Golgi complex. In this region, no polysomes cover the endoplasmic reticulum. The small vesicles are transported by an unknown mechanism and fuse to the Golgi cisternae. Their contents are then packed into secretory granules by the Golgi complex and gradually condense to form the mature secretory granule. At some point between reaching the Golgi complex and the release of Golgi vesicles at the cell surface, proinsulin is cleaved enzymatically to yield insulin plus the C-peptide. Microtubules may play a role in the transport of these granules to the cell surface. Granule extrusion occurs when the cell membrane fuses with the membrane of the granule and the contents of the granule spill into the extracellular space. Here, the contents of the granule dissolve and diffuse into a blood vessel. Evidence has been presented suggesting that a submembranous net of microfilaments participates in mechanical inhibition of the extrusion process until the appropriate stimulus has been received.

The granule membrane is incorporated into the cell membrane and is probably recycled by the cell by means of small endocytotic vesicles (upper left). The secretory processes of the B cell are regulated mainly by the blood glucose level and by autonomic nerve endings. RER, rough endoplasmic reticulum. (Based on data presented by Orci L: A portrait of the pancreatic B cell. *Diabetologia* 1974;**10**:163.)

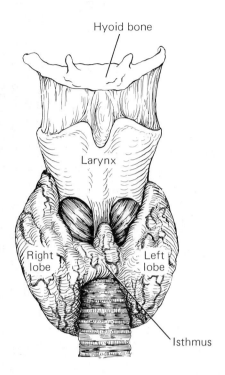

Hyoid bone

Larynx

Right lobe

Left lobe

Isthmus

Figure 22–14. The human thyroid. (Reproduced, with permission, from Ganong WF: *Review of Medical Physiology,* 12th ed. Lange, 1985.)

granules (Fig 22–17). These cells are responsible for the synthesis and secretion of **calcitonin,** a hormone containing 32 amino acids and having a molecular weight of 3500. The effect of calcitonin is to lower blood calcium levels by inhibiting bone reabsorption. Secretion of calcitonin is triggered by an elevation in blood calcium concentration.

Histophysiology

The thyroid is the only endocrine gland whose secretory product is stored in great quantity. This accumulation is unusual in that it occurs in the extracellular colloid. In humans, there is sufficient hormone within the follicles to supply the organism for up to 3 months. Thyroid colloid is composed of a glycoprotein (thyroglobulin) of high molecular weight (660,000). The staining affinity of the follicular colloid varies greatly; it may be either acidophilic or basophilic. Thyroglobulin is also PAS-positive owing to its high carbohydrate content.

The activity of the follicular cells of the thyroid is controlled by the circulating level of TSH (thyrotropin). A rise in the circulating free thyroid hormones inhibits the synthesis of TSH, and when the thyroid hormone level drops the secretion of TSH by the adenohypophysis is stimulated, establishing in this way a homeostatic balance that maintains an adequate quantity of thyroxine and triiodothyronine within the organism (Fig 22–18). TSH secretion is also increased by exposure to cold and is depressed by heat and stressful stimuli. The negative feedback effect of thyroid hormones on TSH secretion may be exerted in part at the hypothalamus but to a greater extent upon

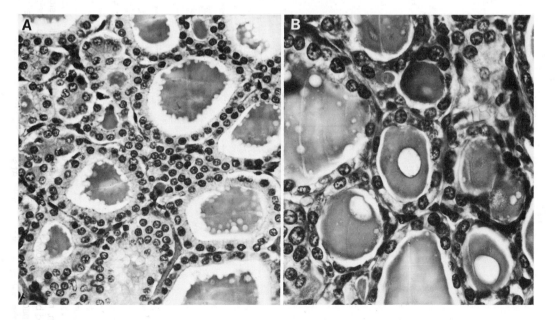

Figure 22–15. Photomicrographs of sections of thyroid glands. The presence of higher epithelial cells indicates that the section on the left is from a more active gland. H&E stain, × 200 *(A)* and 400 *(B).*

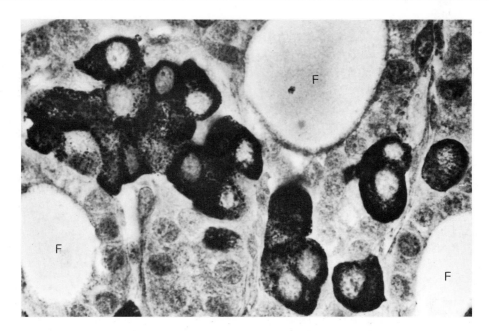

Figure 22–16. Photomicrograph of a dog's thyroid showing its dark-staining parafollicular cells. F indicates the lumen of thyroid follicles. × 800. (Courtesy of F Kameda.)

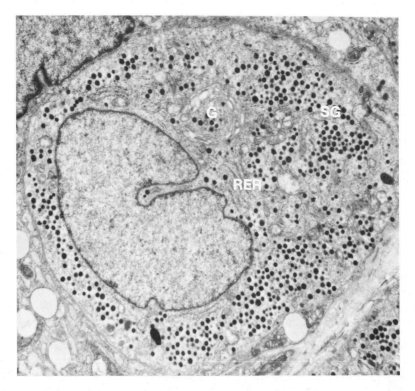

Figure 22–17. Electron micrograph of a calcitonin-producing cell. Observe the small secretory granules (SG) and the scarcity of rough endoplasmic reticulum (RER). G, Golgi region. × 5000.

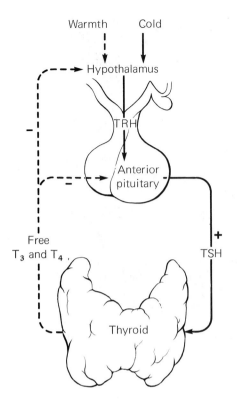

Figure 22–18. Regulation of TSH secretion. Solid arrows indicate stimulation; dashed arrows, inhibition.

the anterior pituitary. A tripeptide has been isolated from the hypothalamus (thyrotropin-releasing hormone, TRH) that stimulates TSH secretion (Fig 22–18).

Synthesis & Accumulation of Hormones by the Follicular Cells

This process takes place in 4 stages, as follows: synthesis of thyroglobulin, uptake of iodide from the blood, activation of the iodide, and iodination of the tyrosyl radicals of thyroglobulin.

These stages are diagrammed in Fig 22–19. They take place in the following manner:

(1) The **synthesis of thyroglobulin** occurs in a manner typical of other protein exporting cells (described in Chapter 4). This process has been studied by radioautographic techniques with the use of tritiated leucine, an amino acid abundant in thyroglobulin (Fig 22–20). Briefly, the secretory pathway is as follows: synthesis of protein in the rough endoplasmic reticulum, addition of carbohydrate in the endoplasmic reticulum and the Golgi complex, and release from formed vesicles at the apical surface of the cell into the lumen of the follicle.

Radioautographic studies performed with the electron microscope show that the addition of the carbohydrate component of thyroglobulin occurs both in the endoplasmic reticulum and the Golgi complex.

Mannose is incorporated within the endoplasmic reticulum, whereas galactose is added to thyroglobulin in the Golgi complex.

(2) The **uptake of circulating iodide** is accomplished in the thyroid by a mechanism of active transport, utilizing the iodide pump, located within the cytoplasmic membrane of the basal region of the follicular cells. This pump is readily stimulated by thyrotropin. The uptake of iodide can be inhibited by certain drugs such as perchlorate and thiocyanate, which act by competing with iodide.

(3) During the **oxidation of iodide,** iodide is oxidized by thyroid peroxidase to an intermediate, which in turn combines in the colloid with the tyrosine residues of thyroglobulin. This process can be blocked by drugs (eg, propylthiouracil and carbimazole) that inhibit the peroxidase-catalyzed iodination of thyroglobulin. Some forms of thyroid dysfunction may be related to a genetic deficiency of peroxidase.

(4) In contrast to the processes described above, **iodination of tyrosine residues** bound to thyroglobulin takes place not inside the follicular cells but in the colloid in contact with the membrane of the apical region of the cells. Initially, a monoiodine compound, monoiodotyrosine (MIT), is formed, followed by the production of the diiodine compound, diiodotyrosine (DIT). Two DIT molecules are then united—the coupling reaction—forming tetraiodothyronine (thyroxine; T_4), which is the main thyroid hormone. Another hormone produced, although on a much smaller scale, is triiodothyronine (T_3), by condensation of MIT with DIT (Fig 22–21). The coupling reaction is an aerobic, energy-requiring one. It is postulated that the union of the iodinated tyrosines is catalyzed by an enzymatic mechanism. For this process to occur normally, thyroglobulin must have the correct spatial configuration. When disease causes the production of abnormal thyroglobulin, this process is blocked, resulting in deficient synthesis of thyroid hormone.

Liberation of T_3 & T_4

When stimulated by TSH, thyroid follicular cells take up colloid by a form of pinocytosis. Folds of apical cytoplasm (lamellipodia) encircle a portion of colloid and bring it into the follicular cell. The pinocytotic vesicles then fuse with lysosomes. The peptide bonds between the iodinated residues and the thyroglobulin molecule are broken by proteases in lysosomes, and T_4, T_3, DIT, and MIT are liberated into the cytoplasm. The free T_4 and T_3 then cross the cell membrane and are discharged into the capillaries. MIT and DIT are not secreted into the blood, since their iodine is removed as a result of the intracellular action of **iodotyrosine dehalogenase.** The products of this enzymatic reaction, iodine and tyrosine, are reused by the follicular cells. T_4 is the most abundant of these compounds, constituting 90% of the circulating thyroid hormone, although T_3 acts more rapidly and is more potent than T_4. In humans, 80 μg/d of free T_4 and 4 μg/d of T_3 are secreted by the thyroid cells into the capillaries.

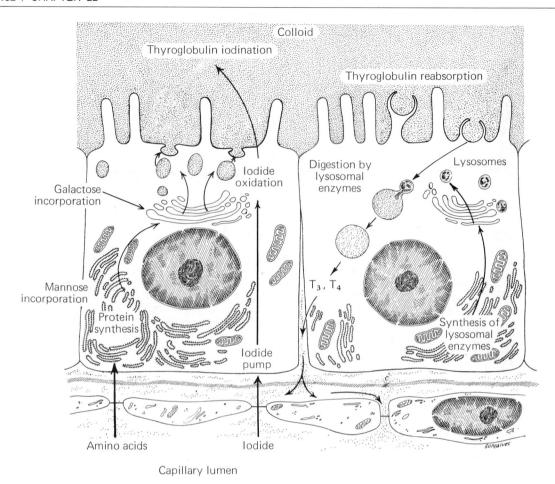

Figure 22–19. Diagram showing the processes of synthesis and iodination of thyroglobulin *(left)* and its reabsorption and digestion *(right).* These events occur in the same cell.

Thyroxine stimulates mitochondrial respiration and oxidative phosphorylation. Since this effect is blocked by dactinomycin, it is dependent on RNA synthesis. T_3 and T_4 increase both the number of mitochondria and the number of their cristae. Mitochondrial protein synthesis is increased, while degradation of their proteins is decreased.

Most of the effects of thyroid hormones are secondary to their effects on basal metabolic rate; they increase the absorption of carbohydrates from the intestine and regulate lipid metabolism. Thyroid hormones also influence body growth and the development of the nervous system during fetal life.

Factors That Affect the Synthesis of Thyroid Hormone

A diet that contains less than 10 μg/d of iodine hinders the synthesis of thyroid hormones. Thyroid hypertrophy as a result of increased TSH secretion causes the disorder known as **iodine deficiency goiter,** which occurs widely in some regions of the world.

The syndrome of adult hypothyroidism is called **myxedema** and may be the result of a number of diseases of the thyroid gland or may be secondary to pituitary or hypothalamic failure. Children who are hypothyroid from birth are called **cretins;** they are characterized by dwarfing and mental retardation.

Hyperthyroidism or thyrotoxicosis may be caused by a variety of thyroid diseases, but the most common form is **Graves' disease** or **exophthalmic goiter.** The levels of TSH are subnormal, and the thyroid hyperfunction in this disease is due to a circulating gamma globulin which exerts effects resembling those of TSH.

THE PARATHYROID GLANDS

The parathyroids are 4 small glands—3 × 6 mm—with a total weight of about 0.4 g. They are situated behind the thyroid gland, one at each end of the upper and lower poles, usually in the capsule that covers the lobes of the thyroid (Fig 22–22). Sometimes they are found embedded in the thyroid gland. The parathyroid glands are derived from pharyngeal pouches—

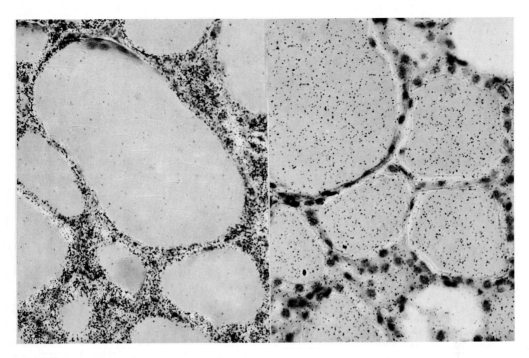

Figure 22–20. Radioautographs of the thyroid glands of rats previously injected with radioactive leucine. *Left:* The tracer was injected 30 minutes before the animal was killed. Observe the radioactivity (dark dots) concentrated mainly over the cells. *Right:* The amino acid was injected 45 days before the animal was killed, and most radioactivity is in the colloid (thyroglobulin). × 385.

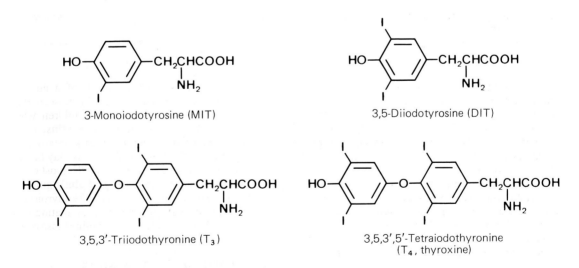

Figure 22–21. Formulas of 3-monoiodotyrosine (MIT) and 3,5-diiodotyrosine (DIT). The condensation of 2 molecules of DIT with the elimination of an alanine residue results in the formation of tetraiodothyronine (T_4; thyroxine). The condensation of one molecule of MIT and one molecule of DIT with the elimination of one alanine residue results in the formation of triiodothyronine (T_3).

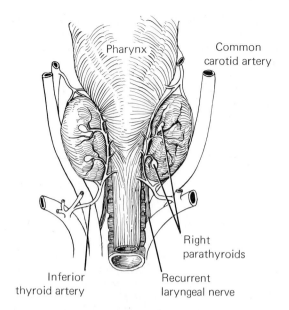

Figure 22–22. The human parathyroid glands, viewed from behind. (Redrawn and reproduced, with permission, from Nordland: The larynx as related to surgery of the thyroid based on an anatomical study. *Surg Gynecol Obstet* 1930;**51**:449; and from *Gray's Anatomy of the Human Body,* 29th ed. Goss CM [editor]. Lea & Febiger, 1973.)

the superior glands from the fourth pouch and the inferior glands from the third. They may be found in the mediastinum, lying beside the thymus, since the parathyroid glands and the thymus originate from the same pharyngeal pouches.

Histology

Each parathyroid gland is contained within a connective tissue capsule. These capsules send septa into the gland, where they merge with the reticular fibers supporting elongated cordlike clusters of secretory cells.

The parenchyma of the parathyroid glands consists of 2 types of cells: the chief or principal cells and the oxyphil cells (Fig 22–23). In hyperplasia, however, a third cell type, the water clear cell, is also seen, but its function is not known.

The **chief cells** are the most numerous in humans. In most other mammals, they are the only parenchymal cells found in the parathyroid gland. They are small (4–8 μm in diameter), polygonal cells, with a vesicular nucleus and a pale-staining, slightly acidophilic cytoplasm. Electron microscopy shows irregularly shaped granules 200–400 nm in diameter in the cytoplasm of the chief cells. They are the secretory granules containing parathyroid hormone, which in the active form is a polypeptide with a molecular weight of 9500. These granules, the number of which varies from one cell to another, are distributed throughout the cytoplasm, but sometimes they are more numerous at the vascular pole of the cell. A prominent Golgi

complex is situated adjacent to the nucleus. Rough endoplasmic reticulum and free ribosomes are present. Small ovoid or spherical mitochondria and lipofuscin pigment bodies are also evident. Masses of glycogen granules occur and are especially large in resting or inactive chief cells.

In humans, **oxyphil cells** begin to appear at about age 7 and increase in number with age. They too are polygonal in shape, but they are larger (6–10 μm in diameter) than chief cells; their nuclei are smaller and stain more densely; and their cytoplasm contains many acidophilic granules (Fig 22–23). The electron microscope reveals that these granules are mitochondria with abundant cristae. The function of the oxyphil cell is uncertain.

Cells with structural characteristics intermediate between chief and oxyphil cells are also seen, suggesting that they are transitions of a single cell type. With increasing age, replacement of secretory cells by adipocytes occurs. Adipose cells can constitute over 50% of the gland in older individuals.

Histophysiology

Parathyroid glands are essential for life. They secrete parathyroid hormone, which controls the concentration of calcium and phosphate ions in the blood. A plasma calcium level of about 10 mg/dL is normal. If calcium levels are lowered, neuromuscular transmission is severely affected.

Decrease in blood calcium stimulates the parathyroid gland to secrete its hormone. In turn, parathy-

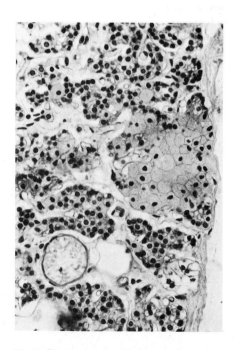

Figure 22–23. Photomicrograph of a section of the parathyroid gland. Observe a group of large, acidophilic oxyphil cells at the middle right portion. × 220. (Courtesy of J James.)

roid hormone acts on the cells of bone tissue, increasing the number of osteoclasts and promoting in this way the reabsorption of the calcified bone matrix and the release of calcium into the blood. Increase in the concentration of calcium in the blood suppresses the production of parathyroid hormone. Calcitonin from the thyroid gland also influences osteoclasts by inhibiting their resorptive action on bone and liberation of calcium; thus calcitonin lowers blood calcium and increases osteogenesis.

In addition to increasing the concentration of calcium, parathyroid hormone reduces the concentration of phosphate in the blood. This effect is a consequence of an increase in the excretion of phosphate in urine. Parathyroid hormone diminishes the absorption of phosphate from the glomerular filtrate at the level of the kidney tubules. There is also strong evidence that parathyroid hormone increases absorption of calcium from the gastrointestinal tract and that vitamin D is necessary for this effect.

In **hyperparathyroidism,** blood phosphate is low and blood calcium is increased. This frequently produces a pathologic deposit of calcium in several organs such as the kidneys and arteries. Bones are decalcified and become subject to fractures. The bone disease caused by hyperparathyroidism is characterized by multiple bone cysts and is known as **osteitis fibrosa cystica.**

Hypoparathyroidism causes an increase in the concentration of phosphate and a decrease in the concentration of calcium in the blood. The bones become denser and more mineralized. This condition causes spastic contractions of the skeletal muscles and generalized convulsions called tetany. These symptoms are due to the exaggerated excitability of the nervous system caused by the lack of calcium ions in the blood. The administration of calcium or of parathyroid hormone terminates the convulsions—the former much more rapidly.

The secretion of the parathyroid cells is regulated by the blood calcium level and apparently is not directly affected by other endocrine glands or the nervous system.

THE PINEAL BODY

The pineal body is also known as the epiphysis cerebri, or pineal gland. In the adult, it is a flattened, conical organ measuring approximately 5–8 mm in length and 3–5 mm at its greatest width and weighing about 120 mg. It is found in the posterior extremity of the third ventricle, above the roof of the diencephalon, to which it is connected by means of a short stalk.

The pineal is covered by pia mater. Connective tissue septa (containing blood vessels and unmyelinated nerve fibers) originate in the pia mater and penetrate the pineal tissue to surround, along with blood capillaries, the cellular cords and follicles, forming irregular lobules (Fig 22–24).

The pineal body consists of several types of cells but principally pinealocytes and astroglial cells. **Pinealocytes** have a slightly basophilic cytoplasm with large irregular or lobate nuclei and sharply defined nucleoli. When impregnated with silver salts (Del Rio Hortega's method), the pinealocytes appear to have long and tortuous branches reaching out to the vascular connective tissue septa where they end as flattened dilatations. The cytoplasm of the pinealocytes contains a great number of free ribosomes and a small

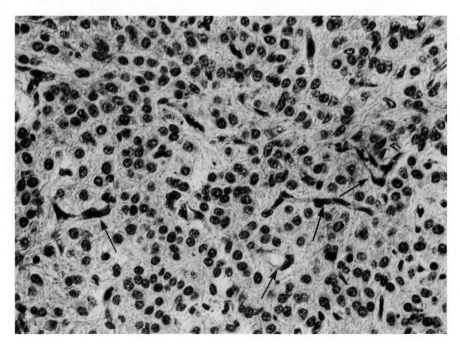

Figure 22–24. Section of a pineal gland. The arrows indicate blood vessels that surround the cellular cords. × 350.

amount of rough endoplasmic reticulum. The Golgi complex and the mitochondria are poorly developed. In addition, one also finds lipid droplets and structures similar to lysosomes. Large numbers of filaments, 5–8 nm in diameter, are abundant in processes of pinealocytes.

The **astroglial cells** of the pineal body are a specific type of cell characterized by elongated nuclei that stain more heavily than those of parenchymal cells. They are observed between the cords of pinealocytes and perivascular areas. These cells have long cytoplasmic processes containing a large number of intermediate filaments 10 nm in diameter and of moderate length.

In addition to the above-mentioned cell types, mast cells are frequently encountered in the pineal body. Mast cells are probably responsible for the high histamine content of this organ.

Age causes an increase in the amount of connective tissue in the pineal body and the formation of calcified bodies (**brain sand**) in the parenchyma of this organ. These calcified bodies are used as a reference point in skull radiology for they appear clearly in x-rays.

Innervation

Silver impregnation reveals nerve fibers throughout the pineal body. When these nerve fibers penetrate the organ, they lose their myelin sheath, the unmyelinated axons ending among pinealocytes (Fig 22–25), and some form synapses. A great number of small vesicles 40 nm in diameter containing norepinephrine are observed in these nerve endings. Serotonin is present also, both in the pinealocytes and in sympathetic nerve terminals. The pineal body is mainly innervated by postganglionic sympathetic fibers (nervus conarii) derived from the superior cervical sympathetic ganglia. Nerves derived from the posterior commissure enter the pineal body via its stalk, but the significance of these nerves is uncertain.

Histophysiology

In spite of the great quantity of research on the pineal gland, its role as an endocrine gland is still a subject of controversy.

The pineal has been claimed at one time or another to be a source of (1) a gonadotropin-releasing hormone; (2) a gonadotropin-inhibiting principle having a structure similar to that of arginine vasotocin; (3) a growth-inhibiting factor; (4) a thyrotropin-releasing hormone; (5) a substance that inhibits the onset of puberty; (6) melatonin, which may inhibit gonadotropin release and causes lightening of amphibian skin; and (7) factors that antagonize the secretion of ACTH and regulate the secretion of aldosterone.

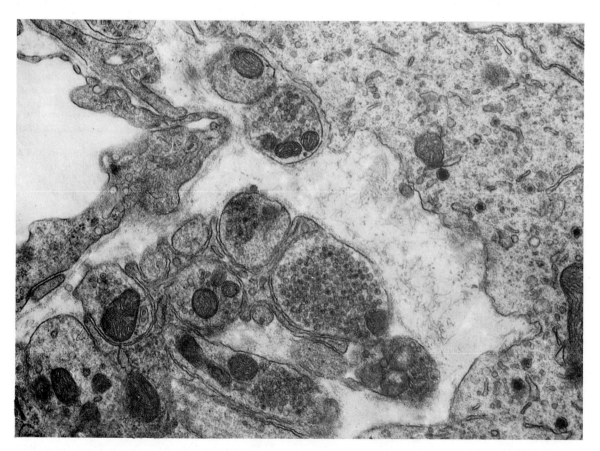

Figure 22–25. Electron micrograph of adrenergic nerve endings in the pineal body. × 32,000. (Courtesy of S Matsushima.)

The hypothesis that has received the widest acceptance is that the pineal acts on the gonads. Whether it secretes hormones into the blood, the cerebrospinal fluid, or both has not been clearly determined.

Melatonin

Melatonin is an indole derivative, isolated from the pineal body of mammals, that induces the aggregation of pigment granules in the melanophores of amphibia. This substance, synthesized only in the pineal, has a 100,000 times stronger effect on melanophores than norepinephrine, which has a similar effect. From this organ has been isolated an enzyme called hydroxyindole-O-methyltransferase, which is capable of methylating N-acetyl-5-hydroxytryptamine and transforming it into melatonin.

The quantity of melatonin and serotonin in the pineal body of rats and humans undergoes diurnal changes according to the alternations of light and dark periods. A diminished activity of hydroxyindole-O-methyltransferase and a consequent inhibition of melatonin synthesis are observed if the rats are maintained in constant illumination.

The first evidence that the pineal body might affect the function of the gonads was the observation that an individual suffering from a destructive tumor of this organ developed precocious puberty and hypertrophy of the gonads. However, the precise role of this organ remains an open question. The mammalian pinealocytes are neuroendocrine transducers, since they respond to a neurotransmitter (ie, norepinephrine) by synthesizing a group of biologically active compounds that modify the function of different endocrine organs.

REFERENCES

Adrenal Gland

Baxter JD, Rousseau GG: Glucocorticoid hormone action: An overview. *Monogr Endocrinol* 1979;**12**:1.

Chester JI, Henderson IW (editors): *General, Comparative and Clinical Endocrinology of the Adrenal Cortex.* Vol 2. Academic Press, 1978.

Christy NP (editor): *The Human Adrenal Cortex.* Harper & Row, 1971.

Coupland RE, Fujita T (editors): *Chromaffin, Enterochromaffin and Related Cells.* Elsevier, 1976.

Gill GN: ACTH regulation of the adrenal cortex. *Pharmacol Ther* [B] 1976;**2**:313.

James VHT (editor): *The Adrenal Gland.* Raven Press, 1979.

Johannisson E: The foetal adrenal cortex in the human: Its ultrastructure at different stages of development and in different functional states. *Acta Endocrinol [Suppl] (Copenh)* 1968;**130**:1.

Lanman JT: The fetal zone of the adrenal gland. *Medicine* 1953;**32**:389.

Long JA, Jones AL: Observations on the fine structure of the adrenal cortex of man. *Lab Invest* 1967;**17**:355.

Pohorecky LA, Wurtman RJ: Adrenocortical control of epinephrine synthesis. *Pharmacol Rev* 1971;**23**:1.

Pollard HB et al: The chromaffin granule and possible mechanisms of exocytosis. *Int Rev Cytol* 1979;**58**:159.

Suzuki T: Physiology of adrenocortical secretion. *Front Horm Res* 1983;**11**:1.

Islets of Langerhans

Cooperstein SJ, Watkins D (editors): *The Islets of Langerhans.* Academic Press, 1981.

Ganong WF: *Review of Medical Physiology,* 12th ed. Lange, 1985.

Like AA: The ultrastructure of the islets of Langerhans in man. *Lab Invest* 1967;**16**:937.

Thyroid Gland

Anast CS: Thyrocalcitonin: A review. *Clin Orthop* 1966;**47**:179.

Bussolati G, Pearse AGE: Immunofluorescence localization of calcitonin in the C cells of pig and dog's thyroid. *J Endocrinol* 1967;**37**:205.

Fujita H: Fine structure of the thyroid cell. *Int Rev Cytol* 1975;**40**:197.

Heimann P: Ultrastructure of the human thyroid: A study of normal thyroid, untreated and treated toxic goiter. *Acta Endocrinol* 1966;**53(Suppl 110)**:5.

Ibrahim MS, Budd GC: An electron microscopic study of the site of iodine binding in the rat thyroid gland. *Exp Cell Res* 1965;**38**:50.

Klinck GH, Oertel JE, Winship I: Ultrastructure of normal human thyroid. *Lab Invest* 1970;**22**:2.

Nunez EA, Gershon MD: Cytophysiology of thyroid parafollicular cells. *Int Rev Cytol* 1978;**52**:1.

Sterling K, Lazarus JH: The thyroid and its control. *Annu Rev Physiol* 1977;**39**:349.

Strum JM, Karnowsky MJ: Cytochemical localization of endogenous peroxidase in the thyroid follicular cells. *J Cell Biol* 1970;**44**:655.

Whur P, Herscovics A, Leblond CP: Radioautographic visualization of the incorporation of galactose-³H and mannose-³H by rat thyroid in vitro in relation to the stages of thyroglobulin synthesis. *J Cell Biol* 1969;**43**:289.

Parathyroid Gland

Gaillard PJ, Talmage RV, Budy AM (editors): *The Parathyroid Glands.* Univ of Chicago Press, 1965.

Gray JK, Cooper CW, Munson PL: Parathyroid hormone. Thyrocalcitonin and the control of mineral metabolism. In: *Endocrine Physiology.* McCann SM (editor). Butterworth, 1974.

Wong ET, Lindall AW: Subcellular location of human parathyroid hormone immunoreactive peptides and preliminary evidence for a precursor to human PTH. *Proc Soc Exp Biol Med* 1975;**148**:387.

Pineal Body

Pelham RW et al: Twenty-four hour cycle of melatonin-like substance in the plasma of human males. *J Clin Endocrinol Metab* 1973;**37**:341.

Reiter RJ (editor): *The Pineal Gland.* Raven Press, 1984.

Tapp E, Huxley M: The histological appearance of the human pineal gland from puberty to old age. *J Pathol* 1972;**108**:137.

23

The Male Reproductive System

The male reproductive system is composed of the testes, genital ducts, accessory glands, and penis. The **testis** has 2 functions—reproductive and hormonal. It is surrounded by a thick capsule of collagenous connective tissue, the **tunica albuginea.** The tunica albuginea is thickened on the posterior surface of the testis to form the **mediastinum testis,** from which fibrous septa penetrate the gland, dividing it into about 250 pyramidal compartments called the **testicular lobules** (Fig 23–1). These septa are incomplete, and

intercommunications frequently exist between the lobules. Each lobule is occupied by 1–4 seminiferous tubules enmeshed in a web of loose connective tissue rich in blood and lymphatic vessels, nerves, and interstitial (Leydig) cells. Seminiferous tubules produce male reproductive cells, the spermatozoa. Interstitial cells secrete testicular androgens (Fig 23–1).

The genital ducts and accessory glands produce secretions that, aided by smooth muscle contractions, propel spermatozoa toward the exterior. These secre-

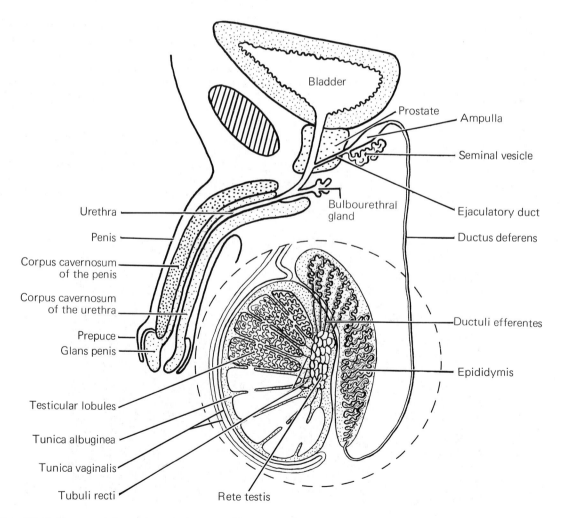

Figure 23–1. Diagram of the male genital system. The testis and the epididymis are in different scales from the other parts of the reproductive system. Observe the communication between the testicular lobules.

tions also provide nutrients for spermatozoa while they are confined to the male reproductive tract. Spermatozoa plus the secretions of the genital ducts and accessory glands comprise the **semen.** The penis is the organ by which semen is introduced into the female reproductive tract.

The testes develop retroperitoneally in the dorsal wall of the abdominal cavity and later are suspended within the scrotum at the ends of the spermatic cords, each carrying with it a serous sac derived from the peritoneum called the **tunica vaginalis** (Fig 23–1). This tunic consists of an outer parietal and an inner visceral layer, covering the tunica albuginea on the anterior and lateral sides of the testis. The scrotum has an important role in maintaining the testes at a temperature below intra-abdominal temperature.

TESTIS

Seminiferous Tubules

Each seminiferous tubule is lined with a complex stratified epithelium and is about 150–250 μm in diameter and 30–70 cm long. The combined length of the tubules of one testis is about 250 m. The convoluted tubules form a network, wherein individual tubules are either blind-ended or branched. At the termination of each tubule, the lumen narrows and the epithelial lining abruptly changes into a simple cuboidal layer of cells. These short segments, known as **straight tubules,** or **tubuli recti,** connect the seminiferous tubules to an anastomosing labyrinth of epithelium-lined channels, the **rete testis.** The rete, present in the connective tissue of the mediastinum, is connected to the cephalic portion of the **epididymis** by 10–20 **ductuli efferentes** (Fig 23–1).

The seminiferous tubules consist of the following components (Figs 23–2 and 23–3): (1) a tunic of fibrous connective tissue; (2) a well-defined basal lamina; and (3) a complex **germinal,** or **seminiferous, epithelium.**

The fibrous **tunica propria** enveloping the seminiferous tubule consists of several layers of fibroblasts. The innermost layer adhering to the basal lamina consists of flattened **myoid cells,** which exhibit smooth muscle characteristics in some species. Myoid cells are not found in humans.

The epithelium consists of 2 types of cells: **Sertoli,** or **supporting, cells** and cells that constitute the **spermatogenic lineage.** The cells of spermatogenic lineage are stacked in 4–8 layers that occupy the space between the basal lamina and the lumen of the tubule. These cells divide several times and finally differentiate, producing spermatozoa. They represent various stages in the continuous process of differentiation of the male germ cells. This phenomenon from start to finish is called **spermatogenesis** and can be divided into 3 phases: (1) **spermatocytogenesis,** during which spermatogonia divide, producing successive generations of cells that finally give rise to **spermatocytes;** (2) **meiosis,** during which the spermatocyte goes through 2 successive divisions, with reduction by half of the number of chromosomes and amount of DNA per cell, producing **spermatids;** and (3) **spermiogenesis,** during which the spermatids go through an elaborate process of cytodifferentiation, producing **spermatozoa.**

The process of spermatogenesis begins with a primitive germ cell, the **spermatogonium,** situated next to the basal lamina. It is a relatively small cell, about 12 μm in diameter, and its nucleus contains pale-staining chromatin (Fig 23–3). The cytoplasm

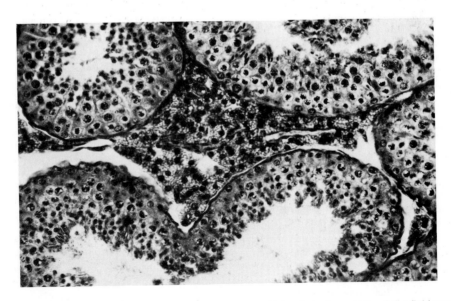

Figure 23–2. Photomicrograph of the testis of a monkey. The interstitial cells in the middle of the field contain vacuoles resulting from the dissolution of lipid droplets during preparation. H&E stain, × 400.

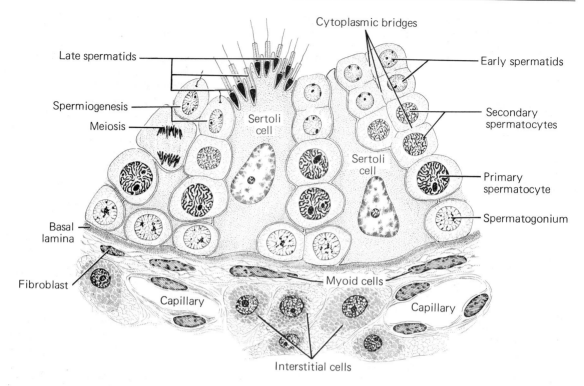

Figure 23–3. Diagram of the structure of a part of a seminiferous tubule and interstitial tissue. This figure does not show the lymphatic vessels found in the connective tissue.

contains a small Golgi complex, spherical mitochondria, and numerous free ribosomes. At sexual maturity, this cell undergoes a series of mitoses, and the newly formed cells can follow one of 2 paths: they can continue, after one or more mitotic divisions, in the same way as the parent cell (the spermatogonium), and thus **type A spermatogonia** become a continuous source of spermatogonia; or they can divide and grow, thus becoming larger than the parent spermatogonium, in which case they are called **type B spermatogonia.** Type B spermatogonia give rise to the **primary spermatocytes.** Soon after their formation, they enter the prophase of the first meiotic division. At the beginning of the prophase of the first meiotic division, the primary spermatocyte has 46 (44 + XY) chromosomes and 4N amount of DNA. (N denotes either the haploid set of chromosomes [23 chromosomes in humans] or the amount of DNA in the haploid set of chromosomes.) In this prophase, the cell passes through 4 stages—leptotene, zygotene, pachytene, and diplotene—and reaches the stage of diakinesis, resulting in the separation of the chromosomes. During these stages of meiosis, crossing over of genes of the chromosomes occurs. Thereafter, the cell enters the metaphase, and in the following anaphase the chromosomes move toward each pole. Since the prophase of this division takes a long time (about 22 days), the majority of cells seen in sections will be in this phase. The primary spermatocytes are the largest cells of the

spermatogenic lineage and are characterized by the presence of chromosomes in different stages of the coiling process within their nuclei. From this first meiotic division there result smaller cells called **secondary spermatocytes** (Fig 23–3) with only 23 chromosomes (22 + X or 22 + Y). This decrease in number (from 46 to 23) is accompanied by a reduction in the amount of DNA per cell (from 4N to 2N). Secondary spermatocytes are difficult to observe in sections of the testis because they remain in interphase very briefly and enter quickly into the second meiotic division, thus being short-lived cells. Division of the secondary spermatocytes results in **spermatids,** cells that contain 23 chromosomes. In this second division, the amount of DNA per cell is reduced by half, forming haploid (1N) cells. This happens because no S phase (DNA synthesis) occurs between the first and second meiotic divisions of the spermatocytes. The meiotic process therefore results in formation of cells with a haploid number of chromosomes. With fertilization, they return to the normal diploid number. It is the meiotic process which, because of the reductional process of cell division, guarantees a constant (fixed) number of chromosomes for the species.

Spermatids are cells resulting from the division of secondary spermatocytes. They can be distinguished by their small size (7–8 μm in diameter), nuclei with areas of condensed chromatin, and juxtaluminal location within the seminiferous tubules (Fig

23–3). Spermatids undergo a complex process of differentiation called **spermiogenesis,** which includes formation of the acrosome, condensation and elongation of the nucleus, development of the flagellum, and loss of much of the cytoplasm. The end result is the mature spermatozoon, which is then released into the lumen of the seminiferous tubule.

Spermiogenesis can be divided into 4 phases (Figs 23–4 and 23–5).

(1) The Golgi phase: The cytoplasm of spermatids contains a prominent Golgi complex near the nucleus, mitochondria, a pair of centrioles, free ribosomes, and tubules of smooth endoplasmic reticulum. Small PAS-positive proacrosomal granules accumulate in the Golgi complex and subsequently coalesce to form a single **acrosomal granule** contained within a membrane-limited **acrosomal vesicle.** The centrioles migrate to a position near the cell surface and opposite the location of the forming acrosome. Formation of the flagellar axoneme is initiated, and the centrioles migrate back toward the nucleus, spinning out the axonemal components as they move.

(2) The cap phase: The acrosomal vesicle and granule spread to cover the anterior half of the condensing nucleus and are now known as the **acrosome** or **acrosomal cap.** The acrosome contains several hydrolytic enzymes such as hyaluronidase, neuraminidase, acid phosphatase, and a protease having trypsinlike activity. Thus, the acrosome serves as a specialized type of lysosome. These enzymes are known to dissociate cells of the corona radiata and to digest

the zona pellucida, structures that surround recently ovulated eggs (Fig 24–3). When spermatozoa encounter ova, the outer membrane of the acrosome fuses with the plasma membrane at multiple sites, liberating the acrosomal enzymes. This process is known as the **acrosomal reaction,** one of the first steps in fertilization.

(3) During the **acrosome phase,** the anterior pole of the cell, containing the acrosome, becomes oriented toward the base of the seminiferous tubule. In addition, the nucleus becomes more elongated and condensed. This process may be facilitated by a cylinder of microtubules, the **manchette,** that surrounds the nucleus. The mitochondria aggregate around the proximal part of the flagellum, forming a thickened region known as the **middle piece.** This disposition of mitochondria is another example of a concentration of these organelles in sites related to cell movement and high energy consumption. Flagellar structure and function are described in Chapter 3. Movement of the flagellum is a result of the interaction among microtubules, ATP, and an ATPase called **dynein. Kartagener's syndrome,** characterized by immotile spermatozoa and consequent infertility, has been described as being due to lack of dynein in the patient's spermatozoa. This disorder is usually coincident with chronic respiratory infections, since a similar deficiency exists in the ciliary axonemes of respiratory epithelial cells. Carbohydrates produced by the glands associated with the male reproductive system and secreted in the seminal fluid are the source of energy

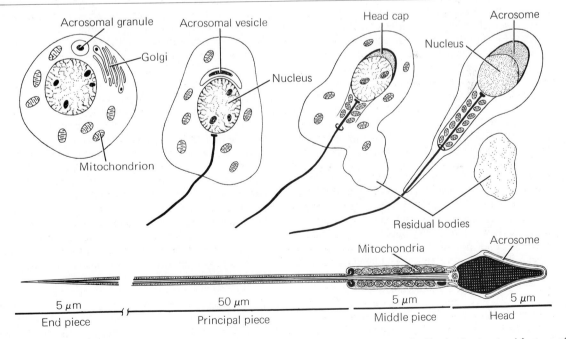

Figure 23–4. *Top:* The principal changes occurring in spermatids during spermiogenesis. The basic structural feature of the spermatozoon is the head, which consists primarily of condensed nuclear chromatin. The reduced volume of the nucleus permits the greater mobility of the sperm and may protect the genome from damage while in transit to the egg. The rest of the spermatozoon is structurally arranged to provide motility. *Bottom:* The structure of a spermatozoon.

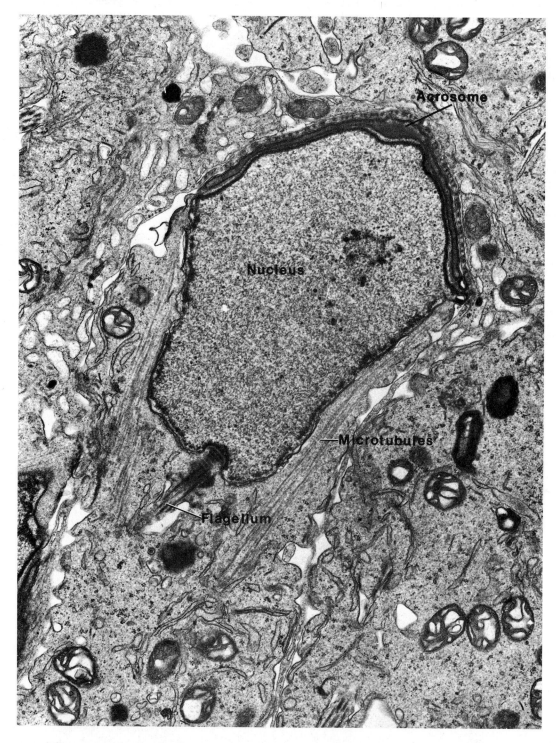

Figure 23–5. Electron micrograph of a mouse spermatid. In the center is its nucleus, covered by the acrosomal head cap. The flagellum can be seen emerging in the lower region below the nucleus. A cylindric bundle of microtubules, the manchette, limits the nucleus laterally. × 15,000. (Courtesy of KR Porter.)

for sperm motility. Among these carbohydrates, the most abundant is the monosaccharide fructose.

(4) In the **maturation phase,** residual cytoplasm is shed and phagocytized by Sertoli cells (Figs 23–4 and 23–10), and the spermatozoa are released into the lumen of the tubule. Mature spermatozoa are shown in Figs 23–4 and 23–6.

During division of the spermatogonia, the resulting cells do not separate completely but remain attached by cytoplasmic bridges. This concept is illustrated in Fig 23–7. The intercellular bridges provide communication between every primary and secondary spermatocyte and spermatid derived from a single spermatogonium. By permitting the interchange of information from cell to cell, these bridges play an important role in coordinating the sequence of events in spermatogenesis. This detail may be of importance in understanding the cycle of the seminiferous epithelium (described below). When the process of spermatogenesis is completed, the sloughing of the cytoplasm and cytoplasmic bridges as residual bodies leads to a separation of the spermatids.

Experimental injection of ³H-thymidine into the testes of volunteers shows that, in men, the changes that occur between the spermatogonia stage and the formation of the spermatozoa take about 64 days.

Besides being a slow process, spermatogenesis occurs neither simultaneously nor synchronously in all of the seminiferous tubules. The process occurs in wavelike fashion, which explains the irregular appearance of the tubules, where each region exhibits a different phase of spermatogenesis. This is why spermatozoa are encountered in some regions of the seminiferous tubules and only spermatids in others. The **cycle of the seminiferous epithelium** refers to the sequence of maturation changes occurring in a given area of the germinal epithelium between 2 successive appearances of a given cell stage. Each cycle in the human lasts 16 ± 1 days, and spermatogenesis ends 4 cycles, or about 64 ± 4.5 days, later. The seminiferous cycle is clearly seen in rodents, in which 12 different stages have been described. In men, 6 stages are known to occur, but their occurrence is not as easily visualized. Fig 23–8 shows the sequence of stages in the human testis.

The **Sertoli cells** are elongated pyramidal cells that partially envelop cells of the spermatogenic series. The bases of the Sertoli cells adhere to the basal lamina, while their apical ends frequently extend into the lumen of the seminiferous tubule. In the light microscope, Sertoli cell outlines appear poorly defined owing to the numerous lateral processes that surround

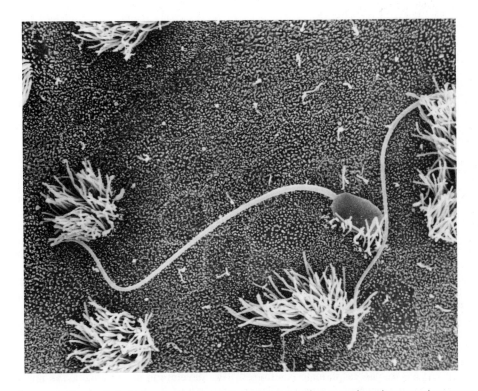

Figure 23–6. Spermatozoon in the uterine cavity of a rodent as seen using scanning electron microscopy. The tufts are ciliated cells. × 2000. (Reproduced, with permission, from Motta P, Andrews PM, Porter KR: *Microanatomy of Cell and Tissue Surfaces: An Atlas of Scanning Electron Microscopy.* Lea & Febiger, 1977. Copyright © Societa Editrice Libraria [Milan].)

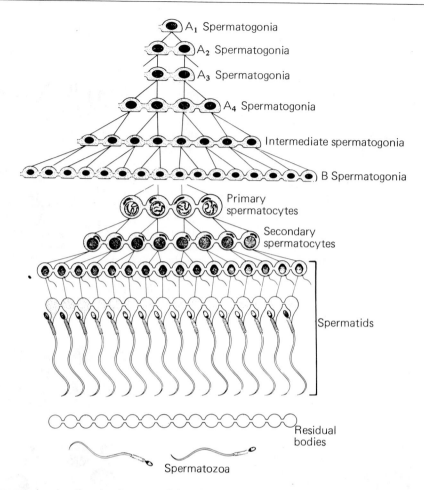

A₁ Spermatogonia

A₂ Spermatogonia

A₃ Spermatogonia

A₄ Spermatogonia

Intermediate spermatogonia

B Spermatogonia

Primary spermatocytes

Secondary spermatocytes

Spermatids

Residual bodies

Spermatozoa

Figure 23–7. Diagram showing the clonal nature of the germ cells. Only the initial spermatogonia divide and produce separate daughter cells. Once committed to differentiation, the cells of all subsequent divisions are connected by intercellular cytoplasmic bridges. Only after they are separated from the residual bodies can the spermatozoa be considered isolated individuals. The actual number of cells is larger than shown in this figure. See the text for the functional implication of the intercellular bridges. (Reproduced, with permission, from Bloom W, Fawcett DW: *A Textbook of Histology,* 10th ed. Saunders, 1975.)

spermatogenic cells (Fig 23–3). Electron microscopic studies reveal that these cells contain abundant smooth endoplasmic reticulum, some rough endoplasmic reticulum, a well-developed Golgi complex, and numerous mitochondria and lysosomes. The elongated nucleus is often triangular in outline, possesses numerous infoldings, and exhibits little heterochromatin. The characteristic well-developed nucleolus has a central oval nucleolonema flanked by 2 basophilic masses of heterochromatin.

Adjacent Sertoli cells are bound together by characteristic occluding junctions found at the level of the spermatogonia. Thus, spermatogonia lie in a **basal compartment** that has free access to materials found in blood. During spermatogenesis, progeny of spermatogonia somehow traverse these junctions and come to lie in the **adluminal compartment.** Here, the more advanced stages of spermatogenesis are protected from

blood-borne products by a **blood-testis barrier** formed by the occluding junctions between Sertoli cells. Spermatocytes and spermatids lie within deep clefts (invaginations) of the lateral and apical margins of the Sertoli cells. As the flagellar tails of the spermatids develop, they appear as tufts extending from the apical ends of the Sertoli cells (Figs 23–3 and 23–9). Sertoli cells are also connected by gap junctions that provide ionic and chemical coupling of the cells, and this may be important in coordinating the cycle of the seminiferous epithelium described above.

Sertoli cells have at least 3 main functions: **(1) Support, protection, and nutritional regulation of the developing spermatozoa.** As mentioned above, the cells of the spermatogenic series are interconnected via cytoplasmic bridges. This network of cells is physically supported by extensive cytoplasmic ramifications of the Sertoli cells. Because spermatocytes, sper-

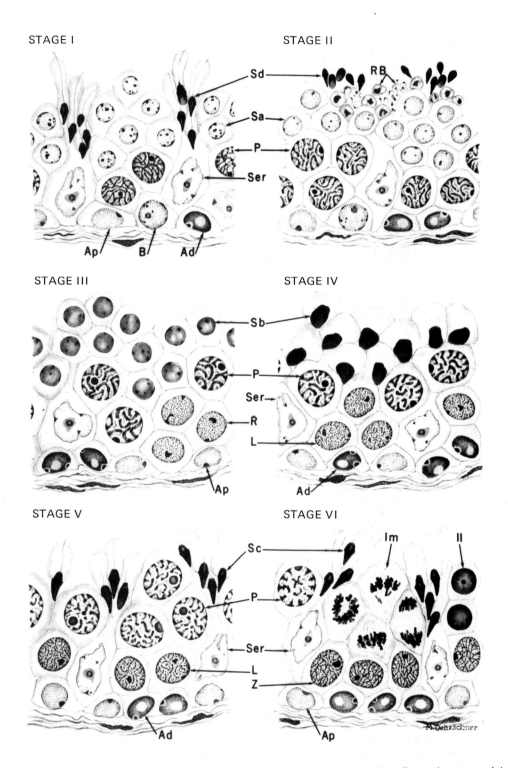

Figure 23–8. Diagrammatic representation of the 6 recognizable cell associations corresponding to the stages of the cycle of the human seminiferous epithelium. Ser, Sertoli cell; Ad and Ap, dark and pale type A spermatogonia; B, type B spermatogonia; R, resting primary spermatocyte; L, leptotene spermatocyte; Z, zygotene spermatocyte; P, pachytene spermatocyte; Im, primary spermatocyte in division; II, secondary spermatocyte in interphase; Sa, Sb, Sc, Sd, spermatids in various stages of differentiation; RB, residual bodies of Regnaud. (Reproduced, with permission, from Clermont Y: *Am J Anat* 1963;**112**:35.)

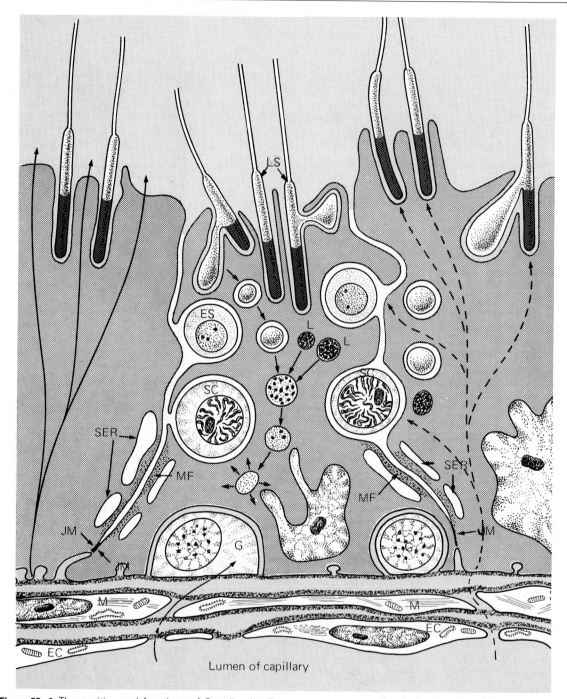

Figure 23–9. The position and functions of Sertoli cells. These cells are bounded by their lateral walls and divide the seminiferous tubules into 2 compartments. The lower part is the basal compartment and comprises the lumen of the blood vessels, the interstitial space, and the regions occupied by the spermatogonia (G). The second (upper) part represents the lumen of the seminiferous tubules as well as the intercellular spaces down to the level of the occluding junctions (JM). This is the adluminal compartment. The arrows pointing to the occluding junctional membrane show the zones where the membranes converge and impede the passage of substances from the first to the second compartment. Above the junctional membranes, specialized regions characterized by the presence of circularly disposed microfilaments (MF) and of cisternae of the smooth endoplasmic reticulum (SER) are seen. The 3 main functions of Sertoli cells are also portrayed. In the cell at left, the arrows indicate the secretion of testicular fluid. In the middle cell, cytoplasmic residual bodies from the forming spermatids undergo phagocytosis and are digested by lysosomes (L). In the cell at right, the dotted arrows indicate the transport of metabolites from the extracellular space to the spermatocytes (SC), and the early (ES) and late (LS) spermatids. Observe that the transport of material from the basal compartment to the lumen and spermatogenic cells passes through the Sertoli cells. Note also the myoid cells (M) and the endothelial cells (EC).

matids, and spermatozoa are isolated from the blood supply by the blood-testis barrier, these spermatogenic cells depend upon the Sertoli cells to mediate the exchange of nutrients and metabolites. The Sertoli cell barrier also protects the developing sperm cells from immunologic attack (discussed below). **(2) Phagocytosis.** During spermiogenesis, excess spermatid cytoplasm is shed as residual bodies. These cytoplasmic fragments are phagocytized and broken down by Sertoli cell lysosomes. **(3) Secretion.** Sertoli cells continuously secrete into the seminiferous tubules a fluid that flows in the direction of the genital ducts and is utilized for sperm transport. Secretion of an androgen-binding protein by Sertoli cells is under the control of FSH and testosterone and serves to concentrate testosterone in the seminiferous tubule, where it is necessary for spermatogenesis. Sertoli cells can convert testosterone to estradiol. They also secrete a peptide called **inhibin,** which suppresses FSH synthesis and release in the anterior pituitary gland.

Sertoli cells in humans and other animals do not divide during the reproductive period. They are extremely resistant to adverse conditions such as infection, malnutrition, or x-ray irradiation and survive these insults much better than cells of the spermatogenic lineage.

In mammals, the release of spermatozoa probably occurs as a result of cellular movements, with the participation of microtubules and microfilaments present in the Sertoli cell apex.

Interstitial Tissue

The spaces between the seminiferous tubules in the testis are filled with accumulations of connective tissue, nerves, blood, and lymphatic vessels. Testicular capillaries are of the fenestrated type and permit the free passage of macromolecules such as the blood proteins. An extensive network of lymphatic vessels is present in the interstitial space, and this explains the similarity of composition between the interstitial fluid and lymph collected from this organ. The connective tissue consists of various cell types, including fibroblasts, undifferentiated connective cells, mast cells, and macrophages. During puberty, an additional cell type becomes apparent that is either rounded or polygonal in shape and has a central nucleus and an eosinophilic cytoplasm rich in small lipid droplets (Figs 23–3 and 23–10). These are the **interstitial,** or **Leydig, cells** of the testis, which have the characteristics of steroid secretory cells described in Chapter 4. These cells produce the male hormone **testosterone,** responsible for the development of the secondary male sex characteristics. Thus, a direct correlation is observed between presence of interstitial cells and production of androgen by the testis. The presence in the interstitial cells of enzymes necessary

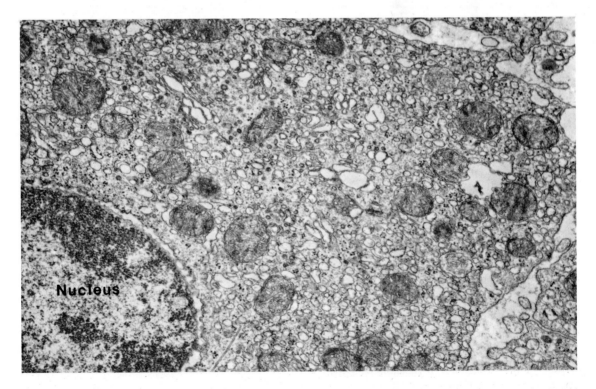

Figure 23–10. Electron micrograph of a section of an interstitial cell from the testis of a rat. There are abundant mitochondria and vesicles of smooth endoplasmic reticulum. × 12,000.

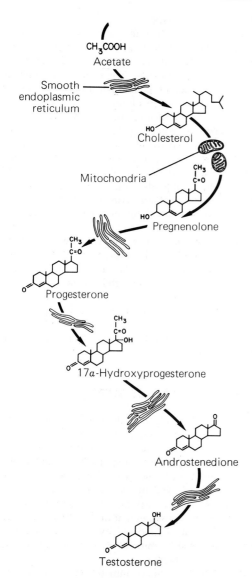

Figure 23–11. A schematic representation of the steps in the conversion of acetate to testosterone. All the enzymes are present in the microsomal fraction (smooth endoplasmic reticulum) except the cholesterol side-chain cleaving enzymes, which are found in the mitochondria. (Reproduced, with permission, from Dym M: The male reproductive system. In: *Histology: Cell and Tissue Biology,* 5th ed. Weiss L (editor). Elsevier, 1983.)

for the synthesis of testosterone has been demonstrated using histochemical and biochemical methods. Cholesterol, stored in lipid droplets or newly synthesized from acetate, is the substrate for side-chain cleaving enzymes located in interstitial cell mitochondria. The product of this reaction is pregnenolone, which is subjected to a series of reactions—culminating in testosterone synthesis—that are mediated by enzymes located in the smooth endoplasmic reticulum (Fig

23–11). Interstitial cell tumors can cause precocious puberty in the male.

The activity and the quantity of the interstitial cells depend on hormonal stimuli. During human pregnancy, placental gonadotropic hormone passes from the maternal blood to the fetus, stimulating the abundant fetal testicular interstitial cells that produce androgenic hormones. The presence of these hormones is required for the embryonic differentiation of the male genitalia. The embryonic interstitial cells remain fully differentiated until up to 4½ months of gestation and then regress, with an associated decrease in testosterone synthesis. They then remain quiescent throughout the rest of the pregnancy and up to the prepubertal period, when they resume testosterone synthesis in response to the stimulus of luteinizing hormone (LH) from the pituitary gland.

Histophysiology of the Testis

Temperature is very important in the regulation of spermatogenesis, and this process occurs only at temperatures below the core body temperature of 37 °C. Testicular temperature is about 35 °C. This is controlled by several mechanisms. A rich venous plexus (the **pampiniform plexus**) surrounds each testicular artery and forms a countercurrent heat exchange system of importance in maintaining a low testicular temperature. Other factors are evaporation of sweat from the scrotum, which contributes to heat loss, and contraction of cremaster muscles of the spermatic cords, which pull the testes into the inguinal canals, where their temperature can be increased.

Failure of descent of the testis (**cryptorchidism**) maintains the testes at the core temperature of 37 °C, which inhibits spermatogenesis. In cases that are not too far advanced, spermatogenesis can occur normally if the testis is moved surgically to the scrotum. Although germ cell proliferation is inhibited by abdominal temperature, testosterone synthesis is not. This explains why individuals with cryptorchidism can be sterile but still develop secondary male characteristics and achieve erection.

Malnutrition, alcoholism, and the action of certain drugs lead to alterations in spermatogonia, with consequent decreased production of spermatozoa. Lack of vitamin E can produce—especially in the rat—total and irreversible destruction of spermatogenic cells, including the spermatogonia, thus resulting in permanent sterility. This has not been observed in men. X-ray irradiation causes destruction of spermatogonia with irreversible sterility. Cadmium salts are quite toxic to the cells of spermatogenic lineage, causing death of those cells and sterility in animals. The drug busulfan acts on the germinal cells, and when administered to pregnant female rats, it promotes the death of the germinal cells of their male offspring. The offspring are therefore sterile, and their seminiferous tubules contain exclusively Sertoli cells.

Without doubt, however, endocrine factors have the most important effect on spermatogenesis. Spermatogenesis depends on the action of the follicle-stimulating (FSH) and luteinizing (LH) hormones of the pituitary gland on the testicular cells. LH acts on the interstitial cells, stimulating the production of testosterone necessary for the normal development of cells of seminal lineage. FSH is known to act on the Sertoli cells, stimulating adenylate cyclase and consequently increasing the presence of cAMP, and promoting the synthesis of **androgen-binding protein** (ABP). This protein combines with testosterone and is secreted into the lumen of the seminiferous tubules (Fig 23–12). Spermatogenesis is inhibited by estrogens and progestogens. The mechanisms of endocrine control are shown in Fig 23–12.

Spermatozoa are transported to the epididymis in an appropriate medium called **testicular fluid** produced by the Sertoli cells and rete testis. This fluid contains steroids, proteins, ions, and androgen-binding protein.

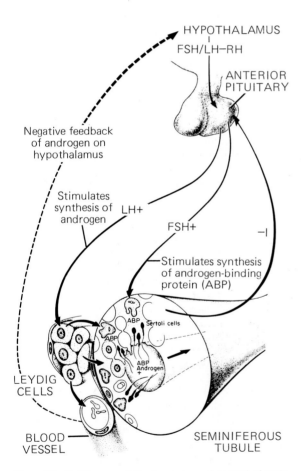

Figure 23–12. Diagram of the hypophyseal control of male reproduction in which luteinizing hormone (LH) acts upon the Leydig cells and follicle-stimulating hormone (FSH) acts upon the seminiferous tubules. A testicular hormone called inhibin (I) inhibits FSH secretion in the pituitary. (Modified and reproduced, with permission, from Bloom W, Fawcett DW: *A Textbook of Histology,* 10th ed. Saunders, 1975.)

Blood-Testis Barrier

The observation that few substances present in blood appear in the testicular fluid suggested the existence of a barrier between the blood and the interior of the seminiferous tubules. The testicular capillaries are of the fenestrated type and permit free passage of large molecules. The occluding junctions between Sertoli cells are responsible for this barrier, which is of importance in protecting male germ cells against blood-borne noxious agents.

Differentiation of spermatogonial cells leads to the appearance of sperm-specific proteins. Since sexual maturity occurs long after the development of immunocompetence, differentiating sperm cells could be recognized as "foreign" and provoke an immune response, which would destroy the germ cells. Consequently, the blood-testis barrier would eliminate any interaction between developing sperm and the immune system. This barrier prevents the passage of immunoglobulins into the seminiferous tubule and would account for the absence of any impairment of fertility in patients whose serum possesses high levels of sperm antibodies. The Sertoli cell barrier therefore functions in protecting the seminiferous epithelium against an autoimmune reaction.

INTRATESTICULAR GENITAL DUCTS

The intratesticular genital ducts are the **tubuli recti** (straight tubules), the **rete testis,** and the **ductuli efferentes** (Fig 23–1). Most seminiferous tubules are in the form of loops, both ends of which join the rete testis by structures known as **tubuli recti.** Straight tubules are recognized by the gradual loss of spermatogenic cells, with only Sertoli cells remaining to form their walls. This segment of the straight tubules is very short and is followed by the main segment consisting of cuboidal epithelium supported by a dense connective tissue sheath.

Straight tubules empty into the **rete testis,** contained within the mediastinum, a thickening of the tunica albuginea. It is a highly anastomotic network of channels lined with cuboidal epithelium.

From the rete testis extend 10–20 **ductuli efferentes** (Figs 23–1 and 23–13). They have an epithelium composed of groups of nonciliated cuboidal cells alternating with ciliated columnar cells. This gives the epithelium a characteristic scalloped appearance. The nonciliated cells reabsorb much of the fluid secreted by the seminiferous tubules. This fluid flow sweeps spermatozoa toward the epididymis. Cilia of the columnar cells beat in the direction of the epididymis, aiding in the transport of spermatozoa. A thin layer of circularly oriented smooth muscle cells is seen outside the basal lamina of the epithelium. The ductuli efferentes gradually fuse to form the **ductus epididymidis** of the epididymis (Fig 23–1).

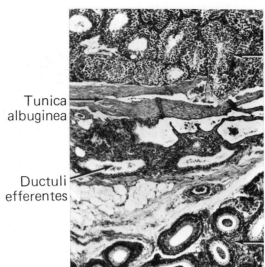

Seminiferous
tubule

Tunica
albuginea

Ductuli
efferentes

Epididymis

Figure 23–13 (at right). Photomicrograph of a section of testis showing the ductuli efferentes, the thick tunica albuginea, and the epididymis. H&E stain, × 80.

EXCRETORY GENITAL DUCTS

The ducts that transport the spermatozoa produced in the testis toward the penile meatus are the ductus epididymidis, the ductus deferens (vas deferens), and the urethra.

The **ductus epididymidis** is a single highly coiled tube about 4–6 meters in length. This long canal forms, with surrounding connective tissue and blood vessels, the body and tail of the **epididymis.** It is lined by pseudostratified columnar epithelium composed of rounded basal cells and columnar principal cells. These cells are supported on a basal lamina surrounded by smooth muscle cells, which probably help to move the sperm along the duct, and by loose connective tissue rich in blood capillaries (Fig 23–14).

The surface of the columnar cells is covered with long and irregular microvilli, called **stereocilia.** Stereocilia have neither basal bodies nor internal microtubules, whereas true cilia have both. When observed with the electron microscope, the principal cells are seen to contain numerous cisternae of rough endoplasmic reticulum in their basal cytoplasm and a large Golgi complex that encircles the nucleus. No secretory granules are present, but there is evidence of endocytosis utilizing coated vesicles. Lysosomes are present

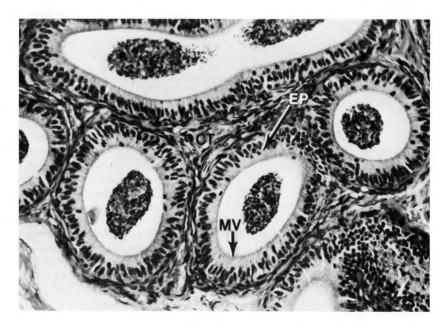

Figure 23–14. Photomicrograph of a section of epididymis showing its structure. Note the epithelium of the ductus epididymidis (EP), the connective tissue (CT), and the microvilli (MV) (stereocilia). H&E stain, × 200.

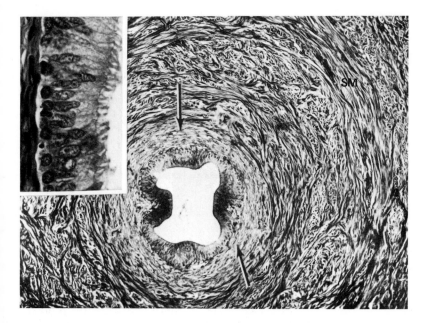

Figure 23–15 (at left). Photomicrograph of a section of ductus deferens. The ductus has a thick wall formed by smooth muscle cells (SM). The arrows point to the thin lamina propria layer. × 16. Observe in the inset the details of the pseudostratified columnar epithelium with stereocilia. Masson's trichrome stain, × 400.

and have been mistaken for secretory granules. Principal cells secrete glycerophosphocholine, which may inhibit **capacitation,** a process that prepares spermatozoa for fertilization. They also produce a glycoprotein that binds firmly to sperm plasma membranes, but the functional significance of this binding is unknown. The epithelium of the ductus epididymidis participates in the uptake and digestion of residual bodies that are eliminated during spermatogenesis. The basal cells are relatively undifferentiated and probably serve as precursors for the principal cells. Surrounding the epithelium is a layer of smooth muscle cells, which gradually increases in thickness along the length of the ductus epididymidis. Peristaltic contractions of these cells serve to propel sperm toward the exterior.

From the epididymis the **ductus (vas) deferens,** a straight tube with a thick, muscular wall, continues toward the prostatic urethra and empties into it (Fig 23–1). It is characterized by a narrow lumen and a thick layer of smooth muscle (Fig 23–15). Its mucosa forms longitudinal folds and is covered along most of its extent by pseudostratified columnar epithelium with stereocilia. Its lamina propria is a layer of connective tissue rich in elastic fibers. The thick muscular layer consists of inner and outer longitudinal layers separated by a circular layer. The ductus deferens forms part of the spermatic cord, which includes the testicular artery, the pampiniform (venous) plexus, and nerves. The spermatic cord is surrounded by longitudinally oriented fibers of skeletal muscle, the cremaster muscle. Before it enters the prostate, the ductus deferens dilates, forming a region called the **ampulla.** In this area, the epithelium becomes thicker and is extensively folded. At the final portion of the ampulla, the seminal vesicles join the duct. From there on, the ductus deferens enters the prostate, opening into the prostatic urethra. The segment entering the prostate is called the **ejaculatory**

duct and has a mucous layer similar to that of the ampulla but without the muscle layer.

ACCESSORY GENITAL GLANDS

The accessory genital glands are the seminal vesicles, the prostate gland, and the bulbourethral glands.

The **seminal vesicles** consist of 2 highly tortuous tubes 15 cm in length. They are not reservoirs for spermatozoa. When the organ is sectioned, the same tube is observed sectioned in different orientations. It has a folded mucosa lined with pseudostratified columnar epithelium that exhibits great individual variations depending on age and other conditions. The epithelium consists of a discontinuous layer of rounded basal cells and a layer of taller superficial cuboidal or low columnar cells, rich in secretory granules. They have ultrastructural characteristics of protein-synthesizing cells (see Chapter 4). The lamina propria of the seminal vesicles is rich in elastic fibers and surrounded by a thin layer of smooth muscle (Fig 23–16). The viscid, yellowish secretion of the seminal vesicles contains unusually high concentrations of fructose, as well as citrate, inositol, prostaglandins, and several proteins. Seventy percent of human ejaculate originates from the seminal vesicles. The height of the epithelial cells of the seminal vesicles and the degree of activity of the secretory processes are testosterone-dependent. In the absence of testosterone, the epithelium of the seminal vesicles atrophies. This atrophy can be reversed by the administration of testosterone.

The **prostate** is a collection of 30–50 branched tubulo-alveolar glands whose ducts empty into the prostatic urethra. The prostate produces prostatic fluid and stores it in its interior for expulsion during ejac-

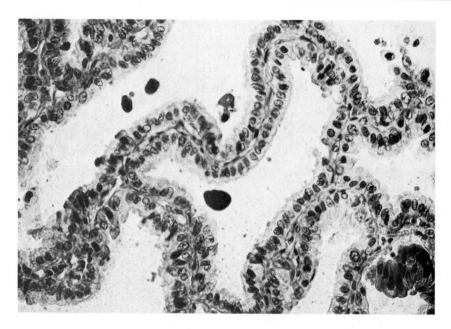

Figure 23–16. Photomicrograph of a section of human seminal vesicle. Masson's trichrome stain, × 300.

ulation. The prostate is surrounded by a fibroelastic capsule rich in smooth muscle. This capsule emits septa that penetrate the gland and divide it into lobes that are indistinct in the adult male. An exceptionally rich fibromuscular stroma surrounds the glands.

The glands of the prostate—**mucosal, submucosal,** and **main glands**—are arranged in 3 concentric areas around the urethra (Fig 23–17). The epithelium is usually simple columnar or pseudostratified, the former being found in the main glands while the latter is characteristic of mucosal and submucosal glands. These cells contain an abundance of rough endoplasmic reticulum, a large Golgi complex, large numbers of secretory granules, and numerous lysosomes. Secretory products of the prostate include amylase;

proteolytic enzymes, including fibrinolysin; citric acid; acid phosphatase; and lipids. Acid phosphatase activity is elevated in the blood of patients with carcinoma of the prostate. Measuring this enzyme activity is important in the diagnosis of this tumor as well as in following the results of therapy.

The main glands contribute most to the volume of the prostatic secretion. For unknown reasons—often after age 40—the mucosal and submucosal glands begin to hypertrophy. This can lead to partial or total obstruction of the urethra. Carcinoma of the prostate, a frequent tumor in older men, usually starts in the main glands. The secretory process of the prostate depends upon dihydrotestosterone.

Small spherical bodies of glycoprotein composition, 0.2–2 mm in diameter, are frequently observed in the lumen of prostatic glands. They are called **prostatic concretions,** or **corpora amylacea** (Fig 23–18). These bodies are often calcified. Their significance is not understood, but their number increases with age.

The **bulbourethral glands** (Cowper's glands), 3–5 mm in diameter, are located proximal to the membranous portion of the urethra and empty into it. They are tubulo-alveolar glands lined with mucus-secreting simple cuboidal epithelium. Skeletal and smooth muscle cells are present in the septa that divide each gland into lobes. The secretion is a clear mucus that acts as a lubricant.

PENIS

The penis consists mainly of 3 cylindric masses of erectile tissue plus the urethra, surrounded exter-

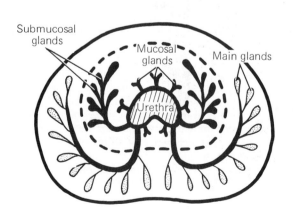

Figure 23–17. Diagram illustrating the position of the prostatic glands.

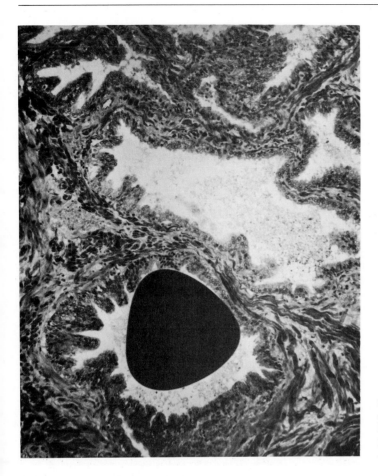

Figure 23–18 (at left). Section of a prostate, showing its epithelium, smooth muscle fibers, and a typical prostatic concretion (corpus amylaceum). H&E stain, × 300.

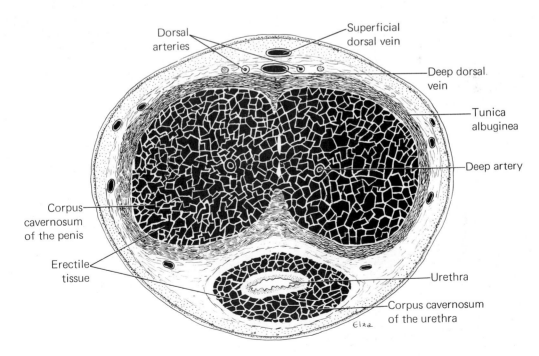

Figure 23–19. Drawing of a transverse section of the penis. (Redrawn and reproduced, with permission, from Leeson TS, Leeson CR: *Histology,* 2nd ed. Saunders, 1970.)

nally by skin. Two of these cylinders—the **corpora cavernosa of the penis**—are placed dorsally. The other, ventrally located, is called the **corpus cavernosum of the urethra,** or corpus spongiosum, and surrounds the urethra. At its end it dilates, forming the **glans penis** (Fig 23–1). The corpora cavernosa are covered by a resistant layer of dense connective tissue, the **tunica albuginea** (Fig 23–19). The corpora cavernosa of the penis and urethra are composed of erectile tissue—venous spaces lined by unfenestrated endothelial cells and separated by trabeculae consisting of connective tissue fibers and smooth muscle cells.

The prepuce is a retractile fold of skin. It contains connective tissue with smooth muscle in its interior. Sebaceous glands are present in the internal fold and in the skin that covers the glans.

Most of the penile urethra is lined with pseudostratified columnar epithelium, but in the glans penis, it becomes stratified squamous epithelium. Mucussecreting **glands of Littre** are found throughout the length of the penile urethra.

The arterial supply of the penis derives from the internal pudendal arteries, which give rise to the deep arteries and the dorsal arteries of the penis. The deep arteries branch to form nutritive arteries and helicine arteries. The former supply oxygen and nutrients to the trabeculae, while the latter empty directly into the cavernous spaces (erectile tissue). Arteriovenous shunts exist between helicine arteries and the deep dorsal vein.

Erection of the penis is due to engorgement of the cavernous spaces with blood. The increased blood flow to this organ is controlled by autonomic neural pathways that are activated by tactile and psychic stimuli. Parasympathetic nerve discharge causes constriction of the arteriovenous shunts and dilation of the helicine arteries. This results in increased blood flow and pressure in the cavernous spaces. Whether the increased pressure also restricts venous outflow remains controversial.

After ejaculation and orgasm have been achieved, parasympathetic activity declines, allowing the penis to return to its flaccid state.

REFERENCES

Afzelius BA et al: Lack of dynein arms in immotile human spermatozoa. *J Cell Biol* 1975;**66**:225.

Brandes D: The fine structure and histochemistry of prostatic glands in relation to sex hormones. *Int Rev Cytol* 1966;**20**:207.

Clermont Y: Renewal of spermatogonia in man. *Am J Anat* 1966;**118**:509.

De Kretser DM: Changes in the fine structure of the human testicular interstitial cells after treatment with human gonadotrophins. *Z Zellforsch Mikrosk Anat* 1967;**83**:344.

Dym M: The fine structure of the monkey Sertoli cell and its role in maintaining the blood-testis barrier. *Anat Rec* 1973;**175**:639.

Dym M: The mammalian rete testes: A morphological examination. *Anat Rec* 1976;**186**:493.

Fawcett DW: The mammalian spermatozoon. *Dev Biol* 1975;**44**:394.

Fawcett DW, Neaves WB, Flores MN: Comparative observations on intertubular lymphatics and the organization of the interstitial tissue of the mammalian testis. *Biol Reprod* 1973;**9**:500.

Hafez ESE, Spring-Mills E (editors): *Accessory Glands of the Male Reproductive Tract.* Ann Arbor Science Publishers, 1979.

Johnson AD, Gomes WR (editors): *The Testis.* Vols 1–4. Academic Press, 1970–1977.

Leeson TS, Leeson CR: The fine structure of cavernous tissue in the adult rat penis. *Invest Urol* 1965;**3**:144.

Nagano T, Suzuki F: Freeze-fracture observations on the intercellular junctions of Sertoli cells and of Leydig cells in the human testis. *Cell Tissue Res* 1976;**166**:37.

Smith MJV: Prostatic corpora amylacea. *Monogr Surg Sci* 1966;**3**:209.

Stambough R, Buckley J: Identification and subcellular localization of the enzymes affecting penetration of the zona pellucida of rabbit spermatozoa. *J Reprod Fertil* 1969;**19**:423.

Steinberger A, Steinberger E (editors): *Testicular Development.* Raven Press, 1979.

Steinberger E: Hormonal control of mammalian spermatogenesis. *Physiol Rev* 1971;**51**:1.

Tindall DJ et al: Structure and biochemistry of the Sertoli cell. *Int Rev Cytol* 1985;**94**:127.

The Female Reproductive System   24

The female reproductive system (Fig 24–1) consists of 2 ovaries, 2 uterine tubes (oviducts), the uterus, the vagina, and the external genitalia. Between menarche and menopause, the system undergoes cyclic changes in structure and functional activity. These modifications are controlled by neurohumoral mechanisms. **Menarche** is the time when the first menses occurs; **menopause** is a variable period during which the cyclic changes become irregular and eventually disappear altogether. In the postmenopausal period there is a slow involution of the reproductive system. In this chapter we shall also study the mammary glands, though they do not belong to the genital system—being, in fact, modified sweat glands—for the reason that they undergo changes directly connected with the functional state of the reproductive system.

THE OVARY

The ovary is an almond-shaped body approximately 3 cm long, 1.5 cm wide, and 1 cm thick. It consists of a **medullary region,** containing a rich vascular bed within a cellular loose connective tissue; and a **cortical region,** where ovarian follicles, containing the oocytes, predominate. There are no sharp limits between the cortical and the medullary regions (Fig 24–2). After about 1 month of embryonic life,

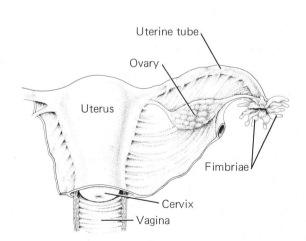

Figure 24–1. Internal organs of the female reproductive system: ovary, fimbriae of infundibulum, uterine tube, uterus, cervix, and vagina.

germ cells **(oogonia)** can be identified in the endodermal yolk sac. They divide mitotically several times while migrating to the genital ridges. Oogonia populate the cortex of the future ovary, and mitotic divisions continue until about the fifth month of fetal life. At this time, each ovary contains over 3 million oogonia. Beginning in the third fetal month, some oogonia enter the prophase of the first meiotic division and become **primary oocytes.** In the human, this process is completed by the end of the seventh month of gestation. During this time, many primary oocytes are lost owing to a degenerative process called **atresia.**

The stroma of the cortical region is composed of characteristic spindle-shaped fibroblasts that respond in a different way to hormonal stimuli than do fibroblasts of other organs. The surface of the ovary is covered by a simple squamous or cuboidal epithelium called **germinal epithelium.** Under the germinal epithelium, the stroma forms a poorly delineated layer of dense connective tissue called the **tunica albuginea.** The tunica albuginea is responsible for the whitish color of the ovary (Fig 24–2).

Ovarian Follicles

Ovarian follicles are embedded in the stroma of the cortex. A follicle consists of an oocyte surrounded by one or more layers of **follicular (granulosa) cells.** Several stages of follicular development are recognized and are described below. The total number of follicles in the 2 ovaries of a normal young adult woman is estimated to be 400,000, but most of them will disappear by atresia during the reproductive years. This follicular regression takes place prior to birth and continues over the entire span of reproductive life. After menopause, only a small number of follicles remain. Atresia may affect any type of follicle from primordial follicles to those that are nearly mature. Since, in general, only one ovum is liberated by the ovaries in each menstrual cycle (average duration: 28 days) and the reproductive life of a woman lasts about 30–40 years, the total number of ova liberated is about 450. All of the other follicles, with their oocytes, fail to mature and degenerate, becoming atretic.

A. Primordial Follicles: The primordial follicles are most numerous before birth. Each consists of a primary oocyte enveloped by only one layer of flattened follicular cells (Fig 24–3).

The oocyte in the primordial follicle is a spherical cell about 25 μm in diameter. Its nucleus is large, is slightly eccentrically situated, and has a large nucleolus. The chromosomes have become greatly un-

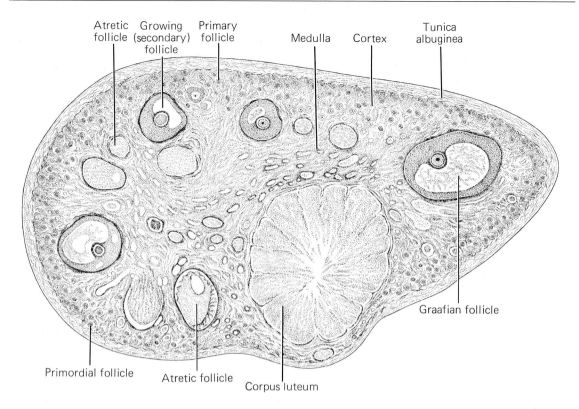

Atretic follicle   Growing (secondary) follicle   Primary follicle   Medulla   Cortex   Tunica albuginea

Graafian follicle

Primordial follicle   Atretic follicle   Corpus luteum

Figure 24–2. Schematic drawing showing the main components of the ovary of an adult woman. (Redrawn and reproduced, with permission, from Copenhaver WM, Bunge RP, Bunge MTS: *Bailey's Textbook of Histology,* 16th ed. Williams & Wilkins, 1972.)

coiled and do not stain intensely. In the cytoplasm, the organelles tend to form a clump adjacent to the nucleus. There are numerous mitochondria, several Golgi complexes, and cisternae of endoplasmic reticulum. In addition, **annulate lamellae,** having the appearance of stacks of segments of the nuclear envelope, are prominent. The squamous follicular cells contain endoplasmic reticulum, mitochondria, and lipid droplets. They are joined to one another by desmosomes. A basal lamina underlies the follicular cells and marks the boundary between the avascular follicle and the surrounding stroma.

B. Growing Follicles: Follicular growth involves mainly the follicular cells but also the primary oocyte and the stroma surrounding the follicle (Figs 24–2, 24–3, and 24–4). Oocyte growth is most rapid during the first part of follicular growth, with this cell reaching a maximum diameter of 125–150 μm. The nucleus enlarges and is now called a **germinal vesicle.** Mitochondria increase in number and become uniformly distributed throughout the cytoplasm; the endoplasmic reticulum hypertrophies; and the Golgi complexes migrate to just beneath the cell surface. Follicular cells form a single layer of cuboidal cells, and the follicle is now called a **unilaminar primary follicle** (Fig 24–3). Follicular cells proliferate by mitosis and form a stratified follicular epithelium or

granulosa layer. The follicle is now called a **multilaminar primary follicle** (Fig 24–3). Gap junctions are now found between follicular cells. A thick, amorphous coat, the **zona pellucida,** composed of at least 3 different glycoproteins, surrounds the oocyte (Figs 24–3, 24–5, and 24–6). It is thought that both the oocyte and follicular cells contribute to the synthesis of the zona pellucida. Filopodia of follicular cells and microvilli of the oocyte penetrate the zona pellucida and make contact with one another via gap junctions (Fig 24–5).

While these modifications are taking place, the stroma immediately around the follicle differentiates to form the **theca folliculi.** This layer subsequently differentiates into the **theca interna** and the **theca externa** (Fig 24–3). The cells of the theca interna are cuboidal and, when completely differentiated, have the same ultrastructural characteristics as cells that produce steroids. These characteristics include abundant profiles of smooth endoplasmic reticulum, mitochondria with tubular cristae, and numerous lipid droplets. Evidence suggests that these cells synthesize androstenedione, which is converted into estradiol by cells of the granulosa. Like all organs of endocrine function, the theca interna is richly vascularized. The theca externa consists mainly of connective tissue. Small vessels penetrate it and supply a rich capillary

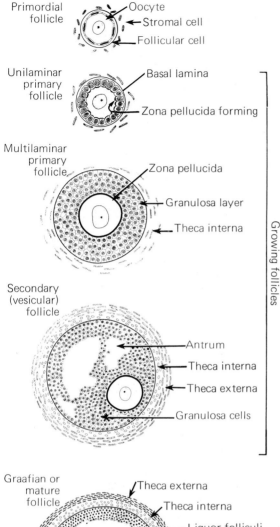

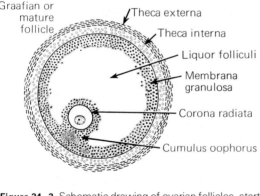

Figure 24–3. Schematic drawing of ovarian follicles, starting with the primordial follicle and ending with mature follicles.

As the follicle grows—mainly owing to the increase in size and number of granulosa cells—accumulations of follicular fluid (**liquor folliculi**) appear between the cells. The cavities that contain this fluid coalesce and finally form only one cavity, the **antrum** (Figs 24–3 and 24–4). These follicles are termed **secondary** (vesicular) **follicles** (Fig 24–3). Follicular fluid contains transudates of plasma and products secreted by follicular cells. Most inorganic ions are present in concentrations similar to those found in plasma. Glycosaminoglycans, several proteins (including steroid-binding proteins), and high concentrations of steroids (progesterone, androgens, and estrogens) are also present. The cells of the granulosa layer are more numerous at a certain point on the follicular wall, forming a small hillock of cells, the **cumulus oophorus,** which contains the oocyte. The cumulus oophorus protrudes toward the interior of the antrum (Fig 24–4). The oocyte grows no more thereafter.

C. Mature Follicles: The mature follicle is about 2.5 cm in diameter and can be seen as a transparent vesicle that bulges from the surface of the ovary. As a result of the accumulation of liquid, the follicular cavity increases in size and the oocyte adheres to the wall of the follicle through a pedicle formed by granulosa cells. Since the granulosa cells do not multiply in proportion to the accumulation of liquid, the granulosa layer becomes thinner.

The granulosa cells forming the first layer around the ovum—and, therefore, in close contact with the zona pellucida—become elongated and form the **corona radiata,** which accompanies the ovum when it leaves the ovary. The corona radiata is still present when the spermatozoon fertilizes the ovum and is retained for some time during the passage of the ovum through the tube.

Ovulation

Ovulation is a process that consists of rupture of the mature follicle with liberation of the ovum which will be caught by the dilated end of the uterine tube. In the human female, only one ovum is usually liberated by the ovary at a time, but 2 or more ova can be expelled at the same time. In the latter case, if 2 or more of the liberated ova are fertilized, there may be more than one fetus (fraternal twins).

Ovulation takes place approximately in the middle of the menstrual cycle, ie, around the 14th day of a 28-day cycle. The mechanism of ovulation is still being investigated. Careful measurements have shown that there is no increase in intrafollicular pressure that could account for follicular rupture. Smooth muscle cells, which are present in the ovarian stroma, are probably not an important factor in ovulation. A current hypothesis invokes increased activity of proteases, such as collagenase and plasmin, which could cause dissolution of connective tissues around the follicle that will ovulate. In any case, a midcycle surge of luteinizing hormone (LH) concentration appears to be indispensable for ovulation.

plexus around the secretory cells of the theca interna. In the granulosa cell layer there are no blood vessels during the stage of follicular growth. The boundary between the 2 thecas is not clear, and the same is true of the boundary between the theca externa and the ovarian stroma. The boundary between the theca interna and the granulosa layer is well defined, since their cells are morphologically different and there is a thick basal lamina between them.

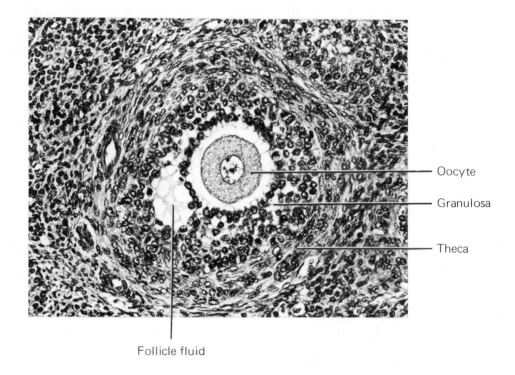

Oocyte

Granulosa

Theca

Follicle fluid

Figure 24 –4. Developing ovarian follicle. In the center of the follicle is an oocyte with a lightly staining nucleus. The limits between the 2 theca layers are not clear. × 320.

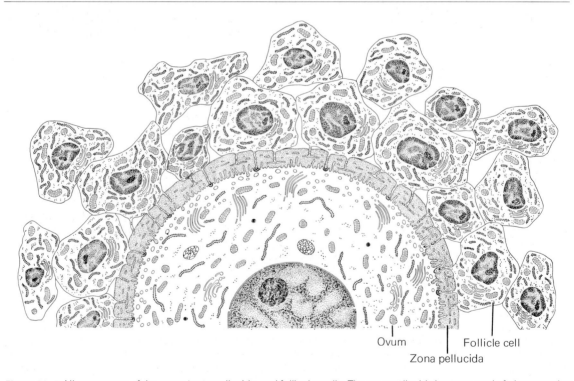

Ovum

Follicle cell

Zona pellucida

Figure 24 –5. Ultrastructure of the ovum, zona pellucida, and follicular cells. The zona pellucida is composed of glycoproteins penetrated by oocyte microvilli and by longer processes from follicular cells. In the cytoplasm of the ovum there are arrays of parallel layers of membranes perforated by pores that resemble the nuclear envelope (annulate lamellae). The nucleus is in prophase of the first meiotic division.

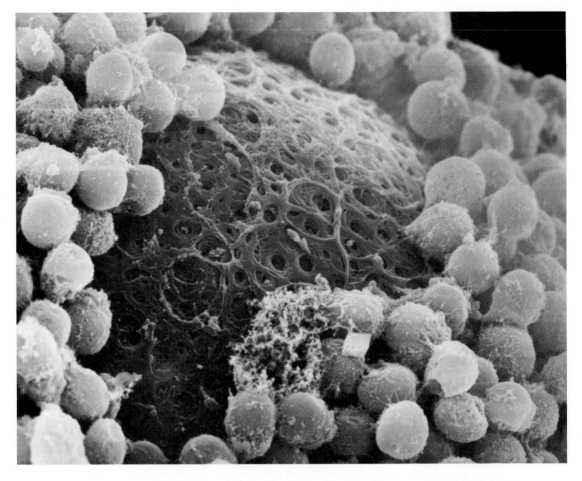

Figure 24–6. Scanning electron micrograph of dog ovary showing an oocyte surrounded by follicular cells. The structure covering the oocyte is the zona pellucida, which appears as an irregular meshwork. × 2950. (Courtesy of C Barros.)

Before ovulation, the ovum—together with the cells of the corona radiata—detaches itself from the wall of the follicle and floats in the follicular fluid. The first maturation division is completed after the increase in LH secretion but before the exit of the ovum from the follicle. An indication of impending ovulation is the appearance on the surface of the follicle of the **stigma,** in which the flow of blood ceases, resulting in a local change in color and translucency of the follicular wall. The germinal epithelium in this area becomes discontinuous, and the stroma becomes thinner. The wall then ruptures and the ovum is expelled from the ovary together with the follicular liquid and blood.

The extremity of the uterine tube that faces the ovary is funnel-shaped and fringed with numerous fingerlike processes called **fimbriae.** At the moment of ovulation, this end is very close to the surface of the ovary and receives the ovum. Owing to the motion of the fimbriae, ciliated cells, and muscular contraction, the ovum enters the infundibulum of the uterine tube, where it is fertilized. Once fertilized, the ovum, now called the **zygote,** begins to undergo cleavage

and is transported to the uterus, a trip that lasts about 5 days. If the ovum is not fertilized within the first 24 hours after ovulation, it begins to degenerate.

Follicular Atresia

Most ovarian follicles undergo a degenerative process called follicular atresia in which follicular cells and oocytes die and are disposed of by phagocytic cells. This process is characterized by cessation of mitosis in the granulosa cells, detachment of granulosa cells from the basal lamina, and death of the oocyte. Although follicular atresia takes place from the time of birth until a few years after the menopause, there are times at which it is particularly intense. Follicular atresia is quite accentuated just after birth, when the effect of maternal hormones ceases, and also during puberty and pregnancy, ie, when marked qualitative and quantitative hormonal modifications take place. The process of atresia may take place during any stage in the development of a follicle.

When atresia starts in a primordial follicle, the outline of the oocyte becomes irregular and the follicular cells become smaller, separating from one an-

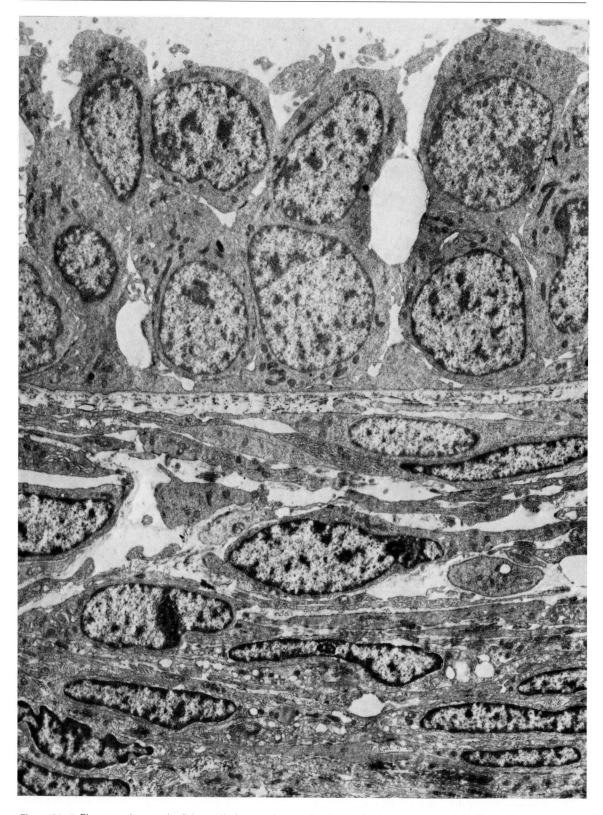

Figure 24–7. Electron micrograph of the wall of a growing ovarian follicle. In the upper part of the figure there are several cuboidal follicular cells. A basal lamina and some reticular fibers separate these cells from the flattened cells of the theca interna. × 6400.

other. The oocyte and the follicular cells start to autolyze, finally leaving a space that is immediately occupied by cells of the ovarian stroma so that no vestige is left.

In growing follicles the degenerative process is basically the same. The zona pellucida is very resistant, becoming wavy and pleated at the onset of the atretic process as a result of the collapse of the follicle, but its material persists longer than the cells of the follicle.

When a follicle in the late stage of growth undergoes atresia, a large quantity of degenerative material is produced that elicits the infiltration and differentiation of macrophages from monocytes carried in the blood by vessels which invade the area of atresia. While removal of the remnants of the follicle in atresia takes place, cells of the ovarian connective tissue that invade the area produce a small amount of collagenous matrix. Later, most vestiges of the follicle disappear, since the collagen is reabsorbed and replaced by typical ovarian stroma, but the theca cells persist as part of the ovarian stroma.

Interstitial Glands

Although granulosa cells and the oocytes undergo degeneration during atresia of the follicles, the theca interna cells frequently persist and become quite active steroid secretors. These active thecal cells are called **interstitial cells**. These cells, which are present from childhood through menopause, are the source of ovarian androgens.

Origin & Maturation of Oocytes

Oocytes are formed during intrauterine life, and their number does not increase after birth. The cells which are precursors of the oocytes are called **primordial germ cells** and originate in the endoderm of the yolk sac. Primordial germ cells migrate to the genital ridge and then into the developing ovary.

Primary follicles as well as growing follicles contain primary oocytes equivalent to primary spermatocytes of the seminiferous tubules (see Chapter 23). These oocytes are in the prophase of the first meiotic division.

The first meiotic division is completed just before ovulation. The chromosomes are equally divided between the daughter cells, but one of the secondary oocytes retains almost all of the cytoplasm. The other becomes the **first polar body,** a very small cell containing the nucleus and a minimal amount of cytoplasm.

Immediately after expulsion of the first polar body and while still in the cortical region of the ovary, the nucleus of the ovum starts the second meiotic division, which stops in metaphase and will only be completed when fertilization has taken place. Fertilization consists of penetration of the ovum by the spermatozoon. The fertilized ovum is called a **zygote.**

The ovum remains viable for an estimated maximum of 24 hours. Penetration by the sperm cell reconstitutes the diploid number of chromosomes typical of the species and serves as a stimulus for the ovum to complete the second meiotic division and cast off the second polar body. When fertilization does not take place, the ovum undergoes autolysis in the uterine tube without completing the second maturation division.

Corpus Luteum

After ovulation, the granulosa cells and those of the theca interna (Fig 24–7) that remain in the ovary form a temporary endocrine gland called the corpus luteum (yellow body) (Fig 24–8). The corpus luteum is localized in the cortical region of the ovary and secretes progesterone and estrogens. Progesterone prevents the development of new ovarian follicles and ovulation.

When the follicular fluid is released, it results in collapse of the follicle's wall so that it becomes folded. Some blood flows into the follicular cavity, where it coagulates and later is invaded by connective tissue cells that originate in the ovarian stroma. This connective tissue, with remnants of blood clot that are gradually removed, remains as the most central part of the corpus luteum.

The granulosa cells do not divide after ovulation. However, they increase greatly in size (20–35 μm in

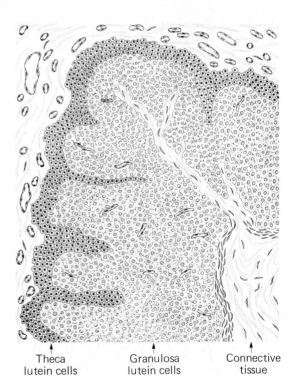

| Theca lutein cells | Granulosa lutein cells | Connective tissue |

Figure 24–8. Drawing of a small portion from a corpus luteum. Granulosa lutein cells derived from the granulosa layer are larger and less darkly stained than the theca lutein cells, which derive from the theca interna.

diameter), comprise about 80% of the parenchyma of the corpus luteum, and are now called **granulosa lutein cells** (Fig 24–8). They possess a hypertrophied Golgi complex, numerous tubules and cisternae of rough and smooth endoplasmic reticulum, rod-shaped mitochondria with lamellar or tubular cristae, and large numbers of lipid droplets. The droplets are often surrounded by cisternae of smooth endoplasmic reticulum. Granulosa lutein cells thus have the characteristics of steroid-secreting cells (Fig 24–9). This is in contrast to their structure in the preovulatory follicle, where they appear to be protein-secreting cells (Fig 24–7).

Cells of the theca interna also contribute to the formation of the corpus luteum by giving rise to **theca lutein cells** (Fig 24–8). These cells are similar in structure to granulosa lutein cells but are smaller (about 15 μm in diameter) and stain more intensely. They are located in the folds of the wall of the corpus luteum.

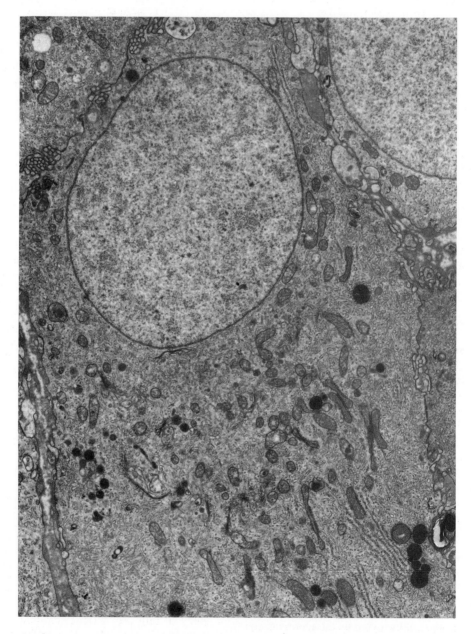

Figure 24–9. Electron micrograph of a human luteal cell. The nucleus contains finely dispersed chromatin, without a visible nucleolus in this section. Observe the marked development of the smooth endoplasmic reticulum. There are also many elongated mitochondria. × 6500. (Reproduced, with permission, from Adams EC, Hertig AT: Studies on the human corpus luteum. *J Cell Biol* 1969;**41**:696.)

The blood capillaries and lymphatics of the theca interna grow into the interior of the corpus luteum and form the rich vascular network of this structure.

The corpus luteum is formed as a consequence of the stimulus provided by luteinizing hormone synthesized by the pars distalis of the pituitary under hypothalamic control. In mice and rats, it has been shown that prolactin (luteotropic hormone, LTH), also secreted by the pars distalis, stimulates the secretion of progesterone by the corpus luteum, but in humans this activity has not been observed. Since the progesterone produced by the corpus luteum has an inhibitory effect on the production of LH; the corpus luteum will soon degenerate unless it receives a stimulus from another source. This inhibitory effect of progesterone on luteinizing hormone production is indirect and mediated through the hypothalamus (Fig 24– 10).

When pregnancy does not occur, the corpus luteum lasts only 10– 14 days; ie, it persists during the second half of the menstrual cycle. After this period, as a result of the lack of luteinizing hormone, it degenerates and disappears. This is the **corpus luteum of menstruation.**

When pregnancy occurs, **chorionic gonadotropin** produced by the placenta will stimulate the corpus luteum, which is maintained for about 6 months and then gradually declines but does not disappear completely and continues to secrete progesterone until the end of pregnancy. This is the **corpus luteum of pregnancy.** It has been shown by immunohistochemistry that the corpus luteum of pregnancy also secretes **relaxin,** a polypeptide hormone that softens the connective tissue of the symphysis pubica, facilitating parturition. The corpus luteum of pregnancy is larger than the corpus luteum of menstruation, sometimes reaching a diameter of 5 cm.

The cells of the corpus luteum of menstruation or of pregnancy undergo degeneration by autolysis, and their cellular remnants are phagocytized by macrophages. The site is occupied by a scar of dense connective tissue forming a **corpus albicans.** The corpus albicans remains for a variable period and is gradually reabsorbed by macrophages of the stroma.

UTERINE TUBE
(Oviduct)

The uterine tube (oviduct, fallopian tube) is a muscular tube (Fig 24– 1) of great mobility, measuring about 12 cm in length. One of its extremities opens into the peritoneal cavity next to the ovary; the other passes through the wall of the uterus and opens into the interior of this organ.

The oviduct is divided into 4 segments, which do not have clear limits. The first segment, the intramural portion **(pars interstitialis),** is situated in the interior of the uterine wall. The second segment, or **isthmus,** is formed by the portion of the tube that is adjacent to the uterus. The third is the **ampulla,** which is more dilated than the isthmus. The fourth segment, the **infundibulum,** is funnel-shaped and situated near the ovary. The free extremity of the infundibulum has a fringe of fingerlike extensions called **fimbriae** (Fig 24– 1).

Histologic Structure

The wall of the oviduct is composed of 3 layers: a mucosa, a muscularis, and a serosa composed of visceral peritoneum (Fig 24– 11).

The mucosa has longitudinal folds that are most numerous in the ampulla. In cross sections, the lumen of the ampulla resembles a labyrinth (Fig 24– 11). These folds become smaller in the segments of the tube that are closer to the uterus. In the intramural portion, the folds are reduced to small bulges in the lumen, so that its internal surface is almost smooth.

The epithelium lining the mucosa is simple columnar and contains 2 types of cells. One is provided with cilia, and the other is devoid of cilia and appears to be secretory (Figs 24– 12 and 24– 13). The 2 types of epithelial cells may be different functional states of a single cell type. Most of the cilia beat toward the uterus, causing movement of the viscous liquid film that covers its surface. This liquid consists mainly of products of secretory cells (peg cells) interspersed

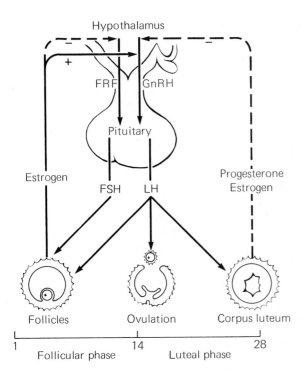

Figure 24–10. Diagram showing the relationships of the hypothalamus, pituitary, and ovaries in the feedback mechanism regulating the secretion of hormones produced during the menstrual cycle. GnRH, gonadotropin-releasing hormone.

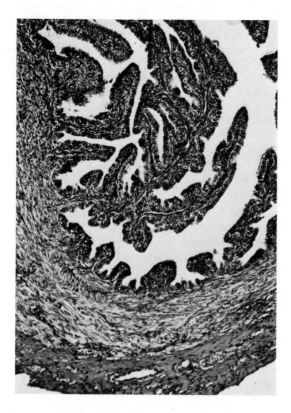

Figure 24–11. Photomicrograph of a cross section through the ampulla of the oviduct. The mucosa projects many folds into the lumen. H&E stain, × 31.

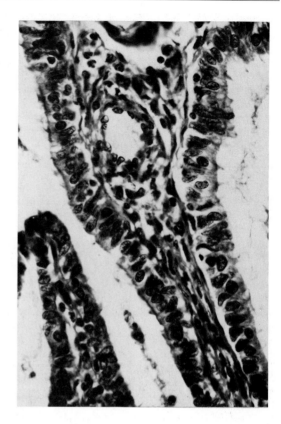

Figure 24–12. Photomicrograph of mucosa of oviduct. The section was made at the level of the ampulla. Masson's stain, × 320.

between ciliated cells. Movement of the film that covers the mucosa of the tube, in conjunction with contractions of the muscle layer, helps to transport the ovum or the embryo toward the uterus and hampers the passage of microorganisms from the uterus to the peritoneal cavity. However, microcinematographic films of the uterine tube lining reveal that some cilia beat toward the ovary. It is believed that these cilia facilitate the movement of the sperm toward the unfertilized egg.

The lamina propria of the mucosa is composed of loose connective tissue. In cases of abnormal nidation, in which the embryo implants itself in the tube (ectopic pregnancy), the lamina propria reacts as does the endometrium, forming numerous decidual cells.

The muscularis is composed of smooth muscle fibers disposed as an inner circular or spiral layer and an outer longitudinal layer.

Histophysiology

The oviduct receives the ovum expelled by the ovary and carries it toward the uterus. Its lumen represents an environment adequate for fertilization, and its secretions contribute to the nutrition of the embryo during the early phases of development.

At the time of ovulation, the oviduct exhibits active movement. The fimbriae of the infundibulum move closer to the surface of the ovary, and the funnel shape of the infundibulum facilitates the recovery of the liberated ovum.

The oviduct undergoes waves of rhythmic contractions, generated by its musculature, which start at the infundibulum and are directed toward the uterus. These waves are important in the movement of the ovum toward the uterus.

The wall of the oviduct is richly vascularized, and its vessels become dilated at the time of ovulation. This gives rigidity and distention to the organ, facilitating its approximation to the ovary.

Fertilization usually takes place at the ampullar-isthmic junction.

UTERUS

The uterus is a pear-shaped organ that consists of a **body** (corpus), which lies above a narrowing of the uterine cavity (the internal os), and a **cervix,** which lies below the internal os. The part of the body of the

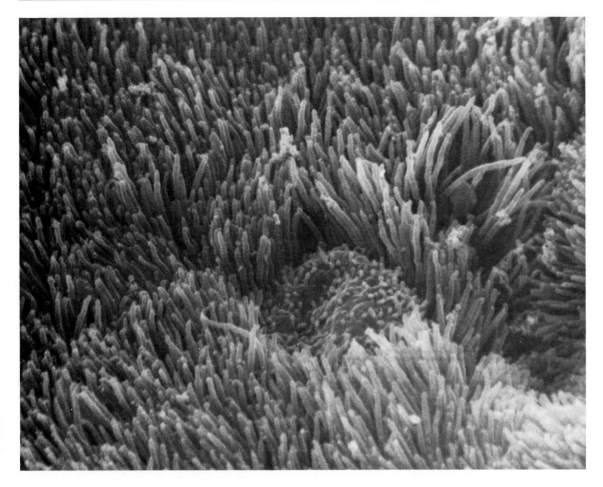

Figure 24–13. Scanning electron micrograph of the lining of an oviduct. Observe the abundant cilia. In the middle is the apex of a secretory cell covered by short microvilli. × 8000. (Courtesy of KR Porter.)

uterus lying above the points of entrance of the uterine tubes is called the **fundus.**

The wall of the uterus is relatively thick and is formed of 3 layers: in different parts of the uterus either an outer **serosa** (connective tissue and mesothelium) or **adventitia** (connective tissue); the **myometrium,** a tunic of smooth muscle; and the **endometrium,** or mucosa of the uterus.

Myometrium

The myometrium is the thickest tunic of the uterus, being composed of bundles of smooth muscle fibers separated by connective tissue. The bundles of smooth muscle form 4 layers that are not well defined. The first and the fourth are composed mainly of fibers disposed longitudinally, ie, parallel to the long axis of the organ. The middle layers contain the larger blood vessels.

During pregnancy, the myometrium goes through a period of great growth. The growth is due to an increase in the number of smooth muscle cells through division of existing smooth muscle cells as well as to hypertrophy. During pregnancy, many smooth muscle cells have ultrastructural characteristics of protein-secreting cells and actively incorporate collagen precursors (^{3}H-proline). The connective tissue fibers of the myometrium are composed of collagen type I and reticular fibers (collagen type III). During pregnancy, there is a significant increase in uterine collagen content.

After pregnancy, there is destruction of some smooth muscle cells, reduction in size of others, and an enzymatic degradation of the collagen. The uterus is reduced in size almost to its prepregnancy dimensions.

Endometrium

The endometrium consists of epithelium and lamina propria containing simple tubular glands that sometimes branch in their deeper portions (near the myometrium). Its epithelial cells are simple columnar and are a mixture of ciliated and secretory cells. The epithelium of the uterine glands is similar to the superficial epithelium, but ciliated cells are rare in the glands.

The connective tissue of the lamina propria is rich in fibroblasts and contains abundant amorphous ground substance. Connective tissue fibers are mostly of the reticular type.

The endometrial layer can be subdivided into 2 zones: (1) the **functionalis,** which constitutes that portion sloughed off at menstruation and replaced during each menstrual cycle; and (2) the **basalis,** that portion of the endometrium retained during menstruation which subsequently provides new epithelium and lamina propria for the renewal of the endometrium. The bases of the uterine glands, which lie deep within the basalis, are the source of the cells that divide and migrate over the exposed connective tissue of the menstrual phase endometrium, thereby providing for the new epithelial lining of the uterus after menstruation.

The blood vessels supplying the endometrium are of special significance in the periodic sloughing of most of this layer. **Arcuate arteries** are circumferentially oriented in the middle layers of the myometrium. From these vessels, 2 sets of arteries arise to supply blood to the endometrium: (1) **straight arteries,** which supply the basalis; and (2) **coiled arteries,** which bring blood to the functionalis.

The Menstrual Cycle

The action of ovarian hormones (estrogens and progesterone) under the stimulus of the anterior lobe of the pituitary causes the endometrium to undergo cyclic structural modifications during the menstrual cycle. The duration of the menstrual cycle is variable but averages 28 days.

Menstrual cycles start usually between 12 and 15 years of age and continue until about age 45 – 50. Since menstrual cycles are a consequence of ovarian modifications related to the production of ova, the female is fertile only during the years when she is having menstrual cycles. This does not mean that sexual activity is terminated by menopause—only that fertility ceases.

For practical purposes, the beginning of the menstrual cycle is taken as the day when menstrual bleeding appears. The menstrual discharge consists of degenerating endometrium mixed with blood from the ruptured blood vessels. The **menstrual phase** is defined as the first to the fourth days of the cycle; the **proliferative phase** is the fifth to the 14th days; and the **secretory phase** is the 15th to the 28th days. The duration of each phase is variable, and the intervals given are only averages.

The menstrual cycle will be described in the following order: proliferative phase, secretory or luteal phase, and menstrual phase. The structural changes that occur during the menstrual cycle are gradual; the clear division of the phases implied in the text has mainly teaching value.

A. Proliferative Phase: After the menstrual phase, the uterine mucosa is reduced to a small band of connective tissue (lamina propria) containing the basal portions of the glands. The epithelial lining and the superficial portion of the lamina propria are sloughed during menstruation. This residual part of the endometrium, which is not shed during menstruation, is the **basalis;** the portion that is sloughed and renewed in each cycle is the **functionalis.**

The proliferative phase is also known as the **follicular phase** because it coincides with development of ovarian follicles and with production of estrogens.

The cells in the bases of the glands proliferate extensively and reconstitute both the glands and surface epithelial lining of the endometrium. Cellular proliferation continues during the entire proliferative phase, and mitoses are observed both in the cells of the epithelial lining and in the glands (Fig 24 – 14). Proliferation of the connective cells and deposition of the ground substance in the lamina propria also occur, with consequent growth of the endometrium as a whole.

At the end of the proliferative phase, the endometrium is 2 – 3 mm thick, and the glands are straight tubules with narrow lumens. The glands consist of simple columnar epithelial cells, 20 – 30 μm tall and 4 – 6 μm wide. During this phase, these cells gradually accumulate more cisternae of rough endoplasmic reticulum, and the Golgi complex increases in size in preparation for their secretory activity. Coiled arteries grow into the regenerating stroma.

B. Secretory or Luteal Phase: This phase starts after ovulation and depends upon progesterone secreted by the corpus luteum. Acting upon glands already developed by the action of estrogen, progesterone stimulates the gland cells to secrete one or more glycoproteins that will be the major source of embryonic nutrition before implantation occurs.

The glands become highly coiled, and the epithelial cells begin to accumulate glycogen below their nuclei. Later, the amount of glycogen diminishes, and glycoprotein secretory products dilate the lumens of the glands. In this phase, the endometrium reaches its maximum thickness (5 mm) as a result of the accumulation of secretions and edema of the stroma. Mitoses are rare during the secretory phase (Fig 24 – 15). The elongation and convolution of the coiled arteries continue and extend into the superficial portion of the endometrium. Progesterone inhibits the contractions of smooth muscle cells of the myometrium that might otherwise interfere with the implantation of the embryo.

C. Menstrual Phase: When fertilization and implantation of the ovum released by the ovary fail to occur, the corpus luteum spontaneously ceases functioning after about 14 days. The levels of progesterone and estrogens in the blood drop rapidly, and the endometrium developed in response to these hormones undergoes involution and is partially shed. If implantation occurs, **human chorionic gonadotropin (hCG)** begins to be synthesized by the developing embryo. This sustains the life of the corpus luteum, and menstruation does not occur.

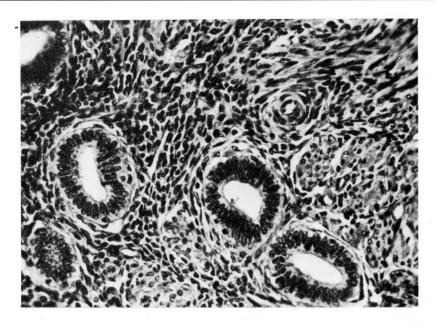

Figure 24–14. Endometrium in the proliferative phase. The epithelial cells of the gland are usually organized as a simple columnar lining, although during the active proliferation phase, the lining may assume a pseudostratified appearance. H&E stain, × 320.

At the end of the secretory phase, the walls of the coiled arteries contract, closing off blood flow and producing ischemia, which leads to death (necrosis) of the endothelium. At this time, rupture of blood vessels above the constrictions takes place, and bleeding begins.

The endometrium becomes partially detached. The amount lost is variable in different women and even in the same woman at different times. At the end of the menstrual phase, the endometrium is almost always reduced to nothing but the basal layer, containing the basal ends of the endometrial glands. Proliferation

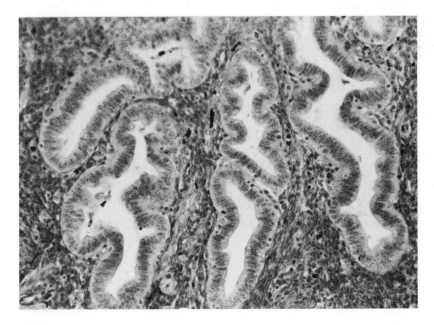

Figure 24–15. Endometrium in the secretory phase (21st day of the menstrual cycle). Uterine glands have a broad lumen with an irregular outline; their lumens are dilated by accumulation of secretory material. H&E stain, × 224.

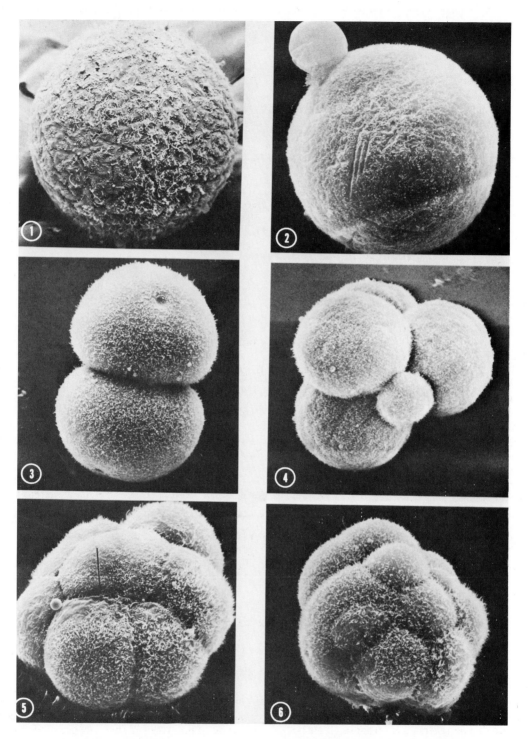

Figure 24–16. Scanning electron micrographs of the surface of an ovum after fertilization and up to the stage of a morula. The zona pellucida has been digested with pronase. *(1)* The ovum of the mouse shortly after its release from an ovarian follicle. The ovum has an intact germinal vesicle at this stage. × 1380. *(2)* Fertilized egg. Note the microvillous surface of the egg and the smooth surface of the first polar body. × 1300. *(3)* Two-cell stage evenly covered with microvilli. × 1320. *(4)* Four-cell stage with microvillous second polar body. × 1870. *(5)* Eight-cell stage. Note smoother regions of membrane where cells come into contact (arrow). × 1400. *(6)* Morula of the mouse. Microvilli are quite numerous, particularly adjacent to the area of cell contact. × 1540. (Reproduced, with permission, from Calarco P: Mammalian preimplantation development. In: *Scanning Electron Microscopy Atlas of Mammalian Reproduction.* Hafez ESE [editor]. Igaku Shoin Ltd, 1975.)

of the gland cells and their migration to the surface initiate the proliferative phase, restarting the cycle.

Uterine Cervix

As previously noted, the **cervix** is the lower, cylindric part of the uterus. This portion differs in histologic structure from the rest of the uterus. The lining consists of a mucus-secreting simple columnar epithelium, but the cervix has few smooth muscle fibers and a large quantity of dense connective tissue. The external aspect of the cervix that bulges into the lumen of the vagina is covered by stratified squamous epithelium.

The mucosa of the cervix contains the mucous **cervical glands,** which are extensively branched. This mucosa does not desquamate during menstruation, although its glands undergo small variations in their structure during the menstrual cycle. When blocking of the ducts of these glands occurs, the retained secretion causes a dilatation that gives rise to **nabothian cysts.** During pregnancy, the cervical mucous glands proliferate and secrete a more viscous and more abundant mucus.

Cervical secretions play a significant role in fertilization of the ovum. At the time of ovulation, the mucous secretions are watery and allow penetration of the uterus by sperm. In the luteal phase or in pregnancy, the progesterone levels alter the mucous secretions so that they become more viscous and prevent the passage of microorganisms, as well as sperm, into the body of the uterus. Dilation of the cervix that precedes parturition is due to intense collagenolysis, a process that promotes the weakening of this organ.

IMPLANTATION

The human ovum is fertilized at the ampullar-isthmic junction of the oviduct, and cleavage of the zygote occurs as it moves passively toward the uterus. Through successive mitoses, a compact collection of cells, the **morula,** covered by the zona pellucida is formed (Fig 24–16). The morula is about the same size as the fertilized ovum (Fig 24–16). The cells that result from segmentation of the zygote are called **blastomeres.** They do not grow in size at this time but serve to divide the zygote into smaller cells that will subsequently differentiate along several pathways.

A cavity at the center of the morula appears as a result of the gradual accumulation of liquid transferred from the lumen of the oviduct; the cells form a fluid-filled sphere, the **blastocyst.** The blastomeres arrange themselves in a peripheral layer **(trophoblast)** that is thickened at one point where a collection of cells remains **(inner cell mass)** and bulges into the cavity. This stage of development corresponds approximately to the fourth or fifth day after ovulation. At this time, the embryo reaches the uterus. The blastocyst remains in the lumen of the uterus for 2 or 3 days and comes into contact with the surface of the endometrium, immersed in the secretion of the endometrial glands.

In the blastocyst stage, the zona pellucida becomes thinner and disappears, allowing cells of the trophoblast, which have the capacity to invade the mucosa, to come into direct contact with the endometrium. Immediately thereafter, the cells of the trophoblast begin to multiply, thus ensuring, with the help of the endometrium, the nourishment of the embryo. The inner cell mass, from which the body of the embryo will originate, grows slightly during this phase.

Implantation, or **nidation,** involves penetration through the uterine epithelium, with little sign of necrosis (Fig 24–17). This type of **interstitial** implantation occurs in humans and a few other mammals. The process starts around the seventh day, and on about the ninth day after ovulation the embryo is totally submerged in the endometrium from which it will receive protection and nourishment during pregnancy.

Implantation takes place when the endometrium is in the secretory phase. The uterine glands contain glycoproteins and glycogen; the vessels are dilated; and the lamina propria is slightly swollen.

During implantation, the trophoblast differentiates into 2 layers, the **syncytiotrophoblast** and the **cytotrophoblast** (Figs 24–17 and 24–18). The former, a multinucleated syncytial external layer, arises by the fusion of mononucleated cytotrophoblasts. The cytotrophoblast consists of an irregular layer of mononucleated ovoid cells (Langhans cells) immediately under the syncytiotrophoblast.

The surface of the syncytiotrophoblast has irregular microvilli, and the superficial cytoplasm contains vesicles delimited by smooth membranes. This suggests the existence of an intense process of pinocytosis in the syncytiotrophoblast, possibly related to the transfer of material from the maternal circulation to the fetus. More deeply, the cytoplasm of the syncytiotrophoblast shows an abundance of both rough and smooth endoplasmic reticulum, a well-developed Golgi complex, and numerous mitochondria. These ultrastructural characteristics are consistent with the role attributed to the syncytiotrophoblast in the secretion of chorionic gonadotropin (a glycoprotein hormone), placental lactogen (a protein hormone), and estrogen and progesterone (steroids). The syncytiotrophoblast contains lipid droplets whose composition (as determined by cytochemical methods) is compatible with the presence of cholesterol, the immediate precursor of steroid hormones.

The syncytiotrophoblasts delineate extracytoplasmic cavities. These cavities increase in size and communicate with one another, resulting in a spongy structure (Fig 24–17). Thus, **lacunae** are formed, lined with syncytiotrophoblast. The lytic activity of the syncytiotrophoblast causes the rupture of both arterial and venous maternal blood vessels, with overflow of blood into these lacunar spaces. Blood flows from the arterial vessels to the lacunae and from there to the veins.

After implantation of the embryo, the endometrium goes through profound changes and is called

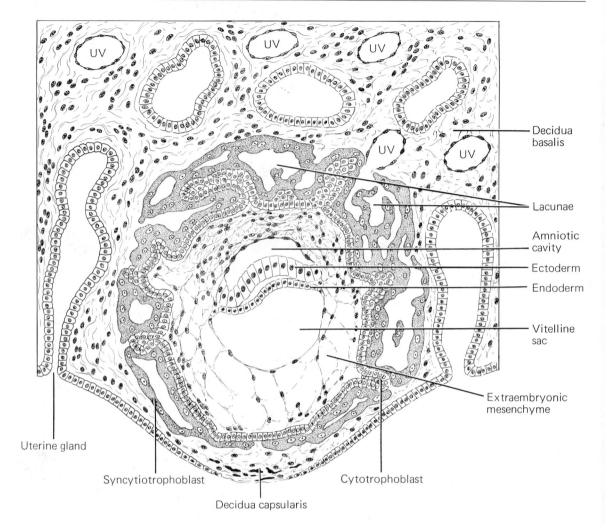

Figure 24–17. Schematic drawing of a human embryo at 12 days, showing the relationships between the embryo and the endometrium (which after implantation is called the decidua). UV, uterine vessels, one of which opens into a lacuna, filling those spaces with blood.

the **decidua.** Cells of the stroma become enlarged and polygonal and are called decidual cells. The decidua can be divided into **decidua basalis,** situated between the embryo and the myometrium; **decidua capsularis,** between the embryo and the lumen of the uterus; and **decidua parietalis,** which is the remainder of the decidua (Fig 24–19).

The trophoblast in contact with the decidua capsularis develops only to a slight extent, since its nutrition is deficient. Growth of the trophoblast in the part of the embryo facing the myometrium is assured by the maternal blood, and its growth is rapid. From this part of the trophoblast, elongated projections, **primary villi,** are formed. Their main characteristic is that they are composed only of cytotrophoblasts and an external syncytiotrophoblast lining. During this stage of embryonic development, an extraembryonic mesenchyme appears before the intraembryonic one

and contributes to the formation of the fetal membranes and placenta. The extraembryonic mesenchyme plus the trophoblast form the **chorion.** On the side of the **decidua capsularis,** the chorion develops to a very slight extent (**smooth chorion,** or **chorion laeve);** on the side of the decidua basalis, the chorion grows extensively and forms the **chorion frondosum.** The layers of the chorion (beginning at the surface) are (1) syncytiotrophoblast, (2) cytotrophoblast, and (3) extraembryonic mesenchyme.

The mesenchyme, when it invades the primary villi, transforms them into **secondary villi** (Figs 24–18 and 24–20). Within the villi, vessels are formed gradually and later will join those formed in the body of the embryo, establishing a circulation and thus allowing exchange of substances and gases between the fetal and maternal blood (Fig 24–20).

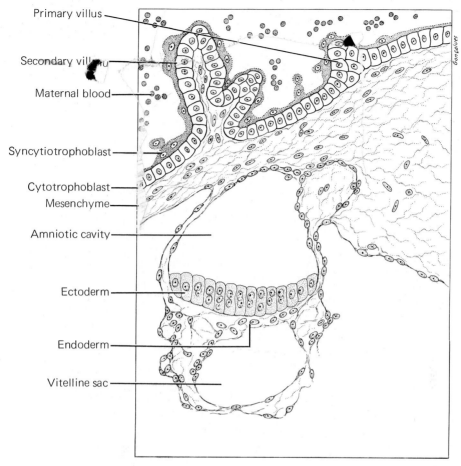

Primary villus

Secondary villus

Maternal blood

Syncytiotrophoblast

Cytotrophoblast

Mesenchyme

Amniotic cavity

Ectoderm

Endoderm

Vitelline sac

Figure 24–18. Human embryo at 15 days. At upper left is shown a chorionic villus protruding into a lacuna containing maternal blood.

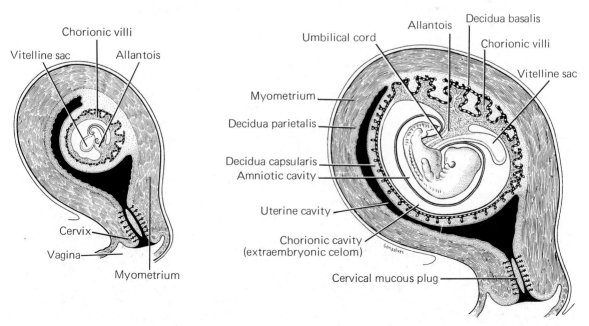

Chorionic villi

Vitelline sac

Allantois

Myometrium

Cervix

Vagina

Myometrium

Umbilical cord

Allantois

Decidua basalis

Chorionic villi

Vitelline sac

Myometrium

Decidua parietalis

Decidua capsularis

Amniotic cavity

Uterine cavity

Chorionic cavity
(extraembryonic celom)

Cervical mucous plug

Figure 24–19. Schematic drawings showing formation of the 3 regions of decidua and the chorionic villi.

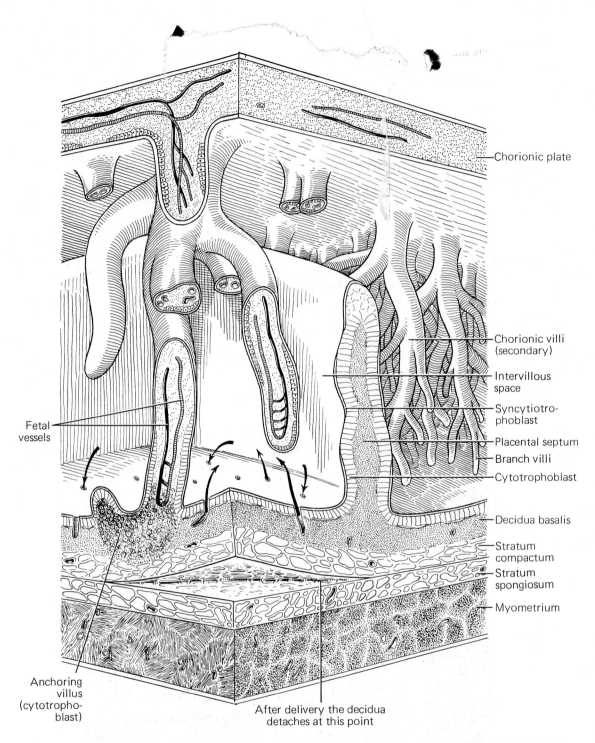

Figure 24–20. Schematic drawing of placental structure. Arrows indicate the blood flow from decidual arteries to intervillous space and back to decidual veins. This direction is determined by the difference in pressure between arterial and venous blood. (Redrawn and reproduced, with permission, from Duplessis GDT, Haegel P: *Embryologie.* Masson, 1971. [English edition © Springer-Verlag, 1972; Chapman & Hall, 1972; Masson, 1972.])

PLACENTA

The placenta is a temporary organ found only in eutherian mammals and is the site where physiologic exchanges between the mother and the fetus occur. It consists of a fetal part (chorion) and a maternal part (decidua basalis).

The placenta is the only organ composed of cells derived from 2 different individuals. The boundary between maternal and fetal tissues is marked by extracellular products of necrosis referred to as **fibrinoid.** Since the embryo and mother are of different genetic constitution, there should be an immunologic attack by the maternal organism against the "foreign" implanting embryo. Why this does not occur remains an active area of investigation.

Fetal Part

The fetal part of the placenta consists of the chorion. It has a **chorionic plate** at the point where the **chorionic villi** arise—the secondary villi already described. These villi consist of a connective tissue core derived from the extraembryonic mesenchyme surrounded by the syncytiotrophoblast and the cytotrophoblast (Fig 24–21). The syncytiotrophoblast remains until the end of pregnancy, but the cytotrophoblast disappears gradually during the second half of pregnancy. The cytotrophoblast undergoes extensive proliferation and concomitant cell fusion during early placentation. However, in the second half of pregnancy, proliferation slows while fusion continues, which results in a loss of the cytotrophoblast cells, since they become incorporated into the growing syncytium.

The chorionic villi may be either free or anchored to the decidua basalis. Both have the same structure, but the free ones do not reach the decidua, whereas the anchored chorionic villi become embedded within the decidua basalis. The surface of the villi is bathed with blood from the lacunae of the basal decidua and is the site where the exchange of substances between fetal and maternal blood occurs.

Maternal Part

The maternal part of the placenta—the decidua basalis—supplies arterial blood for the lacunae situated between the secondary villi and receives venous blood from these lacunae. Although the maternal blood vessels are opened during implantation, the fetal vessels contained in the secondary villi remain intact. Fetal blood and maternal blood do not mix except, on rare occasions, at the end of pregnancy. During this period, the cytotrophoblast is no longer continuous and the capillaries of the villi are close to the surface, and a very slight exchange of blood cells may occur. At that time, the walls of the fetal capillaries are separated from the maternal blood only by the syncytiotrophoblast.

During pregnancy, cells from the connective tissue stroma of the decidua basalis and a lesser number of cells from the decidua parietalis and decidua capsularis form the **decidual cells.** These large, slightly basophilic cells have many profiles of rough endoplasmic reticulum, long mitochondria, and membrane-limited granules contained in club-shaped projections of the cell surface. The nucleus is lightly stained and contains a prominent nucleolus. Decidual cells are more numerous during the first half of pregnancy. These cells

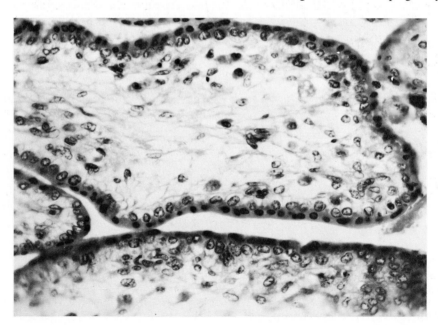

Figure 24–21. Photomicrograph of a chorionic villus in the second half of pregnancy. The syncytiotrophoblast is a continuous layer at the surface. Cytotrophoblast cells form a discontinuous layer just beneath the syncytiotrophoblast. H&E stain, × 320.

secrete prolactin, which is similar but not identical to pituitary prolactin. The significance of this secretory activity is unknown.

At the end of a full-term pregnancy, the placenta has the shape of a disk. The umbilical cord usually arises at the center of the placenta and forms a connection between the fetal and placental circulations.

Histophysiology

Fetal venous blood reaches the placenta through the 2 umbilical arteries, which branch, ultimately giving rise to the vessels of the chorionic villi. In these villi, the fetal blood receives oxygen, loses its CO_2, and returns to the fetus through the umbilical vein.

Since the chorionic villi are submerged in maternal blood, the fetal blood remains isolated by the following structures that form the **placental barrier:** (1) the endothelium of fetal capillaries, (2) the basal lamina of these capillaries, (3) the mesenchyme in the interior of the villus, (4) the basal lamina of the trophoblast, (5) the cytotrophoblast (during the first half of pregnancy), and (6) the syncytiotrophoblast.

The placenta is permeable to several substances, and normally it transfers oxygen, water, electrolytes, carbohydrates, lipids, proteins, vitamins, hormones, antibodies, and some drugs from maternal blood to fetal blood. CO_2, water, hormones, and residual products of metabolism are transferred from fetal blood to the maternal blood.

The placenta is also an endocrine organ, producing hormones such as chorionic gonadotropin, chorionic thyrotropin, chorionic corticotropin, estrogens, and progesterone. It also secretes a protein hormone called human placental lactogen (hPL), which has lactogenic and growth-stimulating activity. All of these hormones are synthesized by the syncytiotrophoblast. Examination of sections of placenta treated with fluorescent antigonadotropin antibody shows fluorescence in the syncytiotrophoblast but not in the cytotrophoblast.

Radioautographic studies after injection of radioactive thymidine show that the cells of the cytotrophoblast multiply actively and incorporate themselves into the syncytiotrophoblast. This indicates that the syncytiotrophoblast grows as a result of growth and mitotic activity of the cytotrophoblast.

VAGINA

The wall of the vagina is devoid of glands and consists of 3 layers: a **mucosa,** a **muscular layer,** and an **adventitia.** The mucus found in the lumen of the vagina comes from the glands of the uterine cervix.

The epithelium of the mucous layer is stratified squamous and has a thickness of 150–200 μm. Its cells may contain a small amount of keratohyalin. However, intense keratinization with change of the cells into keratin plates, as in typical keratinized epithelia, does not occur (Fig 24–22). Under the stimulus of estrogen, the vaginal epithelium synthesizes and accumulates a large quantity of glycogen, which is deposited in the lumen of the vagina when the vaginal cells desquamate. Bacteria in the vagina metabolize glycogen and form lactic acid, which is responsible for the usually low pH of the vagina.

The lamina propria of the vaginal mucosa is composed of loose connective tissue that is very rich in elastic fibers. Among the cells present, one can find lymphocytes and neutrophils in relatively large quantities. During certain phases of the menstrual cycle, these 2 types of leukocytes invade the epithelium and

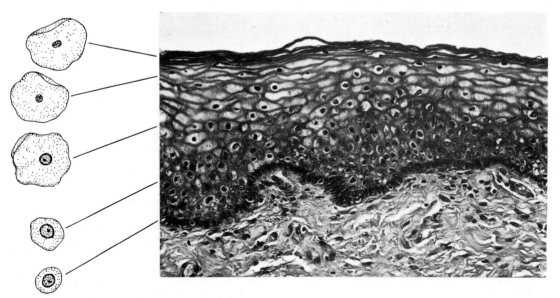

Figure 24–22. Photomicrograph of a section of vaginal mucosa and drawings of the cells found in various epithelial layers. Masson's stain, × 250.

pass into the lumen of the vagina. The lamina propria lacks glands but exhibits a rich vascularization which is the source of the fluid exudate that seeps through the squamous epithelium during sexual stimulation. The vaginal mucosa is virtually devoid of sensory nerve endings, and the few naked nerve endings that do exist are probably pain fibers.

The muscular layer of the vagina is composed mainly of longitudinal bundles of smooth muscle fibers. There are some circular bundles, especially in the innermost part (next to the mucosa).

Outside the muscular layer, a coat of dense connective tissue, the **adventitia,** rich in thick elastic fibers, unites the vagina with the surrounding tissues. The great elasticity of the vagina is related to the large number of elastic fibers in the connective tissues of its wall. In this connective tissue are an extensive venous plexus, nerve bundles, and groups of nerve cells.

EXTERNAL GENITALIA

The female external genitalia, or vulva, consists of the **clitoris, labia minora, labia majora,** and some glands that open into the vestibulum, a space enclosed by the labia minora.

The urethra and the ducts of the vestibular glands open into the vestibulum. The 2 **glandulae vestibulares majores,** or **glands of Bartholin,** are situated one on each side of the vestibulum. These glands are homologous to the bulbourethral glands in the male. The **glandulae vestibulares minores** are more numerous than the glands of Bartholin and are scattered, occurring with greater frequency around the urethra and clitoris. All of the glandulae vestibulares secrete mucus.

The clitoris and the penis are of homologous embryonic origin and histologic structure. The clitoris is formed by 2 erectile bodies ending in a rudimentary **glans clitoridis** and a prepuce. The clitoris is covered with stratified squamous epithelium.

The labia minora are folds of skin with a core of spongy connective tissue permeated by elastic fibers. The stratified squamous epithelium which covers them has cells and a thin keratinized layer on the surface, and sebaceous and sweat glands are present on both surfaces.

The labia majora are folds of skin and contain a large quantity of adipose tissue and a thin layer of smooth muscle. Their inner surface has a histologic structure similar to that of the labia minora. The external surface is covered by skin and coarse, curly hair. Sebaceous and sweat glands are numerous on both surfaces.

The external genitalia are abundantly supplied with sensory tactile nerve endings including Meissner's and Pacini's corpuscles, which contribute to the physiology of sexual arousal.

ENDOCRINE INTERRELATIONSHIPS

Female reproductive function is regulated through certain nuclei of the hypothalamus. Nerve cells in the hypothalamus produce and introduce into the portal blood vessels specific polypeptides that act on the anterior lobe of the pituitary to liberate gonadotropins; these gonadotropins in turn stimulate the secretion of ovarian hormones (estrogens and progesterone) (Fig 24–23). The hypothalamic localization of the ovarian hormone control mechanism might explain why strong, nonspecific cerebral stimuli occasionally affect reproductive function—''boarding school amenorrhea,'' pseudocyesis, etc.

The developing ovarian follicle synthesizes **estrogens,** and the corpus luteum synthesizes estrogens and **progesterone.** The main source of estrogens in the human ovarian follicle seems to be granulosa cells that have all the enzymes necessary to convert cholesterol to **estradiol-17β.** Estradiol found in blood is produced mainly by theca interna cells of the follicle. Estradiol is rapidly converted to **estrone,** which is further metabolized to **estriol,** probably in the liver. Estradiol is the most potent estrogen of the 3 compounds.

The pituitary gonadotropins, follicle-stimulating hormone (FSH) and luteinizing hormone (LH), are produced under the control of a single ''releasing hormone'' (GnRH) liberated by the hypothalamus. FSH stimulates the growth of the ovarian follicles and the formation of estrogens. It is important to note that at any particular time in the cycle, the ovary possesses follicles in all stages of growth. The release of FSH does not promote the formation of a graafian follicle from a primordial follicle during one cycle. The most immediate effect of FSH is probably the maturation of existing late primary or secondary follicles. LH promotes ovulation and the formation of the corpus luteum through differentiation of granulosa cells that remain in the follicle after expulsion of the ovum (Fig 24–23).

The ovary also acts on the pituitary directly and through the hypothalamus. Estrogen inhibits the secretion of FSH and stimulates the secretion of LH. The production of LH is inhibited by progesterone. Just prior to mid cycle, estrogen secretion reaches a peak and causes a brief surge of LH secretion. Luteinizing hormone promotes ovulation, maturation of the oocyte, and formation of the corpus luteum. As the secretion of LH is inhibited by progesterone produced by the corpus luteum, this structure is soon deprived of the pituitary stimulus (LH) necessary for its functioning, and consequently it degenerates.

When fertilization and implantation occur, syncytiotrophoblast cells synthesize the chorionic gonadotropins that stimulate and maintain the function of the corpus luteum during pregnancy.

In rats and mice, the corpus luteum is sensitive to prolactin. In these species, prolactin stimulates secretion by an already formed corpus luteum. There is no evidence that prolactin has any influence on the

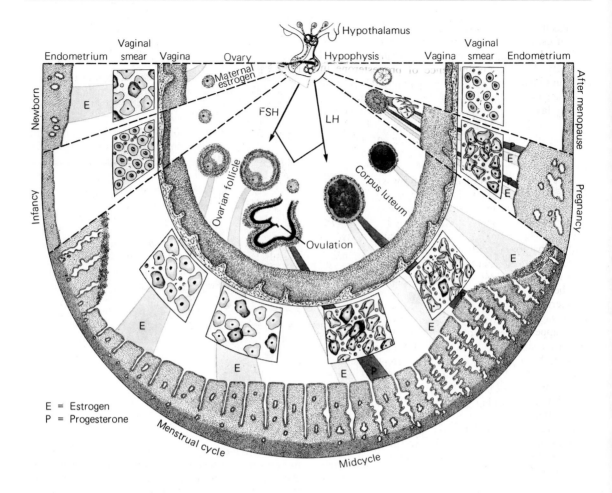

Figure 24–23. Functional changes relating to the hypothalamus, pituitary, ovary, vaginal epithelium, and endometrium. E, estrogen; P, progesterone. (Modified and redrawn from FH Netter, MD.)

human corpus luteum. In humans, prolactin initiates and maintains milk secretion by mammary glands already stimulated by estrogens and progesterone.

EXFOLIATIVE CYTOLOGY

Exfoliative cytology is the study of the characteristics of cells that normally desquamate from various surfaces of the body. Cytologic examination of the vaginal mucosa gives important data on hormonal balance and allows early detection of some types of cancer of the female genital system.

The cells to be examined are taken from the vagina together with the secretions contained there; they are spread on a slide, fixed, and stained by special techniques such as the Shorr trichrome technique, acridine orange, etc. Cells from the epithelium of the vagina predominate in this type of preparation.

In the fully mature vaginal mucosa, 5 types of cells are easily identifiable: (1) cells of the internal portion of the basal layer (called basal cells), (2) cells

of the external portion of the basal layer (called parabasal cells), (3) cells of the intermediate layers, (4) precornified cells, and (5) cornified cells (Figs 24–22 and 24–23).

Under the stimulus of estrogens, the vaginal epithelium becomes thicker, with a larger number of cellular layers. Partial keratinization of the most superficial cells also occurs. The superficial keratinized cells are characterized by a dense, shrunken (pyknotic) nucleus and an acidophilic cytoplasm (keratin is an acidophilic protein). These cells predominate in the smears of estrogen-stimulated vaginal secretions. They have the shape of a plate, since they represent the most superficial elements of stratified squamous epithelium. This appearance is so characteristic of the action of the estrogens that the percentage of acidophilic cells in a smear is a reliable index of estrogenic stimulation. Cytologic smears reveal not only quantitative changes in estrogen concentration but also the effect of progesterone. In the normal menstrual cycle, by day 6 most of the cells are from the intermediate layer, are polygonal in shape, and contain basophilic cytoplasm. At the time of ovulation, under the influence of estrogen, most of the cells are from the precornified layer but 20% or more are fully cornified cells. By day 20, the influence of progesterone in addition to estrogen can be clearly noted. There is an increased number of desquamated cells of the intermediate layers. In contrast to the clearly outlined and separated cells of the proliferative phase, during the secretory phase a loss of cellular outline and clumping can be seen. Almost all of the cells have again become basophilic.

The above characteristics of the progesterone effect are more prominent during pregnancy.

Hormonal deficiency during menopause causes attenuation of the vaginal epithelium, with no keratinized cells. The vaginal smear cells are mainly spherical basal or parabasal cells with basophilic cytoplasm whose large nuclei contain dispersed chromatin. The same type of vaginal smear is obtained during the prepubertal state.

Internal basal cells—those from the deepest layer of the vaginal epithelium—rarely desquamate. This does happen after childbirth but is not due to the trauma caused by expulsion of the fetus, as one might suppose, because it occurs as well in women who have had abdominal deliveries (cesarean operation). The internal basal cells appear on the smear as a result of the intense shedding of the vaginal epithelium that occurs after delivery, which in turn is a consequence of the sudden decline of the hormonal levels of the placenta and ovaries. These cells are small, spherical, and basophilic and have large nuclei with dispersed chromatin (Fig 24–22).

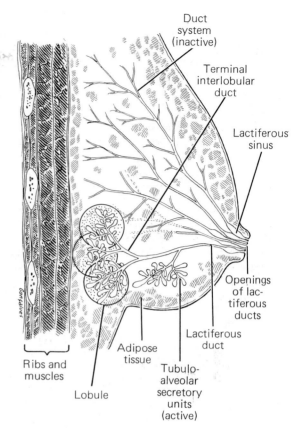

Figure 24–24. Schematic drawing of female breast showing the mammary glands with ducts that open in the nipple. The outlines of the lobules do not exist in vivo but are for instructional purposes. The stippling indicates the loose intralobular connective tissue.

MAMMARY GLANDS

Each mammary gland consists of 15–25 lobes of the compound tubulo-alveolar type whose function is to secrete milk to nourish newborns (Fig 24–24). Each lobe is separated from the others by dense connective tissue and much adipose tissue and is really a gland in itself with its own excretory duct. These excretory **lactiferous ducts,** 2–4.5 cm long, emerge independently in the **nipple,** which has 15–25 openings, each about 0.5 mm in diameter. The histologic structure of the mammary glands varies according to sex, age, and physiologic status.

Embryonic Breast Development

The mammary glands appear in a 6-week-old human embryo as a pair of thickenings of the epidermis, the **milk lines.** They extend from the forelimb to the hindlimb on the ventral side of the fetus. The caudal parts of the milk lines regress early in development. In the thoracic region of a second-trimester fetus, 15–25 ingrowths of the epithelium penetrate the underlying connective tissue and give rise to the future lactiferous ducts. Most of the remainder of each milk line degenerates.

In newborns of both sexes, the glands have a diameter of 3.5–9 mm and consist of ducts that may be swollen with secretory material. Secretion of a fluid by neonates is not unusual, since these glands are affected by placental and maternal hormones.

Breast Development During Puberty

Before puberty, mammary glands are composed of lactiferous sinuses and several branches of these sinuses called lactiferous ducts.

The development of mammary glands in females during puberty constitutes one of the secondary sex characteristics. During this period, the breasts increase in size and develop a prominent nipple. In males, the breasts normally remain flattened.

Breast enlargement during puberty is the result of accumulation of adipose tissue and collagenous connective tissue. Increased branching of lactiferous ducts also plays a minor role. Proliferation of the lactiferous ducts and accumulation of fat are due to an increase in the amount of ovarian estrogens during puberty.

Breast Structure in Adult Women

During puberty, the lactiferous ducts extend their growth and branch extensively. At the tips of the smallest ducts **(terminal interlobular ducts),** the characteristic structure of the adult female gland—the **lobule**—is developed (Fig 24–24). A lobule consists of several **intralobular** ducts emptying into one terminal interlobular duct. Each lobule is embedded in loose cellular intralobular connective tissue. Separating the lobules is a denser, less cellular interlobular connective tissue.

Near the opening of the nipple, the lactiferous ducts dilate to form the lactiferous sinuses (Fig 24–24). The lactiferous sinuses are lined by stratified squamous epithelium at their external openings. Very quickly, this epithelium changes to what appears to be stratified columnar or cuboidal epithelium. Electron microscopic examination has revealed that the cells adjacent to the lumen are ductal epithelial cells, while the cells lying on the basal lamina are closely packed myoepithelial cells. Ductal epithelial cells contain a few mitochondria, occasional cisternae of rough endoplasmic reticulum, many free ribosomes, and a small Golgi complex. The epithelial cells are joined by tight junctions and desmosomes. The myoepithelial cells are spindle-shaped and oriented with their long axes parallel to the length of the duct. The terminal interlobular ducts (Fig 24– 24) consist of simple cuboidal epithelium resting on basal lamina and a discontinuous layer of myoepithelial cells.

In the intralobular connective tissue surrounding the alveoli are some lymphocytes and plasma cells. Toward the end of pregnancy, the plasma cell population increases significantly and is responsible for the secretion of immunoglobulins (secretory IgA) that confer passive immunity on the newborn.

During the menstrual cycle, small alterations in the histologic structure of these glands are observed, ie, proliferation of cells of the ducts at about the time of ovulation. These changes coincide with the period during which circulating estrogen is at its peak. Greater hydration of connective tissue in the premenstrual phase produces breast enlargement.

The **nipple** has a conical shape. Its color may be pink, light brown, or dark brown. Externally, it is covered by keratinized stratified squamous epithelium continuous with that of the adjacent skin. The skin around the nipple constitutes the **areola.** The color of the areola changes from pink to dark brown during pregnancy owing to local accumulation of melanin. After delivery, the areola may become lighter in color but never returns to its original shade. The epithelium of the nipple rests on a layer of connective tissue rich in smooth muscle fibers. These fibers are disposed in circles around the deeper lactiferous ducts and parallel to them where they enter the nipple. The nipple is abundantly supplied with sensory nerve endings.

The Breasts During Pregnancy

The mammary glands undergo intense growth during pregnancy as a result of proliferation of **alveoli** within lobules. Alveoli are spherical collections of epithelial cells that become the active milk-secreting structures in lactation. Alveolar cells contain a basally placed nucleus surrounded by numerous cisternae of rough endoplasmic reticulum. The ribosomes attached to the rough endoplasmic reticulum account for the basophilia of this part of the alveolar cell. A supranuclear Golgi complex is present, and mitochondria and lysosomes are scattered throughout the cytoplasm. At this time, a few fat droplets, not surrounded by a membrane, can be seen in the apical cytoplasm of

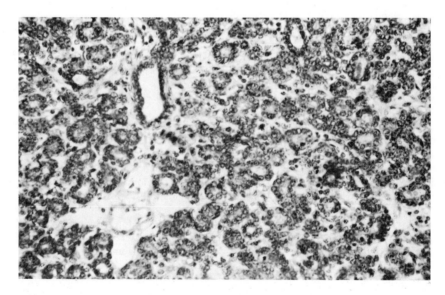

Figure 24 –25. Photomicrograph of a mammary gland during pregnancy. There is intense proliferation of the alveoli. No secretion is seen. H&E stain, × 200.

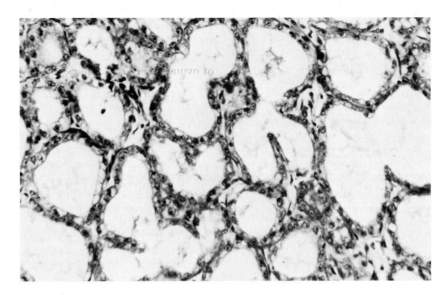

Figure 24–26. Photomicrograph of a lactating mammary gland. The alveoli are distended by the secretion (milk) accumulated in their lumens. H&E stain, × 200.

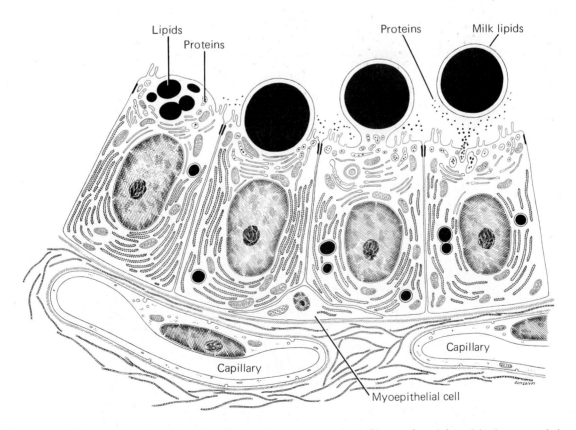

Figure 24–27. Schematic drawing of alveolar cells from the mammary gland. Observe from left to right the accumulation and extrusion of milk lipids and proteins. The proteins are released through exocytosis, while lipid extrusion involves apocrine secretion.

alveolar cells. Also present are a few membrane-limited secretory vacuoles containing one to several dense aggregates of milk proteins. The number of secretory vacuoles and fat droplets greatly increases in lactation (see below). Four to 6 stellate myoepithelial cells encompass each alveolus; they are found between the alveolar epithelial cells and the basal lamina. These cells possess numerous actin-containing microfilaments and an elaborate meshwork of intermediate (7–11 nm in diameter) filaments composed of cytokeratins (see Chapter 4). The amounts of connective tissue stroma and adipose tissue, relative to the parenchyma, decrease considerably. Despite this growth process, there are few signs of secretion until late in pregnancy (Fig 24–25).

Growth of the mammary glands during pregnancy occurs as a result of the synergistic action of several hormones, mainly estrogen, progesterone, prolactin, and human placental lactogen. These hormones stimulate the growth of the secretory parts (alveoli) of the mammary glands.

During pregnancy, the quantity of estrogen increases, since this hormone is also produced by the placenta. The amount of progesterone also increases, as this steroid is produced first by the corpus luteum (which remains active during early pregnancy) and later by the placenta.

The Breasts During Lactation

Milk is produced by the epithelial cells of the alveoli and accumulates in their lumens and inside the lactiferous ducts (Fig 24–26). The secretory cells become small and low cuboidal, and their cytoplasm contains spherical droplets of various sizes containing mainly neutral triglycerides. These lipid droplets pass out of the cells into the lumen and in the process are enveloped with a portion of the apical cell membrane (Fig 24–27). This is one of the few examples of apocrine secretion (see Chapter 4). Lipids constitute 4% of human milk.

Besides the lipid droplets, which are at the apical pole of the secretory cell, one can see a large number of membrane-limited vacuoles containing granules composed of caseins as well as other milk proteins. The synthesis of milk proteins occurs on ribosomes associated with the rough endoplasmic reticulum,

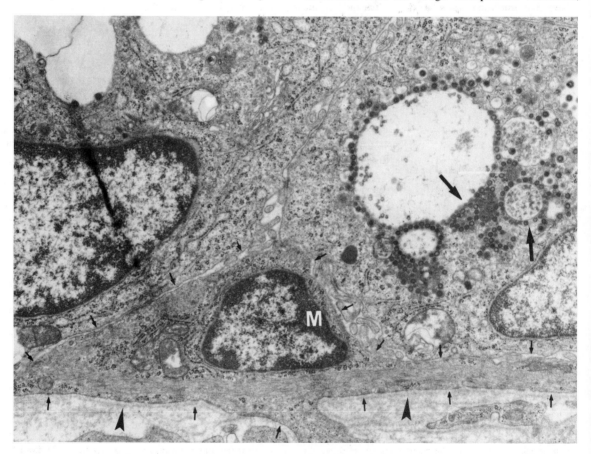

Figure 24–28. Electron micrograph of mouse mammary gland. A myoepithelial cell (M) is seen in the lower part of the picture and is outlined by small arrows. The myoepithelial cell is contained within the basal lamina that surrounds the secretory cells (arrowheads). In this species, but not in women, the secretory cells contain numerous virus particles (large arrows). × 17,500. (Reproduced, with permission, from Junqueira LCU, Salles LMM: *Ultra-Estrutura e Função Celular.* Edgard Blücher, 1975.)

which is abundant in the basal part of the cell; they pass through the Golgi complex and accumulate at the apical pole in membrane-bound vesicles. Milk proteins include several caseins, α-lactalbumin, and immunoglobulin A. These proteins are released by exocytosis (Fig 24–27). Proteins constitute approximately 1.5% of human milk.

Lactose, the sugar of milk, is synthesized from glucose and galactose. α-Lactalbumin is a regulatory subunit of lactose synthase. Lactose constitutes about 7% of human milk.

The first secretion to appear after birth is called **colostrum**. It contains less fat and more protein than regular milk and is rich in antibodies (predominantly secretory IgA) that provide some degree of passive immunity to the newborn, especially within the gut lumen.

When a woman is breast-feeding, the nursing action of the child stimulates tactile receptors in the nipple, resulting in liberation of the posterior pituitary hormone **oxytocin**. This hormone causes contraction of myoepithelial cells (Fig 24–28) in alveoli and ducts, resulting in ejection of milk **(milk ejection reflex)**. Negative emotional stimuli, such as frustration, anxiety, or anger, can inhibit the liberation of oxytocin, thus preventing the milk ejection reflex.

Postlactational Regression of the Breasts

With cessation of breast feeding (weaning), most alveoli that developed during pregnancy undergo degeneration. This includes sloughing of whole cells as well as autophagic reabsorption of cellular components. Myoepithelial cells and the basal lamina persist and are reutilized in the next pregnancy.

Senile Involution of the Breasts

After menopause, involution of the mammary glands is characterized by reduction in size and atrophy of their secretory portions and, to a certain extent, of the ducts. Atrophic changes also occur in the interlobular connective tissue.

Breast Cancer

About 9% of all women born in the USA will develop breast cancer at some time during their lives. Most of these cancers arise from epithelial cells of the lactiferous ducts (carcinomas). If these cells metastasize to the lungs, brain, or bone, breast carcinoma becomes a major cause of death. Early detection (self-examination) and treatment will reduce the mortality rate from breast cancer.

REFERENCES

Adams EC, Hertig AT: Studies on the human corpus luteum. 1. Observations on the ultrastructure of development and regression of the luteal cells during the menstrual cycle. 2. Observations on the ultrastructure of the luteal cells during pregnancy. *J Cell Biol* 1969;**41**:696, 716.

Baker TG, Franchi LL: The fine structure of oogonia and oocytes in human ovaries. *J Cell Sci* 1967;**2**:213.

Banarjee MR: Responses of mammary cells to hormones. *Int Rev Cytol* 1976;**47**:1.

Dirksen ER, Satir P: Ciliary activity in the mouse oviduct as studied by transmission and scanning electron microscopy. *Tissue Cell* 1972;**4**:389.

Enders AC: Fine structure of anchoring villi of the human placenta. *Am J Anat* 1968;**122**:419.

Enders AC: Formation of the syncytium from cytotrophoblast in the human placenta. *Obstet Gynecol* 1965;**25**:378.

Enders AC, Schlafke SJ: Cytological aspects of trophoblast-uterine interaction in early implantation. *Am J Anat* 1969;**125**:1.

Ferenczy A et al: Scanning electron microscopy of the human Fallopian tube. *Science* 1972;**175**:783.

Fisher ER: Ultrastructure of the human breast and its disorders. *Am J Clin Pathol* 1976;**66**:291.

Gulyas BJ: Fine structure of the luteal tissue. Pages 238–254 in: *Ultrastructure of Endocrine Cells and Tissues*. Motta PM (editor). Martinus Nijhoff, 1984.

Guraya SS: Recent advances in the morphology, histochemistry and biochemistry of the developing mammalian ovary. *Int Rev Cytol* 1977;**51**:49.

Haddad A, Nagai MET: Radioautographic study of glycoprotein biosynthesis and renewal in the ovarian follicles of mice and the origin of the zona pellucida. *Cell Tissue Res* 1977;**177**:347.

Hertig AT: The primary human oocyte: Some observations on the fine structure of Balbiani's vitelline body and the origin of the annulate lamellae. *Am J Anat* 1968;**122**:107.

Hertig AT, Adams EC: Studies on the human oocyte and its follicle. 1. Ultrastructural and histochemical observations on the primordial follicle stage. *J Cell Biol* 1967;**34**:647.

Hertig AT, Rock J, Adams EC: A description of 34 human ova within the first 17 days of development. *Am J Anat* 1956;**98**:435.

Jones RE (editor): *The Vertebrate Ovary*. Plenum Press, 1978.

Junqueira LCU et al: Morphologic and histochemical evidence for the occurrence of collagenolysis and for the role of neutrophilic polymorphonuclear leukocytes during cervical dilation. *Am J Obstet Gynecol* 1980;**138**:273.

Long JA: Corpus luteum of pregnancy in the rat: Ultrastructural and cytochemical observations. *Biol Reprod* 1973;**8**:87.

Mathieu P, Rahier J, Thomas K: Localization of relaxin in human gestational corpus luteum. *Cell Tissue Res* 1981;**219**:213.

Moseman HW: *Comparative Morphology of the Mammalian Ovary*. Univ of Wisconsin Press, 1973.

Motta PM, Hafez ESE (editors): *Biology of the Ovary*. Martinus Nijhoff, 1980.

Nagato T et al: A scanning electron microscope study of myoepithelial cells in exocrine glands. *Cell Tissue Res* 1980;**209**:1.

Nemanic MK, Pitelka DR: A scanning electron microscope study of the lactating mammary gland. *J Cell Biol* 1971;**48**:410.

Peters H, McNatty KP: *The Ovary: A Correlation of Structure and Function in Mammals*. Granada Publishing, 1980.

Pitelka DR, Hamamoto ST: Ultrastructure of the mammary secretory cell. In: *Biochemistry of Lactation*. Mepham TB (editor). Elsevier, 1983.

Ross R, Klebanoff SJ: Fine structural changes in uterine smooth muscle and fibroblasts in response to estrogens. *J Cell Biol* 1967;**32**:27.

Segal SJ: The physiology of human reproduction. *Sci Am* (Sept) 1974;**231**:52.

Tersakis J: The ultrastructure of normal human first trimester placenta. *J Ultrastruct Res* 1963;**9**:268.

Villee DB: Development of endocrine function in the human placenta and fetus. *N Engl J Med* 1969;**281**:473.

Vorherr H: *The Breast: Morphology, Physiology and Lactation.* Academic Press, 1974.

Weiss G, O'Byrne EM, Steinetz BG: Relaxin: A product of the human corpus luteum of pregnancy. *Science* 1976;**194**:948.

Wynn RM (editor): *Biology of the Uterus.* Plenum Press, 1977.

Yoshida Y: Ultrastructure and secretory function of the syncytial trophoblast of human placenta in early pregnancy. *Exp Cell Res* 1964;**34**:305.

Zuckerman S, Weir BJ (editors): *The Ovary,* 2nd ed. Vol 1. General Aspects. Academic Press, 1977.

Index